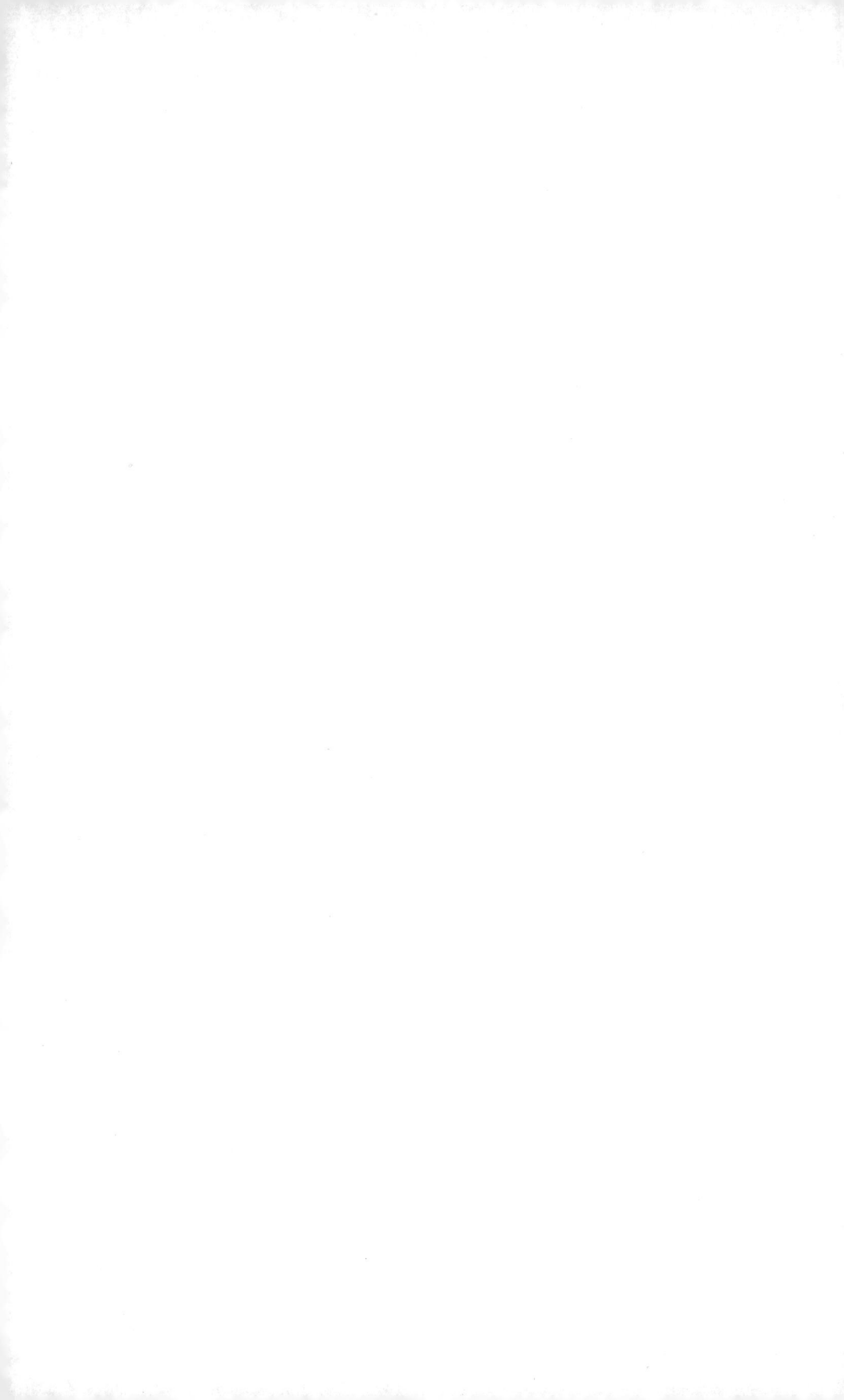

MOLECULAR BASIS OF THYROID CANCER

Cancer Treatment and Research
Steven T. Rosen, M.D., *Series Editor*

Klastersky, J. (ed): *Infectious Complications of Cancer.* 1995. ISBN 0-7923-3598-8.
Kurzrock, R., Talpaz, M. (eds): *Cytokines: Interleukins and Their Receptors.* 1995. ISBN 0-7923-3636-4.
Sugarbaker, P. (ed): *Peritoneal Carcinomatosis: Drugs and Diseases.* 1995. ISBN 0-7923-3726-3.
Sugarbaker, P. (ed): *Peritoneal Carcinomatosis: Principles of Management.* 1995. ISBN 0-7923-3727-1.
Dickson, R.B., Lippman, M.E. (eds.): *Mammary Tumor Cell Cycle, Differentiation and Metastasis.* 1995. ISBN 0-7923-3905-3.
Freireich, E.J, Kantarjian, H. (eds): *Molecular Genetics and Therapy of Leukemia.* 1995. ISBN 0-7923-3912-6.
Cabanillas, F., Rodriguez, M.A. (eds): *Advances in Lymphoma Research.* 1996. ISBN 0-7923-3929-0.
Miller, A.B. (ed.): *Advances in Cancer Screening.* 1996. ISBN 0-7923-4019-1.
Hait , W.N. (ed.): *Drug Resistance.* 1996. ISBN 0-7923-4022-1.
Pienta, K.J. (ed.): *Diagnosis and Treatment of Genitourinary Malignancies.* 1996. ISBN 0-7923-4164-3.
Arnold, A.J. (ed.): *Endocrine Neoplasms.* 1997. ISBN 0-7923-4354-9.
Pollock, R.E. (ed.): *Surgical Oncology.* 1997. ISBN 0-7923-9900-5.
Verweij, J., Pinedo, H.M., Suit, H.D. (eds): *Soft Tissue Sarcomas: Present Achievements and Future Prospects.* 1997. ISBN 0-7923-9913-7.
Walterhouse, D.O., Cohn, S. L. (eds.): *Diagnostic and Therapeutic Advances in Pediatric Oncology.* 1997. ISBN 0-7923-9978-1.
Mittal, B.B., Purdy, J.A., Ang, K.K. (eds): *Radiation Therapy.* 1998. ISBN 0-7923-9981-1.
Foon, K.A., Muss, H.B. (eds): *Biological and Hormonal Therapies of Cancer.* 1998. ISBN 0-7923-9997-8.
Ozols, R.F. (ed.): *Gynecologic Oncology.* 1998. ISBN 0-7923-8070-3.
Noskin, G. A. (ed.): *Management of Infectious Complications in Cancer Patients.* 1998. ISBN 0-7923-8150-5.
Bennett, C. L. (ed.): *Cancer Policy.* 1998. ISBN 0-7923-8203-X.
Benson, A. B. (ed.): *Gastrointestinal Oncology.* 1998. ISBN 0-7923-8205-6.
Tallman, M.S., Gordon, L.I. (eds): *Diagnostic and Therapeutic Advances in Hematologic Malignancies.* 1998. ISBN 0-7923-8206-4.
von Gunten, C.F. (ed): *Palliative Care and Rehabilitation of Cancer Patients.* 1999. ISBN 0-7923-8525-X
Burt, R.K., Brush, M.M. (eds): *Advances in Allogeneic Hematopoietic Stem Cell Transplantation.* 1999. ISBN 0-7923-7714-1.
Angelos, P. (ed.): *Ethical Issues in Cancer Patient Care* 2000. ISBN 0-7923-7726-5.
Gradishar, W.J., Wood, W.C. (eds): *Advances in Breast Cancer Management.* 2000. ISBN 0-7923-7890-3.
Sparano, Joseph A. (ed.): *HIV & HTLV-I Associated Malignancies.* 2001. ISBN 0-7923-7220-4.
Ettinger, David S. (ed.): *Thoracic Oncology.* 2001. ISBN 0-7923-7248-4.
Bergan, Raymond C. (ed.): *Cancer Chemoprev*ention. 2001. ISBN 0-7923-7259-X.
Raza, A., Mundle, S.D. (eds): *Myelodysplastic Syndromes & Secondary Acute Myelogenous Leukemia* 2001. ISBN: 0-7923-7396.
Talamonti, Mark S. (ed.):*Liver Directed Therapy for Primary and Metastatic Liver Tumors.* 2001. ISBN 0-7923-7523-8.
Stack, M.S., Fishman, D.A. (eds): *Ovarian Cancer.* 2001. ISBN 0-7923-7530-0.
Bashey, A., Ball, E.D. (eds): *Non-Myeloablative Allogeneic Transplantation.* 2002. ISBN 0-7923-7646-3.
Leong, Stanley P.L. (ed.): *Atlas of Selective Sentinel Lymphadenectomy for Melanoma, Breast Cancer and Colon Cancer.* 2002. ISBN 1 4020 7013 6.
Andersson, B., Murray D. (eds): *Clinically Relevant Resistance in Cancer Chemotherapy.* 2002. ISBN 1-4020-7200-7.
Beam, C. (ed.): *Biostatistical Applications in Cancer Research.* 2002. ISBN 1-4020-7226-0.
Brockstein, B., Masters, G. (eds): *Head and Neck Cancer.* 2003. ISBN 1-4020-7336-4.
Frank, D.A. (ed.): *Signal Transduction in Cancer.* 2003. ISBN 1-4020-7340-2.
Figlin, Robert A. (ed.): *Kidney Cancer.* 2003. ISBN 1-4020-7457-3.
Kirsch, Matthias; Black, Peter McL. (ed.): *Angiogenesis in Brain Tumors.* 2003. ISBN 1-4020-7704-1.
Keller, E.T., Chung, L.W.K. (eds): *The Biology of Skeletal Metastases.* 2004. ISBN 1-4020-7749-1.
Kumar, Rakesh (ed.): *Molecular Targeting and Signal Transduction.* 2004. ISBN 1-4020-7822-6.
Verweij, J., Pinedo, H.M. (eds): *Targeting Treatment of Soft Tissue Sarcomas.* 2004. ISBN 1-4020-7808-0.
Finn, W.G., Peterson, L.C. (eds.): *Hematopathology in Oncology.* 2004. ISBN 1-4020-7919-2.
Farid, N., (ed.): *Molecular Basis of Thyroid Cancer.* 2004. ISBN 1-4020-8106-5.

MOLECULAR BASIS OF THYROID CANCER

Edited by

NADIR R. FARID
Osancor Biotech, Inc., Watford WD17 3BY Herts
United Kingdom

KLUWER ACADEMIC PUBLISHERS
Boston / New York / Dordrecht / London

Distributors for North, Central and South America:
Kluwer Academic Publishers
101 Philip Drive, Assinippi Park
Norwell, Massachusetts 02061 USA
Telephone (781) 871-6600 Fax (781) 681-9045
E-Mail: Kluwer@wkap.com

Distributors for all other countries:
Kluwer Academic Publishers Group
Post Office Box 322
3300 AH Dordrecht, THE NETHERLANDS
Telephone 31 786 576 000 Fax 31 786 576 254
E-Mail: services@wkap.nl

   Electronic Services <http://www.wkap.nl>

Library of Congress Cataloging-in-Publication Data

Molecular basis of thyroid cancer / edited by Nadir R. Farid
   p. ; cm. – (Cancer treatment and research ; v. 122)
   Includes index.
   ISBN 1-4020-8106-5 (alk. paper)
     1. Thyroid gland–Cancer–Molecular aspects.   I. Farid,
   Nadir R.   II. Series.
   [DNLM: 1. Cell Transformation, Neoplastic–genetics.
   2. Thyroid Neoplasms–genetics.
   WK 270 M718 2004]
   RC280.T6M64 2004
   616.99'444–dc22   2004051535

Copyright © 2004 by Kluwer Academic Publishers

All rights reserved. No part of this work may be reproduced, stored in a retrieval system, or transmitted in
any form or by any means, electronic, mechanical, photocopying, microfilming, recording, or otherwise,
without the written permission from the Publisher, with the exception of any material supplied
specifically for the purpose of being entered and executed on a computer system, for exclusive use by the
purchaser of the work.

Permission for books published in Europe: permissions@wkap.nl
Permissions for books published in the United States of America: permissions@wkap.com

Printed on acid-free paper.
Printed in the United States of America.

The Publisher offers discounts on this book for course use and bulk purchases.
For further information, send email to <Laura.Walsh@wkap.com>.

CONTENTS

Preface   vii

1. The origin of cancer   1
   EVAN Y. YU AND WILLIAM C. HAHN

2. The pathology of thyroid cancer   23
   SYLVIA L. ASA

3. Thyroid lymphomas   69
   RUNJAN CHETTY

4. Molecular events in follicular thyroid tumors   85
   TODD G. KROLL

5. Molecular epidemiology of thyroid cancer   107
   MARTIN SCHLUMBERGER

6. Growth factors and their receptors in the genesis and treatment of thyroid cancer   121
   SHEREEN EZZAT

7. Biology of Ras in thyroid cells   131
   JUDY L. MEINKOTH

8. P53 and other cell cycle regulators   149
   NADIR R. FARID

9. Abnormalities of nuclear receptors in thyroid cancer   165
   SHEUE-YANN CHENG

10. Matrix metalloproteinases in thyroid cancer   179
    YUFEI SHI AND MINJING ZOU

11. The molecular pathways induced by radiation and leading to thyroid carcinogenesis   191
    YURI E. NIKIFOROV

12. TRK oncogenes in papillary thyroid carcinoma   207
    ANGELA GRECO, EMANUELA ROCCATO AND MARCO A. PIEROTTI

13. Thyroidal iodide transport and thyroid cancer   221
    ORSOLYA DOHÁN AND NANCY CARRASCO

14. Molecular signaling in thyroid cancer   237
    NICHOLAS J. SARLIS AND SALVATORE BENVENGA

15. Gene expression in thyroid tumors   265
    LASZLO PUSKAS AND NADIR R. FARID

16. Animal models of thyroid carcinogenesis   273
    CARSTEN BOLTZE

17. Diagnostic molecular markers in thyroid cancer   295
    MATTHEW D. RINGEL

18. Thyroid cancer imaging   317
    T.T.H PHAN, P.L. JAGER, K.M. VAN TOL, T. P. LINKS

19. Past, presence and future of thyroid-stimulating hormone (TSH) superactive analogs   345
    MARIUSZ W. SZKUDLINSKI

20. Pathobiology of antineoplastic therapy in undifferentiated thyroid cancer   357
    KENNETH B. AIN

21. Gene therapy for thyroid cancer   369
    YUJI NAGAYAMA

22. Familial papillary thyroid carcinoma   381
    CARL D. MALCHOFF AND DIANA M. MALCHOFF

23. RET activation in medullary carcinomas   389
    MARCO A. PIEROTTI, ELENA ARIGHI, DEBORA DEGL'INNOCENTI AND
    MARIA GRAZIA BORRELLO

24. From genes to decisions   417
    LOIS M. MULLIGAN

PREFACE

Thyroid cancer is the fastest growing cancer in the U.S., especially among women. Given the relative success we have had in its treatment, there is a need to capitalize on it by better understanding the factors that underpin this malignancy, and exploring better strategies for diagnosis, treatment, and follow-up. To do so, we must take full advantage of the revolution in modern biology.

This comprehensive volume addresses the needs of a broad readership. Against a backdrop of the complexity of the origins of cancer, pathology of thyroid tumors, including lymphomas, is discussed, as are molecular genetic lesions associated with spontaneous and radiation-related thyroid tumors, diagnostic tests available to surmise tumor subtypes (including a review of the potential of DNA micro arrays), advances in therapeutics (including recombinant hTSH superagonists, allowing for better treatment of well differentiated thyroid carcinoma and its imaging), and combinations of drugs that might influence the course of poorly differentiated and anaplastic thyroid cancer. In this book, we glimpse into the promise of gene therapy in the future management of otherwise lethal anaplastic and poorly differentiated thyroid tumors. The molecular genetics of medullary thyroid cancer is considered in depth, and malignancy is used as a showcase for genetic prediction and counseling.

The Molecular Basis of Thyroid Cancer is an indispensable companion for endocrinologists (particularly those with an interest in thyroid cancer), thyroid surgeons, nuclear medicine physicians, molecular oncologists, clinical biochemists, and those in biotechnology intent on the innovation of better diagnosis and therapy of cancer.

I am fortunate and privileged to be the editor of *The Molecular Basis of Thyroid Cancer*. I compiled a list of top scientists based on their areas of expertise in thyroid cancer whom I hoped would contribute, and received enthusiastic and positive responses. Their chapters are superb.

Throughout this project I have been supported and advised by two wonderful individuals from Kluwer: the untiring Maureen Tobin, editorial assistant and Laura Walsh, editor. They have made the task of putting this book together a pleasure.

Nadir R. Farid

1. THE ORIGIN OF CANCER

EVAN Y. YU, M.D. AND WILLIAM C. HAHN, M.D., Ph.D.

Dana-Farber Cancer Institute and Brigham and Women's Hospital, Harvard Medical School, Boston, MA 02115

INTRODUCTION

Cancer is a complex genetic disease. Work over the past fifty years confirms that the genetic alterations found associated with human cancers impair the function of pathways critical to controlling cell growth and differentiation. In aggregate, these genetic mutations allow a malignant cell to acquire a set of biologic attributes leading to autonomous proliferation and metastatic spread. Despite this paradigm, the precise nature and timing of each of the events that conspire to program the malignant cell remain incompletely understood.

Although familial cancer syndromes are responsible for only a minority of human cancers, the study of these kindreds has facilitated our understanding of cancer genetics. In many such syndromes, individuals inherit one defective, predisposing allele in the germline, and only later in life do they acquire a second loss of function mutation. As first described by Knudson, this "two hit" hypothesis helps explain such inherited cancer syndromes such as retinoblastoma and Wilms' tumors (1). Although the tumors in these patients express mutations in specific inherited genes, the finding that these tumors also harbor a myriad of other genetic changes indicates that further alteration by somatic mutation are required for tumor development(2).

However, the majority of human cancers lack a readily definable predisposing genetic defect and appear to be the result of a concert of acquired genetic alterations. Work from many laboratories, using both patient-derived material and experimental cancer models, have begun to define these malignant genetic mechanisms.

In spontaneously arising human cancers, we still cannot determine the exact number and nature of genetic alterations involved in the process of transformation from a normal cell to a malignant one. Since cancer encompasses more than 100 different types of malignant diseases with great heterogeneity of clinical characteristics, every tumor could hypothetically be completely unique. Thus, cancers, in general, could harbor an undecipherable number of genetic and epigenetic changes leading to their development.

Alternatively, pathogenesis of human cancers may be dependent on a distinct set of genetic and biochemical alterations that apply uniformly to most if not all human tumors. These changes may alter the functions of specific pathways involved in important biological functions and facilitate malignant transformation, endowing cells with specific changes in cell physiology, termed "acquired capabilities," ensuring their survival and continued success (3). In particular, cancer cells generate their own mitogenic signals, proliferate without limits, resist cell cycle arrest, evade apoptosis, induce angiogenesis, and eventually devise mechanisms for invasion and metastasis.

GENETIC REQUIREMENTS FOR CANCER

Epidemiologic analyses have shown that four to six rate-limiting events must occur before a tumor becomes clinically apparent (4,5). The changes that must occur are genetic and/or epigenetic in nature. Most of these events result from somatic mutations that occur infrequently or are induced by carcinogen exposure, and only in aggregate do they lead to the tumorigenic state.

The colorectal carcinoma model

In a seminal series of studies, Vogelstein and his colleagues described a stepwise genetic history of colorectal tumors (6). Since colorectal carcinoma develops intraluminally and tissue is readily available for examination, specific histopathological alterations that occur in cancer development are readily observed in different stages. By studying tissue derived from specific histopathologic stages, ranging from normal colonic epithelium to frank carcinoma, they catalogued genetic alterations specific for each stage, thereby developing a model that dissected an accumulation of separate genetic mutations that could in combination lead to malignancy (7,8).

A vast majority of early adenomatous polyps were found to exhibit an inactivated mutant form of the tumor suppressor gene, adenomatous polyposis coli (*APC*) (9). Alterations in this gene had been previously shown to be responsible for Familial Adenomatous Polyposis (FAP) (10,11). However, patients with germline mutations of *APC* have a greater risk for but do not necessarily develop colorectal cancer. In addition to the germline mutation, somatic mutation of the wild-type *APC* allele must also occur (9,12).

When they investigated intermediate size adenomas, they found that approximately half carry activating mutant *RAS* oncogenes (6,13). Interestingly, normal colonic epithelium harboring *RAS* mutations alone, do not lead to neoplasia (14), and these cells may eventually succumb to apoptosis (15), suggesting that other genetic alterations are necessary for *RAS* mutation to contribute to tumor formation. In a subset of larger

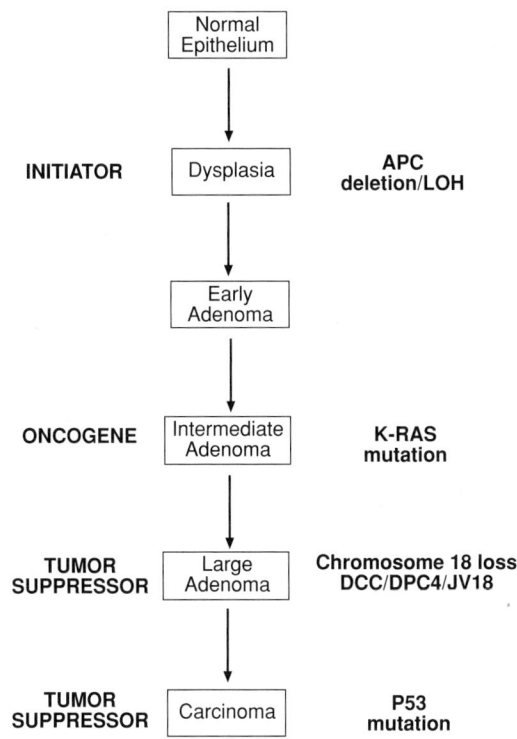

Figure 1. Genetic Model of Colorectal Carcinoma Development. Multiple genetic alterations are found at different stages of development from pre-malignant lesions on to frank carcinoma. These genetic lesions may represent necessary alterations to progress to the next developmental phase toward cancer.

adenomas, alteration of a chromosome 18-associated tumor suppressor gene such as *DCC*, *DPC4*, or *JV18*, were common. Finally, 80% of colorectal carcinomas show evidence of genetic alterations of the *P53* tumor suppressor gene (16). Surprisingly, however, patients with Li-Fraumeni syndrome, who have germline mutations of *P53*, do not have a higher risk of colorectal cancer development and do not even tend to develop polyposis (17). Thus, although both *P53* and *RAS* play individual roles in colon cancer pathogenesis, these observations suggest that oncogenesis cannot be accomplished by a random accumulation of mutations. The order of alteration, as well as the necessity for an initiator like *APC* deletion, may both be important determinants for formation of the resultant tumor (Figure 1).

These observations provide evidence that the history of human cancer follows a stepwise progression of genetic events. This model, however, demonstrates only one of many potential pathways to the neoplastic state.

While these observations in colorectal cancer certainly suggest that all cancers progress through a similar series of ordered events, no other human cancer has been similarly mapped, and abundant evidence indicates that specific mutations differ among particular cancers. Understanding the combination of events required in each type of human cancer remains an important goal of future studies.

EXPERIMENTAL MODELS

Initial studies of human cancer cells were limited to samples obtained from tumor biopsy specimens. To facilitate further study, cells from these tumors were frequently adapted into cell lines that grow in culture (18). These cell lines are useful for many purposes, however, it is impossible to determine the order or even a set of defined genetic or biochemical changes that lead to neoplastic development. Complicating matters further is the high likelihood that additional genetic alterations are acquired over time through propagation in culture.

Recently, transcriptional profiling has been helpful in evaluating the simultaneous expression of thousands of genes in particular cancers or cancer cell lines (19,20). Unfortunately, while these studies have provided us with tools to better classify cancers, they have not yet yielded insight into the functionally important gene expression changes required for cancer growth. It is still impossible from these analyses to determine which genes have true functional roles in the transformation to the malignant state. Thus, a complementary approach to studying the genetic alterations necessary to form a tumor is to transform normal cells, *in vitro*, by serially introducing multiple oncogenes. An alternative method of cancer modeling is through the production of genetically altered mice harboring specific alterations associated with human cancer.

Rodent cell transformation

In rodent systems, single oncogenes fail to transform primary cells without the presence of prior predisposing mutations (21,22). In contrast, two introduced oncogenes convert embryonic rodent cells to a tumorigenic phenotype (23,24). These observations indicated that the conversion of normal cells into cancer cells requires multiple genetic changes to occur.

Collaborating oncogenes that induced transformation in these cultured rodent primary cells included *Myc/Ras* or *E1a/ras* (23,24). Further confirmation of this collaboration through transgenic mouse experiments occurred when a *Ras* or a *Myc* transgene was placed under the control of mammary- or prostate- specific promoters (25,26). Dysplasia in promoter specific organs developed at high rates in the transgenic mice expressing single oncogenes, but frank tumors did not develop unless mice expressed both transgenes. These findings support the concept that specific oncogenes collaborate to aid in tumor development *in vivo*, as well as in cultured cells.

Barriers to human cellular immortalization

While two oncogenes appeared to suffice to transform rodent cells, the transformation of primary human cell lines proved to be more complex. This difference is in part because human cells require more genetic alteration to bypass the barriers of immortalization (Figure 2). When normal human cells are grown in culture, their proliferative potential is limited and they eventually enter an irreversible, quiescent state, termed mortality stage 1 (M1) or replicative senescence (27). Although these cells are still viable, they can no longer be stimulated to divide. The exact trigger for entry into replicative

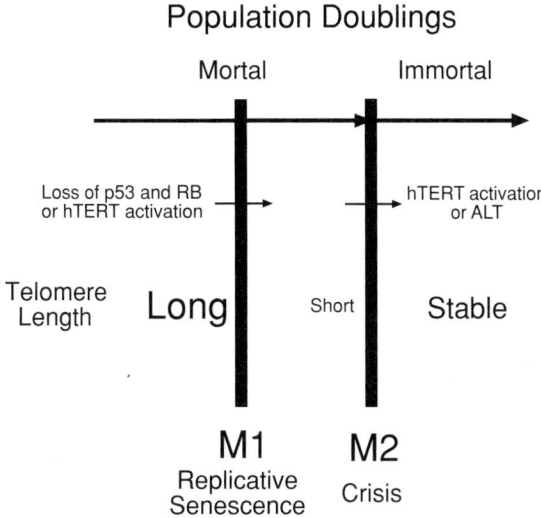

Figure 2. Barriers to Human Cellular Immortalization. Normal passage of cells is halted at MI unless this barrier is bypassed by p53 and RB inactivation or hTERT expression. These cells can then continue dividing until their telomeres become critically short at M2. hTERT expression or ALT allows telomere length stabilization and cellular immortalization.

senescence is still unclear, although there are a variety of stimuli that have a role in this process (28).

Pre-senescent cells can be experimentally manipulated to bypass replicative senescence through ectopic expression of certain genes. Expression of *hTERT*, the catalytic subunit of telomerase is capable of bestowing some but not all primary cells with immortality (29,30). Another mechanism of bypassing this first proliferative barrier is through simultaneous abrogation of the *P53* tumor suppressor and retinoblastoma (*RB*) pathways (28). Expression of viral oncoproteins, such as SV40 large T antigen (31) or human papillomavirus E6 and E7 oncoproteins (32), which bind to and inactivate p53 and RB (33), respectively, offer experimental methods of achieving this dual inactivation.

Cells that lack telomerase overexpression but that express the above mentioned viral oncoproteins, may then undergo another 10–20 population doublings before they encounter mortality stage 2 (M2) or crisis. Here the vast majority of cells have short telomeres (34), display karyotypic abnormalities (35), and die by apoptosis (36). Since in culture telomeres shorten by 50-100 base pairs during each cell replication (37), ongoing passage allows telomeres to shorten to a critical length. This results in an inability to protect the ends of chromosomes, leading to genomic instability and triggering crisis (38).

Rare variants, approximately 1 in 10 million cells, emerge from crisis, and have infinite proliferative capability (31). These cells typically exhibit stable telomere lengths and express the *hTERT* gene with preserved activity (38), which is felt to be expressed at low levels in normal cells (39). These findings have been corroborated by observations in post-senescent, pre-crisis cells that avoid crisis and proliferate indefinitely after transduction with *hTERT* (40–42). However, a subgroup of cells may become immortal without significant *hTERT* or telomerase expression (43,44). These cells have a separate mechanism of telomere length maintenance, termed alternative lengthening of telomeres (ALT), which likely involves recombination (45).

Human cell transformation

The observations that suggested that human cell immortalization is more complex than rodent cell immortalization also complicated attempts for experimental transformation of human cells. From this set of observations, Sager and her colleagues postulated that the senescence program is a barrier to cancer development (46,47). Recent work, however, has begun to identify combinations of genetic alterations that suffice to confer human cellular transformation.

Thus, specifically targeting each of the barriers of immortalization by introduction of the SV40 Early Region, which encodes the large T oncoprotein, in combination with the *hTERT* gene into normal human fibroblasts and kidney cells suffice for immortalization (48,49). Since the SV40 Early Region also encodes for small t oncoprotein, subsequent transduction with oncogenic *RAS* results in the ability to develop tumors in immunocompromised mice, hence transformation. Additional studies have revealed this combination of genetic alterations to be sufficient to transform multiple cell types, including cells of mammary (50), lung (51), prostate, ovarian, mesothelial (52), endothelial, and neuroectodermal (53) origin. Thus, it is necessary to understand the roles of these basic genetic elements involved in transformation in regards to the critical pathways that they effect. For example, the large T oncoprotein may functionally inactivate the p53 and RB pathways, but the inactivation of these two pathways may in sum not equal the effects of the oncoprotein alone, as there may be additional functions gained with large T. Thus, a myriad of other genetic mutations that lead down similar or parallel paths may also bestow specific "acquired capabilities," leading to similar functional endpoints or the neoplastic phenotype.

MOLECULAR CHANGES

Experimental evidence has allowed the delineation of a few crucial pathways in human primary cell transformation. Although there are many important cellular capabilities, allowing a normal cell to bypass cell cycle arrest checkpoints, escape apoptosis, guard against crisis, and provide its own mitogenic signals, may be sufficient to allow for transformation to the oncogenic phenotype. These basic genetic elements may be generalized to most human cancers, however, specific alterations that contribute to oncogenesis are found in some cancers, such as thyroid cancer. These well-defined specific molecular alterations involved both in thyroid-specific and general malignant transformation are described below.

The *P53* tumor suppressor gene

Perhaps one of the most common alterations in human cancers is mutation of the *P53* pathway, found altered in most, if not all, human cancers (54). Loss of wild-type p53 protein expression, in conjunction with gain-of-function from mutant proteins (55), contribute to acquisition of specialized cell properties, such as proliferative and survival advantages. p53 performs these tasks by acting as a transcription factor induced in response to DNA damage, hypoxia, or oncogene activation (54,56). This, in turn, initiates a program of gene regulation leading down at least two major separate pathways, one for cell cycle arrest to allow time to repair damaged DNA and another for apoptosis to trigger the cell to euthanize (54,57).

Wild-type p53 protein may act as a cellular defense mechanism through its effects on cell cycle arrest and apoptosis, both major obstacles to tumor formation. Cells that are unable to arrest and correct DNA damage have increased potential to develop genetic instability with ongoing replication. At the same time, survival of a neoplastic cell, also includes evasion of apoptosis, preventing the cell-suicide program from taking an antitumor effect. Thus, abrogation of wild-type p53 function, may be sufficient in some tumor types to dismantle the apoptotic machinery (58). However, in other tumors, specific components of the apoptotic cascade, such as bcl-2 (59), Akt (60), or caspases (61), must also be inactivated.

p53 regulates a number of genes involved in the cell cycle. One of these proteins, $p21^{CIP1}$, is upregulated by p53 and inhibits the cyclin dependent kinases, resulting in G1 cell cycle checkpoint arrest. Another is Hdm2, a negative regulator of p53, which is also positively regulated by p53 protein itself (Figure 3). Hdm2 physically binds p53

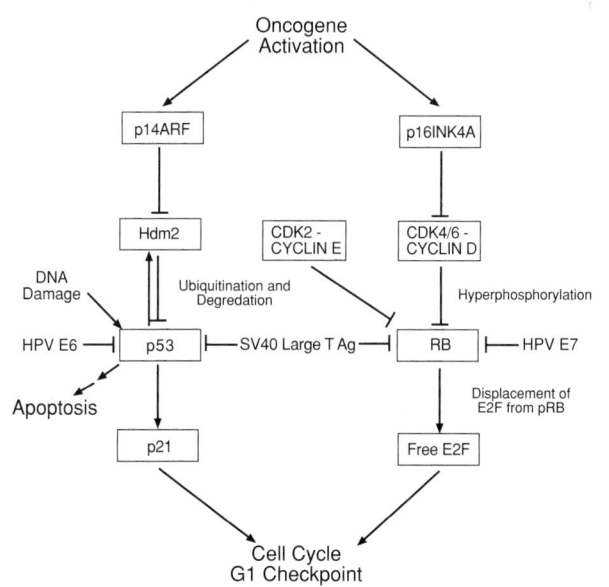

Figure 3. The P53 and RB tumor suppressor pathways. These are both central molecular pathways that are often dysregulated in cancer. Each of these tumor suppressors are regulated by multiple proteins, and disruption can occur at any of these points in human cancer. The role of p53 in apoptosis entails a complex pathway that is not shown on this diagram. Arrows signify activation of the target while blunt lines act in an inhibitory fashion.

protein, inhibiting its activity as a transcriptional factor, meanwhile catalyzing p53 ubiquitination which marks it for proteasomal degradation (62) Hdm2 is itself regulated by $P14^{ARF}$, another tumor suppressor whose protein product binds to and inactivates Hdm2 (63).

While *P53* may be directly mutated in over half of all human cancers, in some tumors no *P53* mutation is observed, yet other genes in the pathway are altered. For example, Hdm2 can be overexpressed and antagonize p53 protein function in a variety of cancers, including B-cell lymphomas (64), melanomas (65), and breast cancers (66). Other tumors harbor $P14^{ARF}$ deletions or suppression by methylation, permitting Hdm2 to remain active and drive the degradation of p53 (63,67). Thus, a various array of genetic and biochemical alterations can converge to enforce a common resultant phenotype, aiding in tumor development and progression.

As will be described in greater detail elsewhere, in thyroid carcinoma, *P53* alterations have been found more frequently in both poorly differentiated and undifferentiated thyroid carcinomas (68). Thus, p53 may have a role in the dedifferentiation process. A combination of mutation (69), loss of heterozygosity (70), and overexpression (71,72), presumably from decreased degradation, have all been found in thyroid cancer, again declaring the importance of this critical pathway. (See Chapter 8).

The retinoblastoma (RB) protein

Regulation of passage through the G_1 checkpoint of the cell cycle is one of the most important roles of the retinoblastoma protein (73). In its hypophosphorylated form, this protein inhibits cellular commitment to mitosis by blocking cell cycle entry into S-phase. In that state, it is bound to various members of the E2F family of proteins (74). These RB-E2F complexes can inhibit gene transcription by multiple methods: (1) Interfering the ability of free E2Fs' to act as transcriptional factors for cyclin E, cyclin A, and multiple other genes necessary for DNA replication (75) (2) Actively recruiting histone deacetylases (HDACs) (76) and other chromatin remodeling factors to E2F responsive promoters (77).

RB inactivation is a crucial step in allowing a cell to pass the G_1 checkpoint and continue through the cell cycle (Figure 3). Normally, one of the cyclin D subtypes (D1, D2, or D3) assembles with one of the cyclin-dependent kinases, CDK4 or CDK6, and cyclin E binds to CDK2. These active holoenzymes phosphorylate RB proteins. Once in a hyperphosphorylated state, RB is unable to bind E2F or HDACs, and releases the repression on genes required for S-phase entry.

Several other tumor suppressor genes also contribute to the phosphorylation status of pRB. For instance, $p16^{INK4A}$ inhibits the activity of cyclin D-dependent kinases to prevent RB phosphorylation and halt cell division (78). The cyclin E-CDK2 complex is inhibited by both $p21^{CIP1}$ (79) and $p27^{KIP1}$ (80). However, when a strong mitogenic stimulus is present, increased cyclin D1 tends to complex with CDK4, and this combination sequesters $p27^{KIP1}$. This leaves cyclin E-CDK2 free from $p27^{KIP1}$ inhibition to phosphorylate and inactivate RB. E2F, as a result, dissociates from hyperphosphorylated RB and acts as a transcription factor for a number of responder genes, including cyclin E. The transcription of these responder genes are required for cell cycle progression through the G1 restriction checkpoint, facilitating cellular division.

Like *P53*, mutations in *RB* or its associated tumor suppressor genes occur frequently, and disabling this pathway may be required for the formation of human cancer cells (81,82). For example, loss of function mutations of *RB* also can be found in osteosarcomas and lung cancers, particularly small cell tumors (81). Although *RB* mutations do occur in non-small cell lung carcinomas, they appear to be present in approximately 20–30% of cases as compared to 80% of the small cell subtype (75). However, p16^{INK4A} loss is evident in over half of all non-small cell lung cancers. Inactivation of *P16^{INK4A}*, by genetic lesions or by methylation, disrupts the RB pathway in a large array of other cancers, including pancreatic, breast, glioblastoma multiforme, and T cell ALL (67,75). Cyclin D1 overexpression drives the cell cycle forward and can also substitute for RB inactivation, as noted in breast cancers (83) and mantle cell lymphomas, where there is juxtaposition of the cyclin D1 gene with the immunoglobulin heavy chain promoter enhancer via a t(11:14) translocation (75). Cyclin E overexpression in breast cancers have also been noted and may help drive past the *RB* inhibition checkpoint in G1 (84). Finally, in many cervical cancers, human papillomaviruses (HPV) E7 oncoprotein sequesters and tags RB for degradation (85). Even in those cervical carcinomas that do not express HPV E7, *RB* somatic mutation is detectable. Alterations in the *RB* pathway seem to be mutually exclusive, as usually only one component of the pathway is mutated or lost; nonetheless, convergence on the loss of growth suppression by RB does seem to exist in the majority of human cancers (81).

However, the role of the *RB* in human thyroid cancer remains unclear. Although there are several human immunohistochemical studies (86–88) that remain inconclusive as well as studies evaluating *E2f* and *Rb* in rodents (89–91), definitive molecular evidence for the role of *RB* in human thyroid cancers is lacking. (See Chapter 8).

Mitogenic stimuli and oncogenic *RAS*

Normal and cancer cells differ in their innate ability to proliferate in the absence of mitogenic stimulation. The presence of surrounding growth factors are crucial for the continued proliferation of normal human cells. Cancer cells, in contrast, have reduced their dependence on external stimuli due to the activation of oncogenic mutations that generate constitutively active mitogenic signals (92). For example, alterations in growth-factor receptors, such as *HER2/NEU* amplification in breast cancer (93,94) or epidermal growth factor receptor mutation in most carcinomas (95), function as autonomous growth stimuli.

In human thyroid cancer, multiple activating receptors have been implicated in disease pathogenesis. Characteristic chromosomal rearrangements linking the promoter and amino-terminus domains of unrelated gene(s) to the carboxy-terminus of the *RET* gene result in a constitutively active chimeric receptor, termed (RET/PTC). This event may initiate papillary thyroid cancers (96). Constitutive activation of this mutant kinase promotes interaction with SHC adaptor proteins, intermediates in the *RAS* signaling pathway (97). Although rare, another early event in papillary thyroid cancers, may involve rearrangements of specific TRK tyrosine kinase receptors (98).

Both epidermal growth factor receptor (EGFR) and its ligands, epidermal growth factor (EGF) and transforming growth factor alpha (TGF-α), are also widely expressed in both normal thyroid and thyroid neoplastic tissue (99,100); however, EGF has a higher binding affinity for neoplastic thyroid tissue when compared to normal tissue (101). EGF and its receptor stimulate proliferation of thyroid cancer cells and enhance invasion (102), suggesting their potential role in malignant progression.

Multiple intracellular protein networks exist downstream of growth factor receptors that can become constitutively active in a mutated state, conferring a growth-inducing effect. As discussed above, introduction of one of these aberrant signals, *H-RAS*, turns an activating switch on and facilitates malignant transformation to previously immortalized human and rodent primary cells. (See Chapter 7).

Various RAS proteins, members of a large superfamily of low-molecular-weight GTP-binding proteins, control several crucial signaling pathways that regulate cell proliferation. Their ability to effect downstream intracellular signaling proteins first rely on post-translational farnesylation to localize the *RAS* protein to the cell membrane. Then the ratio of biologically active RAS-GTP to inactive RAS-GDP depends upon the presence and activity of various guanine nucleotide exchange factors (GEFs) and their antagonists, GTPase activating proteins (GAPs) (103).

Multiple effector pathways lay immediately downstream of *RAS* (Figure 4). The RAF family of proteins, which can trigger a cascade of phosphorylating events through the mitogen-activated protein kinase (MAPK) pathway, leads to cell cycle progression. There is resultant ERK-mediated transcriptional upregulation of angiogenic factors, and increased capability for invasiveness through expression of matrix metalloproteinases. Through RAS stimulation of phosphatidylinositol 3-kinases (PI3Ks), RAC, which is a Rho family protein, can also increase invasiveness through its effects on the actin cytoskeleton. PI3K also triggers a strong anti-apoptotic survival signal through Akt/protein kinase B (PKB). Much like Akt, RALGDS, which is activated by RAS, inhibits the Forkhead transcription factors of the FoxO family which have a role in cell cycle arrest through induction of p27^{KIP1} and apoptosis through the expression of BIM and FAS ligand (104). Finally, phospholipase C (PLC) is another RAS effector which promotes activation of protein kinase C and calcium mobilization (105). Alterations in the RAS proteins or their downstream effectors can therefore have the potential to lead to constitutively active signals, aiding the oncogenic phenotype. (See Chapter 7).

Activating point mutations of *RAS* occur in approximately 20% of human tumors, most frequently in pancreatic, thyroid, colorectal, and lung carcinomas, obviating the requirement for the neoplastic cells to encounter external growth stimuli (106,107) In general human cancer and thyroid cancer cells, somatic *RAS* mutations seem to be an early event. These activating mutations are frequently found in follicular thyroid carcinomas and occasionally papillary thyroid carcinoma (108).

Three members of the *RAS* family, *K-RAS* (around 85% of total), which is ubiquitously expressed, *N-RAS* (about 15%), and *H-RAS* (less than 1%), are commonly found to be activated by mutation in human tumors (109). These point mutations all prevent GAP induced GTPase activity, leaving RAS in its active, GTP-bound form. GAP deletion also leads to a similar resultant RAS activation; *NF1* or neurofibromin

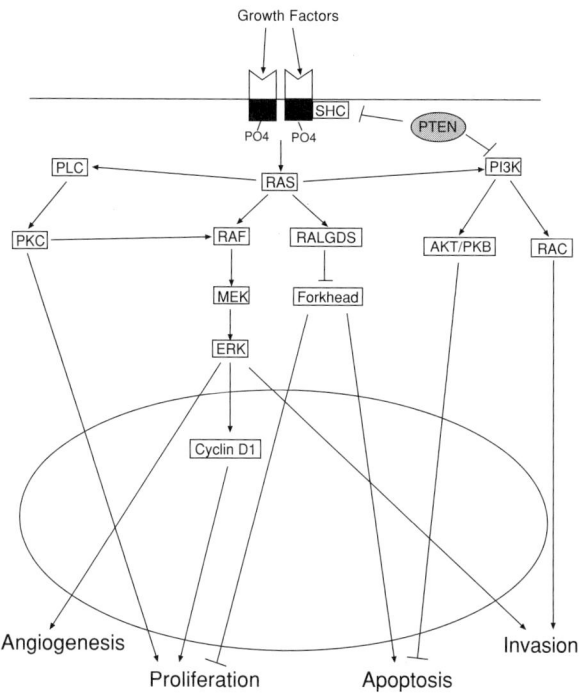

Figure 4. Downstream Mediators of *RAS*. The RAS family of proteins lead down multiple signal transduction networks to not only effect a mitogenic stimulus, but also to provide other important cellular capabilities important for cancer cells. These signaling pathways can lead to cell survival, angiogenic potential, and invasion.

loss is an example of this phenomenon and leads to benign and occasionally malignant tumors of neural crest origin (110). These single point mutations in *RAS* contribute to many of the "acquired capabilities" of cancer cells, including dysregulated growth, inappropriate survival, invasiveness, and angiogenesis (111).

In many cancers that lack *RAS* mutations, downstream effectors of RAS signaling are frequently altered, leading to acquisition of a similar set of neoplastic attributes (105). Mutations of the *BRAF* gene were initially found to be present in around 66% of melanomas and also approximately 12% of colon cancers (112). Recently, two unique somatic mutations of the *BRAF* gene have been identified in papillary thyroid carcinoma (113,114), and they offer genetic evidence for constitutive activation of the RET/PTC-RAS-BRAF signaling pathway (113). Amplification of the *P110α* gene results in *PI3K* activation in 40% of ovarian tumors, while one of its downstream targets, AKT2, can also be amplified in breast and ovarian carcinomas (115). Finally, the *PTEN* tumor suppressor gene, acts as a phosphatase on specific downstream targets of PI3K, such as AKT, inactivating that pathway; *PTEN* deletions occurs in 30–40% of human cancers (116). Altogether, in human cancers the RAS proteins are not only central mediators of both upstream growth factor receptors, but also their downstream targets play critical cellular roles, bestowing constitutively active mitogenic signals as well as multiple other important functions for oncogenesis.

Telomeres and telomerase

Telomeres are terminal structures at the ends of each eukaryotic chromosome and are composed of guanine rich, DNA 5′-TTAGGG-3′ repeats, as well as multiple DNA-binding proteins (117,118). At the end of each telomere is a single stranded 3′ overhang (119–121) that forms a large secondary loop structure, termed a T-loop (122). Telomeric DNA is maintained by telomerase, a RNA-dependent, DNA polymerase (123). Telomerase is composed of multiple subunits, two of which are crucial for enzymatic function, the RNA component (hTERC) and catalytic component (hTERT) (124) hTERT is the rate limiting component of the holoenzyme, as hTERT expression is restricted solely to cells that demonstrate telomerase enzymatic activity (125).

One of the main functions of telomeres are to protect the ends of chromosomes from forming illegitimate fusions, which would lead to genetic instability (126–128). Many DNA damage-associated proteins, such as the MRE11 complex (129) and Ku 70/80 (130,131) bind to telomere associated proteins. Thus, it has also been hypothesized that the telomere may serve as a cap, guarding the chromosome end from recognition as damaged DNA (132,133).

Both telomere length and maintenance are associated with human cell lifespan, genetic instability, senescence, immortalization, and transformation. In approximately 90% of human tumors, telomere maintenance and replicative immortality may be achieved through activation of telomerase; the remaining tumors may be maintained through "alternative lengthening of telomeres" (ALT), a telomerase-independent mechanism (134). Interestingly, studies examining malignant transformation in ALT cells lacking *P53* and *RB* function, but expressing oncogenic RAS, confirm that malignant transformation is impossible even with stable telomere lengths unless hTERT is ectopically introduced (135). Thus, 3′ overhang and T-loop maintenance by hTERT may have a role in the mechanism of transformation (136). Additionally, hTERT itself may serve some physical capping function that may be important for malignant transformation. Finally, it remains possible that hTERT has some either direct or indirect role in regulation of other important gene(s) that are critical for transformation.

In thyroid cancer, the correlation of telomere length to telomerase activity is poor, implying that there are other mechanisms that regulate telomere dynamics (137). However, most thyroid cancer cells do have sustained telomere length and have assayable telomerase activity while telomerase negative cell telomeres are likely maintained through ALT (138). Thus, similar to other types of cancers, telomere length is also important for thyroid cancer; although hTERT function and telomerase activity in thyroid cancer require further delineation of their mechanism(s) in cancer pathogenesis.

GENETIC INSTABILITY

Although the above discussed molecular alterations and their regulatory pathways are crucial to the development of a neoplastic cell, one additional hallmark may be necessary to achieve a malignant state. This cardinal feature is genetic instability, which likely allows a cell to more rapidly acquire additional neoplastic attributes through the stepwise accumulation of mutations.

When the homeostatic mechanisms that guard the integrity of chromosomes are disrupted, additional genetic alterations may accumulate that lead to further deleterious effects. Though the various components of DNA damage detection, signaling, and repair mechanisms (139) are poorly understood, the operation of this repair machinery is incompletely understood, the adequate operation of this repair machinery is integral in preventing the survival of aberrant cells with neoplastic potential. An abnormal level of genetic instability is consistently found in many tumors (140). This instability, however, can be at either a DNA sequence level or at the level of the chromosome, in the form of aneuploidy.

Cytogenetic deformities are not an absolute finding in human cancers, as subtle DNA sequence changes can occasionally suffice to predispose to tumor formation. For instance, mutations in DNA mismatch repair genes, such as *MSH2* or *MLH1* (141), give rise to instability at the nucleotide sequence level since common replication errors can no longer be properly repaired. These tumors demonstrate microsatellite instability, which is detectable as short DNA sequence repeats seen scattered throughout the genome (142,143). These markers identify tumors that typically have two to three times as many single nucleotide mutations as compared to normal cells or cancers of the same histology but are mismatch repair proficient (144,145)

Different sets of proteins recognize and repair various types of physical DNA lesions. For instance, ultraviolet light induces adjacent pyrimidine dimerization, affecting DNA transcription and replication. Such events are repaired by the nucleotide excision repair proteins (NER) (146). In contrast, double-strand breaks (DSBs) develop in response to ionizing radiation, oxidative stress, or the stalling of replication forks at sites of DNA damage (147). These DSBs can only be repaired by homologous recombination or non-homologous end-joining (148). Thus, the cell must have unique mechanisms to recognize low levels of DNA damage at any location in the genome and shuttle the specific repair proteins required for that type of lesion. Examples include the *Xeroderma pigmentosum* group C protein involved in NER (146), MUTS proteins which bind to mismatched bases (149), and the Ku heterodimer which binds to DSBs (150). If these repair mechanisms are not in proper order, a dividing cell could improperly segregate, and depending on the type of lesion, possibly result in aneuploidy.

One important feature for a DNA damage response is the slowing or arrest of the defective cell at specific DNA damage checkpoint (151,152). This serves to delay important cell cycle transitions until repair has occurred. In human cells, the *ATR/ATM* signaling network, which can together detect a wide variety of DNA lesions through genomic surveillance during DNA replication, has a large role in this action. *ATR* disruption is lethal; *ATM* defects are not, although they are responsible for ataxia telangiectasia, which causes hypersensitivity to agents causing DSBs and increases cancer risk (152) *ATR*, when necessary, is likely to be the initiator of a global DNA damage response by activating downstream proteins like CHK1, CHK2, and RAD53. This leads to cell-cycle arrest, chromatin modulation, and further upregulation of other repair pathway proteins (139).

Alterations in DNA damage pathways, conferring genetic instability, may be early events in tumorigenesis, as is the case in microsatellite instability tumors. A heterogeneous population of cells will undergo a selective process in regards to instability. Cells with excess instability accumulate increasing amounts of DNA damage with continued proliferation eventually surpassing the threshold of viability, succumbing to apoptosis. Other cells with either too little or no genetic instability, halt at the natural barriers to immortalization. Certain cells with the appropriate amount of instability develop a survival and proliferative advantage by selecting out the right set of mutations, typically an accumulation of oncogenes and tumor suppressor genes that are now no longer able to be repaired (153). This eventually leads to clonal outgrowth and tumor formation.

ANGIOGENESIS, INVASION, AND METASTASIS

Although the initiating event in oncogenesis is not reliant upon angiogenesis, the continued success and maintainence of a tumor depends upon the utilization of this system for sustenance and eventual dissemination. In general, a solid tumor cannot grow successfully beyond 2 mm in diameter without neovascularization through the switch to the angiogenic phenotype (154,155). Thus, a tumor must acquire its own blood supply by developing new vascular structures that connect directly with existing host vasculature.

Angiogenesis is achieved by the secretion of proangiogenic factors, namely vascular endothelial growth factor (VEGF), angiopoetins, and basic fibroblast growth factors (bFGF); alternatively, the down-regulation of antiangiogenic proteins, such as endostatin, angiostatin, and thrombospondin-1 (TSP-1), also have a similar effect (155,156). These proteins signal to a complex array of downstream signaling proteins that cooperate to facilitate the overall regulation of angiogenesis. Unfortunately, this molecular circuitry remains poorly understood at this time.

An example of how tightly tumor angiogenesis may be tied to the other crucial pathways involved in tumorigenesis, is the intricate involvement of the p53 protein. Not only is p53 involved in G1 cell cycle regulation and apoptosis, but it also has a role in the regulation of angiogenesis, mainly through its interactions with TSP-1. The wild-type p53 protein can act on *TSP-1* promoter sequences and stimulate endogenous TSP-1 production (157). Since TSP-1 is a potent inhibitor of angiogenesis, wild-type *P53* gene expression loss, coincides with the switch to the angiogenic phenotype. Additionally, mutant p53 cells have been shown to upregulate VEGF (158), perhaps the most potent proangiogenic agent.

Invasion and metastasis are the final steps in tumor progression, but a unified set of responsible genetic elements has yet to be identified. Studies have described target genes that may be intimately involved in tumor migration, such as matrix metalloproteinases (159), however, the discovery of integral pathways to invasion and metastasis require further study. Just as studies have led to the discovery of common pathways for cell cycle progression, apoptosis, and autonomous growth stimulation, the discovery of a "metastasis pathway" could have utility for better understanding and treatment of cancers.

BEYOND CANCER GENOMES

To date, genetic alterations are still the easiest changes in cancer cells to detect and study experimentally. In the future, successful sequencing of an entire human cancer cell genome will certainly yield more important information for the further study of cancer. However, even with this data, many important alterations will be missed, since not all changes occur at the DNA sequence level and are instead occurring at a non-genetic level. For example, both epigenetic phenomena and post-translational modifications have critical roles in the regulation of important cellular capabilities that contribute to the neoplastic phenotype.

Epigenetic alterations

Alterations in gene expression that do not involve mutations of DNA sequences are epigenetic events. These arise during cell development and proliferation and serve as an additional method of adaptation to environmental and selective pressures. It has become clear in recent years, that epigenetic changes have an impact to the development of human cancers through silencing of tumor suppressors and DNA damage elements, chromosomal instability, and even activation of oncogenes (160,161).

Hypermethylation-mediated silencing of tumor suppressor genes may be important for tumor development since, among other advantages, it tends to lead to a selective cellular growth advantage (160,161). Methylation of cytosine residues at CpG dinucleotides occurs, and 70–80% of these dinucleotides are heavily methylated in human cells (162). Long GC-rich stretches of DNA in the human genome, termed CpG islands, are often uniquely associated with flanking genes and are protected from modification (163). These normally unmethylated CpG islands may become methylated in cancer cells, resulting in loss of expression of the flanking genes (160). This form of methylation-induced silencing affects tumor suppressors genes such as *CDH1* (164) and *P16* (165), both implicated in cancer development. Epigenetic alterations found in familial and non-hereditary forms of breast and colon cancer offer further supportive evidence for the role of methylation in neoplastic formation (166).

Although the exact mechanism of abnormal epigenetic changes leading to neoplasia is unknown, likely candidates include changes in expression of the key enzymes that regulate DNA methylation, such as the DNA methyltransferases (DNMTs). Overexpression of *DNMT* mRNA levels have been found in malignancies of various histological origin, including lung (167), colon (168,169), and ovarian (170) cancer cells. Further evidence is the fact that overexpression of DNMT1 leads to de novo methylation of CpG islands (171), and can facilitate cellular transformation (172,173).

CONCLUSIONS

The development of human cancer is a complex process that entails the alteration of multiple cell physiologic functions. Although possibilities for genetic and/or epigenetic alterations are innumerable, common principles have recently been delineated that ensure the success of any cell exhibiting a malignant phenotype. The specific pathways and principles discussed above are known to contribute in an intimate manner to this process, but the foundation is just being set.

At this time, the study of cancer is frequently performed through experimentation with artificial cell lines or genetically altered and transformed primary cells. Although useful, it is still impossible to know the exact conditions and order of events that occur *in vivo* during metamorphosis to a neoplastic cell. Perhaps, in the future, when better cancer cell models are developed, we will define cancer by a set of distinct pathways intersecting with common principles.

Thyroid carcinomas, in particular, offer excellent models for studying cancer in general, as they offer a broad spectrum of tumor subtypes. For instance, both papillary and follicular tumors tend to be well-differentiated and may have utility in studying early genetic lesions involved in neoplastic formation. Anaplastic tumors offer the other end of the differentiation spectrum. Medullary thyroid carcinomas are associated with the MEN2 familial syndrome and supply another model to study genetic predisposition to cancer.

In the following chapters, the specific molecular defects involved in thyroid cancers will be discussed in detail. These defects may be specific for different subsets of thyroid carcinomas, but they typically lead into unifying pathways that phenotypically result in specific "acquired capabilities" for the cells. It is important to recognize these molecular changes, not only to gain greater understanding of the origin of thyroid cancers, but also to use this information for superior drug development and treatment.

Early stage thyroid cancer is standardly treated and often cured by surgical resection. However, advanced stage disease is still incurable, and current treatment measures with chemotherapy have not been shown to significantly improve morbidity or mortality. Thus, identifying these important molecular changes may one day lead to the development of new targeted therapies that can be readily tested in the metastatic setting.

REFERENCES

1. Knudson, A. G. Antioncogenes and human cancer. *Proc Natl Acad Sci* **90**, 10914–10921 (1993).
2. Knudson, A. G. Two genetic hits (more or less) to cancer. *Nat Rev Cancer* **1**, 157–162 (2001).
3. Hanahan, D., Weinberg, R. A. The hallmarks of cancer. *Cell* **100**, 57–70 (2000).
4. Armitage, P., Doll, R. The age distribution of cancer and a multi-stage theory of carcinogenesis. *Br J Cancer* **8**, 1–12 (1954).
5. Renan, M. J. How many mutations are required for tumorigenesis? Implications from human cancer data. *Mol Carcinog* **7**, 139–146 (1993).
6. Vogelstein, B., Fearon, E. R., Hamilton, S. R., et al. Genetic alterations during colorectal-tumor development. *N Engl J Med* **319**, 525–532 (1988).
7. Fearon, E. R., Vogelstein, B. A genetic model for colorectal tumorigenesis. *Cell* **1990**, 759–767 (1990).
8. Kinzler, K. W., Vogelstein, B. Lessons from hereditary colorectal cancer. *Cell* **87**, 159–170 (1996).
9. Ichii, S., Horii, A., Nakatsuru, S., et al. Inactivation of both APC alleles in an early stage of colon adenomas in a patient with familial adenomatous polyposis (FAP). *Hum Mol Genet* **1**, 387–390 (1992).
10. Groden, J., Thliveris, A., Samowitz, W., et al. Identification and characterization of the familial adenomatous polyposis coli gene. *Cell* **66**, 589–600 (1991).
11. Nishisho, I., Nakamura, Y., Miyoshi, Y., et al. Mutations of chromosome 5q21 genes in FAP and colorectal cancer patients. *Science* **253**, 665–669 (1991).
12. Levy, D. B., Smith, K. J., Beazer-Barclay, Y., et al. Inactivation of both APC alleles in human and mouse tumors. *Cancer Res* **54**, 5953–5958 (1994).
13. Shibata, D., Schaeffer, J., Li, Z. H., et al. Genetic heterogeneity of the c-K-ras locus in colorectal adenomas but not in adenocarcinomas. *J Natl Cancer Inst* **85**, 1058–1063 (1993).

14. Jen, J., Powell, S. M., Papadopoulos, N., et al. Molecular determinants of dysplasia in colorectal lesions. *Cancer Res* **54**, 5523–5526 (1994).
15. Shpitz, B. H. K., Medline, A., Bruce, W. R., et al. Natural history of aberrant crypt foci. *Dis Colon Rectum* **39**, 763–767 (1996).
16. Baker, S. J., Preisinger, A. C., Jessup, J. M., et al. p53 gene mutations occur in combination with 17p allelic deletions as late events in colorectal tumorigenesis. *Cancer Res* **50**, 7717–7722 (1990).
17. Garber, J. E., Goldstein, A. M., Kantor, A. F., et al. Follow-up study of twenty-four families with Li-Fraumeni syndrome. *Cancer Res* **51**, 6094–6607 (1991).
18. Masters, J. R. Human cancer cell lines; fact and fantasy. *Nat Rev Mol Cell Biol* **1**, 233–236 (2000).
19. Golub, T. R., Slonim, D. K., Tamayo, P., et al. Molecular classification of cancer: class discovery and class prediction by gene expression monitoring. *Science* **286**, 531–537 (1999).
20. Yeang, C. H., Ramaswamy, S., Tamayo, P., et al. Molecular classification of multiple tumor types. *Bioinformatics* **17: Suppl 1**, S316–S322 (2001).
21. Newbold, R. F., Overell, R. W., Connell, J. R. Induction of immortality is an early event in malignant transformation of mammalian cells by carcinogens. *Nature* **299**, 633–635 (1982).
22. Newbold, R. F., Overell, R. W. Fibroblast immortality is a prerequisite for transformation by EJ c-HA-ras oncogene. *Nature* **304**, 648–651 (1983).
23. Land, H., Parada L. F., Weinberg, R. A. Tumorigenic conversion of primary embryo fibroblasts requires at least two cooperating oncogenes. *Nature* **304**, 596–602 (1983).
24. Ruley, H. E. Adenovirus early region 1A enables viral and cellular transforming genes to transform primary cells in culture. *Nature* **304**, 602–606 (1983).
25. Sinn, E., Muller, W., Pattengale, P., et al. Coexpression of MMTV/v-Ha-ras and MMTV/c-myc genes in transgenic miceL synergistic action of oncogenes in vivo. *Cell* **49**, 465–475 (1987).
26. Thompson, T. C., Southgate, J., Kitchener, G., Land, H. Multistage carcinogenesis induced by ras and myc oncogenes in a reconstituted organ. *Cell* **56**, 917–930 (1989).
27. Hayflick, L., Moorhead, P. S. The serial cultivation of human diploid cell strains. *Exp Cell Res* **25**, 585–621 (1961).
28. Shay, J. W., Wright, W. E., Werbin, H. Defining the molecular mechanisms of human cell immortalization. *Biochim Biophys Acta* **1072**, 1–7 (1991).
29. Bodnar, A. G., Ouellette, M., Frolkis, M., et al. Extension of life-span by introduction of telomerase into normal human cells. *Science* **279**, 349–352 (1998).
30. Kiyono, T., Foster, S. A., Koop, J. I., et al. Both Rb/p16INK4a inactivation and telomerase activity are required to immortalize human epithelial cells. *Nature* **396**, 84–88 (1998).
31. Shay, J. W., Wright, W. E. Quantitation of the frequency of immortalization of normal human diploid fibroblasts by SV40 large T-antigen. *Exp Cell Res* **184**, 109–118 (1989).
32. Shay, J. W., Pereira-Smith, O. M., Wright, W. E. A role for both RB and p53 in the regulation of human cellular senescence. *Exp Cell Res* **196**, 33–39 (1991).
33. Ali, S. H., DeCaprio, J. A. Cellular transformation by SV40 large T antigen: Interaction with host proteins. *Semin Cancer Biol* **11**, 15–23 (2001).
34. Wei, W., Sedivy, J. M. Differentiation between senescence (M1) and crisis (M2) in human fibroblast cultures. *Exp Cell Res* **253**, 519–522 (1999).
35. Stewart, N., Bacchetti, S. Expression of SV40 large T antigen, but not small t antigen, is required for the induction of chromosomal aberrations in transformed human cells. *Virology* **180**, 49–57 (1991).
36. Macera-Bloch, L., Houghton, J., Lenahan, M., et al. Termination of lifespan of SV40-transformed human fibroblasts in crisis is due to apoptosis. *J Cell Physiol* **190**, 332–344 (2002).
37. Harley, C. B., Futcher, A. B., Gredier, C. W. Telomeres shorten during ageing of human fibroblasts. *Nature* **345**, 458–460 (1990).
38. Counter, C. M., Avilion, A. A., Le Feuvre, C. E., et al. Telomere shortening associated with chromosome instability is arrested in immortal cells which express telomerase activity. *EMBO J* **11**, 1921–1929 (1992).
39. Masutomi, K., Yu, E. Y., Khurts, S., et al. Telomerase maintains telomere structure in normal human cells. *Cell* **114**, 241–253 (2003).
40. Counter, C. M., Hahn, W. C., Wei, W., et al. Dissociation among in vitro telomerase activity, telomere maintenance, and cellular immortalization. *Proc Natl Acad Sci USA* **95**, 14723–14728 (1998).
41. Halvorsen, T. L., Leibowitz, G., Levine, F. Telomerase activity is sufficient to allow transformed cells to escape from crisis. *Mol Cell Biol* **19**, 1864–1870 (1999).
42. Zhu, J., Wang, H., Bishop, J. M., Blackburn, E. H. Telomerase extends the lifespan of virus-transformed human cells without net telomere lengthening. *Proc Natl Acad Sci* **96**, 3723–3728 (1999).

43. Bryan, T. M., Englezou, A., Gupta, J., et al. Telomere elongation in immortal human cells without detectable telomerase activity. *EMBO J* **14**, 4240–4248 (1995).
44. Murnane, J. P., Sabatier, L., Marder, B. A., et al. Telomere dynamics in an immortal human cell line. *EMBO J* **13**, 4953–4962 (1994).
45. Dunham, M. A., Neumann, A. A., Fasching, C. L., et al. Telomere maintenance by recombination in human cells. *Nat Genet* **26**, 447–450 (2000).
46. O'Brien, W., Stenman, G., Sager, R. Suppression of tumor growth by senescence in virally transformed human fibroblasts. *Proc Natl Acad Sci USA* **83**, 8659–8663 (1986).
47. Sager, R. Senescence as a mode of tumor suppression. *Environ Health Perspect* **93**, 59–62 (1991).
48. Hahn, W. C., Counter, C. M., Lundberg, A. S., et al. Creation of human tumour cells with defined genetic elements. *Nature* **400**, 464–468 (1999).
49. Hahn, W. C., Dessain, S. K., Brooks, M. W., et al. Enumeration of the simian virus 40 early region elements necessary for human cell transformation. *Mol Cell Biol* **22**, 2111–2123 (2002).
50. Elenbaas, B., Spirio, L., Koerner, F., et al. Human breast cancer cells generated by oncogenic transformation of primary mammary epithelial cells. *Genes Dev* **15**, 50–65 (2001).
51. Lundberg, A. S., Randell, S. H., Stewart, S. A., et al. Immortalization and transformation of primary human airway epithelial cells by gene transfer. *Oncogene* **21**, 4577–4586 (2002).
52. Yu, J., Boyapati, A., Rundell K. Critical role for SV40 small-t antigen in human cell transformation. *Virology* **290**, 192–198 (2001).
53. Rich, J. N., Guo, C., McLendon, R. E., et al. A genetically tractable model of human glioma formation. *Cancer Res* **61**, 3556–3560 (2001).
54. Levine, A. J. p53, The cellular gatekeeper for growth and division. *Cell* **88**, 323–331 (1997).
55. Dittmer, D., Pati, S., Zambetti, G., et al. Gain of function mutations in p53. *Nat Genet* **4**, 42–46 (1993).
56. Lowe, S. W. Activation of p53 by oncogenes. *Endocr Relat Cancer* **6**, 45–48 (1999).
57. Giaccia, A. J., Kastan, M. B. The complexity of p53 modulation: emerging patterns from divergent signals. *Genes Dev* **12**, 2973–2983 (1998).
58. Shen, Y., White, E. p53-Dependent apoptosis pathways. *Adv Cancer Res* **82**, 55–84 (2001).
59. Yin, X. M., Oltvai, Z. N., Veis-Novack, D. J., et al. Bcl-2 gene family and the regulation of programmed cell death. *Cold Spring Harb Symp Quant Biol* **59**, 387–393 (1994).
60. Datta, S. R., Brunet, A., Greenberg, M. E. Cellular survival: a play in three Akts. *Genes Dev* **13**, 2905–2927 (1999).
61. Thornberry, N. A., Lazebnik, Y. Caspases: enemies within. *Science* **281**, 1312–1316 (1998).
62. Juven-Gershon, T., Oren, M. Mdm2: the ups and downs. *Mol Med* **5**, 71–83 (1999).
63. Sherr, C. J. The INK4a/ARF network in tumour suppression. *Nat Rev Mol Cell Biol* **2**, 731–737 (2001).
64. Sanchez-Aguilera, A., Sanchez-Beato, M., Garcia, J. F., et al. p14(ARF) nuclear overexpression in aggressive B-cell lymphomas is a sensor of malfunction of the common tumor suppressor pathways. *Blood* **99**, 1411–1418 (2002).
65. Polsky, D., Bastian, B. C., Hazan, C., et al. HDM2 protein overexpression, but not gene amplification, is related to tumorigenesis of cutaneous melanoma. *Cancer Res* **61**, 7642–7646 (2001).
66. Ho, G. H., Calvano, J. E., Bisogna, M., et al. Genetic alterations of the p14ARF-hdm2-p53 regulatory pathway in breast carcinoma. *Breast Cancer Res Treat* **65**, 225–232 (2001).
67. Sharpless, N. E., Depinho, R. A. The INK4A/ARF locus and its two gene products. *Curr Opin Genet Dev* **9**, 22–30 (1999).
68. Gimm, O. Thyroid cancer. *Cancer Lett* **163**, 143–156 (2001).
69. Fagin, J. A., Matsuo, K., Karmakar, D. J., et al. High prevalence of mutations of the p53 gene in poorly differentiated human thyroid carcinomas. *J Clin Invest* **91**, 179–184 (1993).
70. Ito, T., Seyama, T., Mizuno, T., et al. Genetic alterations in thyroid tumor progression: association with p53 gene mutations. *Jpn J Cancer Res* **84**, 526–531 (1993).
71. Dobashi, Y., Sakamoto, A., Sugimura, M., et al. Overexpression of p53 as a possible prognostic factor in human thyroid carcinoma. *Am J Surg Pathol* **17**, 375–381 (1993).
72. Donghi, R., Longoni, A., Pilotti, P., et al. Gene p53 mutations are restricted to poorly differentiated and undifferentiated carcinomas of the thyroid gland. *J Clin Invest* **91**, 1753–1760 (1993).
73. Kaelin, W. G. J. Functions of the retinoblastoma protein. *Bioessays* **21**, 950–958 (1999).
74. Dyson, N. The regulation of E2F by pRB-family proteins. *Genes Dev* **12**, 2245–2262 (1998).
75. Sherr, C. J., McCormick, F. The RB and p53 pathways in cancer. *Cancer Cell* **2**, 103–112 (2002).

76. Rayman, J. B., Takahashi, Y., Indjeian, V. B., et al. E2F mediates cell cycle-dependent transcriptional repression in vivo by recruitment of an HDAC1/mSin3B corepressor complex. *Genes Dev* **16**, 933–947 (2002).
77. Ogawa, H., Ishiguro, K., Gaubatz, S., et al. A complex with chromatin modifiers that occupies E2F- and Myc-responsive genes in Go cells. *Science* **296**, 1132–1136 (2002).
78. Roussel, M. F. The INK4 family of cell cycle inhibitors in cancer. *Oncogene* **18**, 5311–5317 (1999).
79. LaBaer, J., Garrett, M. D., Stevenson, L. F., et al. New functional activities for the p21 family of CDK inhibitors. *Genes Dev* **11**, 847–862 (1997).
80. Cheng, M., Olivier, P., Diehl, J. A., et al. The p21^{CIP1} and p27^{KIP1} CDK "inhibitors" are essential activators of cyclin D-dependent kinases in murine fibroblasts. *EMBO J* **18**, 1571–1583 (1999).
81. Sellers, W. R., Kaelin, W. G. Role of the retinoblastoma protein in the pathogenesis of human cancer. *J Clin Oncol* **15**, 3301–3312 (1997).
82. Hahn, W. C., Weinberg, R. A. Modeling the molecular circuitry of cancer. *Nat Rev Cancer* **2**, 331–341 (2002).
83. Sicinski, P., Weinberg, R. A. A specific role for cyclin D1 in mammary gland development. *J Mammary Gland Biol Neoplasia* **2**, 335–342 (1997).
84. Jacks, T., Weinberg, R. A. The expanding role of cell cycle regulators. *Science* **280**, 1035–1036 (1998).
85. zur Hausen, H. Papillomaviruses and cancer: from basic studies to clinical applications. *Nat Rev Cancer* **2**, 342–350 (2002).
86. Ito, Y., Yoshida, H., Uruno, T., et al. p130 expression in thyroid neoplasms; its linkage with tumor size and dedifferentiation. *Cancer Lett* **192**, 83–87 (2003).
87. Anwar, F., Emond, M. J., Schmidt, R. A., et al. Retinoblastoma expression in thyroid neoplasms. *Mod Pathol* **13**, 562–569 (2000).
88. Holm, R., Nesland, J. M. Retinoblastoma and p53 tumour suppressor gene protein expression in carcinomas of the thyroid gland. *J Pathol* **172**, 267–272 (1994).
89. Harvey, M., Vogel, H., Lee, E. Y., et al. Mice deficient in both p53 and Rb develop tumors primarily of endocrine origin. *Cancer Res* **55**, 1146–1151 (1995).
90. Coxon, A. B., Ward, J. M., Geradts, J., et al. RET cooperates with RB/p53 inactivation in a somatic multi-step model for murine thyroid cancer. *Oncogene* **17**, 1625–1628 (1998).
91. Lee, E. Y., Cam, H., Ziebold, U., et al. E2F4 loss suppresses tumorigenesis in Rb mutant mice. *Cancer Cell* **2**, 463–472 (2002).
92. McCormick, F. Signalling networks that cause cancer. *Trends Cell Biol* **9**, M53-M56 (1999).
93. Press, M. F., Jones, L. A., Godolphin, W., et al. HER-2/neu oncogene amplification and expression in breast and ovarian cancers. *Prog Clin Biol Res* **354A**, 209–221 (1990).
94. Ross, J. S., Fletcher, J. A. HER-2/neu (c-erb-B2) gene and protein in breast cancer. *Am J Clin Pathol* **112 Suppl 1**, S53–S67 (1999).
95. Kuan, C. T., Wikstrand, C. J., Bigner, D. D. EGF mutant receptor vIII as a molecular target in cancer therapy. *Endocr Relat Cancer* **8**, 83–96 (2001).
96. Viglietto, G., Chiappetta, G., Martinez-Tello, F. J., et al. RET/PTC oncogene activation is an early event in thyroid carcinogenesis. *Oncogene* **11**, 1207–1210 (1995).
97. Asai, N., Murakami, H., Iwashita, T., Takahashi, M. A mutation at tyrosine 1062 in MEN2A-Ret and MEN2B-Ret impairs their transforming activity and association with shc adaptor proteins. *J Biol Chem* **271**, 17644–17649 (1996).
98. Pierotti, M. A., Bongarzone, I., Borrello, M. G., et al. Rearrangements of TRK proto-oncogene in papillary thyroid carcinomas. *J Endocrinol Investig* **18**, 130–133 (1995).
99. van der Laan, B. F., Freeman, J. L., Asa, S. L. Expression of growth factors and growth factor receptors in normal and tumorous human thryroid tissues. *Thyroid* **5**, 67–73 (1995).
100. Lemoine, N. R., Hughes, C. M., Gullick, W. J., et al. Abnormalities of the EGF receptor system in human thyroid neoplasia. *Int J Cancer* **49**, 558–561 (1991).
101. Duh, Q. Y., Gum, E. T., Gerend, P. L., et al. Epidermal growth factor receptors in normal and neoplastic thyroid tissue. *Surgery* **98**, 1000–1007 (1985).
102. Hoelting T., S., A. E., Clark O. H., et al. Epidermal growth factor enhances proliferation, migration, and invasion of follicular and papillary thyroid cancer in vitro and in vivo. *J Clin Endocrinol Metab* **79**, 401–408 (1994).
103. Campbell, S. L., Khosravi-Far, R., Rossman, K.L. Increasing complexity of Ras signaling. *Oncogene* **17**, 1395–1413 (1998).
104. De Ruiter, N. D., Burgering B. M., Bos J. L. Regulation of the Forkhead transcription factor AFX by Ral-dependent phosphorylation of threonines 447 and 451. *Mol Cell Biol* **21**, 8225–8235 (2001).

105. Downward, J. Targeting ras signalling pathways in cancer therapy. *Nat Rev Cancer* **3**, 11–22 (2003).
106. Bos, J. L. Ras oncogenes in human cancer: a review. *Cancer Res* **49**, 4682–4689 (1989).
107. Ellis, C. A., Clark, G. The importance of being K-ras. *Cell Signal* **12**, 425–434 (2000).
108. Namba, H. R., S. A., Fagin, J. A. Point mutations of ras oncogenes are an early event in thyroid tumorigenesis. *Mol Endocrinol* **4**, 1474–1479 (1990).
109. Lowy, D. R., Willumsen, B. M. Function and regulation of ras. *Annu Rev Biochem* **62**, 851–891 (1993).
110. Weiss, B., Bollag, G., Shannon, K. Hyperactive Ras as a therapeutic target in neurofibromatosis type 1. *Am J Med* **89**, 14–22 (1999).
111. Shields, J. M., Pruitt, K., McFall, A., et al. Understanding Ras: 'it ain't over 'til it's over'. *Trends Cell Biol* **10**, 147–154 (2000).
112. Davies, H., Bignell, G. R., Cox, C., et al. Mutations of the BRAF gene in human cancer. *Nature* **417**, 949–954 (2002).
113. Kimura, E. T., Nikiforova, M. N., Zhu, Z., et al. High prevalence of BRAF mutations in thyroid cancer: Genetic evidence for constitutive activation of the RET/PTC-RAS-BRAF signaling pathway in papillary thyroid carcinomas. *Cancer Res* **63**, 1454–1457 (2003).
114. 114. Cohen, Y., Xing, M., Mambo, E., et al. BRAF mutation in papillary thyroid carcinoma. *J Natl Cancer Inst* **95**, 625–627 (2003).
115. Bellacosa, A., de Feo, D., Godwin, A. K., et al. Molecular alterations of the AKT2 oncogene in ovarian and breast carcinomas. *Int J Cancer* **64**, 280–285 (1995).
116. Simpson, L., Parsons, R. PTEN: life as a tumor suppressor. *Exp Cell Res* **264**, 29–41 (2001).
117. McEachern, M. J., Krauskopf, A., Blackburn, E. H. Telomeres and their control. *Annu Reve Genet* **34**, 331–358 (2000).
118. Moyzis, R. K., Buckignham, J. M., Cram, L. S., et al. A highly conserved repetitive DNA sequence, (TTAGGG)n, present at the telomeres of human chromosomes. *Proc Natl Acad Sci* **85**, 6622–6626 (1988).
119. Henderson, E. R., Blackburn, E. H. An overhanging 3' terminus is a conserved feature of telomeres. *Mol Cell Biol* **9**, 345–348 (1989).
120. McElligott, R., Wellinger, R. J. The terminal DNA structure of mammalian chromosomes. *EMBO J* **16**, 3705–3714 (1997).
121. Wright, W. E., Tesmer, V. M., Huffman, K. E., et al. Normal human chromosomes have long G-rich telomeric overhangs at one end. *Genes Dev* **11**, 2801–2809 (1997).
122. Griffith, J. D., Comeau, L., Rosenfield, S., et al. Mammalian telomeres end in a large duplex loop. *Cell* **97**, 503–514 (1999).
123. Greider, C. W., Blackburn, E. H. A telomeric sequence in the RNA of Tetrahymena telomerase required for telomere repeat synthesis. *Nature* **337**, 331–337 (1989).
124. Nakamura, T. M., Cech, T. R. Reversing time: Origin of telomerase. *Cell* **92**, 587–590 (1998).
125. Nakamura, T. M., Morin, G. B., Chapman, K. B., et al. Telomerase catalytic subunit homologs from fission yeast and human. *Science* **277**, 955–959 (1997).
126. Karlseder, J., Broccoli, D., Dai, Y., et al. p53- and ATM-dependent apoptosis induced by telomeres lacking TRF2. *Science* **283**, 1321–1325 (1999).
127. Blasco, M. A., Lee, H. W., Hande, M. P., et al. Telomere shortening and tumor formation by mouse cells lacking telomerase RNA. *Cell* **91**, 25–34 (1997).
128. Hahn, W. C., Stewart, S. A., Brooks, M. W., et al. Inhibition of telomerase limits the growth of human cancer cells. *Nat Med* **5**, 1164–1170 (1999).
129. Zhu, X. D., Kuster, B., Mann, M., et al. Cell-cycle-regulated association of RAD50/MRE11/NBS1 with TRF2 and human telomeres. *Nat Genet* **25**, 347–352 (2000).
130. Hsu, H. L., Gilley, D., Galande, S. A., et al. Ku acts in a unique way at the mammalian telomere to prevent end joining. *Genes Dev* **14**, 2807–2812 (2000).
131. Hsu, H. L., Gilley, D., Blackburn, E. H., et al. Ku is associated with the telomere in mammals. *Proc Natl Acad Sci USA* **96**, 12454–12458 (1999).
132. Kirk, K. E., Harmon, B. P., Reichardt, I. K., et al. Block in anaphase chromosome separation caused by a telomerase template mutation. *Science* **275**, 1478–1481 (1997).
133. de Lange, T. Protection of mammalian telomeres. *Oncogene* **21**, 532–540 (2002).
134. Bryan, T. M., Englezou, A., Dalla-Pozza, L., et al. Evidence for an alternative mechanism for maintaining telomere length in human tumors and tumor-derived cell lines. *Nat Med* **3**, 1271–1274 (1997).
135. Stewart, S. A., Hahn, W. C., O'Connor, B. F., et al. Telomerase contributes to tumorigenesis by a telomere length-independent mechanism. *Proc Natl Acad Sci USA* **99**, 12606–12611 (2002).

136. Blasco, M. A., Hahn, W. C. Evolving views of telomerase and cancer. *Trends Cell Biol* **13**, 289–294 (2003).
137. Jones, C. J., Soley, A., Skinner, J. W., et al. Dissociation of telomere dynamics from telomerase activity in human thyroid cancer cells. *Exp Cell Res* **240**, 333–339 (1998).
138. Matthews, P., Jones, C. J., Skinner, J., et al. Telomerase activity and telomere length in thyroid neoplasia: biological and clinical implications. *J Pathol* **194**, 183–193 (2001).
139. Rouse, J., Jackson, S. P. Interfaces between the detection, signaling, and repair of DNA damage. *Science* **297**, 547–551 (2002).
140. Lengauer, C., Kinzler, K. W., Vogelstein, B. Genetic instability in colorectal cancers. *Nature* **386**, 623–627 (1997).
141. Peltomaki, P., de la Chapelle, A. Mutations predisposing to hereditary nonpolyposis colorectal cancer. *Adv Cancer Res* **71**, 93–119 (1997).
142. Ionov, Y., Peinado, M. A., Malkhosyan, S., et al. Ubiquitous somatic mutations in simple repeated sequences reveal a new mechanism for colonic carcinogenesis. *Nature* **363**, 558–561 (1993).
143. Thibodeau, S. N., Bren, G., Schaid, D. Microsatellite instability in cancer of the proximal colon. *Science* **260**, 816–819 (1993).
144. Parsons, R., Li, G. M., Longley, M. J., et al. Hypermutability and mismatch repair deficiency in RER+ tumor cells. *Cell* **75**, 1227–1236 (1993).
145. Eshleman, J. R., Lang, E. Z., Bowerfind, G. K., et al. Increased mutation rate at the hprt locus accompanies microsatellite instability in colon cancer. *Oncogene* **10**, 33–37 (1995).
146. de Laat, W. L., Jaspers, N. G., Hoeijmakers, H. J. Molecular mechanism of nucleotide excision repair. *Genes Dev* **13**, 768–785 (1999).
147. Kuzminov, A. Collapse and repair of replication forks in Escherichia coli. *Mol Microbiol* **16**, 373–384 (1995).
148. Featherstone, C., Jackson, S. P. DNA double-strand break repair. *Curr Biol* **9**, R759–761 (1999).
149. Jiricny, J. Eukaryotic mismatch repair: an update. *Mutat Res* **409**, 107–121 (1998).
150. Smith, G. C., Jackson, S. P. The DNA-dependent protein kinase. *Genes Dev* **13**, 916–934 (1999).
151. Lowndes, N. F., Murguia, J. R. Sensing and responding to DNA damage. *Curr Opin Genet Dev* **10**, 17–25 (2000).
152. Abraham, R. T. Cell cycle checkpoint signaling through the ATM and ATR kinases. *Genes Dev* **15**, 2177–2196 (2001).
153. Cahill, D. P., Kinzler, K. W., Vogelstein, B., Lengauer, C. Genetic instability and darwinian selection in tumours. *Trends Cell Biol* **9**, M57–60 (1999).
154. Folkman, J. The role of angiogenesis in tumor growth. *Semin Cancer Biol* **3**, 65–71 (1992).
155. Hanahan D, F. J. Patterns and emerging mechanisms of the angiogenic switch during tumorigenesis. *Cell* **86**, 353–364 (1996).
156. Fidler, I. J., Singh, R. K., Yoneda, J., et al. Critical determinants of neoplastic angiogenesis. *Cancer J* **6: Suppl 3**, S225–S236 (2000).
157. Dameron, K. M., Volpert, O. V., Tainsky, M. A., et al. Control of angiogenesis in fibroblasts by p53 regulation of thrombospondin-1. *Science* **265**, 1582–1584 (1994).
158. Kieser, A., Weich, H. A., Brandner, G., et al. Mutant p53 potentiates protein kinase C induction of vascular endothelial growth factor expression. *Oncogene* **9**, 963–969 (1994).
159. Egeblad, M. New functions for the matrix metalloproteinases in cancer progression. *Nat Rev Cancer* **2**, 161–174 (2002).
160. Jones, P. A., Baylin, S. B. The fundamental role of epigenetic events in cancer. *Nat Rev Genet* **3**, 415–428 (2002).
161. Esteller, M., Herman, J. G. Cancer as an epigenetic disease: DNA methylation and chromatin alterations in human tumours. *J Pathol* **196**, 1–7 (2002).
162. Ehrlich, M. Amount and distribution of 5-methylcytosine in human DNA from different types of tissues or cells. *Nucleic Acids Res* **10**, 2709–2721 (1982).
163. Antequera, F., Bird, A. Number of CpG islands and genes in human and mouse. *Proc Natl Acad Sci USA* **90**, 11995–11999 (1993).
164. Grady, W. M., Willis, J., Guilford, P. J., et al. Methylation of the CDH1 promoter as the second genetic hit in hereditary diffuse gastric cancer. *Nat Genet* **26**, 16–17 (2000).
165. Myohanen, S. K., Baylin, S. B., Herman, J. G. Hypermethylation can selectively silence individual p15ink4A alleles in neoplasia. *Cancer Res* **58**, 591–593 (1998).
166. Esteller, M., Fraga, M. F., Guo, J., et al. DNA methylation patterns in herditary human cancers mimic sporadic tumorigenesis. *Hum Mol Genet* **10**, 3001–3007 (2001).

167. Belinsky, S. A., Nikula, K. J., Baylin, S. B., Issa, J. P. Increased cytosine DNA methyltransferase activity is target-cell-specific and an early event in lung cancer. *Proc Natl Acad Sci USA* **93**, 4045–4050 (1996).
168. Issa, J. P., Vertino, P. M., Wu, J., et al. Increased cytosine DNA-methyltransferase activity during colon cancer progression. *J Natl Cancer Inst* **85**, 1235–1240 (1993).
169. de Marzo, A. M., Marchi, V. L., Yang, E. S., et al. Abnormal regulation of DNA methyltransferase expression during colorectal carcinogenesis. *Cancer Res* **59**, 3855–3860 (1999).
170. Ahluwalia, A., Hurteau, J. A., Bigsby, R. M., Nephew, K. P. DNA methylation in ovarian cancer. II. Expression of DNA methyltransferases in ovarian cancer cell lines and normal ovarian epithelial cells. *Gynecol Oncol* **82**, 299–304 (2001).
171. Vertino, P. M., Yen, R. W., Gao, J., Baylin, S. B. De novo methylation of CpG island sequences in human fibroblasts overexpressing DNA (cytosine-5-)-methyltrensfererase. *Mol Cell Biol* **16**, 4555–4565 (1996).
172. Wu, J., Issa, J. P., Herman, D. E., et al. Expression of an exogenous eukaryotic DNA methyltransferase gene induces transformation of NIH 3T3 cells. *Proc Natl Acad Sci USA* **90**, 8891–8895 (1993).
173. Bakin, A. V., Curran, T. Role of DNA 5-methylcytosine transferase in cell transformation by fos. *Science* **283**, 387–390 (1999).

2. THE PATHOLOGY OF THYROID CANCER

SYLVIA L. ASA

Professor, Department of Laboratory Medicine & Pathobiology, University of Toronto;
Pathologist-in-Chief, University Health Network and Toronto Medical Laboratories;
Freeman Centre for Endocrine Oncology, Mount Sinai & Princess Margaret Hospitals;
Toronto, Ontario Canada

Thyroid nodules are extremely common in the general population; it has been estimated that about 20% of the population has a palpable thyroid nodule and approximately 70% has a nodule that can be detected by ultrasound (1). The prevalence of thyroid nodules is greater in women than in men, and multiple nodules are more common than solitary nodules.

The differential diagnosis of the thyroid nodule includes numerous entities, non-neoplastic and neoplastic, benign and malignant (2–5). The pathologist has an important role to play in their evaluation. The use of fine needle aspiration biopsy has significantly improved our ability to identify specific high-risk disorders and to facilitate their management in an expeditious and cost-effective manner. Patients who require surgery for further confirmation of the disease process rely upon the pathologist to correctly characterise their nodule and pathologists are actively involved in research to clarify the pathogenesis of thyroid disease.

While some of these entities are readily diagnosed based on specific features seen in a routine slide stained with conventional dyes, the morphologic evaluation of many of these lesions is fraught with controversy and diagnostic criteria are highly variable from Pathologist to Pathologist (6). Nevertheless, histology remains the gold standard against which we measure outcomes of cytology, intraoperative consultations, molecular and other studies, and it represents the basis on which we determine patient management and the efficacy of various therapies. Unfortunately, no current morphologic criteria provide adequate information to predict outcome for many follicular nodules of thyroid.

Advances in our understanding of the molecular basis of thyroid cancer will allow more accurate characterisation of specific subtypes of neoplasia and malignancy even on single cells obtained at fine needle aspiration biopsy. This should further enhance the usefulness of this technique and better guide the management of patients with a thyroid nodule.

THYROID FOLLICULAR HYPERPLASIA AND NEOPLASIA

Follicular nodules are the most commonly encountered problems in the surgical pathology of the thyroid. These lesions can be classified along the full spectrum of thyroid pathology from hyperplastic nodules to benign follicular adenomas and malignant follicular carcinomas.

Nodular goitre

Sporadic nodular goitre is characterised by numerous follicular nodules with heterogeneous architecture and cytology, features that have suggested a hyperplastic rather than neoplastic pathogenesis (7–10). The gland may be distorted by multiple bilateral nodules and can achieve weights of several hundred to a thousand grams, but this disorder is often identified as a dominant nodule in what clinically appears to be an otherwise normal gland. Histologically, the nodules are irregular; some are poorly circumscribed while others are surrounded by scarring and condensation of thyroid stroma, creating the appearance of complete encapsulation. They are composed of follicles of variable size and shape. Some follicles are large, with abundant colloid surrounded by flattened, cuboidal or columnar epithelial cells, often with cellular areas composed of small follicles lined by crowded epithelium with scant colloid in a small lumen, alone or pushing into large colloid-filled follicles as "Sanderson's polsters" (Figure 1). There may be focal necrosis, haemorrhage with haemosiderin deposition and cholesterol clefts, fibrosis, and granulation tissue; these degenerative changes are usually found in the centre of large nodules, creating stellate scars.

The morphologic classification of cellular follicular nodules in nodular glands can be extremely difficult. Hyperplasia may be extremely difficult to distinguish from neoplasia. Classical guidelines that allow distinction of a hyperplastic nodule from a follicular adenoma include the following: (i) multiple lesions suggest hyperplasia whereas a solitary lesion is likely to be neoplastic, (ii) a poorly encapsulated nodule is likely hyperplastic; a well developed capsule suggests a neoplastic growth, (iii) variable architecture reflects a polyclonal proliferation whereas uniform architecture suggests a monoclonal neoplastic growth, (iv) cytologic heterogeneity suggests hyperplasia; monotonous cytology is characteristic of neoplasia, (v) the presence of multiple lesions in hyperplasia means that areas similar to the lesion in question will be present in the adjacent gland; in contrast, neoplasms have a distinct morphology compared with the surrounding parenchyma, (vi) classically hyperplastic nodules are said not to compress the surrounding gland whereas neoplasms result in compression of the adjacent parenchyma. For the most part, large nodules in multinodular glands tend to be incompletely encapsulated and poorly demarcated from the internodular tissue. However, in some glands, large encapsulated lesions with relatively monotonous architecture

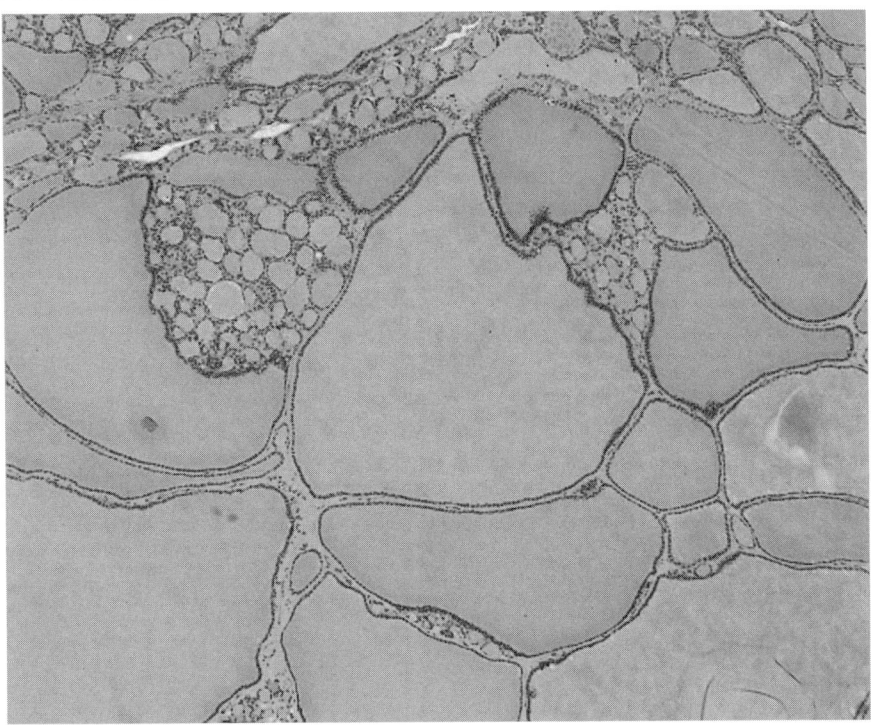

Figure 1. A hyperplastic nodule of thyroid is characterized by architectural and cytologic heterogeneity, usually with abundant colloid and often with subfollicle formation within larger follicles.

and cytology make distinction of hyperplasia from adenoma difficult. Many pathologists have applied nonspecific terms such as "adenomatoid nodules" to describe such lesions.

The pathophysiology of nodule formation remains poorly understood. The aetiology of this disorder has long remained elusive, since the goitres do not appear to be TSH-dependent (9). The work of Stüder suggests that the initial proliferation is a polyclonal one involving cells that are intrinsically more rapidly growing than their neighbours (7,10,11). While the stimulus for growth is not certain, high levels of circulating thyroid growth-stimulating immunoglobulins (TGI) and defects in T suppressor cell function have been documented in patients with sporadic nodular goitre (12,13), implicating autoimmunity in the pathogenesis of this disease. Drexhage and colleagues (12) compared immunoglobulin preparations of patients who have goitrous Graves' disease with those of patients who have sporadic nodular goitre and have found that the former are approximately 10-fold more potent in inducing growth than the latter. It has been postulated that the weaker stimuli result in proliferation of only the most sensitive of the heterogeneous follicular epithelial cell population, hence the nodularity, and that "toxic" nodular goitre results from preferential replication of cells which are highly responsive to TSH stimulation (14,15). These data implicating an autoimmune pathogenesis explain the presence of chronic inflammation that is usually focally associated with nodular hyperplasia.

In contrast, molecular studies have indicated that the dominant nodules of multinodular goitres are monoclonal proliferations, and therefore represent benign neoplasms (8,16,17). It may be that these represent true adenomas arising in the background of a hyperplastic process that is mediated by growth stimulating immunoglobulins. Moreover, most hyperfunctioning nodules are also now thought to represent clonal benign neoplasms with activating mutations of the TSH receptor or Gsα (18–22). The evidence of clonal proliferation in sporadic nodular goitre and the identification of ras mutations as early events in morphologically classified hyperplastic nodules in this disorder (23) indicates that the thyroid is a site for the hyperplasia-neoplasia sequence. Nevertheless, clinical experience has shown us that the vast majority of these lesions remain entirely benign.

Follicular adenoma

Solitary follicular nodules have been unequivocally shown to be monoclonal (24,25,26) and in the absence of invasive behaviour or of markers of papillary carcinoma, these lesions are considered to be benign. Follicular adenomas are described as solitary encapsulated follicular lesions that exhibit a uniform architectural and cytologic pattern. However, the inclusion of nodules in sporadic nodular goitre in this category alters these criteria.

On aspiration cytology, the diagnosis of "follicular lesion" covers both follicular adenoma and follicular carcinoma, which are difficult if not impossible to distinguish because the diagnostic criteria do not rest on cytologic characteristics. The aspirate of a follicular lesion is usually cellular with follicular cells in sheets or microfollicular arrangements. The follicular cells are monotonous with elongated, bland nuclei and micronucleoli. Worrisome features include nuclear crowding, altered polarity, pleomorphism, macronucleoli and coarse chromatin. The main practical role of cytology is to distinguish a colloid nodule or papillary carcinoma from a follicular neoplasm.

Follicular adenomas are well delineated and usually thickly encapsulated neoplasms that can be classified histologically according the size or presence of follicles and degree of cellularity, each adenoma tending to have a consistent microscopic pattern (Figure 2). The subclassification of follicular adenomas into simple, microfollicular, trabecular, oxyphil, atypical, papillary and signet ring cell types has no prognostic significance.

Atypical adenomas are highly cellular tumours with unusual gross and/or histologic appearances that suggest the possibility of malignancy but these tumours lack evidence of invasion. They may have necrosis, infarction, numerous mitoses or unusual cellularity. Many so-called "atypical adenomas" are indeed papillary carcinomas. The distinction of an encapsulated follicular variant papillary carcinoma from follicular adenoma relies on cytologic characteristics. The presence of the cytologic features of papillary carcinoma described below should indicate that diagnosis, despite lack of invasion. Whether some follicular nodules classified histologically as adenomas have the biologic potential to become carcinoma is not clear; aneuploid cell populations

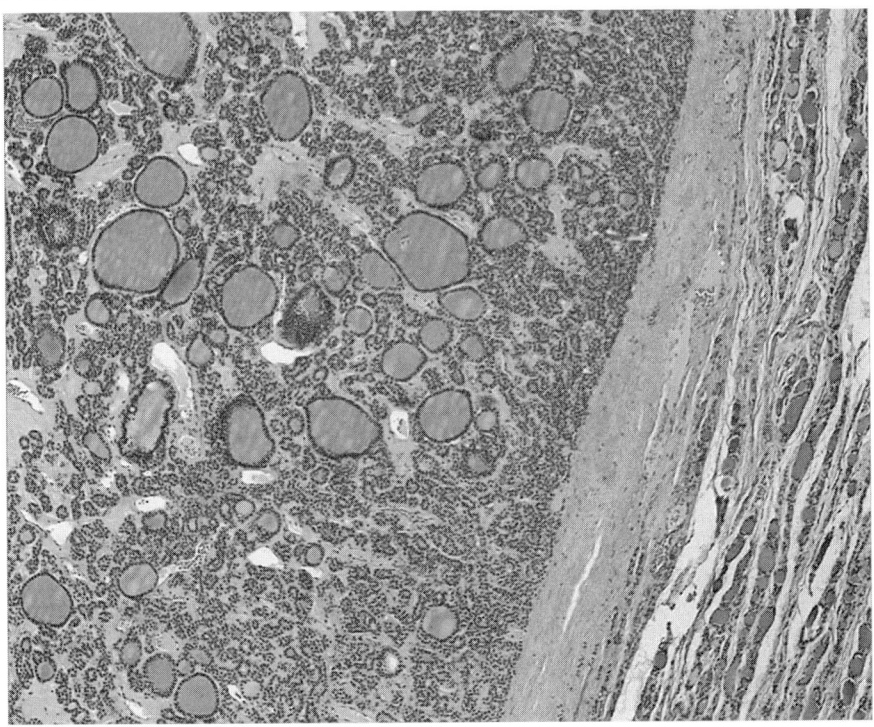

Figure 2. A follicular adenoma is usually well delineated and often surrounded by a thick fibrous capsule. The lesion is generally characterized by uniformity of architecture and cytology.

have been described in a significant percentage of these lesions, suggesting that some of these may represent carcinoma in situ.

Follicular carcinoma

Follicular adenoma and most follicular carcinomas are indistinct with respect to their clinical presentation, radiographic appearance, cytologic findings and microscopic features. In most cases, the parenchymal component of both tumour types is essentially the same histomorphologically. The distinction between these two conditions has been considered possible only by recognition of invasion or metastasis. As indicated above, some encapsulated follicular adenomas exhibit evidence of aneuploidy and may in fact represent in situ follicular carcinomas.

Nuclear and cellular atypia and mitotic figures may be present in adenomas as well as in carcinomas and therefore cytologic characteristics are not helpful. Most follicular tumours are composed of cells with nuclei that are round to oval with uniformly speckled chromatin; the nuclei are evenly spaced and lack the crowded, overlapping appearance found in papillary carcinoma. As stated previously, these lesions cannot be

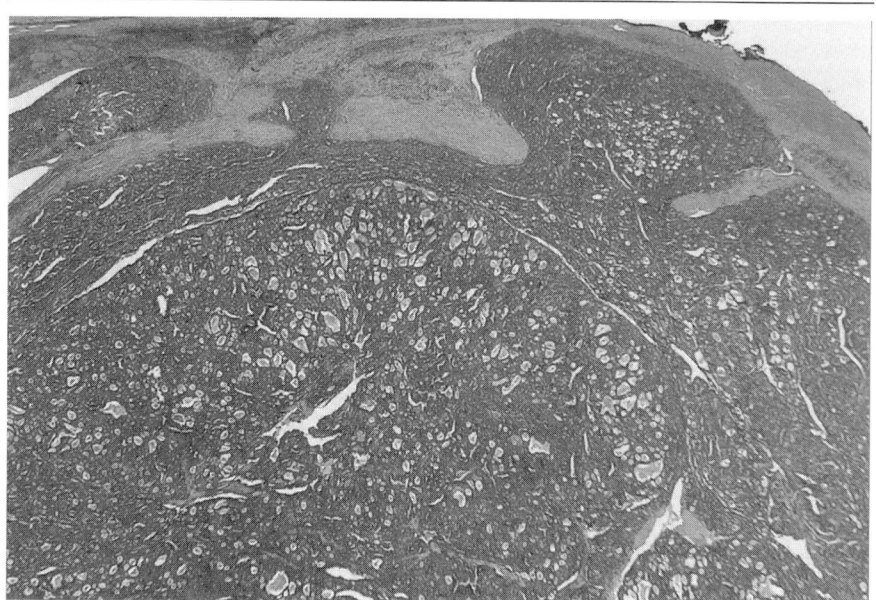

Figure 3. The distinction of follicular carcinoma from follicular adenoma relies on unequivocal evidence of invasive behaviour, as in the multifocal mushrooming capsular penetration exhibited by this lesion.

diagnosed as benign or malignant by fine needle aspiration; the diagnosis should be restricted to "follicular lesion".

Follicular carcinoma can only be diagnosed by the pathologist on high quality sections of well-fixed tissues that demonstrate capsular and/or vascular invasion (Figure 3). At the time of intraoperative consultation, frozen section will reveal only a very small number of these lesions, since the likelihood of identifying microinvasive foci on a single frozen section are low. The use of multiple frozen sections is not cost effective in the evaluation of these lesions (27).

Follicular carcinomas are divided into groups that reflect the biology of tumour growth and metastasis. *Widely invasive follicular carcinomas*, which are usually identifiable as invasive grossly, and certainly are not difficult to recognise as invasive microscopically, carry a poor prognosis with a 25–45% ten year survival (28,29). However, such lesions tend to be insular carcinomas (see below). In contrast, the more common scenario is that of minimal capsular invasion and patients with these tumors have an excellent prognosis. The diagnosis of follicular neoplasms requires very careful and thorough examination of the entire capsule of the follicular neoplasm by the pathologist (30). *Minimally invasive follicular carcinoma* is identified by invasion through but not widely beyond the capsule. Borderline lesions include those with invasion into the capsule beyond the bulk of the lesion but not through the full thickness of the capsule or situations in which islands of tumor are trapped within a capsule, associated with perpendicular rupture of collagen. The finding of nests, cords, or individual tumour cells within a tumour capsule leads some pathologists to the diagnosis of minimally invasive follicular carcinoma, however, this may represent an artefact in a patient who has undergone fine needle aspiration biopsy, with trapping by fibrosis or displacement of tumour cells into the capsule. The pathologist is therefore advised to carefully search for evidence of fine needle aspiration biopsy in the adjacent tissue. This would include finding focal haemorrhage, deposition of haemosiderin-laden macrophages, the presence of granulation tissue and/or fibrosis, all of which would indicate a needle biopsy site and the possibility of artifactual invasion rather than genuine invasion.

The concept of unencapsulated follicular carcinoma was raised by the identification of tumours that lack a capsule. In one report of four such cases, one patient developed metastases, and this gave rise to citations of a 25% metastatic rate by such lesions (31). However, this has not been substantiated in larger series and this concept has largely been abandoned.

Patients with minimally invasive follicular carcinomas are on average about 10 years younger than those with widely infiltrative carcinomas and since traces of capsule are found in about 24% of widely invasive lesions, it is possible that encapsulated follicular carcinoma is a precursor of the widely invasive lesion (32). Minimally invasive carcinomas have ten year survival rates of 70–100% (33) and therefore some argue that this disease does not warrant the painstaking search for microscopic invasion that distinguishes it from follicular adenoma. Nevertheless, the investigators that have reported these promising data have treated their patients for carcinoma rather than for benign disease (34).

Vasculoinvasive follicular carcinomas are aggressive and require management accordingly. While vascular invasion is more reliable for the diagnosis of malignancy, again the criteria are vague. Vascular invasion cannot be evaluated within the tumour and therefore again the circumference of the lesion is the site that warrants careful examination. Bulging of tumour under endothelium does not qualify as vascular invasion if the endothelium is intact. Nests of tumour cells within an endothelial lumen generally are accepted as representing invasion, however, it is recognised that artefactual implantation of tumour cells into blood vessels can occur during the surgical procedure or sectioning. Therefore, invasive tumour cells infiltrating the wall of an endothelial-lined space and thrombus adherent to intravascular tumour are required to distinguish true invasion from artefact.

Elastin stains are of little value in assessing vascular invasion, since the involved vessels are usually thin-walled veins with little if any elastic tissue. Immunohistochemical markers such as factor-8 related antigen, type IV collagen, CD31 and CD34 can be used to improve the recognition of vascular invasion in follicular carcinoma.

It is obvious that the diagnosis of malignancy in well-differentiated encapsulated follicular tumours rests on subjective criteria. The search for objective markers of malignancy has yielded only one candidate thus far; HBME-1, a marker of mesothelial cells, is immunohistochemically detected in 40% of thyroid follicular malignancies of papillary or follicular differentiation (35–37) and has been used successfully in cytology studies as well as histopathologic evaluation (Figure 4) of thyroid nodules (36,37). Recent studies have advocated the use of galectin-3 as another marker of malignancy

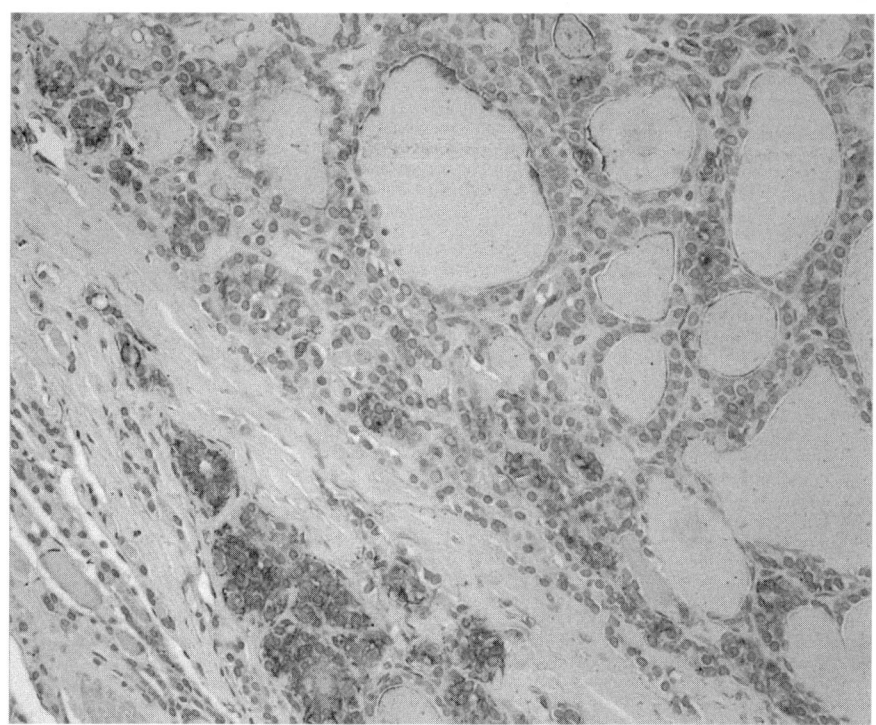

Figure 4. Immunoreactivity for HBME-1 is a feature of thyroid malignancies of epithelial cell derivation, such as this follicular carcinoma with superficial capsular invasion.

(38–40). While this marker also stains normal, hyperplastic and inflamed thyroid tissue, positivity in malignancies is more diffuse and strong. These data should limit the application of this technique for cytology but this has not been widely recognized (41).

Another molecular marker with application to follicular carcinoma is a gene rearrangement that involves the thyroid transcription factor Pax 8 and the peroxisome proliferator-activated receptor γ (PPARγ) gene (42). Normal thyroid follicular cells express Pax 8 at high levels; this transcription factor is essential for thyroid development, involved in regulating expression of the endogenous genes encoding thyroglobulin, thyroperoxidase, and the sodium/iodide symporter. PPARγ, a transcription factor that is implicated in the inhibition of cell growth and promotion of cell differentiation, is also expressed by normal thyroid follicular epithelium. However, this in-frame rearrangement results in a fusion protein that likely interferes with the normal function of both differentiating factors, thereby explaining its potential role in thyroid tumorigenesis. The rearrangement is most reliably detected using fluorescence in situ hybridization (FISH) technology to identify the translocation of the two genes that are normally localized on chromosomes 2q13 (Pax 8) and 3p25 (PPARγ). The presence of overexpressed

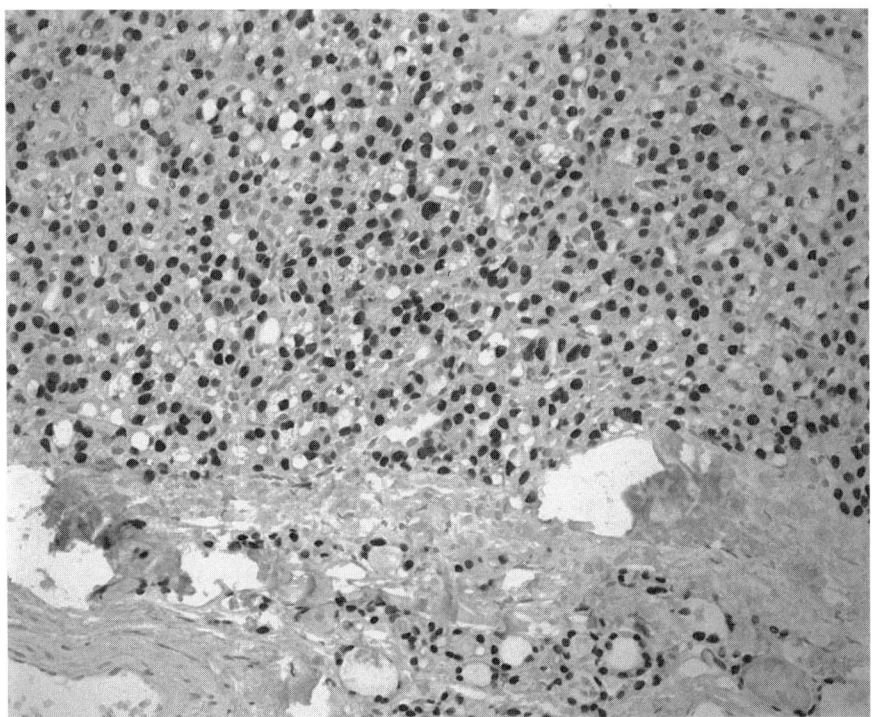

Figure 5. Overexpression of PPAR-γ due to a Pax 8-PPAR-γ gene rearrangement is detectable by immunohistochemistry. This finding has been correlated with aggressive behaviour, usually with vascular invasion.

protein can also be identified using immunostains for PPARγ where strong nuclear staining identifies tumours harboring a translocation (Figure 5). Although follicular carcinomas of thyroid are rare (43), and the numbers of cases studied has been small, it appears to be a useful tool for the diagnosis of malignancy in thyroid follicular lesions, particularly to predict vascular spread and aggressive behaviour (44).

DNA aneuploidy is a well-recognised feature of human malignant tumors and it was initially hoped that ploidy analyses could help to distinguish adenomas from carcinomas of the thyroid. However, it has now been recognised that about 27% of follicular adenomas are aneuploid and about 40% of follicular carcinomas are diploid (45). Therefore such measurements are of limited diagnostic value for the individual patient. In contrast, however, ploidy may be a useful adjunct in determining prognosis.

The significance of this diagnosis must be interpreted in light of clinical data that assess the behaviour of this disorder. The dominant determinant of cause-specific mortality in patients with follicular carcinoma is the presence of distant metastases (46–48). Most studies have indicated that morbidity and mortality for patients with non-metastatic encapsulated follicular carcinoma is very low and correlates better with patient age than with any other parameter. Some have suggested that capsular invasion alone does not alter the incidence of distant metastases or cancer-related death (33).

Since the incidence of follicular carcinoma is low (43), most investigators still advocate total thyroidectomy and radioactive iodine therapy (34,49,50). The rationale for total thyroidectomy is not bilateral carcinoma; multifocal disease in follicular carcinoma is exceedingly rare and the identification of occult papillary carcinoma in the contralateral lobe is not an indication for further surgery (51). The only logical rationale for completion thyroidectomy is to allow selective uptake of radioactive iodine by metastatic tumour deposits rather than by residual thyroid gland. Uptake of radioactive iodine by distant metastases is a favourable prognostic factor and is improved by pretherapeutic total thyroidectomy, resulting in improved survival (52–54). In contrast, external beam radiotherapy is not thought to be of use in patients with differentiated thyroid carcinoma, apart from those with locally advanced tumours such as widely invasive follicular carcinomas that involve extrathyroidal soft tissues of the neck and cannot be completely resected (54).

The last few decades have seen a decrease in the incidence of follicular thyroid carcinoma, probably due to dietary iodine supplementation (43). However, misdiagnosis of this tumour continues. Benign lesions, such as partly encapsulated hyperplastic nodules or nodules exhibiting pseudoinvasion after fine needle aspiration (55), are often overdiagnosed as malignant; papillary carcinomas with follicular architecture are often misinterpreted as follicular carcinoma. The clinical features, pathophysiology and biological behaviour of follicular cancer differ significantly from those of the entities with which it is often confused. Only careful histopathologic classification will allow correct evaluation of treatment options and prognosis.

PAPILLARY LESIONS OF THYROID

Hyperplastic nodules and adenomas with papillary architecture

The "papillary hyperplastic nodule" of the thyroid is usually identified in girls, usually teenagers in and around the age of menarche. These present as solitary nodules and it is unusual for them to be associated with clinical hyperfunction, although that might occur. These lesion are distinguished from papillary carcinoma in that they are totally encapsulated, often show central cystic change, have subfollicle formation in the centres of broad oedematous papillae, and do not show nuclear features of papillary carcinoma (Figure 6). Although one analysis of clonality has suggested that these are polyclonal hyperplasias (56), the detection of Gsα or TSH receptor activating mutations in such nodules suggests that they are neoplasms (18–22). Their behaviour is almost always benign. Some have advocated the name "papillary adenoma" for these tumours; while scientifically appropriate, this term carries historical connotations that some feel are unacceptable (5).

In adults, one can have a similar histologic appearance in a "hot" nodule, that is, a thyroid nodule that is associated with clinical toxicity or subclinical hyperthyroidism and iodine uptake on scan. These lesions may be solitary but are often seen in the setting of sporadic nodular goitre (see above).

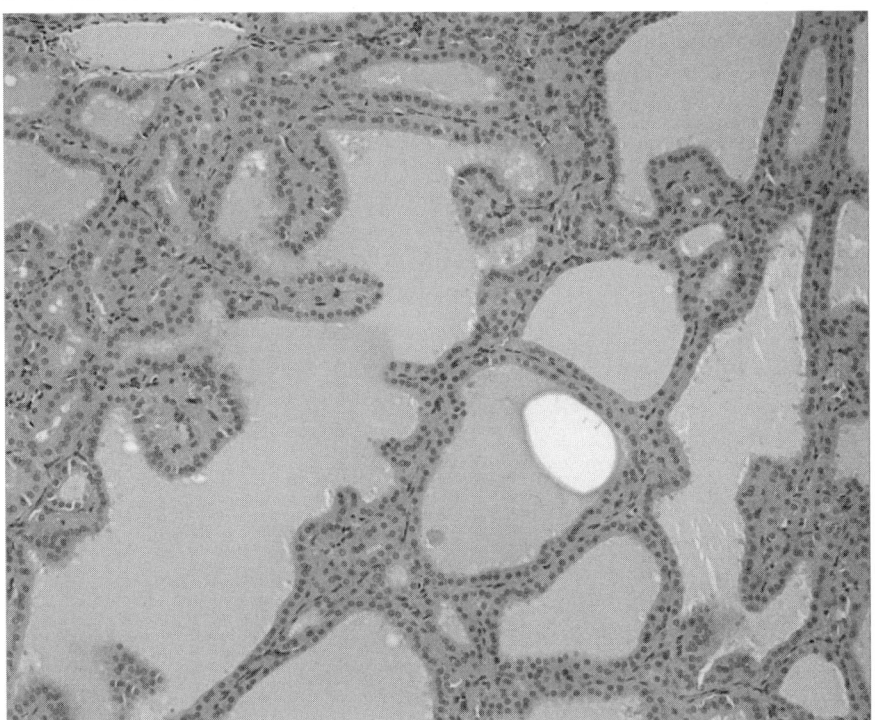

Figure 6. A benign adenoma with true papillary architecture has an organized centripedal orientation of the papillae that are lined by cells with bland nuclei that lack the atypia of papillary carcinoma.

On fine needle aspiration and on histologic evaluation, particularly at frozen section, papillary hyperplastic nodules or adenomas can be very alarming and lead to a false positive diagnosis of papillary carcinoma. Indeed, these entities give rise to well formed papillae but on higher magnification, the cytologic criteria for the diagnosis of papillary carcinoma, including powdery nuclear chromatin, multiple micro- and/or macronucleoli, intranuclear cytoplasmic inclusions, and linear chromatin grooves (57), are lacking.

Papillary carcinoma

Papillary carcinoma comprises at least 80% of thyroid epithelial malignancies diagnosed in regions of the world where goitres are not endemic. The terminology is misleading; papillary carcinomas can exhibit papillary architecture (Figure 7) but they may also have follicular (Figure 8) or mixed papillary and follicular patterns (58–62). It is now recognised that the diagnosis of papillary carcinoma is based on what the WHO has described as "a distinctive set of nuclear characteristics" (63). In contrast to true follicular carcinomas, these lesions are usually more indolent and most have an excellent prognosis with a 20 year survival rate of 90% or better (64,65).

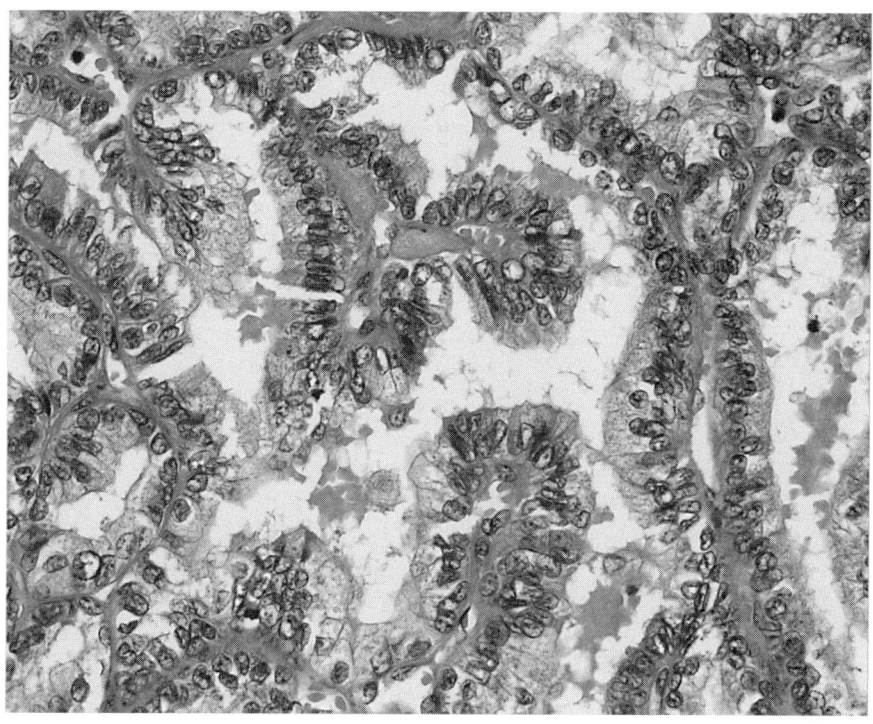

Figure 7. Papillary carcinoma was named as such because many of these lesions have complex papillary architecture. The papillae are lined by crowded cells with nuclear atypia.

The defining nuclear features are readily seen on cytology of fine needle aspirates as well as on histologic sections (Figure 9). They include an alteration of the size and the roundness of the normal follicular cell nucleus to one that is large and oval. Due to peripheral margination of chromatin, the centre of the nucleus has an empty appearance, which when pronounced has been termed "ground glass" (66). The chromatin and nucleolus are pushed to the edge of the nucleus. The nuclear contour is strikingly irregular, resulting in a "crumpled paper" appearance, intranuclear cytoplasmic pseudoinclusions and nuclear grooves (67,68). No one specific feature is absolutely diagnostic of papillary carcinoma; a constellation or combination of nuclear features is required for the diagnosis.

Papillary carcinomas may be multifocal; this has been interpreted as reflective of intraglandular lymphatic dissemination, but the identification of such microcarcinomas in up to 24% of the population (69) and the detection of different clonal rearrangements in multifocal lesions (70) support the interpretation of multifocal primary lesions in most patients. Nevertheless, when these lesions do invade, they show preference for lymphatic involvement with a high percentage of regional lymph node metastases.

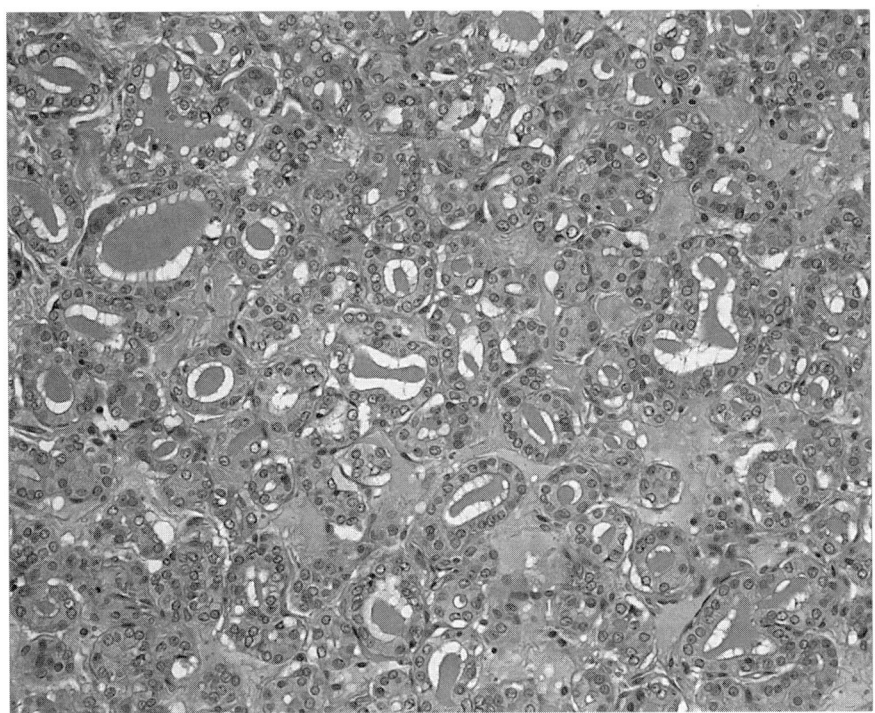

Figure 8. Papillary carcinoma may have partial or complete follicular architecture. The follicles usually harbour hypereosinophilic colloid that has peripheral scalloping. The nuclei exhibit characteristic atypia.

Metastases beyond the neck are unusual in common papillary carcinoma and probably only occur in about 5 to 7% of cases.

The most useful prognostic markers in papillary carcinoma are patient variables, tumour size and extent of disease (28,29,53,71). Patients under the age of 45 usually have an excellent prognosis; in contrast those over 45 years of age generally have a poorer outlook. Sex has also been said in the past to be an important determinant of tumour biology but more recent studies have suggested that there is no major difference in the behaviour of papillary carcinoma in men compared to women. Tumour size is exceedingly important (72). Tumours less than 1 cm are common and appear to be different biologically than larger tumours (73–75); a recent study has shown that occult papillary carcinomas are identified in up to 24% of the population in thyroids that are removed for non-malignant or unrelated disease (69). In contrast, tumours greater than 1 cm are thought to be of clinical significance and those larger than 3 cm generally have a poorer prognosis than do smaller tumours. The presence of cervical lymph node metastasis, whether microscopic or identified clinically, is thought to increase the risk of recurrence of disease but has been shown to have no impact on mortality.

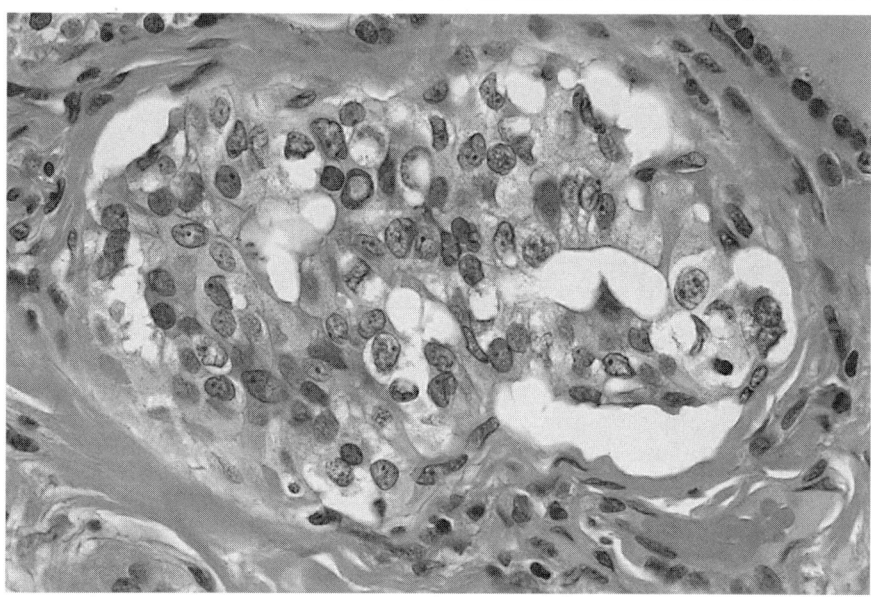

Figure 9. The nuclear features of papillary carcinoma encompass clearing of nucleoplasm and peripheral margination of chromatin, prominent and often multiple nucleoli, and irregular nuclear contours that result in formation of linear grooves and cytoplasmic pseudoinclusions.

Extrathyroidal extension, in contrast, predicts a worse prognosis and the presence of distant metastases is the hallmark of an aggressive tumour that will bear the potential for high mortality.

Grossly, papillary carcinomas vary in size from microcarcinomas (also called small, tiny, occult and minute), which are defined as lesions measuring less than 1 cm (usually 4 to 7 mm) to large neoplasms that extend extrathyroidally beyond the thyroid capsule into surrounding soft tissue. The bulk of clinical papillary carcinomas are intrathyroidal tumours confined within the capsule of the thyroid and may have an encapsulated appearance (this is usual for the follicular variant) or an irregularly infiltrative appearance. One can see gross cystic change but usually papillary carcinoma is a firm tumor and some are calcified or even ossified.

Microscopically, papillary carcinomas classically are composed of papillae but virtually all contain follicular elements. Ghosts of dead papillae or infarcted papillae calcify with a concentric whorled pattern that is characteristic of psammoma bodies (Figure 10); these are found in 40 to 50% of classical papillary carcinomas, either in the tumour stroma or in the surrounding non-tumourous thyroid, but they are distinctively uncommon in lesions with follicular architecture.

Inflammatory infiltrates within papillary carcinomas and in the surrounding thyroid parenchyma have been noted by several authors, although the prognostic significance of this is not clear (76,77). Some people have postulated that this inflammatory infiltrate

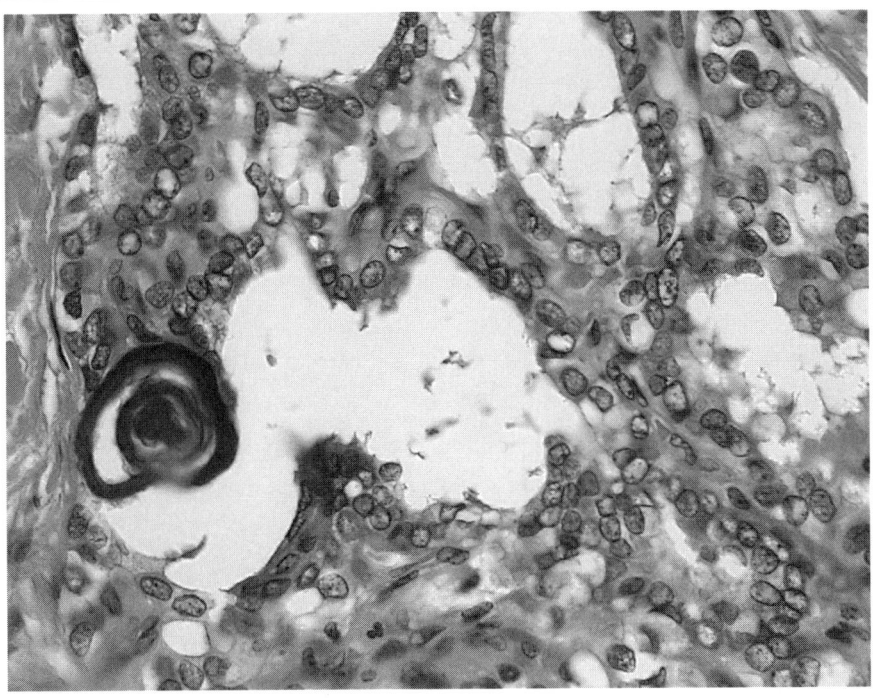

Figure 10. A minority of papillary carcinomas form psammoma bodies, concentric calcifications.

may indicate host-tumour immune interactions that are responsible for the general indolence of this type of thyroid carcinoma (76).

Variants

Although there are reports to the contrary, the exact histological variant of papillary carcinoma usually cannot be predicted from the appearance of the fine needle aspirate (78). Nevertheless, the histologic distinctions, which are characteristic (3,5,63,79–81), are of prognostic value.

Papillary microcarcinoma (75), *cystic and encapsulated variants of papillary carcinoma* (82) have an apparently better prognosis than usual papillary carcinoma.

The follicular variant has been recognized more frequently in the past 20 years (5,63,83,84). It has either been misdiagnosed as follicular carcinoma or underdiagnosed as follicular adenoma or atypical adenoma. Any lesion with follicular architecture and characteristic nuclear features of papillary carcinoma should be classified as this tumor. Infiltrating areas and metastases may exhibit a more striking papillary appearance and may even have psammoma bodies. It is unclear what the ultimate biological and clinical behaviour of follicular variant is, since some of these may be underdiagnosed as atypical adenomas and it is likely that the initial reports of this tumour included the aggressive biological spectrum of this variant.

The presence of cytologic atypia may raise the possibility of papillary carcinoma without being sufficiently convincing for unequivocal diagnosis. In some cases the changes may be induced by previous needle biopsy. The presence of haemorrhage, granulation tissue and hemosiderin laden-macrophages, inflammation and foreign body giant cells and even foreign material should point to this possibility. There may be calcification that can be mistaken for psammoma bodies. Various metaplastic changes occur. These changes have been described with the acronym WHAFFT which stands for *"Worrisome Histological Alterations Following FNA of Thyroid"* (55). The diagnosis of papillary carcinoma should not be made in this situation unless the lesion is entirely unequivocal.

In cases where the features are suggestive of papillary carcinoma but not entirely diagnostic, specific markers of this tumour as well as other markers if malignancy may be useful. A proportion of malignancies of thyroid follicular epithelium stain for HBME-1 (35–37) and some investigators have advocated the use of galectin-3 as a marker of thyroid carcinoma (38–41). Stains for high molecular weight cytokeratins may be useful. This technique, also considered controversial in the past, has recently been shown to be useful when applied to paraffin sections with microwave antigen retrieval (85). The results of these studies indicate that moderate to strong diffuse staining is confined to papillary carcinoma (Figure 11) whereas follicular neoplasms and hyperplastic nodules are negative or show only focal staining in areas of reaction to degeneration or previous fine needle aspiration biopsy. Nevertheless, only approximately 60% of papillary carcinomas are positive; a positive stain is therefore helpful, but negative stains are unable to assist in the diagnostic process.

The diagnosis of this entity has been further advanced by the recognition of a family of gene rearrangements that are specific to papillary carcinoma (86). The *ret*/PTC oncogenes (1 through 15, depending on the site of rearrangement, reviewed in (87)) are the result of DNA damage with rearrangements that transpose various cellular genes adjacent to the gene encoding the intracellular tyrosine kinase domain of the *ret* protooncogene (88–92). The rearrangements result in constitutive tyrosine kinase activation and translocation of the fusion protein to the cytoplasm (93). Animal models have shown the tumorigenicity of these fusion proteins (94–96); the rearrangements are common in radiation-induced tumors (97–101) but are also found in sporadic papillary carcinomas (102–105) and appear to be an early event in tumour development (106). Immunohistochemical staining with antisera directed against the carboxy terminus of *ret* allows rapid and clinically useful detection of this marker of papillary carcinoma which is present in almost 80% of occult papillary microcarcinomas and approximately 50% of clinically detected lesions (70). Again, a negative stain is not useful, however, the combination of high molecular weight cytokeratins and *ret* provides a set of immunohistochemical markers that aids in the diagnosis of papillary carcinoma in equivocal cases (107). At the moment, antisera or antibodies to *ret* offer inconsistent detection of these rearrangements and molecular diagnostics using RT-PCR remain the gold standard of this diagnostic tool. This methodology has been applied to FNA specimens when collected in suspension (108) and application of this technique enhances the cytological diagnosis of papillary carcinoma.

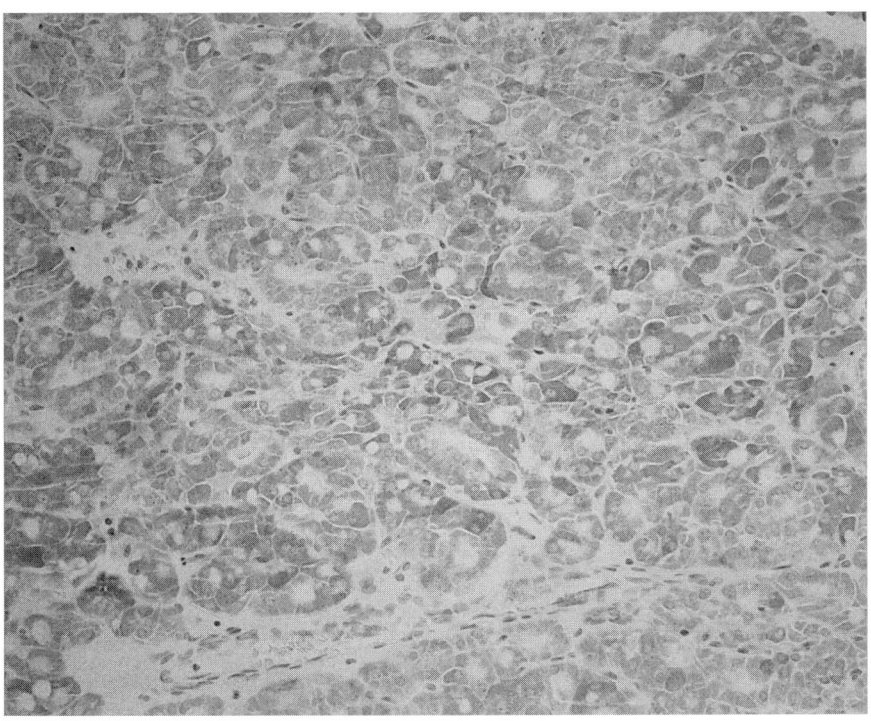

Figure 11. A diffuse cytoplasmic staining pattern for high molecular weight cytokeratins and cytokeratin-19 are the hallmark of papillary carcinomas of all types.

An unusual variant of papillary carcinoma is the *hyalinizing trabecular tumour*. This tumour was originally described by pioneers such as Zipkin in 1905 (109), Masson in 1922 (110), and Ward et al. in 1982 (111). The terminology "hyalinizing trabecular adenoma" (HTA) was defined by Carney et al. in 1987 (112). This lesion has also been designated "paraganglioma-like adenoma of thyroid" (PLAT) by Bronner et al (113) because of its unusual histologic pattern (Figure 12). Since the original descriptions, a malignant counterpart, hyalinizing trabecular carcinoma (HTC), has been described (114–116) and both HTA and HTC are now incorporated under the umbrella of hyalinizing trabecular tumors (HTT). Their main importance lies in the fact that they are sometimes mistaken for other entities such as paraganglioma or medullary carcinoma (112). Immunohistochemical stains for neuroendocrine markers will easily discriminate between HTT and paraganglioma or medullary carcinoma. However, it was noted that many features of HTT were also seen in papillary carcinoma; both lesions are of thyroid follicular epithelial origin and therefore both express thyroglobulin; several cases of HTT have been reported in patients with Hashimoto's thyroiditis or who have had a history of neck irradiation (117); HTT can co-exist with papillary carcinoma (5); HTT can often exhibit papillary carcinoma-like histologic features such as

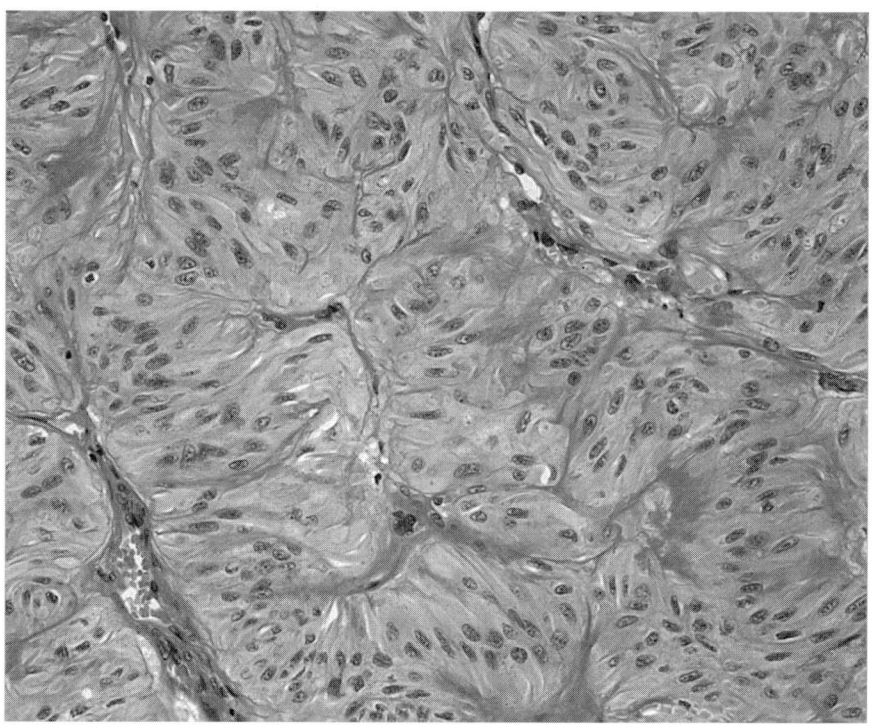

Figure 12. The hyalinizing trabecular tumour of thyroid is characterized by elongated spindle-shaped cells with hyaline cytoplasm, as well as stromal hyaline fibrosis. The tumour cells exhibit the nuclear atypia of papillary carcinoma.

psammoma-body formation, and characteristic nuclear changes including elongation, hypochromasia, grooves and pseudoinclusions (112). Based on these observations, a number of authors have hypothesized that these two entities are related and may in fact share a similar pathogenesis (118). These lesions are generally well delineated tumors characterised architecturally by trabecular and nesting architecture and elongated tumor cells which can have abundant pale eosinophilic cytoplasm and scattered "yellow bodies" (112,113,117,119). There is perivascular hyaline fibrosis and the cytoplasmic hyaline is usually identified as cytoplasmic filaments of cytokeratin. Occasional cases are immunoreactive for S100 protein. Most importantly, the tumour cells harbour large clear nuclei with irregular and elongated contours, grooves and inclusions as well as micronucleoli, features of papillary carcinoma. Application of *ret*/PTC analysis identified rearrangements in these lesions at a rate identical to that found in other papillary carcinomas (120,121) and many pathologists now consider this to be a variant of papillary carcinoma. However, some continue to maintain that these are distinct lesions (122,123).

The *diffuse sclerosis variant* occurs in young individuals and often presents as goitre without a specific mass lesion (124–127). This tumour microscopically involves thyroid

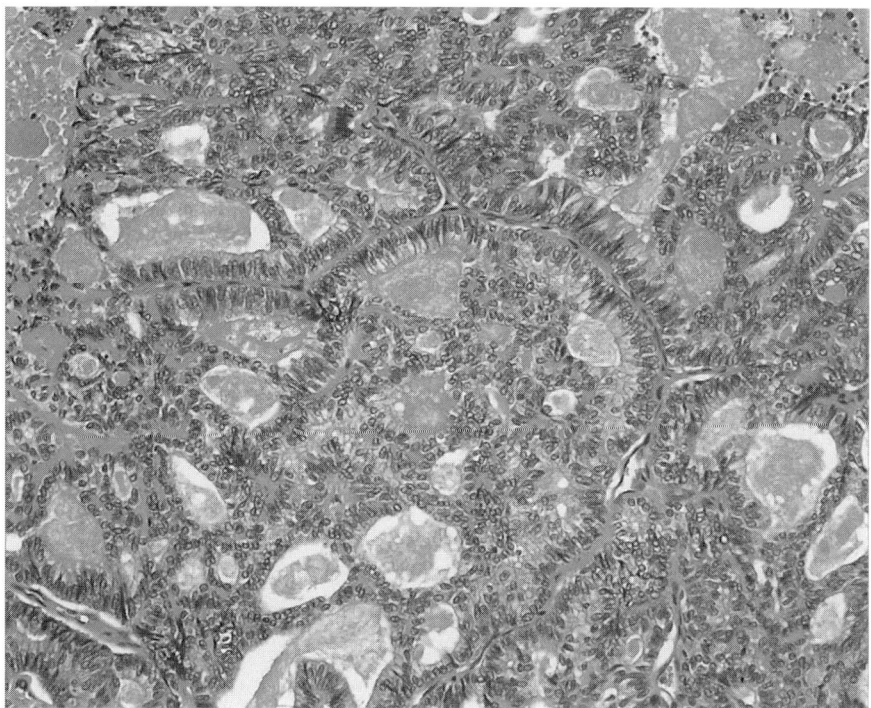

Figure 13. Patients with a family history of familial adenomatous polyposis and a germline mutation of the APC gene develop a type of papillary thyroid carcinoma that is characterized by a prominent cribriform and/or morular architecture.

lymphatics, exhibits squamous metaplasia and forms numerous psammoma bodies, giving it a very gritty appearance when examined grossly. These tumours almost always have lymph node metastases at presentation and 25% have lung metastases as well. It is interesting that about 10% of the paediatric thyroid cancers that occurred following the Chernobyl nuclear accident in 1986 were of the diffuse sclerosis type (128).

An unusual variant of papillary thyroid carcinoma known as the *cribriform-morular variant* has been identified in patients who harbour mutations of the APC gene that is responsible for familial adenomatous polyposis (FAP) syndrome (25,62,129). These lesions have unusual architecture as their name implies; they exhibit intricate admixtures of cribriform, follicular, papillary, trabecular, and solid patterns of growth (Figure 13), with morular or squamoid areas. Cribriform structures are prominent. The tumor cells are generally cuboidal or tall, with nuclear pseudostratification. Vascular and capsular invasion are common in these lesions, and while they may exhibit lymph node metastasis, there are no data to suggest that they have worse outcomes than other conventional forms of papillary carcinoma. They harbour *ret*/PTC gene rearrangements and do not exhibit loss of heterozygosity of the normal allele of the APC gene to explain an independent mechanism of tumorigenesis. Alterations in the APC

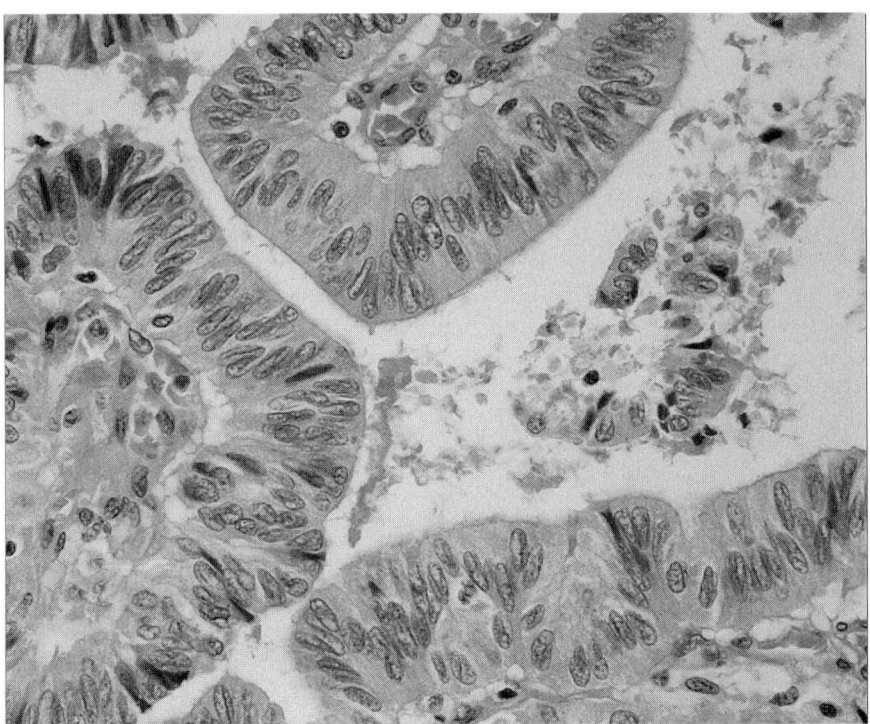

Figure 14. Tall cell papillary carcinoma is composed of a majority of tumour cells that have a height-to-width ratio that exceeds 3:1. These lesions are usually more aggressive than conventional papillary carcinomas.

gene are not thought to underlie the more common sporadic thyroid carcinomas (130,131).

Aggressive variants of papillary carcinoma include *the tall cell variant* and probably related lesions, the *trabecular and columnar cell variant* (132–137). The tall cell variant is defined as a tumor composed of cells that have a height to width ratio that exceeds 3:1 (Figure 14). They usually have complex papillary architecture and may show focal tumor cell necrosis. Tall cells generally have abundant eosinophilic cytoplasm. Columnar cells are similar to tall cells but generally are more crowded with pseudostratification and resemble endometrial lining. The two cell types tend to be found in the same tumours. Tumors that exhibit this feature in more than 30% of the tumor mass generally tend to occur in older individuals with a median age at diagnosis of 20 years older than usual papillary carcinoma, are often large lesions greater than 5 cm and often extend extrathyroidally (134). In addition to lymphatic invasion, vascular invasion is not uncommonly found in these lesions. Tumor mortality rates vary up to 25% for tall cell tumors and 90% for columnar cell carcinoma (136,138).

The management of the less aggressive forms of papillary thyroid carcinoma is controversial. Most experts advocate total thyroidectomy and radioactive iodine therapy (34,50). The rationale for total thyroidectomy is twofold, based on the frequency of bilateral carcinoma and on the need for enhancement of uptake of radioactive iodine by metastatic tumor deposits rather than residual thyroid tissue. However, as shown by the studies of Sugg et al (70), the identification of occult papillary carcinoma in the contralateral lobe is usually not attributable to intrathyroidal dissemination, which would justify further surgery for local disease. Therefore, the major indications for total thyroidectomy are the enhancement of uptake of radioactive iodine and the more sensitive use of thyroglobulin to detect persistent disease (52–54). The controversy involves the management of patients with low risk clinical and pathological parameters; some have advocated less aggressive management with unilateral thyroidectomy and no radioiodine therapy in this setting (49). Recent studies have identified potential markers of those more aggressive tumors that will metastasise to local lymph nodes, including loss of nuclear p27 and upregulation of cyclin D1 (139–141) and these may prove valuable to stratify patients for completion thyroidectomy and radioiodine therapy, but more studies are needed to validate these data. Since there are no controlled clinical trials that address this issue, the answer remains an empirical one. As for follicular carcinoma, external beam radiotherapy is not used in patients with papillary thyroid carcinoma, apart from those with locally advanced tumors that involve extrathyroidal soft tissues of the neck and cannot be completely resected (54,71).

HÜRTHLE CELL LESIONS

Hürthle cells in the thyroid represent a misnomer in that Dr. Hürthle originally described the parafollicular cell. The first description of oxyphilic cells in the thyroid is actually attributed to Askenazy. However, the term Hürthle cell is ingrained in the literature and it is unlikely that the historical error will even be corrected.

The Hürthle cell is derived from the follicular epithelium by metaplasia and possesses the capacity to produce thyroglobulin (142). Morphologically, Hürthle cells are characterised by large size, polygonal to square shape, distinct cell borders, voluminous granular and eosinophilic cytoplasm, prominent nucleus with "cherry-pink" macronucleoli. With the Papanicolau stain, the cytoplasm may be orange, green or blue. By electron microscopy, the cytoplasmic granularity is produced by large mitochondria filling the cell, consistent with oncocytic transformation (143,144). Hürthle cells have been studied by enzyme histochemistry and have been shown to contain a high level of oxidative enzymes (145,146). Somatic mutations and sequence variants of mitochondrial DNA (mtDNA) have been identified in oncocytic thyroid carcinomas (147,148). Similar changes have been found in the nontumorous thyroid tissue of patients with oncocytic neoplasms (148), suggesting that certain polymorphisms predispose to this cytologic alteration.

Hürthle cells are sometimes considered to be a cause of concern in needle biopsies (57). When they are not the major component in a thyroid aspirate, they are not diagnostic of any given lesion. Hürthle cells are found in patients with thyroiditis as well as in several forms of thyroid neoplasia. Confusion and concern also arises with the histologic diagnosis of Hürthle cell nodules in the thyroid. Hürthle cell nodules found in the setting of thyroiditis or nodular goitre may be hyperplastic. Those lesions that arise in otherwise normal glands are usually encapsulated and are considered to be neoplastic. They can have microfollicular, macrofollicular, trabecular or solid architecture. On occasion, especially with the solid pattern and since these lesions can be extremely vascular, they may resemble medullary thyroid carcinomas and it may be necessary to resort to immunoperoxidase stains for thyroglobulin and calcitonin to obtain the correct diagnosis.

Hürthle cell adenomas and Hürthle cell follicular carcinomas are diagnosed when more than 75% of a lesion is composed of this cell type; the criteria for the diagnosis of lesions that are composed predominantly of Hürthle cells are the same as those applied to follicular lesions that do not contain Hürthle cells (149). The diagnosis of Hürthle cell papillary carcinoma (see below) is possible when the minimal cytologic criteria for papillary carcinoma are present (150).

FNA of Hürthle cell tumors may cause them to partially or totally infarct (151). This probably occurs because of the high metabolic activity of these cells and the delicate blood supply of these lesions that may readily become inadequate after direct trauma. A solitary tumor of the thyroid which occurs in a patient without thyroiditis and which is purely or predominantly composed of Hürthle cells on FNA should be excised, since Hürthle cell tumors show an average of 30% malignancy rate based on histology (149).

Hürthle cell hyperplasia

Hürthle cells are found in the thyroid in a variety of conditions and therefore are not specific for any particular disease. Individual cells, follicles or groups of follicles may show Hürthle cell features in irradiated thyroids, in ageing thyroids, in nodular goitre and in thyroiditis as well as in long-standing autoimmune hyperthyroidism (142). One can see these cells in chronic lymphocytic thyroiditis, in Graves' disease and in nodular goitre, where one can often find an entire nodule composed of oncocytes.

Hürthle cell adenoma and carcinoma

For many years it was felt that all Hürthle cell neoplasms of the thyroid (Figure 15) should be considered malignant since it was felt that the histology could not predict clinical behaviour. However, numerous studies have indicated that the criteria that apply to all follicular neoplasms of the thyroid also distinguish malignant from benign Hürthle cell lesions (149,152–158) . The larger the Hürthle cell lesion, however, the more likely it is to show invasive characteristics; a Hürthle cell tumour which is 4 cm or greater has an 80% chance of showing histologic evidence of malignancy (149). Nuclear atypia, which is the hallmark of the Hürthle cell, multinucleation, and mitotic activity are not useful to predict prognosis and therefore should not be used as diagnostic criteria for malignancy.

A subgroup of Hürthle cell neoplasm has been described which show some atypical features including marked nuclear anaplasia, mitoses, spontaneous infarction and

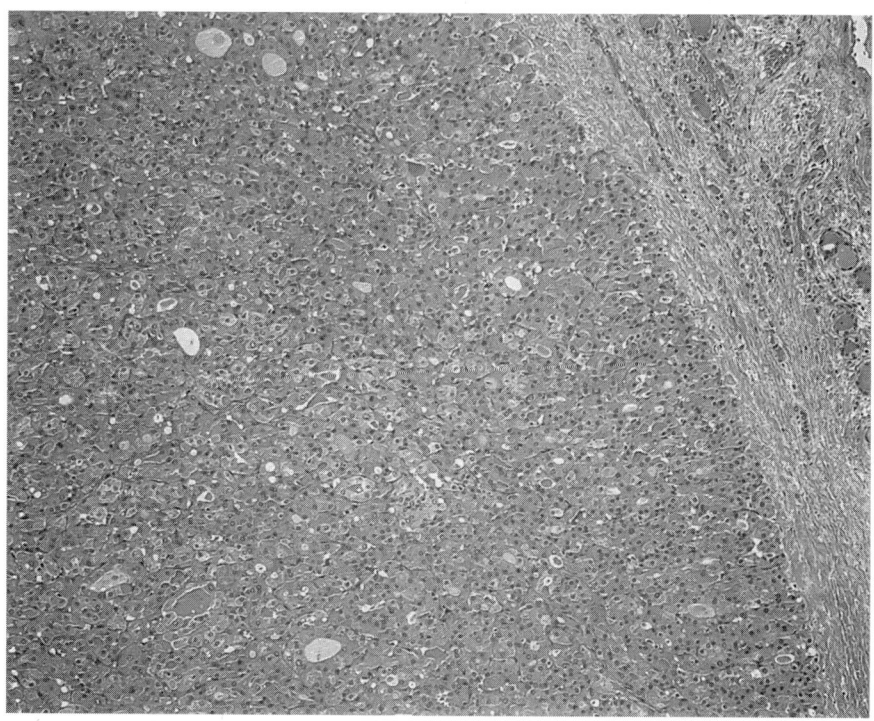

Figure 15. Hürthle cell tumours of thyroid are usually well delineated or encapsulated lesions in which more than 75% of the tumor cells have abundant eosinophilic granular cytoplasm due to the accumulation of spherulated and dilated mitochondria. These cells are derived from follicular epithelium and the criteria used to classify them should be identical to those used for non-oncocytic lesions.

trapping of tumor cells within the capsule in the absence of a preoperative FNA. Some authors have called these "atypical Hürthle cell adenoma" or "tumour of indeterminate malignancy". The great majority of these behave in a clinically benign fashion.

Flow cytometric analyses document aneuploid cell populations in 10 to 25% of Hürthle cell neoplasms that are clinically and histologically classified as adenomas (159–161). Virtually all of these tumours behave in a benign fashion after excision. Among histologically confirmed carcinomas, patients with thyroid tumors that have diploid DNA content tend to have a better prognosis than those with aneuploid values (159,161,162). Oncocytic neoplasms show frequent chromosomal DNA imbalance, with numerical chromosomal alterations being the dominant feature (163). Activating ras mutations are infrequent in oncocytic tumors (163).

The management of Hürthle cell carcinoma is controversial (155,156,164–167). In most institutions patients undergo total thyroidectomy followed by radioactive iodine. Iodine uptake by these lesions tends to be poor. External beam radiotherapy is advocated only for locally invasive disease.

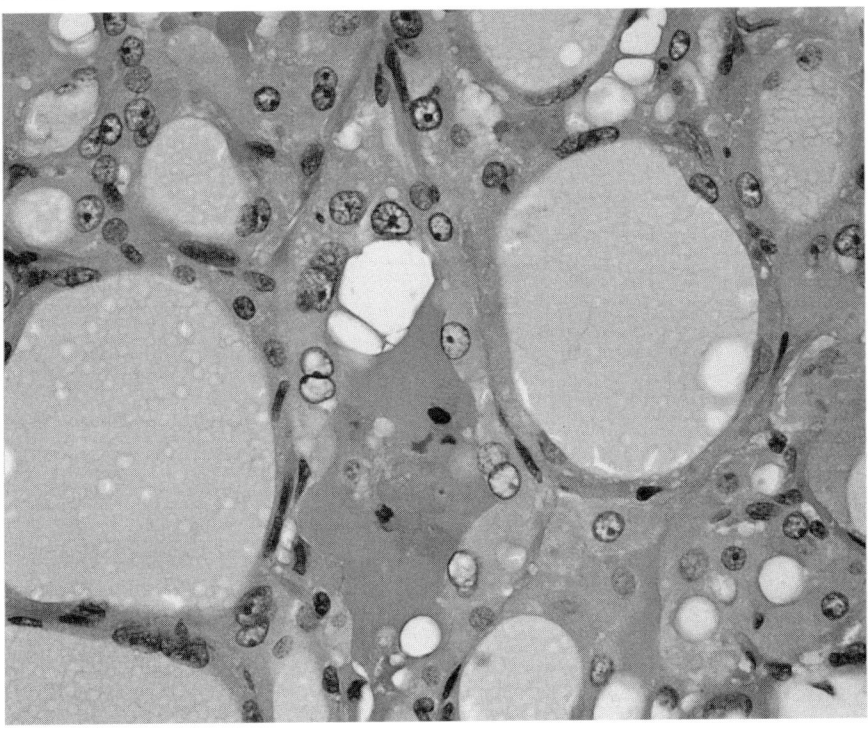

Figure 16. Oncocytic tumours with or without papillae that exhibit the nuclear features of papillary carcinoma represent Hürthle cell or oncocytic papillary carcinomas. This is an example of a follicular lesion that was not invasive, mimicking adenoma, but that harboured a ret/PTC gene rearrangement and metastasized to a local lymph node.

Hürthle cell papillary carcinoma

Many Hürthle cell tumors, whether benign or malignant, show papillary change which is really a pseudopapillary phenomenon, since Hürthle cell neoplasms have only scant stroma and may fall apart during manipulation, fixation and processing.

True oxyphilic or Hürthle cell variant of papillary carcinoma has been reported to comprise from 1 to 11% of all papillary carcinomas (144,168–173). These tumors have papillary architecture, but are composed predominantly or entirely of Hürthle cells (144,174). The nuclei may exhibit the characteristics of usual papillary carcinoma (169,175) (Figure 16), or they may instead resemble the pleomorphic nuclei of Hürthle cells, being large, hyperchromatic and pleomorphic (63,170). The clinical behaviour of this rare subtype is controversial; some authors have reported that they behave like typical papillary carcinomas (63,150,172,174,175), while others maintain that the Hürthle cell morphology confers a more aggressive behaviour (176,177) with higher rates of 10 year tumor recurrence and cause-specific mortality (170). This suggestion of aggressive behaviour may be attributed to inclusion of tall cell variant papillary carcinoma in the group of Hürthle cell carcinomas.

One morphologic subtype of Hürthle cell papillary carcinoma which, because of a characteristic cystic change and extensive lymphocytic infiltration into the cores of the papillae of the tumour, has a striking histological resemblance to papillary cystadenoma lymphomatosum of the salivary gland and has been called "Warthin-like tumour of the thyroid" (178). This lesion occurs in the setting of chronic lymphocytic thyroiditis, predominantly in women, and is associated with a similar prognosis to usual papillary carcinoma.

The diagnosis of Hürthle cell follicular variant papillary carcinoma remains controversial. Many of these lesions have been diagnosed in the past as Hürthle cell adenoma, however, reports of aggressive behaviour suggested that this diagnosis could not be trusted (156,179). The application of *ret*/PTC analysis by RT-PCR allowed recognition of a follicular variant of Hürthle cell papillary carcinoma as a group of lesions with no invasive behaviour at the time of diagnosis but that harboured a *ret*/PTC gene rearrangement (180,181). Many of these lesions exhibit irregularity of architecture with hypereosinophilic colloid and nuclear features of papillary carcinoma, but these can be obscured by the hyperchromasia and prominent nucleoli of oncocytic change. Nevertheless, they can be recognised when there is a high index of suspicion and with the addition of immunohistochemistry for HBME-1, galectin-3, CK19 and ret or by RT-PCR studies of ret rearrangements. These tumours have the potential to metastasise (182), explaining the occurrence of malignancy in patients with a histopathological diagnosis of adenoma.

Nodules associated with hashimoto's thyroiditis

In 1912, Hashimoto described a well-defined clinicopathologic syndrome consisting of goitre, hypothyroidism, and lymphocytic thyroiditis. It is now generally accepted that the form of lymphocytic thyroiditis known as Hashimoto's thyroiditis is of autoimmune aetiology (183,184). Patients have antibodies to thyroglobulin and to thyroid peroxidase (also know as "microsomal antigen") (185). Some patients also have antibodies to a colloid component other than thyroglobulin "second colloid antigen") and, occasionally, to thyroid hormones. Patients with this disorder are most often women (female-male ratio is 10:1) between 30 and 50 years of age. They typically develop a diffuse, lobulated, asymmetrical, nontender goitre. Most patients with long-standing disease are hypothyroid. Occasionally there is a transient episode of hyperthyroidism known as "Hashitoxicosis" early in the course of the disease; this has been attributed to release of stored hormone during tissue destruction or to stimulation by antibodies to the TSH receptor (185).

The presence of thyroid growth-stimulating immunoglobulins (TGI) in these patients and/or compensatory TSH excess due to tissue destruction and hypothyroidism have been implicated in the development of hyperplastic nodules that present as discrete masses in patients with this disorder. Aspiration of these lesions yields an admixture of epithelial cells and inflammatory cells (57). The hallmark is the Hürthle cell, a follicular epithelial cell that is characterised by abundant granular cytoplasm and a nucleus often with prominent "cherry pink" nucleolus. The background is composed of small and large lymphocytes, plasma cells, germinal centre fragments and macrophages with or without tangible bodies. Follicular cells and colloid are usually scant but may show nuclear atypia with irregular nuclear contours and prominent grooves.

The appearance of the thyroid involved by Hashimoto's thyroiditis is variable. The gland is usually enlarged and can weigh more than 200 g. It is composed of firm, lobulated, rubbery tissue with a homogeneous, pale grey, fleshy cut surface that lacks colloid translucence and resembles lymphoid tissue. Microscopically, the gland is diffusely infiltrated by mononuclear inflammatory cells, including lymphocytes, plasma cells, immunoblasts, and macrophages. Lymphoid follicles contain well-formed germinal centres. The glandular epithelium exhibits variable degrees of damage. Residual follicles are either atrophic, with sparse colloid and flattened epithelium or exhibit oxyphilic metaplasia, the accumulation of abundant eosinophilic granular cytoplasm characteristic of Hürthle cells (142). Follicular epithelial cells may also exhibit marked cytologic atypia that can be characterised by irregular nuclear membranes, grooves and even clearing of nucleoplasm. These features which in the face of inflammation are considered reactive, mimic papillary carcinoma (3,5). Areas of squamous metaplasia may be found (186). As the disease evolves, fibrosis becomes more conspicuous and in some patients, there is progression to the "fibrous variant" with less prominent lymphocytic infiltration, more prominent squamous metaplasia, and intense fibrosis that almost totally replaces thyroid tissue (187).

The nodules that usually precipitate surgical intervention are cellular areas composed of follicles with variable colloid storage. It is not uncommon for them to be composed predominantly of Hürthle cells and they may be difficult to distinguish from adenomas. The cytologic atypia that resembles that of papillary carcinoma and the fibrosis that can trap follicular epithelium create difficult diagnostic problems. The distinction of thyroid cancer from a reactive process or hyperplasia can be extremely difficult. Application of special techniques is particularly important in this setting. Stains such as HBME-1, galectin-3, CK 19 and ret can be of assistance.

Recent data indicate that glands with Hashimoto's disease express *ret*/PTC gene rearrangements (188). In the author's experience, this is the case when there are nodules of Hürthle cells or micropapillary carcinomas in the tissue submitted for examination, but not if these lesions are carefully excluded from the inflamed tissue examined (70). In general, *ret*/PTC expression in Hürthle cell nodules in this setting identifies gene rearrangements that correlate with other features of papillary carcinoma.

Sudden and rapid enlargement of a nodule in a patients with Hashimoto's thyroiditis may indicate the development of primary thyroid lymphoma which occurs usually in this setting.

POORLY DIFFERENTIATED (INSULAR) CARCINOMA

Poorly differentiated or insular carcinoma is a tumour of follicular cell origin which mimics the architecture of medullary thyroid carcinoma (189–191). The tumour may

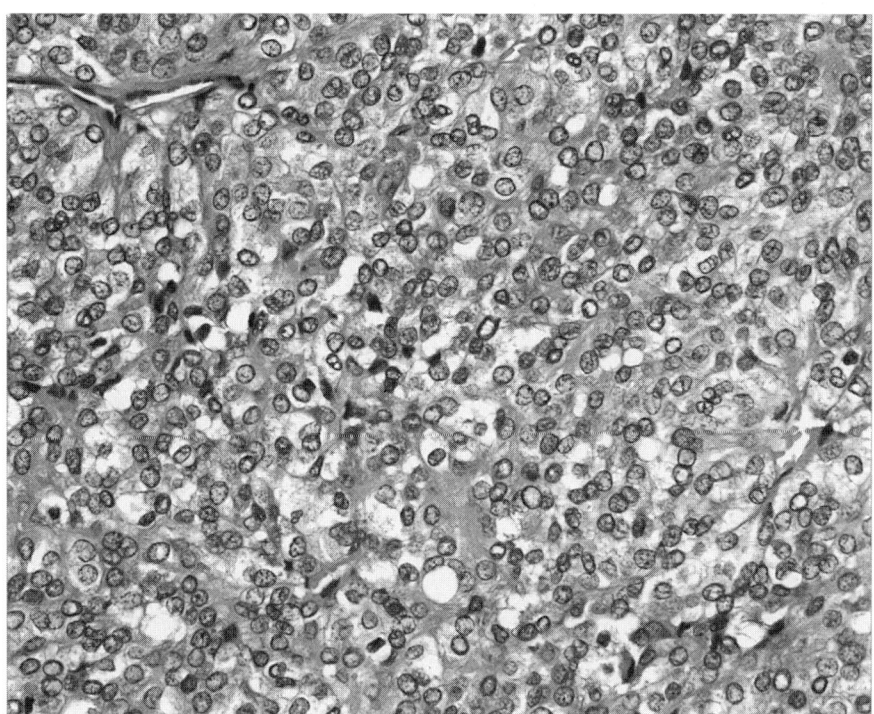

Figure 17. Insular or poorly differentiated carcinoma derived from follicular epithelium can mimick medullary carcinoma since it has a solid nesting architecture. Individual tumour cell necrosis is usually present.

have a central nidus that is encapsulated but usually the lesion exhibits frank capsular invasion and forms satellite nodules in the surrounding thyroid. The tumour architecture is characterised by large well-defined solid nests; it is largely devoid of follicular architecture and devoid of colloid (Figure 17). The tumor cells are usually small and uniform in size and there is a variable degree of mitotic activity. Sclerosis can mimic amyloid, however, congo red stains are negative and immunohistochemical stains for calcitonin, chromogranin and CEA are negative. In contrast the tumors are uniformly positive for thyroglobulin, confirming the follicular cell differentiation of this neoplasm. In contrast to anaplastic carcinomas, there is little pleomorphism and no bizarre, giant, or multinucleated cells are found, however, mitotic activity is identified. Single cell necrosis is a defining feature, but geographic necrosis is unusual.

Insular carcinoma behaves in an aggressive fashion and is often lethal. This is the lesion that most often is identified in cases that have been diagnosed as "widely invasive follicular carcinoma". Most aggressive Hürthle cell lesions show insular growth and focal tumor cell necrosis. Vascular invasion and or metastases are frequent at the time of diagnosis. Insular carcinoma therefore occupies a position both morphologically and biologically between differentiated papillary or follicular carcinoma and anaplastic thyroid carcinoma. These tumors are not uncommonly found associated with well differentiated carcinoma (either papillary or follicular) and the insular growth is thought to represent a dedifferentiation phenomenon. Since this entity has only been recognised relatively recently and the clinical literature does not include studies of this tumor type as a separate entity, appropriate clinical management remains to be established.

Clear cell carcinoma is a rare finding in the thyroid and raises important differential diagnoses. The identification of any clear cell lesion should alert the pathologist to the possibility of metastasis, particularly from renal or adrenal tumors (5). However, primary clear cell tumors of thyroid follicular cells occur and are thought to be due to accumulation of glycogen, lipid or even mucin (5). Proof that these represent follicular cells is obtained from thyroglobulin and TTF-1 staining. The term "clear cell tumor" should be restricted to lesions in which more than 75% of the tumor cells show this change.

ANAPLASTIC CARCINOMA

Anaplastic or undifferentiated carcinoma accounts for 5% to 10% of all primary malignant tumors of the thyroid (192) but in many centres this is decreasing with earlier detection of disease. These tumors are rapidly growing, with massive local invasion that usually overshadows the early metastases, most frequently to lung, adrenals and bone (4,5). They are highly lethal with a 5 year survival rate of 7.1% (193) and a mean survival period of 6.2 to 7.2 months (193,194).

Microscopically, anaplastic carcinomas exhibit wide variation. Three general patterns are recognised but most tumours manifest mixed morphology:

The most common type is the *giant cell variant*; as the name suggests, these tumors are composed predominantly of large cells with abundant amphophilic or eosinophilic, often granular cytoplasm and bizarre, often multiple, hyperchromatic nuclei (Figure 18). Some have round, densely acidophilic intracytoplasmic hyaline globules. These tumors grow in solid sheets; artefactual tissue fragmentation may simulate an alveolar pattern.

The squamoid variant is composed of large, moderately pleomorphic epithelial cells that form nests, resembling squamous carcinoma (Figure 19). They may even form keratin pearls.

Spindle cell anaplastic carcinomas have a fascicular architecture and dense stromal collagen with spindle-shaped tumor cells. They may resemble fibrosarcoma; the presence of scattered atypical cells and inflammatory infiltrates may suggest malignant fibrous histiocytoma. Prominent vascularization may suggest hemangioendothelioma (3,5,195).

In all three variants, mitotic figures and atypical mitoses are frequent. There is usually extensive necrosis and in some cases, necrosis may be so extensive that the only viable tumour is around blood vessels. Inflammatory infiltrates are associated with necrosis and the osteoclast-like giant cells that are occasionally found in these tumors have been shown by immunohistochemical studies to be reactive cells of monocytic/histiocytic lineage (196,197).

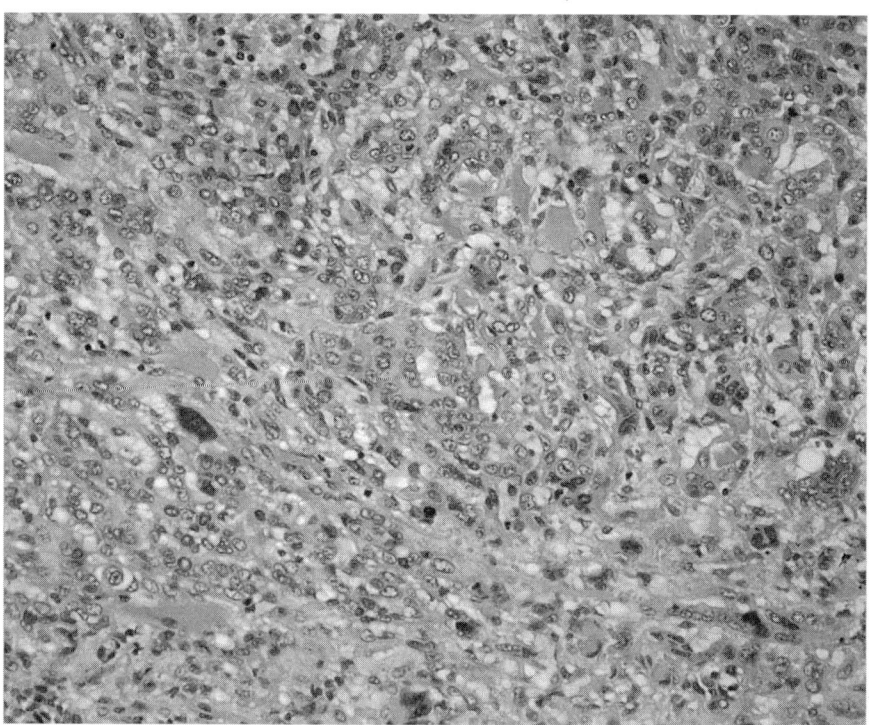

Figure 18. Anaplastic carcinoma may arise in differentiated carcinoma; it is characterized by anaplastic giant cells, prominent mitoses and geographic necrosis (not shown).

Anaplastic carcinomas are highly infiltrative. Malignant cells usually grow between residual thyroid follicles and invade skeletal muscle, adipose tissue and other perithyroidal structures. Blood vessel invasion and thrombosis with or without tumour cell involvement is frequent.

The appearances of anaplastic carcinoma on FNA are quite varied and reflect the histologic type with giant cells or squamoid cells or spindle cells. There is high cellularity, with necrosis, acute inflammation and marked cellular pleomorphism. Mitoses are often atypical and no colloid is seen.

Immunohistochemistry is useful in only a limited fashion in the diagnosis of these lesions. Most anaplastic carcinomas do not contain convincing reactivity for thyroglobulin and the few that are positive have only a weak or focal reaction (194,197–201). This staining must be interpreted carefully, since it may reflect trapped nontumorous follicles or follicular cells, and since thyroglobulin is known to diffuse into non-follicular cells (5). The epithelial nature of the tumor cells can be verified with stains for cytokeratins but again most undifferentiated lesions are negative for this marker. Squamoid areas may exhibit reactivity for high molecular weight keratins and/or epithelial membrane antigen (EMA) (194,197–199). CEA reactivity may be found in the centre of squamous

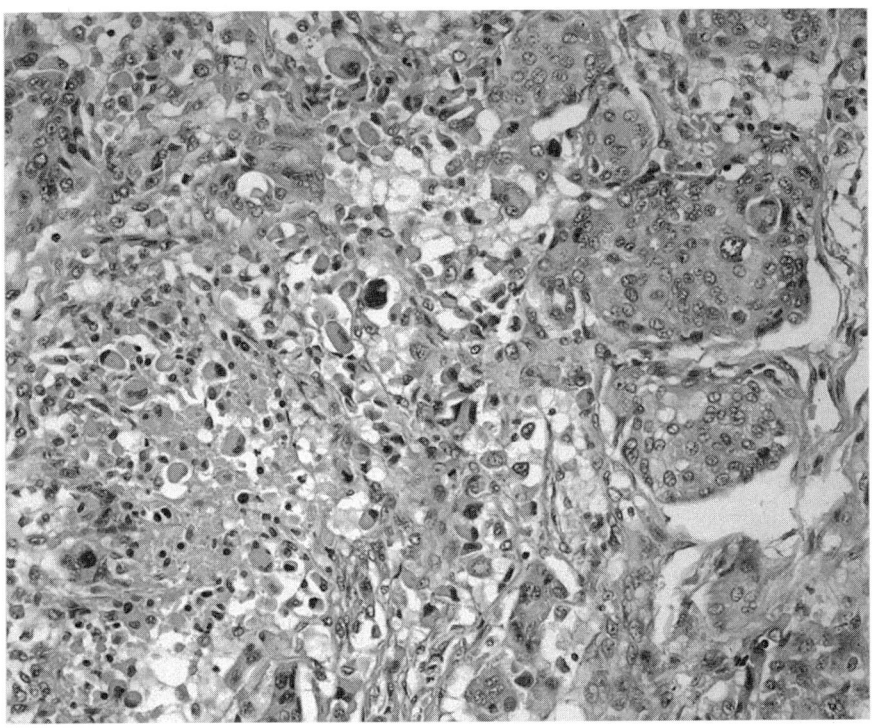

Figure 19. Some anaplastic carcinomas exhibit rhabdoid and/or sqamous morphology.

nests (194,197). Anaplastic tumours have been reported to be positive for calcitonin, but this finding should alter the diagnosis to that of medullary carcinoma (5).

p53 mutations are common in anaplastic thyroid carcinomas (202–208); since mutated forms of this tumour suppressor gene have prolonged half lives, the application of immunohistochemistry has yielded positive results in these tumours (209,210). (Chapter 8).

By electron microscopy (196,198,201,211,212), there may be formation of intercellular junctions, microvilli, and basal lamina, providing evidence of epithelial differentiation. However, many tumors do not exhibit evidence of any differentiation. Their large nuclei have prominent nucleoli and clumped chromatin; usually the cytoplasm contains only poorly developed rough endoplasmic reticulum, scattered dense bodies, lipid droplets, numerous free ribosomes, mitochondria and lysosomes. Intermediate filaments (keratin or vimentin) may form filamentous whorls that correspond to the acidophilic hyaline globules seen by light microscopy. Secretory granules are not seen in these tumours.

Most anaplastic thyroid carcinomas are aneuploid on flow cytometry; this abnormality correlates with poor outcome (162).

Some tumors do not exhibit immunohistochemical or ultrastructural markers that allow classification as epithelial malignancies. Nevertheless, the diagnosis of anaplastic carcinoma should be favoured for pleomorphic lesions in older patients if they arise in the thyroid.

Small cell carcinomas and lymphomas constitute a common source of diagnostic error, often misclassified as anaplastic carcinomas (3,5,195,198). The former are usually poorly differentiated medullary carcinomas, which can also mimic giant cell or spindle cell anaplastic carcinomas; the latter are readily identified by staining for leukocyte common antigen (LCA) and other markers of lymphoid cells. Rarely, primary intrathyroidal thymoma may be mistaken for anaplastic carcinoma (213,214).

The reported association between well-differentiated thyroid carcinoma and anaplastic carcinoma ranges from 7% to 89% of cases, however, the lower figures are likely underestimates, attributable to inadequate sampling (3,193,194,198,215–217). The data suggest that anaplastic carcinoma originates most often in an abnormal thyroid; the tumor has a higher incidence in regions of endemic goitre and a history of goitre is reported in over 80% of cases (3,193). As stated above, nodular goitre is often the site of monoclonal proliferation, the first step in the hyperplasia-neoplasia sequence. However, it is difficult to document transformation of a benign lesion to a malignant tumor. Insular carcinoma appears to be intermediate in the spectrum, and may represent a transition form (190,217). The association of papillary carcinoma, particularly the more aggressive tall cell variant, with anaplastic tumors has also been described (3,217,218). Thyroid carcinomas can exhibit an entire spectrum of differentiation through insular to anaplastic foci. The significance of microscopic insular or anaplastic change is controversial; some people have suggested that focal microscopic dedifferentiation does not alter prognosis but others have shown that this finding alone is statistically significant as a marker of aggressive behaviour.

The factors underlying dedifferentiation in thyroid tumors remain to be established; age and radiation have been implicated (219,220). Clearly, the vast majority of well differentiated thyroid lesions do not undergo such transformation. A pattern of genetic mutations resulting in oncogene activation or loss of tumour suppressor gene activity has been proposed to correlate with the stepwise progression from adenoma to carcinoma and through the dedifferentiation process in thyroid (202,203).

MEDULLARY CARCINOMA

Medullary carcinoma of the thyroid comprises 5–10% of all thyroid carcinomas (5). This lesion is usually readily recognised because of its unusual cytologic and histologic features but sometimes special investigation is required to distinguish it from follicular lesions or other tumours, including lymphomas and/or anaplastic carcinomas.

The aspirate from medullary carcinoma has a variable appearance. The cells may be spindle-shaped, columnar or plasmacytoid; they may even exhibit oncocytic or clear cell morphology. Nucleoli and nuclear pseudoinclusions are often seen. Amyloid is identified in up to 60% of cases as homogeneous, spherical or rod-shaped extracellular material which polarises with the Pap stain or the Congo Red stain. The diagnosis is confirmed by immunostaining for calcitonin or the demonstration of secretory granules on electron microscopy.

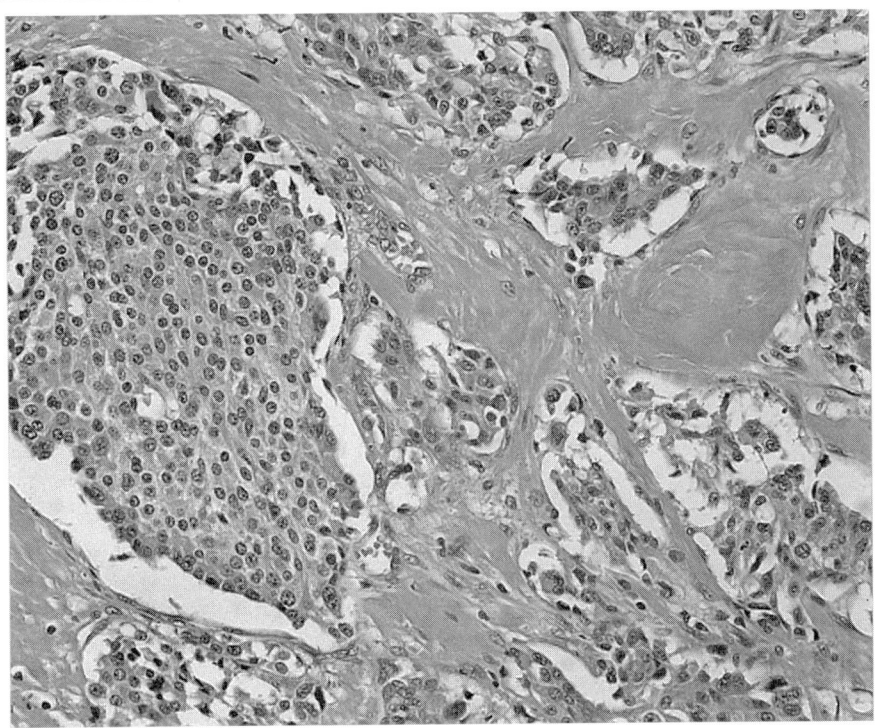

Figure 20. Medullary carcinoma of thyroid is derived from the calcitonin-producing C cells that are neuroendocrine cells. These lesions are composed of solid nests of epithelial cells with poorly defined cell borders. They often have stromal fibrosis and occasionally there is deposition of intensely eosinophilic material, amyloid, derived from the calcitonin precursor molecule.

Medullary carcinoma has a wide range of histologic appearances (2,221). Typically, the tumors are composed of sheets or more usually nests of round, polyhedral or spindle-shaped cells which may exhibit palisading at the periphery (Figure 20). The stroma is vascular. There may be prominent amyloid in the stroma, which, when present, provides a helpful diagnostic marker. However, although amyloid is present in more than half of these tumours, it may be intracytoplasmic and difficult to identify without a high index of suspicion. In addition, amyloid may also be present in occasional non-medullary thyroid carcinomas (222).

Sometimes, fixation artefact produces a pseudopapillary appearance; areas of true papillary architecture may also be found and the distinction of such lesions from papillary carcinoma can be difficult (223). A pseudofollicular appearance frequently results from entrapped nonneoplastic thyroid follicles or rounded masses of amyloid and true glandular variants have been described. Dedifferentiation results in a small cell tumour morphology, which can mimic lymphoma. Oncocytic features may predominate and make the distinction of medullary from oncocytic follicular carcinoma difficult.

Foreign body giant cells may be associated with amyloid deposits and calcification may be identified. These features may result in difficult differential diagnosis. True psammoma bodies are generally not seen in these tumours but have been reported.

Staining for amyloid can be helpful. Congo Red staining is typical and the apple-green birefringence with polarised light is diagnostic. Nevertheless, as indicated, some follicular tumors may also contain amyloid stroma.

Immunohistochemical staining represents the gold standard for the diagnosis of medullary thyroid carcinoma. These tumours express cytokeratins, chromogranin A, and NSE, but the most specific diagnostic marker is calcitonin. The number of calcitonin-positive cells varies from case to case, but the diagnosis should be questioned in the absence of calcitonin staining. The amyloid in these tumours often stains for calcitonin, likely because the amyloid protein represents deposition of a precursor of the calcitonin molecule.

These tumours also stain for carcinoembryonic antigen (CEA) and the inverse relationship between the intensity of staining for calcitonin and that for CEA may be prognostically significant: tumors containing few calcitonin-positive cells and abundant CEA immunoreactivity are said to have a worse prognosis than the well differentiated tumours with strong calcitonin immunoreactivity (224,225). CEA is not identified in follicular thyroid tumors; occasional reports of positivity are attributable to use of antibodies that react with non-specific cross-reacting antigens (226). Therefore CEA positivity indicates the presence of medullary thyroid carcinoma or other lesions such as metastatic carcinomas or thymic carcinomas.

Medullary thyroid carcinomas also produce a number of other peptides including somatostatin, derivatives of the proopiomelanocortin molecule (ACTH, MSH, ß-endorphin and enkephalin), serotonin, glucagon, gastrin, cholecystokinin, VIP, bombesin, and α-HCG (5,227–229). Calcitonin gene-related peptide (CGRP) is also identified in normal C-cells as well as medullary thyroid carcinomas. Individual tumours may express a variety of these various hormones but none have been shown to correlate with altered prognosis (230).

Ultrastructural examination confirms the presence of cells that do not form desmosomes but do show complex interdigitations of cell membranes. The cytoplasm contains characteristic membrane-bound secretory granules which usually are numerous and variable in size.

The importance of distinguishing this tumour from follicular lesions is two-fold. The first is for diagnostic classification and management considerations in the individual patient. These tumors do not preferentially take up iodine and therapy with radioactive iodine is not indicated; in contrast, expression of somatostatin receptors by some of these tumors (231) makes the octreoscan a feasible diagnostic tool to localise the primary lesion and to identify metastatic deposits (232) and somatostatin analoges may have applications in the management of disseminated disease (233). The other aspect of management involves the implications for both the patient and members of his/her family, since many of these tumours are hereditary (234).

The inherited forms of medullary carcinoma are of three types: familial medullary thyroid carcinoma alone (FMTC), multiple endocrine neoplasia (MEN) type IIA in which MTC is associated with pheochromocytomas, and MEN IIB in which the thyroid and adrenal proliferative disorders are associated with mucosal ganglioneuromas and a Marfanoid habitus. The inheritance of all three syndromes was mapped to the pericentromeric region of chromosome 10 by linkage analysis (235–237). Subsequently, mutations in exons 10 and 11 of the *ret* proto-oncogene in patients with FMTC or MEN IIA and at codon 918 in MEN IIB (238,239) have provided a more accurate marker of germline mutation and predisposition to this disease (240). Current recommendations suggest that family members of FMTC and MEN IIA kindreds have genetic screening early in life and affected members should undergo total thyroidectomy at around the age of 5 years. This age was chosen because of the early onset of medullary thyroid carcinoma in these familial forms of the disease; metastatic tumour has been found in patients as young as 6 years of age. Affected children with MEN IIB undergo surgery even earlier (241, Chapter 24).

Sporadic medullary carcinomas also may have mutations of *ret* in the same codons as the familial disorders (239,242); the mutation involved may have prognostic value (243). The presence of *ret* mutations in sporadic tumours indicates the importance of analysing DNA from white blood cells to establish that a mutation is germ line, therefore potentially hereditary. Other oncogenes and tumor suppressor genes have not been implicated in the pathogenesis of MCT: *ras* mutations are rare, c-*myc*, and c-*erb*B are not amplified (244,245), and p53 mutations are not found in these tumors (246).

Familial forms of medullary thyroid carcinoma usually result in multicentric disease as well as multicentric C-cell hyperplasia (247). Many definitions of C-cell hyperplasia have been offered, all requiring immunohistochemistry since C cells cannot be reliably recognised with routine histologic stains. Quantitation of C cells as well as geographic mapping throughout the gland must be performed (247,248). C cells are usually limited to the central portion of the junction between the upper and middle thirds of the lateral lobes where they are generally distributed singly rather than in clusters. Increased numbers of C cells (>7 cells per cluster), complete follicles surrounded by C cells, and distribution of cells beyond this geographic location are indicative of C-cell hyperplasia. The presence of C-cell hyperplasia usually indicates an inherited disorder rather than a sporadic lesion, however, C-cell hyperplasia can also be associated with chronic hypercalcemia, thyroid follicular nodular disease, and thyroiditis (249–252).

The identification of oncogenic activation of *ret* in familial C cell disease has raised questions about the term "C cell hyperplasia". In this disorder, unlike other familial cancer syndromes that result from inactivation of tumour suppressor genes, each affected member is born with an activated oncogene. Theoretically, then, every C cell has already undergone transformation, since it does not appear to require a second hit to knock out protective mechanisms. If this proves to be true, it will suggest that the term "C cell hyperplasia" is a misnomer, since each C cell with its activated oncogene is a transformed cell that represents a site of neoplastic potential. This remains to be proven, however, and the mechanism of tumorigenesis in C cells of the thyroid, as it unfolds, will shed further light on the biology of neoplasia.

MIXED FOLLICULAR-C CELL LESIONS

Although controversial, mixed follicular-parafollicular cell carcinomas do occur (253); these rare monomorphous tumours are composed of cells showing dual differentiation (254,255). Composite tumors are composed of two intermixed well differentiated components, one showing thyroglobulin immunoreactivity and either papillary or follicular architecture and cytology, the other with calcitonin and CEA immunopositivity (81,256). The diagnosis of a mixed or composite tumor can be convincing only in cases where metastatic disease is identified, since the identification of thyroglobulin and calcitonin in a primary intrathyroidal tumor may represent the identification of a typical medullary thyroid carcinoma with trapped nontumorous elements containing thyroglobulin, or phagocytosis of thyroglobulin by medullary carcinoma cells. Moreover, the two tumours may occur separately in the same gland and metastasise together to a regional node (257,258).

CONCLUSION

Thyroid nodules are common and their management can be difficult and controversial. Clearly, the pathologist has an important role to play in their evaluation. The use of fine needle aspiration biopsy has significantly improved our ability to identify specific high risk disorders and to facilitate their management in an expeditious and cost-effective manner. Patients who require surgery for further confirmation of the disease process rely upon the pathologist to correctly characterize their nodule and pathologists are actively involved in research to clarify the pathogenesis of thyroid disease. There are other areas of thyroid pathology that have seen uniform advances in our understanding of the pathobiology of disease. Most experts accept tall cell or columnar morphology as predictive of more aggressive variants of papillary carcinoma. The recognition of insular carcinomas as an intermediate category of "poorly differentiated carcinoma" has been validated by clinical and molecular studies. The biology of familial genetic alterations in medullary carcinoma has revolutionised patient care. Advances in our understanding of the molecular basis of thyroid cancer will allow more accurate characterization of specific subtypes of neoplasia and malignancy even on single cells obtained at fine needle aspiration biopsy. This should further enhance the usefulness of this technique and better guide the management of patients with a thyroid nodule.

REFERENCES

1. Ezzat S, Sarti DA, Cain DR, Braunstein GD. Thyroid incidentalomas. Prevalence by palpation and ultrasonography. Arch Intern Med 1994; 154:1838–1840.
2. Hedinger C, Williams ED, Sobin LH. The WHO histological classification of thyroid tumors: A commentary on the second edition. Cancer 1989; 63:908–911.
3. LiVolsi VA. Surgical Pathology of the Thyroid. Philadelphia, P.A.: W.B. Saunders, 1990.
4. Murray D. The thyroid gland. In: Kovacs K, Asa SL, editors. Functional Endocrine Pathology. Boston: Blackwell Science, 1998: 295–380.
5. Rosai J, Carcangiu ML, DeLellis RA. Tumors of the Thyroid Gland. Atlas of Tumor Pathology, Third Series, Fascicle 5. Washington, D.C.: Armed Forces Institute of Pathology, 1992.
6. Lloyd RV, Erickson LA, Sebo TJ. Diagnosis of follicular variant of papillary carcinoma by a panel of endocrine pathologists. Lab Invest , 106A. 2003.

7. Studer H, Peter H-J, Gerber H. Natural heterogeneity of thyroid cells: The basis for understanding thyroid function and nodular goiter growth. Endocr Rev 1989; 10:125–135.
8. Aeschimann S, Kopp PA, Kimura ET et al. Morphological and functional polymorphism within clonal thyroid nodules. J Clin Endocrinol Metab 1993; 77:846–851.
9. Studer H, Ramelli F. Simple goiter and its variants: Euthyroid and hyperthyroid multinodular goiters. Endocr Rev 1982; 3:40–61.
10. Peter HJ, Gerber H, Studer H, Smeds S. Pathogenesis of heterogeneity in human multinodular goiter. A study on growth and function of thyroid tissue transplanted onto nude mice. J Clin Invest 1985; 76:1992–2002.
11. Studer H, Hunziker HR, Ruchti C. Morphologic and functional substrate of thyrotoxicosis caused by nodular goiters. Am J Med 1978; 65:227–234.
12. Drexhage HA, Bottazzo GF, Bitensky L, Chayen J, Doniach D. Evidence for thyroid growth-stimulating immunoglobulin in some goitrous thyroid diseases. Lancet 1980; 2:287–292.
13. Van der Gaag RD, Drexhage HA, Wiersinga WM et al. Further studies on thyroid growth-stimulating immunoglobulins in euthyroid nonendemic goiter. J Clin Endocrinol Metab 1985; 60:972–979.
14. Studer H, Peter H-J, Gerber H. Toxic nodular goitre. J Clin Endocrinol Metab 1985; 14:351–372.
15. Wiener JD, Van der Gaag RD. Autoimmunity and the pathogenesis of localized thyroid autonomy (Plummer's disease). Clin Endocrinol 1985; 23:635–642.
16. Apel RL, Ezzat S, Bapat B, Pan N, LiVolsi VA, Asa SL. Clonality of thyroid nodules in sporadic goiter. Diag Mol Pathol 1995; 4:113–121.
17. Bamberger AM, Bamberger CM, Barth J, Heidorn K, Kreipe H, Schulte HM. Clonal composition of thyroid nodules from patients with multinodular goiters: Determination by X-chromosome inactivation analysis with M27beta. Experimental and Clinical Endocrinology (Leipzig) suppl.1, 73. 1993.
18. Lyons J, Landis CA, Harsh G. Two G protein oncogenes in human endocrine tumors. Science 1990; 249:635–639.
19. Porcellini A, Ciullo I, Laviola L, Amabile G, Fenzi G, Avvedimento VE. Novel mutations of thyrotropin receptor gene in thyroid hyperfunctioning adenomas. Rapid identification by fine needle aspiration biopsy. J Clin Endocrinol Metab 1994; 79:657–661.
20. van Sande J, Parma J, Tonacchera M, Swillens S, Dumont J, Vassart G. Genetic basis of endocrine disease. Somatic and germline mutations of the TSH receptor gene in thyroid disease. J Clin Endocrinol Metab 1995; 80:2577–2585.
21. Parma J, Duprez L, Van SandemH et al. Diversity and prevalence of somatic mutations in the thyrotropin receptor and Gs alpha genes as a cause of toxic thryoid adenomas. J Clin Endocrinol Metab 1997; 82:2695–2701.
22. Krohn D, Fuhrer D, Holzapfel H, Paschke R. Clonal origin of toxic thyroid nodules with constitutively activating thyrotropin receptor mutations. J Clin Endocrinol Metab 1998; 83:180–184.
23. Ezzat S, Zheng L, Kholenda J, Safarian A, Freeman JL, Asa SL. Prevalence of activating *ras* mutations in morphologically characterized thyroid nodules. Thyroid 1996; 6:409–416.
24. Hicks DG, LiVolsi VA, Neidich JA, Puck JM, Kant JA. Clonal analysis of solitary follicular nodules in the thyroid. Am J Pathol 1990; 137:553–562.
25. Cetta F, Toti P, Petracci M et al. Thyroid carcinoma associated with familial adenomatous polyposis. Histopathology 1997; 31(3):231–236.
26. Namba H, Matsuo K, Fagin JA. Clonal composition of benign and malignant human thyroid tumors. J Clin Invest 1990; 86:120–125.
27. Bronner MP, Hamilton R, LiVolsi VA. Utility of frozen section analysis on follicular lesions of the thyroid. Endocr Pathol 1994; 5:154–161.
28. Treseler PA, Clark OH. Prognostic factors in thyroid carcinoma. Surg Oncol Clin N Am 1997; 6:555–598.
29. Clark OH. Predictors of thyroid tumor aggressiveness. West J Med 1996; 165:131–138.
30. Yamashina M. Follicular neoplasms of the thyroid. Total circumferential evaluation of the fibrous capsule. Am J Surg Pathol 1992; 16:392–400.
31. Kahn NF, Perzin KH. Follicular carcinoma of the thyroid: An evaluation of the histologic criteria used for diagnosis. Pathol Annu 1983; 1:221–253.
32. Jorda M, Gonzalez-Campora R, Mora J, Herrero-Zapatero A, Otal C, Galera H. Prognostic factors in follicular carcinoma of the thyroid. Arch Pathol Lab Med 1993; 117:631–635.
33. van Heerden JA, Hay ID, Goellner JR et al. Follicular thyroid carcinoma with capsular invasion alone: A nonthreatening malignancy. Surgery 1992; 112:1130–1138.

34. Harness JK, Thompson NW, McLeod MK, Eckhauser FE, Lloyd RV. Follicular carcinoma of the thyroid gland: Trends and treatment. Surgery 1984; 96:972–980.
35. Miettinen M, Karkkainen P. Differential reactivity of HBME-1 and CD15 antibodies in benign and malignant thyroid tumours. Preferential reactivity with malignant tumours. Virchows Arch 1996; 429:213–219.
36. Sack MJ, Astengo-Osuna C, Lin BT, Battifora H, LiVolsi VA. HBME-1 immunostaining in thyroid fine-needle aspirations: a useful marker in the diagnosis of carcinoma. Mod Pathol 1997; 10:668–674.
37. van Hoeven KH, Kovatich AJ, Miettinen M. Immunocytochemical evaluation of HBME-1, CA 19-9, and CD-15 (Leu-M1) in fine-needle aspirates of thyroid nodules. Diagn Cytopathol 1997; 18:93–97.
38. Fernandez PL, Merino MJ, Gomez M et al. Galectin-3 and laminin expression in neoplastic and non-neoplastic thyroid tissue. J Pathol 1997; 181:80–86.
39. Orlandi F, Saggiorato E, Pivano G et al. Galectin-3 is a presurgical marker of human thyroid carcinoma. Cancer Res 1998; 58:3015–3020.
40. Cvejic D, Savin S, Paunovic I, Tatic S, Havelka M, Sindinovic J. Immuhohistochemical localization of galectin-3 in malignant and benign human thyroid tissue. Anticancer Res 1998; 18:2637–2642.
41. Inohara H, Honjo Y, Yoishii T et al. Expression of galectin-3 in fine-needle aspirates as a diagnostic marker differentiating benign from malignant thyroid neoplasms. Cancer 1999; 85:2475–2484.
42. Kroll TG, Sarraf P, Pecciarini L et al. PAX8-PPARγ1 fusion oncogene in human thyroid carcinoma. Science 2000; 289(5483):1357–1360.
43. LiVolsi VA, Asa SL. The demise of follicular carcinoma of the thyroid gland. Thyroid 1994; 4:233–235.
44. Nikiforova MN, Biddinger PW, Caudill CM, Kroll TG, Nikiforov YE. PAX8-PPAR gamma rearrangement in thyroid tumors: RT-PCR and immunohistochemical analyses. Am J Surg Pathol 2002; 26(8):1016–1023.
45. Zedenius J, Auer G, Bäckdahl M et al. Follicular tumors of the thyroid gland: Diagnosis, clinical aspects and nuclear DNA analysis. World J Surg 1992; 16:589–594.
46. Samaan NA, Schultz PN, Haynie TP, Ordonez NG. Pulmonary metastasis of differentiated thyroid carcinoma: Treatment results in 101 patients. J Clin Endocrinol Metab 1985; 65:376–380.
47. DeGroot LJ, Kaplan EL, Shukla MS, Salti G, Straus FH. Morbidity and mortality in follicular thyroid cancer. J Clin Endocrinol Metab 1995; 80:2946–2953.
48. Mizukami Y, Michigishi T, Nonomura A et al. Distant metastases in differentiated thyroid carcinomas: A clinical and pathologic study. Hum Pathol 1990; 21:283–290.
49. Shah JP, Loree TR, Dharker D, Strong EW. Lobectomy versus total thyroidectomy for differentiated carcinoma of the thyroid: a matched-pair analysis. Am J Surg 1993; 166:331–335.
50. Singer PA, Cooper DS, Daniels GH et al. Treatment guidelines for patients with thyroid nodules and well-differentiated thyroid cancer. American Thyroid Association. Arch Intern Med 1996; 156:2165–2172.
51. Pasieka JL, Thompson NW, McLeod MK, Burney RE, Macha M. The incidence of bilateral well-differentiated thyroid cancer found at completion thyroidectomy. World J Surg 1992; 16:711–717.
52. Benker G, Olbricht Th, Reinwein D et al. Survival rates in patients with differentiated thyroid carcinoma. Influence of postoperative external radiotherapy. Cancer 1990; 65:1517–1520.
53. Mazzaferri EL, Jhiang SM. Long-term impact of initial surgical and medical therapy on papillary and follicular thyroid cancer. Am J Med 1994; 97:418–428.
54. Tsang RW, Brierley JD, Simpson WJ, Panzarella T, Gospodarowicz MK, Sutcliffe SB. The effects of surgery, radioiodine, and external radiation therapy on the clinical outocme of patients with differentiated thyroid carcinoma. Cancer 1998; 82:375–388.
55. LiVolsi VA, Merino MJ. Worrisome histologic alterations following fine needle aspiration of the thyroid. Pathol Annu 1994; 29(2):99–120.
56. Namba H, Ross JL, Goodman D, Fagin JA. Solitary polyclonal autonomous thyroid nodule: A rare cause of childhood hyperthyroidism. J Clin Endocrinol Metab 1991; 72:1108–1112.
57. Kini SR. Thyroid. 2 ed. New York: Igaku-Shoin Ltd., 1996.
58. Vickery AL. Thyroid papillary carcinoma. Pathological and philosophical controversies. Am J Surg Pathol 1983; 7:797–807.
59. Rosai J, Zampi G, Carcangiu ML, Pupi A, et al. Papillary carcinoma of the thyroid. Am J Surg Pathol 1983; 7:809–817.
60. Vickery AL, Carcangiu ML, Johannessen JV, et al. Papillary carcinoma. Semin Diagn Pathol 1985; 2:90–100.
61. LiVolsi VA. Papillary neoplasms of the thyroid. Pathologic and prognostic features. Am J Clin Pathol 1992; 97:426–434.

62. Soravia C, Sugg SL, Berk T et al. Familial adenomatous polyposis-associated thyroid cancer. Am J Pathol 1999; 154:127–135.
63. Hedinger C, Williams ED, Sobin LH. Histological typing of thyroid tumours. World Health Organization International Histological Classification of Tumours. 2 ed. Berlin: Springer-Verlag, 1988.
64. Hay ID. Papillary thyroid carcinoma. Endocrinol Metab Clin North Am 1990; 19:545–576.
65. Mazzaferri E, Jhiang S. Long-term follow-up impact of initial surgical and medical therapy on papillary and follicular thyroid cancer. Am J Med 1994; 97:418–428.
66. Hapke MR, Dehner LP. The optically clear nucleus. A reliable sign of papillary carcinoma of the thyroid? Am J Surg Pathol 1979; 3:31–38.
67. Chan JKC, Saw D. The grooved nucleus: A useful diagnostic criterion of papillary carcinoma of the thyroid. Am J Surg Pathol 1986; 10:672–679.
68. Deligeorgi-Politi H. Nuclear crease as a cytodiagnostic feature of papillary thyroid carcinoma in fine-needle aspiration biopsies. Diagn Cytopathol 1987; 3:307–310.
69. Fink A, Tomlinson G, Freeman JL, Rosen IB, Asa SL. Occult micropapillary carcinoma associated with benign follicular thyroid disease and unrelated thyroid neoplasms. Mod Pathol 1996; 9(8):816–820.
70. Sugg SL, Ezzat S, Rosen IB, Freeman J, Asa SL. Distinct multiple ret/PTC gene rearrangements in multifocal papillary thyroid neoplasia. J Clin Endocrinol Metab 1998; 83:4116–4122.
71. Brierley JD, Panzarella T, Tsang RW, Gospodarowicz MK, O'Sullivan B. A comparison of different staging systems predictability of patient outcome. Thyroid carcinoma as an example. Cancer 1997; 79:2414–2423.
72. Noguchi M, Tanaka S, Akiyama T, et al. Clinicopathological studies of minimal thyroid and ordinary thyroid cancers. Jpn J Surg 1984; 13:110–117.
73. Harach HR, Franssila KO, Wasenius V-M. Occult papillary carcinoma of the thyroid. A "normal" finding in Finland. A systematic autopsy study. Cancer 1985; 56:531–538.
74. Yamashita H, Nakayama I, Noguchi S et al. Thyroid carcinoma in benign thyroid diseases. An analysis from minute carcinoma. Acta Pathol Jpn 1985; 35(4):781–788.
75. Yamashita H, Noguchi S, Murkama N, et al. Prognosis of minute carcinoma of the thyroid. Follow-up study of 48 patients. Acta Pathol Jpn 1986; 36:1469–1475.
76. Schröder S, Schwarz W, Rehpenning W, Löning T, Böocker W. Dendritic/Langerhans cells and prognosis in patients with papillary thyroid carcinomas. Am J Clin Pathol 1988; 89:295–300.
77. Volpé R. Immunology of human thyroid disease. In: Volpé R, editor. Autoimmune diseases of the endocrine system. Boca Raton: CRC Press, 1990: 73–240.
78. Leung CS, Hartwick RWJ, Bédard YC. Correlation of cytologic and histologic features in variants of papillary carcinoma of the thyroid. Acat Cytol 1993; 37:645–650.
79. Hawk WA, Hazard JB. The many appearances of papillary carcinoma of the thyroid. Cleve Clin Q 1976; 43:207–216.
80. Chan JK. Papillary carcinoma of the thyroid: classical and variants. Histol Histopathol 1990; 5:241–257.
81. Mizukami Y, Michigishi T, Nonomura A et al. Mixed medullary-follicular carcinoma of the thyroid occurring in familial form. Histopathology 1993; 22:284–287.
82. Evans HL. Encapsulated papillary neoplasms of the thyroid. A study of 14 cases followed for a minimum of 10 years. Am J Surg Pathol 1987; 11:592–597.
83. Chen KTK, Rosai J. Follicular variant of thyroid papillary carcinoma: A clinicopathologic study of six cases. Am J Surg Pathol 1977; 1:123–130.
84. Tielens ET, Sherman SI, Hruban RH, et al. Follicular variant of papillary thyroid carcinoma; a clinicopathologic study. Cancer 1994; 73:424–431.
85. Raphael SJ, Apel RL, Asa SL. Detection of high-molecular-weight cytokeratins in neoplastic and non-neoplastic thyroid tumors using microwave antigen retrieval. Mod Pathol 1995; 8:870–872.
86. Santoro M, Carlomagno F, Hay ID et al. Ret oncogene activation in human thyroid neoplasms is restricted to the papillary cancer subtype. J Clin Invest 1992; 89:1517–1522.
87. Tallini G, Asa SL. RET oncogene activation in papillary thyroid carcinoma. Adv Anat Pathol 2001; 8(6):345–354.
88. Fusco A, Grieco M, Santoro M et al. A new oncogene in human thyroid papillary carcinomas and their lymph-nodal metastases. Nature 1987; 328:170–172.
89. Pierotti MA, Santoro M, Jenkins RB et al. Characterization of an inversion on the long arm of chromosome 10 juxtaposing D10S170 and RET and creating the oncogenic sequence RET/PTC. Proc Natl Acad Sci USA 1992; 89:1616–1620.
90. Minoletti F, Butti Mg, Coronelli S et al. The two genes generating RET/PTC3 are localized in chromosomal band 10q11.2. Genes, Chromosomes & Cancer 1994; 11:51–57.

91. Sozzi G, Bongarzone I, Miozzo M et al. A t(10;17) translocation creates the RET/PTC2 chimeric transforming sequence in papillary thyroid carcinoma. Genes, Chromosomes & Cancer 1994; 9: 244–250.
92. Jhiang SM, Mazzaferri EL. The ret/PTC oncogene in papillary thyroid carcinoma. J Lab Clin Med 1994; 123:331–337.
93. Ishizaka Y, Shima H, Sugimura T, Nagao M. Detection of phosphorylated ret/TPC oncogene product in cytoplasm. Oncogene 1992; 7:1441–1444.
94. Jhiang SM, Sagartz JE, Tong Q et al. Targeted expression of the ret/PTC1 oncogene induces papillary thyroid carcinomas. Endocrinology 1996; 137:375–378.
95. Santoro M, Chiappetta G, Cerrato A et al. Development of thyroid papillary carcinomas secondary to tissue-specific expression of the RET/PTC1 oncogene in transgenic mice. Oncogene 1996; 12:1821–1826.
96. Powell DJJr, Russell J, Nibu K et al. The RET/PTC3 oncogene: metastatic solid-type papillary carcinomas in murine thyroids. Cancer Res 1998; 58:5523–5528.
97. Klugbauer S, Lengfelder E, Demidchik EP, Rabes HM. High prevalence of RET rearrangement in thyroid tumors of children from Belarus after the Chernobyl reactor accident. Oncoogene 1995; 11:2459–2467.
98. Nishisho I, Rowland JM, Bove KE, Monforte-Munoz H, Fagin JA. Distinct pattern of ret oncogene rearrangements in morphological variants of radiation-induced and sporadic thyroid papillary carcinoma in children. Cancer Res 1997; 57:1690–1694.
99. Klugbauer S, Lengfelder E, Demidchik EP, Rabes HM. A new form of RET rearrangement in thyroid carcinomas of children after the Chernobyl reactor acident. Oncogene 1996; 13:1099–1102.
100. Fugazzola L, Pierotti MA, Vigano E, Pacini F, Vorontsova TV, Bongarzone I. Molecular and biochemical analysis of RET/PTC4, a novel oncogenic rearrangement between RET and ELE1 genes, in a post-Cherynobyl papillary thyroid cancer. Oncogene 1996; 13:1093–1097.
101. Klugbauer S, Demidchik EP, Lengfelder E, Rabes HM. Detection of a novel type of RET rearrangement (PTC5) in thyroid carcinomas after Chernobyl and analysis of the involved RET-fused gene RFG5. Cancer Res 1998; 58:198–203.
102. Williams GH, Rooney S, Thomas GA, Cummins G, Williams ED. RET activation in adult and childhood papillary thyroid carcinoma using a reverse transcriptase-polymerase chain reaction approach on archival-nested material. Br J Cancer 1996; 74:585–589.
103. Jhiang SM, Caruso DR, Gilmore E et al. Detection of the PTC/retTPC oncogene in human thyroid cancers. Oncogene 1992; 7:1331–1337.
104. Sugg SL, Zheng L, Rosen IB, Freeman JL, Ezzat S, Asa SL. ret/PTC-1,-2 and -3 oncogene rearrangements in human thyroid carcinomas: Implications for metastatic potential? J Clin Endocrinol Metab 1996; 81:3360–3365.
105. Mayr B, Brabant G, Goretzki P, Ruschoff J, Dietmaier W, Dralle H. ret/Ptc-1, -2, and -3 oncogene rearrangements in human thyroid carcinomas: implications for metastatic potential? J Clin Endocrinol Metab 1997; 82:1306–1307.
106. Viglietto G, Chiappetta G, Martinez-Tello FJ et al. RET/PTC oncogene activation is an early event in thyroid carcinogenesis. Oncogene 1995; 11:1207–1210.
107. Cheung CC, Ezzat S, Freeman JL, Rosen IB, Asa SL. Immunohistochemical diagnosis of papillary thyroid carcinoma. Mod Pathol 2001; 14(4):338–342.
108. Cheung CC, Carydis B, Ezzat S, Bedard YC, Asa SL. Analysis of ret/PTC gene rearrangements refines the fine needle aspiration diagnosis of thyroid cancer. J Clin Endocrinol Metab 2001; 86(5):2187–2190.
109. Zipkin P. Hyalinahniliche collagene kugeln als produkte epitelialer zellen in malignen strumen. Virchows Arch 1905; 182:374–406.
110. Masson P. Cancers thyroidiens a polarite alternative. Bull Cancer 1922; 11:350–355.
111. Ward JV, Murray D, Horvath E, Kovacs K, Bauman A. Hyaline cell tumor of the thyroid with massive accumulation of cytoplasmic microfilaments. Laboratory Investigation 46, 88A. 1982.
112. Carney JA, Ryan J, Goellner JR. Hyalinizing trabecular adenoma of the thyroid gland. Am J Surg Pathol 1987; 11:583–591.
113. Bronner MP, LiVolsi VA, Jennings TA. PLAT: Paraganglioma-like adenomas of the thyroid. Surg Pathol 1988; 1:383–389.
114. Sambade C, Franssila K, Cameselle-Teijeiro J, Nesland J, Sobrinho-Simoes M. Hyalinizing trabecular adenoma: A misnomer for a peculiar tumor of the thyroid gland. Endocr Pathol 1991; 2:83–91.
115. Molberg K, Albores-Saavedra J. Hyalinizing trabecular carcinoma of the thyroid gland. Hum Pathol 1994; 25:192–197.

116. McCluggage WG, Sloan JM. Hyalinizing trabecular carcinoma of the thyroid gland. Histopathology 1996; 28:357–362.
117. Katoh R, Jasani B, Williams ED. Hyalinizing trabecular adenoma of the thyroid. A report of three cases with immunohistochemical and ultrastructural studies. Histopathology 1989; 15:211–224.
118. Li M, Carcangiu ML, Rosai J. Abnormal intracellular and extracellular distribution of base membrane material in papillary carcinoma and hyalinizing trabecular tumors of the thyroid: implication for deregulation secretory pathways. Hum Pathol 1997; 28:1366–1372.
119. Chan JKC, Tse CCH, Chiu HS. Hyalinizing trabecular adenoma-like lesion in multinodular goitre. Histopathology 1990; 16:611–614.
120. Cheung CC, Boerner SL, MacMillan CM, Ramyar L, Asa SL. Hyalinizing trabecular tumor of the thyroid: a variant of papillary carcinoma proved by molecular genetics. Am J Surg Pathol 2000; 24(12):1622–1626.
121. Papotti M, Volante M, Giuliano A et al. RET/PTC activation in hyalinizing trabecular tumors of the thyroid. Am J Surg Pathol 2000; 24(12):1615–1621.
122. Hirokawa M, Carney JA, Ohtsuki Y. Hyalinizing trabecular adenoma and papillary carcinoma of the thyroid gland express different cytokeratin patterns. Am J Surg Pathol 2000; 24(6):877–881.
123. Hirokawa M, Carney JA. Cell membrane and cytoplasmic staining for MIB-1 in hyalinizing trabecular adenoma of the thyroid gland. Am J Surg Pathol 2000; 24(4):575–578.
124. Chan JKC, Tsui MS, Tse CH. Diffuse sclerosing variant of papillary carcinoma of the thyroid: a histological and immunohistochemical study of three cases. Histopathology 1987; 11:191–201.
125. Carcangiu ML, Bianchi S. Diffuse sclerosing variant of papillary thyroid carcinoma: Clinicopathologic study of 15 cases. Am J Surg Pathol 1989; 13:1041–1049.
126. Soares J, Limbert E, Sobrinho-Simoes M. Diffuse sclerosing variant of papillary thyroid carcinoma. A clinicopathologic study of 10 cases. Path Res Pract 1989; 185:200–206.
127. Fujimoto.Y., Obara T, Ito Y, et al. Diffuse sclerosing variant of papillary carcinoa of the thyroid. Cancer 1990; 66:2306–2312.
128. Nikiforov Y, Gnepp DR. Pediatric thyroid cancer after the Chernobyl disaster: Pathomorphologic study of 84 cases (1991–1992) from the Republic of Belarus. Cancer 1994; 74:748–766.
129. Cameselle-Teijeiro J, Chan JK. Cribiform-morular variant of papillary carcinoma: a distinct variant representing the sporadic counterpart of familial adenomatous polyposis-associated with thyroid carcinoma. Mod Pathol 1999; 12:400–411.
130. Zeki K, Spambalg D, Sharifi N, Gonsky R, Fagin JA. Mutations of the adenomatous polyposis coli gene in sporadic thyroid neoplasms. J Clin Endocrinol Metab 1994; 79:1317–1321.
131. Colletta G, Sciacchitano S, Palmirotta R et al. Analysis of adenomatous polyposis coli gene in thyroid tumours. Br J Cancer 1994; 70(6):1085–1088.
132. Flint A, Davenport RD, Lloyd RV. The tall cell variant of papillary carcinoma of the thyroid gland. Arch Pathol Lab Med 1991; 115:169–171.
133. Hicks MJ, Batsakis JG. Tall cell carcinoma of the thyroid gland. Ann Otol Rhinol Laryngol 1993; 102:402–403.
134. Van den Brekel MWM, Hekkenberg RJ, Asa SL, Tomlinson G, Rosen IB, Freeman JL. Prognostic features in tall cell papillary carcinoma and insular thyroid carcinoma. Laryngoscope 1997; 107:254–259.
135. Sobrinho-Simoes M, Nesland JM, Johannessen JV. Columnar cell carcinoma: another variant of poorly differentiated carcinoma of the thyroid. Am J Clin Pathol 1988; 89:264–267.
136. Evans HL. Columnar-cell carcinoma of the thyroid. A report of two cases of an aggressive variant of thyroid carcinoma. Am J Clin Pathol 1986; 85:77–80.
137. Akslen L, Varhaug JE. Thyroid carcinoma with mixed tall cell and columnar cell features. Am J Clin Pathol 1990; 94:442–445.
138. Johnson TL, Lloyd RV, Thompson NW, Beierwaltes WH, Sisson JC. Prognostic implications of the tall cell variant of papillary thyroid carcinoma. Am J Surg Pathol 1988; 12:22–27.
139. Khoo ML, Ezzat S, Freeman JL, Asa SL. Cyclin D1 protein expression predicts metastatic behavior in thyroid papillary microcarcinomas but is not associated with gene amplification. J Clin Endocrinol Metab 2002; 87(4):1810–1813.
140. Khoo ML, Beasley NJ, Ezzat S, Freeman JL, Asa SL. Overexpression of cyclin D1 and underexpression of p27 predict lymph node metastases in papillary thyroid carcinoma. J Clin Endocrinol Metab 2002; 87(4):1814–1818.

141. Khoo ML, Freeman JL, Witterick IJ et al. Underexpression of p27/Kip in thyroid papillary microcarcinomas with gross metastatic disease. Arch Otolaryngol Head Neck Surg 2002; 128(3):253–257.
142. Friedman NB. Cellular involution in thyroid gland: significance of Hürthle cells in myxedema, exhaustion atrophy, Hashimoto's disease and reaction in irradiation, thiouracil therapy and subtotal resection. J Clin Endocrinol 1949; 9:874–882.
143. Nesland JM, Sobrinho-Simoes M, Holm R, Sambade MC, Johannessen JV. Hürthle cell lesions of the thyroid: a combined study using transmission electron microscopy, scanning electron microscopy and immunocytochemistry. Ultrastructrual Pathol 1985; 8:131–142.
144. Sobrinho-Simoes M, Nesland JM, Holm R, Sambade MC, Johannessen JV. Hürthle cell and mitochondrion-rich papillary carcinomas of the thyroid gland: An ultrastructural and immunocytochemical study. Ultrastruct Pathol 1985; 8:131–142.
145. Triggs SM, Pearse AGE. Histochemistry of oxidate enzyme systems in the human thyroid with special reference to Askanazy cells. J Pathol Bacteriol 1960; 80:353–358.
146. Clark OH, Gerend PL. Thyrotropin receptor-adenylate cyclase system in Hürthle cell neoplasms. J Clin Endocrinol Metab 1985; 39:719–723.
147. Yeh JJ, Lunetta KL, van Orsouw NJ et al. Somatic mitochondrial DNA (mtDNA) mutations in papillary thyroid carcinomas and differential mtDNA sequence variants in cases with thyroid tumours. Oncogene 2000; 19(16):2060–2066.
148. Maximo V, Soares P, Lima J, Cameselle-Teijeiro J, Sobrinho-Simoes M. Mitochondrial DNA somatic mutations (point mutations and large deletions) and mitochondrial DNA variants in human thyroid pathology: a study with emphasis on Hurthle cell tumors. Am J Pathol 2002; 160(5):1857–1865.
149. Bronner MP, LiVolsi VA. Oxyphilic (Askenasy/Hürthle cell) tumors of the thyroid. Microscopic features predict biologic behavior. Surg Pathol 1988; 1:137–150.
150. Chen KTK. Fine-needle aspiration cytology of papillary Hürthle-cell tumors of thyroid: A report of three cases. Diagn Cytopathol 1991; 7:53–56.
151. Kini SR, Miller JM, Abrash MP, Γαβα A, Johnson T. Post fine needle apsiration biopsy infarction in thyroid nodules. Modern Pathology 1, 48A. 1988.
152. Johnson TL, Lloyd RV, Burney RE, Thompson NW. Hürthle cell thyroid tumors: an immunohistochemical study. Cancer 1987; 59:107–112.
153. Arganini M, Behar R, Wi TC et al. Hürthle cell tumors: a twenty-five year experience. Surgery 1986; 100:1108–1114.
154. Gosain AK, Clark OH. Hürthle cell neoplasms: malignant potential. Arch Surg 1984; 119:515–519.
155. Har-El G, Hadar T, Segal K, Levy R, Sidi J. Hürthle cell carcinoma of the thyroid gland. A tumor of moderate malignancy. Cancer 1986; 57:1613–1617.
156. Thompson NW, Dunn EL, Batsakis JG, Nishiyama RH. Hürthle cell lesions of the thyroid gland. Surg Gynecol Obstet 1974; 139:555–560.
157. Flint A, Lloyd RV. Hürthle cell neoplasms of the thyroid gland. Pathol Annu 1990; 25:37–52.
158. Carcangiu ML, Bianchiu S, Savino D, et al. Follicular Hürthle cell tumors of the thyroid gland. Cancer 1991; 68:1944–1953.
159. McLeod MK, Thompson NW, Hudson JL et al. Flow cytometric measurements of nuclear DNA and ploidy analysis in Hürthle cell neoplasms of the thyroid. Arch Surg 1988; 123:849–854.
160. Ryan J J, Hay ID, Grant CS, Rainwater LM, Farrow GM, Goellner JR. Flow cytometric DNA measurements in benign and malignant Hürthle cell tumors of the thyroid. World J Surg 1988; 12:482–487.
161. Galera-Davidson H, Bobbo M, Bartels PH, Dytch HE, Puls JH, Wied GL. Correlation between automated DNA ploidy measurements of Hürthle cell tumors and their histopathologic and clinical features. Anal Quant Cytol Histol 1986; 8:158–167.
162. Klemi PJ, Joensuu H, Eerola E. DNA aneuploidy in anaplastic carcinoma of the thyroid gland. Am J Clin Pathol 1988; 89:154–159.
163. Tallini G, Hsueh A, Liu S, Garcia-Rostan G, Speicher MR, Ward DC. Frequent chromosomal DNA unbalance in thyroid oncocytic (Hurthle cell) neoplasms detected by comparative genomic hybridization. Lab Invest 1999; 79(5):547–555.
164. Bondeson L, Bondeson A-G, Ljungberg O. Treatment of Hürthle cell neoplasms of the thyroid. Arch Surg 1983; 118:1453.
165. Bondeson L, Bondeson AG, Ljungberg O, Tibblin S. Oxyphil tumors of the thyroid. Ann Surg 1981; 194:677–680.
166. Gundry SR, Burney RE, Thompson NW, Lloyd R. Total thyroidectomy for Hürthle cell neoplasm of the thyroid. Arch Surg 1983; 118:529–532.

167. Watson RG, Brennan MD, Goellner JR, van Heerden JA, McConahey WM, Taylor WF. Invasive Hürthle cell carcinoma of the thyroid: Natural history and management. Pathol Annu 1984; 59:851–855.
168. Gardner LW. Hürthle-cell tumors of the thyroid. Arch Pathol 1955; 59:372–381.
169. González-Campora R, Herrero-Zapatero A, Lerma E, Sanchez F, Galera H. Hürthle cell and mitochondrion-rich cell tumors. A clinicopathologic study. Cancer 1986; 57:1154–1163.
170. Herrera MF, Hay ID, Wu PS et al. Hürthle cell (oxyphilic) papillary thyroid carcinoma: A variant with more aggressive biologic behavior. World J Surg 1992; 16:669–675.
171. Meissner WA, Adler A. Papillary carcinoma of the thyroid. A study of the pathology of two hundred twenty-six cases. Arch Pathol 1958; 66:518–525.
172. Tscholl-Ducommun J, Hedinger C. Papillary thyroid carcinomas. Morphology and Prognosis. Virchows Arch [Pathol Anat] 1982; 396:19–39.
173. Beckner ME, Heffess CS, Oertel JE. Oxyphilic papillary thyroid carcinoma. Am J Clin Pathol 1995; 103:280–287.
174. Hill JH, Werkhaven JA, DeMay RM. Hürthle cell variant of papillary carcinoma of the thyroid gland. Otolaryngol Head Neck Surg 1988; 98:338–341.
175. Berho M, Suster S. The oncocytic variant of papillary carcinoma of the thyroid. A clinicopathologic study of 15 cases. Hum Pathol 1997; 28:47–53.
176. Barbuto D, Carcangiu ML, Rosai J. Papillary Hürthle cell neoplasms of the thyroid gland: A study of 20 cases (abstract). Lab Invest 1990; 62:7A.
177. Wu P-C, Hay ID, Herrmann MA et al. Papillary thyroid carcinoma (PTC), oxyphilic cell type: A tumor misclassified by the World Health Organization (WHO)? Clinical Research 39, 279A. 1991.
178. Apel RL, Asa SL, LiVolsi VA. Papillary Hürthle cell carcinoma with lymphocytic stroma. "Warthin-like tumor" of the thyroid. Am J Surg Pathol 1995; 19:810–814.
179. Grant CS, Barr D, Goellner JR, Hay ID. Benign Hürthle cell tumors of the thyroid: A diagnosis to be trusted? World J Surg 1988; 12:488–495.
180. Cheung CC, Ezzat S, Ramyar L, Freeman JL, Asa SL. Molecular basis of Hurthle cell papillary thyroid carcinoma. J Clin Endocrinol Metab 2000; 85(2):878–882.
181. Chiappetta G, Toti P, Cetta F et al. The RET/PTC oncogene is frequently activated in oncocytic thyroid tumors (Hurthle cell adenomas and carcinomas), but not in oncocytic hyperplastic lesions. J Clin Endocrinol Metab 2002; 87(1):364–369.
182. Belchetz G, Cheung CC, Freeman J, Rosen IB, Witterick IJ, Asa SL. Hurthle cell tumors: using molecular techniques to define a novel classification system. Arch Otolaryngol Head Neck Surg 2002; 128(3):237–240.
183. Volpé R. Lymphocytic (Hashimoto's) thyroiditis. In: Werner SC, Ingbar SC, editors. The Thyroid. New York: Harper and Row, 1978: 996–1008.
184. Jansson R, Karlsson A, Forsum U. Intrathyroidal HLA-DR expression and T lymphocyte phenotypes in Graves' thyrotoxicosis, Hashimoto's thyroiditis and nodular colloid goitre. Clin Exp Immunol 1984; 58:264–272.
185. Asa SL. The pathology of autoimmune endocrine disorders. In: Kovacs K, Asa SL, editors. Functional Endocrine Pathology. Boston: Blackwell Scientific Publications, 1991: 961–978.
186. Dube VE, Joyce GT. Extreme squamous metaplasia in Hashimoto's thyroiditis. Cancer 1971; 27:434–437.
187. Katzmann JA, Vickery AL. The fibrosing variant of Hashimoto's thyroiditis. Hum Pathol 1974; 5:161–170.
188. Wirtschafter A, Schmidt R, Rosen D et al. Expression of the RET/PTC fusion gene as a marker for papillary carcinoma in Hashimoto's thyroiditis. Laryngoscope 1997; 107:95–100.
189. Carcangiu ML, Zampi G, Rosai J. Poorly differentiated ("insular") thyroid carcinoma. A reinterpretation of Langhans' "wuchernde Struma". Am J Surg Pathol 1984; 8:655–668.
190. Sakamoto A, Kasai N, Sugano H. Poorly differentiated carcinoma of the thyroid. A clinicopathologic entity for a high-risk group of papillary and follicular carcinomas. Cancer 1983; 52:1849–1855.
191. Papotti M, Botto Micca F, Favero A, Palestini N, Bussolati G. Poorly differentiated thyroid carcinomas with primordial cell component. A group of aggressive lesions sharing insular, trabecular, and solid patterns. Am J Surg Pathol 1993; 17:291–301.
192. Samaan NA, Ordoñez NG. Uncommon types of thyroid cancer. Endocrinol Metab Clin North Am 1990; 19:637–648.
193. Aldinger KA, Samaan NA, Ibanez M, Hill CS, Jr. Anaplastic carcinoma of the thyroid. A review of 84 cases of spindle and giant cell carcinoma of the thyroid. Cancer 1978; 41:2267–2275.

194. Venkatesh YSS, Ordoñez NG, Schultz PN, Hickey RC, Goepfert H, Samaan NA. Anaplastic carcinoma of the thyroid. A clinicopathologic study of 121 cases. Cancer 1990; 66:321–330.
195. Shvero J, Gal R, Avidor I, Hadar T, Kessler E. Anaplastic thyroid carcinoma. A clinical, histologic, and immunohistochemical study. Cancer 1988; 62:319–325.
196. Gaffey MJ, Lack EE, Christ ML, Weiss LM. Anaplastic thyroid carcinoma with osteoclast-like giant cells. A clinicopathologic, immunohistochemical, and ultrastructural study. Am J Surg Pathol 1991; 15:160–168.
197. Ordóñez NG, El-Naggar AK, Hickey RC, Samaan NA. Anaplastic thyroid carcinoma. Immunocytochemical study of 32 cases. Am J Clin Pathol 1991; 96:15–24.
198. Carcangiu ML, Steeper T, Zampi G, Rosai J. Anaplastic thyroid carcinoma. A study of 70 cases. Am J Clin Pathol 1985; 83:135–158.
199. Hurlimann J, Gardiol D, Scazziga B. Immunohistology of anaplastic thyroid carcinoma. A study of 43 cases. Histopathology 1987; 11:567–580.
200. LiVolsi VA, Brooks JJ, Arendash-Durand B. Anaplastic thyroid tumors. Immunohistology. Am J Clin Pathol 1987; 87:434–442.
201. Pilotti S, Collini P, Del Bo R, Cattoretti G, Pierotti MA, Rilke F. A novel panel of antibodies that segregates immunocytochemically poorly differentiated carcinoma from undifferentiated carcinoma of the thyroid gland. Am J Surg Pathol 1994; 18:1054–1064.
202. Fagin JA. Genetic basis of endocrine disease 3. Molecular defects in thyroid gland neoplasia. J Clin Endocrinol Metab 1992; 75:1398–1400.
203. Farid NR, Shi Y, Zou M. Molecular basis of thyroid cancer. Endocr Rev 1994; 15:202–232.
204. Fagin JA, Matsuo K, Karmakar A, Chen DL, Tang S-H, Koeffler HP. High prevalence of mutations of the p53 gene in poorly differentiated human thyroid carcinomas. J Clin Invest 1993; 91:179–184.
205. Donghi R, Longoni A, Pilotti S, Michieli P, Della Porta G, Piarotti MA. Gene p53 mutations are restricted to poorly differentiated and undifferentiated carcinomas of the thyroid gland. J Clin Invest 1993; 91:1753–1760.
206. Nakamura T, Yana I, Kobayashi T et al. p53 gene mutations associated with anaplastic transformation of human thyroid carcinomas. Jpn J Cancer Res 1992; 83:1293–1298.
207. Ito T, Seyama T, Mizuno T et al. Unique association of p53 mutations with undifferentiated but not with differentiated carcinomas of the thyroid gland. Cancer Res 1992; 52:1369–1371.
208. Wyllie FS, Lemoine NR, Williams ED, Wynford-Thomas D. Structure and expression of nuclear oncogenes in multi-stage thyroid tumorigenesis. Br J Cancer 1989; 60:561–565.
209. Hosal SA, Apel RL, Freeman JL et al. Immunohistochemical localization of p53 in human thyroid neoplasms: correlation with biological behavior. Endocr Pathol 1997; 8:21–28.
210. Jossart GH, Epstein HD, Shaver JK et al. Immunocytochemical detection of p53 in human thyroid carcinomas is associated with mutation and immortalization of cell lines. J Clin Endocrinol Metab 1996; 81:3498–3504.
211. Gaal JM, Horvath E, Kovacs K. Ultrastructure of two cases of anaplastic giant cell tumor of the human thyroid gland. Cancer 1975; 35:1273–1279.
212. Jao W, Gould VE. Ultrastructure of anaplastic (spindle and giant cell) carcinoma of the thyroid. Cancer 1975; 35:1280–1292.
213. Asa SL, Dardick I, Van Nostrand AWP, Bailey DJ, Gullane PJ. Primary thyroid thymoma: a distinct clinicopathologic entity. Hum Pathol 1988; 19:1463–1467.
214. Chan JKC, Rosai J. Tumors of the neck showing thymic or related branchial pouch differentiation: A unifying concept. Hum Pathol 1991; 22:349–367.
215. Nishiyama RH, Dunn EL, Thompson NW. Anaplastic spindle-cell and giant-cell tumors of the thyroid gland. Cancer 1972; 30:113–127.
216. Spires JR, Schwartz MR, Miller RH. Anaplastic thyroid carcinoma. Association with differentiated thyroid cancer. Arch Otolaryngol Head Neck Surg 1988; 114:40–44.
217. van der Laan BFAM, Freeman JL, Tsang RW, Asa SL. The association of well-differentiated thyroid carcinoma with insular or anaplastic thyroid carcinoma: Evidence for dedifferentiation in tumor progression. Endocr Pathol 1993; 4:215–221.
218. Bronner MP, LiVolsi VA. Spindle cell squamous carcinoma of the thyroid: An unusual anaplastic tumor associated with tall cell papillary cancer. Mod Pathol 1991; 4:637–643.
219. Yoshida A, Kamma H, Asaga T et al. Proliferative activity in thyroid tumors. Cancer 1992; 69:2548–2552.
220. Kapp DS, LiVolsi VA, Sanders MM. Anaplastic carcinoma following well-differentiated thyroid cancer: Etiological considerations. Yale J Biol Med 1982; 5:521–528.

221. Uribe M, Fenoglio-Preiser CM, Grimes M, Feind C. Medullary carcinoma of the thyroid gland. Clinical, pathological, and immunohistochemical features with review of the literature. Am J Surg Pathol 1985; 9:577–594.
222. Valenta LJ, Michel-Bechet M, Mattson JC, Singer FR. Microfollicular thyroid carcinoma with amyloid rich stroma, resembling the medullary carcinoma of the thyroid (MCT). Cancer 1977; 39:1573–1586.
223. Harach HR, Williams ED. Glandular (tubular and follicular) variants of medullary carcinoma of the thyroid. Histopathology 1983; 7:83–97.
224. Nelkin BD, de Bustros AC, Mabry M, Baylin SB. The molecular biology of medullary thyroid carcinoma. A model for cancer development and progression. JAMA 1989; 261:3130–3135.
225. Mendelsohn G, Wells SA, Baylin SB. Relationship of tissue carcinoembryonic antigen and calcitonin to tumor virulence in medullary thyroid carcinoma. An immunohistochemical study in early, localized and virulent disseminated stages of disease. Cancer 1984; 54:657–662.
226. Schröder S, Klöppel G. Carcinoembryonic antigen and nonspecific cross-reacting antigen in thyroid cancer. An immunocytochemical study using polyclonal and monoclonal antibodies. Am J Surg Pathol 1987; 11:100–108.
227. Williams ED, Morales AM, Horn RC. Thyroid carcinoma and Cushing's syndrome. A report of two cases with a review of the common features of the non-endocrine tumours associated with Cushing's syndrome. J Clin Pathol 1968; 21:129–135.
228. Birkenhäger JC, Upton GV, Seldenrath HJ, Kreiger DT, Tashjian AHJr. Medullary thyroid carcinoma: ectopic production of peptides with ACTH-like, corticotrophin releasing factor-like and prolactin production-stimulating activities. Acta Endocrinol (Copen) 1976; 83:280–292.
229. Goltzman D, Huang S-N, Browne C, Solomon S. Adrenocorticotropin and calcitonin in medullary thyroid carcinoma: frequency of occurrence and localization in the same cell type by immunohistochemistry. J Clin Endocrinol Metab 1979; 49:364–369.
230. Takami H, Bessho T, Kameya T et al. Immunohistochemical study of medullary thyroid carcinoma: Relationship of clinical features to prognostic factors in 36 patients. World J Surg 1988; 12:572–579.
231. Reubi JC, Chayvialle JA, Franc B, Cohen R, Calmettes C, Modigliani E. Somatostatin receptors and somatostatin content in medullary thyroid carcinomas. Lab Invest 1991; 64:567–573.
232. Lamberts SWJ, Bakker WH, Reubi JC, Krenning EP. Somatostatin-receptor imaging in the localization of endocrine tumors. N Engl J Med 1990; 323:1246–1249.
233. Lamberts SWJ, Krenning EP, Reubi JC. The role of somatostatin and its analogs in the diagnosis and treatment of tumors. Endocr Rev 1991; 12:450.
234. Schimke RN, Hartmann WH. Familial amyloid-producing medullary thyroid carcinoma and pheochromocytoma: A distinct genetic entity. Ann Intern Med 1965; 63:1027–1037.
235. Goodfellow PJ. Mapping the inherited defects associated with multiple endocrine neoplasia type 2A, multiple endocrine neoplasia type 2B, and familial medullary thyroid carcinoma to chromosome 10 by linkage analysis. Endocrinol Metab Clin North Am 1994; 23:177–185.
236. Carson NL, Wu J, Jackson CE, Kidd KK, Simpson NE. The mutation for medullary thyroid carcinoma with parathyroid neoplasia (mTC with PTs) is closely linked to the centromeric region of chromosome 10. Am J Hum Genet 1990; 47:946–951.
237. Nelkin BD, Nakamura N, White RW et al. Low incidence of loss of chromosome 10 in sporadic and hereditary human medullary thyroid carcinoma. Cancer Res 1989; 49:4114–4119.
238. Mulligan LM, Kwok JBJ, Healey CS et al. Germ-line mutations of the *RET* proto-oncogene in multiple endocrine neoplasia type 2A. Nature 1993; 363:458–460.
239. Hofstra RMW, Landsvater RM, Ceccherini I et al. A mutation in the RET proto oncogene associated with multiple endocrine neoplasia type 2B and sporadic medullary thyroid carcinoma. Nature 1994; 367:375–376.
240. Marsh DJ, Robinson BG, Andrew S et al. A rapid screening method for the detection of mutations in the RET proto-oncogene in multiple endocrine neoplasia type 2A and familial medullary thyroid carcinoma families. Genomics 1994; 23:477–479.
241. Brandi ML, Gagel RF, Angeli A et al. Guidelines for diagnosis and therapy of MEN type 1 and type 2. J Clin Endocrinol Metab 2001; 86(12):5658–5671.
242. Santoro M, Rosati R, Grieco M et al. The *ret* proto-oncogene is consistently expressed in human pheochromocytomas and thyroid medullary carcinomas. Oncogene 1990; 5:1595–1598.
243. Zedenius J, Larsson C, Bergholm U et al. Mutations of codon 918 in the RET proto-oncogene correlate to poor prognosis in sporadic medullary thyroid carcinomas. J Clin Endocrinol Metab 1995; 80:3088–3090.

244. Moley JF, Brother MB, Wells SA, Spengler BA, Biedler JL, Brodeur GM. Low frequency of *ras* gene mutations in neuroblastomas, pheochromocytomas, and medullary thyroid cancers. Cancer Res 1991; 51:1596–1599.
245. Yang KP, Castillo SG, Nguyen CV. C-myc, N-ras, c-erb B: lack of amplification or rearrangement in human medullary thyroid carcinoma and a derivative cell line. Anticancer Res 1990; 10:189–192.
246. Yana I, Nakamura T, Shin E. Inactivation of the p53 gene is not required for tumorigenesis of medullary thyroid carcinoma or pheochromocytoma. Jpn J Cancer Res 1992; 83:1113–1116.
247. Wolfe HJ, Melvin KEW, Cervi-Skinner SJ. C-cell hyperplasia preceding medullary thyroid carcinoma. N Engl J Med 1973; 289:437–441.
248. DeLellis RA, Wolfe HJ. The pathobiology of the human calcitonin (C)-cell: a review. Pathol Annu 1981; 16:25–52.
249. Albores-Saavedra J, Monforte H, Nadji M, Morales AR. C-cell hyperplasia in thyroid tissue adjacent to follicular cell tumors. Hum Pathol 1988; 19:795–799.
250. Biddinger PW, Brennan MF, Rosen PP. Symptomatic C-cell hyperplasia associated with chronic lymphocytic thyroiditis. Am J Surg Pathol 1991; 15:599–604.
251. Scopsi L, Di Palma S, Ferrari C, Holst JJ, Rehfeld JF, Rilke F. C-cell hyperplasia accompanying thyroid diseases other than medullary carcinoma: an immunocytochemical study by means of antibodies to calcitonin and somatostatin. Mod Pathol 1991; 4:297–304.
252. Libbey NP, Nowakowski KJ, Tucci JR. C-cell hyperplasia of the thyroid in a patient with goitrous hypothyroidism and Hashimoto's thyroiditis. Am J Surg Pathol 1989; 13:71–77.
253. LiVolsi VA. Mixed Thyroid Carcinoma: A real entity? Lab Invest 1987; 57:237–239.
254. Holm R, Sobrinho-Simoes M, Nesland JM, Johannessen J-V. Concurrent production of calcitonin and thyroglobulin by the same neoplastic cells. Ultrastruct Pathol 1986; 10:241–248.
255. Holm R, Sobrinho-Simoes M, Nesland JM, Sambade C, Johannessen J-V. Medullary thyroid carcinoma with thyroglobulin immunoreactivity. A special entity? Lab Invest 1987; 57:258–268.
256. Apel RL, Alpert LC, Rizzo A, LiVolsi VA, Asa SL. A metastasizing composite carcinoma of the thyroid with distinct medullary and papillary components. Arch Pathol Lab Med 1994; 118:1143–1147.
257. González-Cámpora R, Lopez-Garrido J, Martin-Lacave I, Miralles-Sánchez EJ, Villar JL. Concurrence of a symptomatic encapsulated follicular carcinoma, an occult papillary carcinoma and a medullary carcinoma in the same patient. Histopathology 1992; 21:380–382.
258. Pastolero GC, Coire CI, Asa SL. Concurrent medullary and papillary carcinomas of thyroid with lymph node metastases. Am J Surg Pathol 1996; 20:245–250.

3. THYROID LYMPHOMAS

RUNJAN CHETTY, MB BCH, FRCPATH, FRCPA, FRCPC, DPHIL (OXON)
Department of Laboratory Medicine and Pathobiology,
University of Toronto,
University Health Network/Toronto Medical Laboratories,
Toronto, Canada

INTRODUCTION AND HISTORICAL ASPECTS

Primary thyroid lymphomas have been recognised for many years and have been documented from the 1940s and 1950s. It was deemed to be important to recognise this entity "for it seems that about a third of the cases may be treated successfully with X-rays, followed by maintained thyroid medication" (1). Thus, the importance of separating lymphomas from its mimics, namely, chronic thyroiditis and small cell carcinoma, was evident at an early stage because of the therapeutic implications. Indeed, the histological difficulty in separating lymphoma from chronic thyroiditis and small cell carcinoma, no doubt led to the under-diagnosis of lymphoma. Even 50 years and more ago, certain peculiarities of thyroid lymphoma were apparent to pathologists: the predilection for elderly women, long survival and the tendency for similar lesions to occur in the gastrointestinal tract. These lymphomas were so characteristic that Brewer and Orr coined the term "struma reticulosa" to describe them (2). The fact that primary and secondary lymphomas could occur in the thyroid was accepted and sporadic papers on the subject, including the occasional large review, appeared in the literature (3). It was not until the early 1980s that primary lymphomas of the thyroid gland came under scrutiny again and was the centre of intense research. The introduction of the mucosa associated lymphoid tissue (MALT) concept led to the critical examination of primary thyroid lymphomas and similar appearing lymphomas with the seminal work of Isaacson and Wright responsible for the crystallization and clarification of the pathogenesis and morphology of these lymphomas (4–6). It is now clear that MALT and lymphomas arising from these sites share morphological, immunophenotypic and molecular features to the extent that MALT-lymphomas can metastasize from one MALT site to another.

INCIDENCE

Lymphomas occurring primarily in the thyroid are decidedly uncommon, accounting for about 5% of all thyroid malignancies (7–10). This figures increases to 10% of thyroid malignancies in certain geographic locales where antecedent chronic thyroiditis is common (10, 11). Primary thyroid lymphomas constitute 2.5 to 7% of all extranodal lymphomas (12–14).

It is stated that 25 to 100% of thyroid lymphomas arise against a background of thyroiditis, either chronic lymphocytic or Hashimoto's thyroiditis (15–18). This association is so strong that the relative risk of a patient with chronic thyroiditis developing lymphoma of the thyroid is 40 to 80 times greater than the general population (14, 19, 20). The lymphomas evolve after a prolonged period, usually 20 to 30 years after the onset of chronic lymphocytic thyroiditis (14).

CLINICAL PRESENTATION

Women are more frequently affected than men with a ratio of 2.5 to 8.4: 1. Most patients are in the 50 to 80 year age range. There is usually rapid enlargement of an already existing goitre, and the mass may extend extra-thyroidally. The rapid growth and extent of invasion may result in dysphagia, hoarseness and dyspnoea (3, 16, 21). Thyroid function is usually normal but hypothyroidism has been documented in a minority of cases (11, 22). If hypothyroidism is present, it is usually due to the preexisting thyroiditis and not due to the obliteration of thyroid parenchyma by the lymphomatous infiltrate. Very rare cases of hyperthyroidism have been encountered where rapid destruction of thyroid follicles with release of colloid and thyroid hormone into the circulation, have been implicated as causative (23, 24).

NOMENCLATURE AND TERMINOLOGY

In the last 10 or so years lymphoma classification has undergone a major revision with the appearance of the Revised European-American Lymphoma (REAL) classification (25–27) and the subsequent World Health Organization (WHO) update, refinement and minor modification of the REAL classification (28–34). After Isaacson and Wright brought the concept of MALT and lymphomas arising therefrom to prominence, the terms MALT lymphoma or lymphoma arising in MALT or "MALT-oma" have been used. The advent of the REAL/WHO classifications led to a re-appraisal, and these peculiar and characteristic lymphomas were categorized as: extra-nodal marginal zone B-cell lymphomas (MZBL) of MALT-type. This is the prototype lymphoma occurring primarily in the thyroid. Variants and other common related lymphomas will be discussed.

TYPES OF PRIMARY THYROID LYMPHOMA

As mentioned above the most morphologically distinctive and recognizable (but not necessarily the commonest variant encountered) primary lymphoma is MZBL of

Table 1. Staging of primary thyroid lymphomas

Stage IE: Primary thyroid lymphoma (PTL) with or without perithyroidal soft tissue extension,
Stage IIE: PTLs with involvement of lymph nodes on the same side of the diaphragm,
Stage IIIE: PTLs with involvement of lymph nodes on both sides of the diaphragm,
Stage IV E: PTLs with dissemination to other extranodal sites.

MALT type. Others seen include: MZBL of MALT type with large cell (blastic) transformation (mixed MZBL and diffuse large B cell lymphoma [DLBCL]), DLBCL without MZBL and a miscellaneous, heterogenous group usually consisting of single case reports of a wide variety of lymphomas that can occur in lymph nodes and any other extranodal site. These include: Hodgkin's disease, follicular lymphoma, intravascular lymphomatosis, anaplastic large cell lymphoma and T-cell lymphomas (35–42). These will not be dealt with, as their occurrence in the thyroid is the same as any other extra-nodal site or lymph node for that matter.

The high-grade lesions: mixed MZBL/DLBCL and DLBCL without MZBL are the commonest histological types of primary thyroid lymphoma that are encountered (36, 42).

STAGING

The recommended staging system is Musshoff's modification of the Ann Arbor staging system (36). See Table 1. Over 90% of patients present as stages IE or IIE.

PATHOLOGY

Gross pathology

Enlargement of the thyroid gland, either rapidly or slowly, is the commonest gross manifestation (Figure 1). This is often accompanied by extrathyroidal extension into surrounding soft tissue and skeletal muscle. The lymphomatous gland varies in its naked eye appearance: fleshy, tan, white, grey or red with a fish-flesh appearance, firm or soft, multinodular, lobulated or with diffuse deposits, solid or cystic. The cut surface may be smooth, bulging or lobular. Foci of hemorrhage and necrosis may be present imparting a mottled or variegated appearance to the cut surface. Lymphomatous involvement of the gland ranges from 0.5 to 19.5 cm (36). Uninvolved thyroid tissue, if present, may show the macroscopic features of the associated lymphocytic thyroiditis: beige in color with fibrosis and lobular accentuation. Obviously, none of these gross features are specific to lymphoma of the thyroid gland.

LIGHT MICROSCOPY

MZBL of MALT type

This type of lymphoma is probably the most histologically distinct and recognizable of all the primary thyroid lymphomas. The constituent cells are slightly larger than centrocytes and are called "centrocyte-like" cells in view of this resemblance. These cells have condensed chromatin, slightly irregular nuclear contours but are rarely, if ever, cleaved (Figure 2). The centrocyte-like cells have a propensity for permeating thyroid follicle epithelial cells giving rise to the histological hallmark of MALT lymphomas,

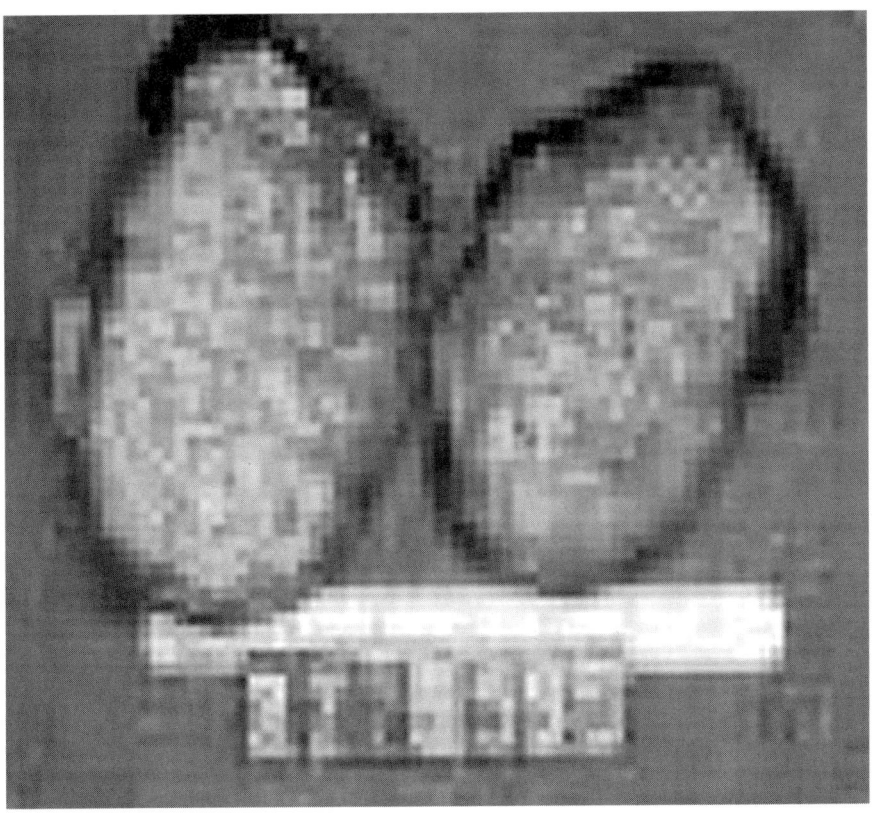

Figure 1. Gross illustration of a thyroid gland infiltrated by a lymphoma: enlarged, fleshy gland that is tan coloured.

the so-called "lymphoepithelial lesion" (Figures 3 & 4). Not only are the centrocyte-like cells seen insinuating between thyroid follicle cells but they are also found in between thyroid follicles within the stroma. The thyroid follicles bearing lymphoepithelial lesions vary in appearance from being relatively intact (Figure 5) to showing marked atrophy and destruction (Figure 6). In the more severe lymphoepithelial lesions, the follicles are markedly attenuated and may not be seen on H&E sections. Tombstones or the occasional residual epithelial cell may only be visible with a cytokeratin stain as a remnant of a previous follicle (Figure 5). Sometimes the centrocyte-like cells traverse the thyroid follicle cells and come to occupy the centres of the follicles displacing/kern-1ptreplacing the colloid, so-called "stuffed follicles" or what Derringer and colleagues have dubbed, "MALT balls" (36) (Figure 7). Other cellular components that are present in MZBL of MALT type include: plasma cells, mature, round, slightly elongated or lymphoplasmacytoid lymphocytes, monocytoid B-lymphocytes and centroblastic appearing cells (Figure 8). Indeed, the occasional eosinophil and histiocyte

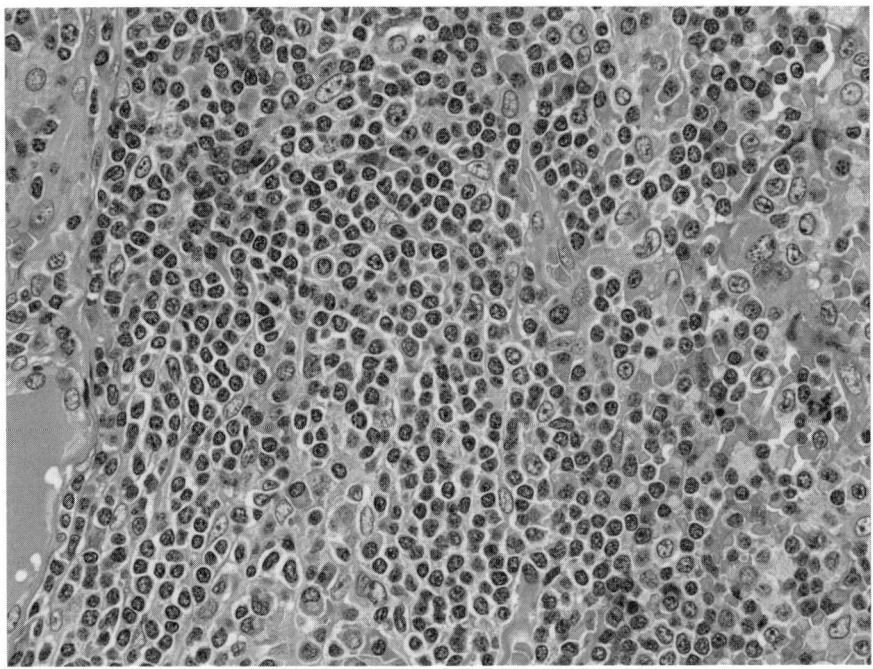

Figure 2. Centrocyte-like cells are the dominant cell type in MZBL of MALT-type. They are slightly larger than mature centrocytes and have a slightly irregular, but not cleaved, nuclear contour.

may also be present. The infiltrate between thyroid follicles is typically heterogenous and the centrocyte-like cells almost exclusively participate and form lymphoepithelial lesions. However, plasma cells can form a major component of the infiltrate and can in some instances be the dominant cell type. The plasma cells are mainly mature in morphology although bi-nucleate forms and those harboring Russell and Dutcher bodies have been encountered. The plasma cells rarely, if ever, permeate the thyroid follicle epithelium and tend to have a para-follicular distribution (Figure 9). This may be so marked in some instances that there almost appears to be a "compartmentalization" of the plasma cells away from the centrocyte-like cells and they appear as a separate infiltrate. In general, they are admixed together. The monocytoid B-cell component, made up of uniform small to intermediate cells with characteristic abundant eosinophilic to clear cytoplasm, occurs in clusters of varying size. Centroblastic cells, larger cells with vesicular chromatin and prominent nucleoli, are found scattered in amongst the other cellular constituents (Figure 10). They are not the dominant cell type nor do they form cohesive aggregates in MZBL of MALT type.

Reactive lymphoid follicles are also a common feature in this type of lymphoma (Figure 11). These are found within the neoplastic infiltrate and are not related to the associated lymphocytic thyroiditis. The follicles warrant careful examination to separate

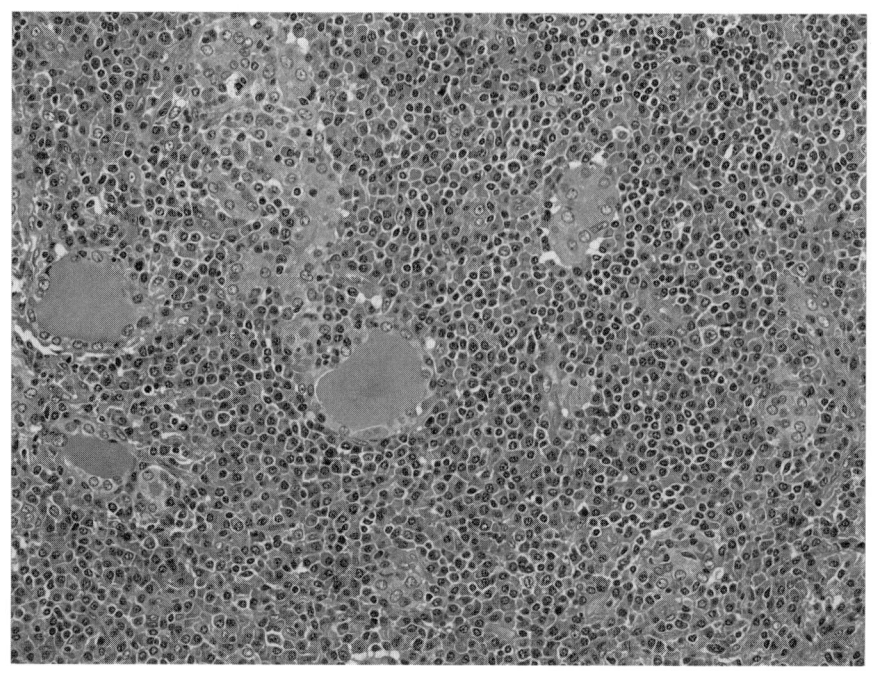

Figure 3. The centrocytes-like cells home into the thyroid follicles, traverse the epithelial cells and form lymphoepithelial lesions.

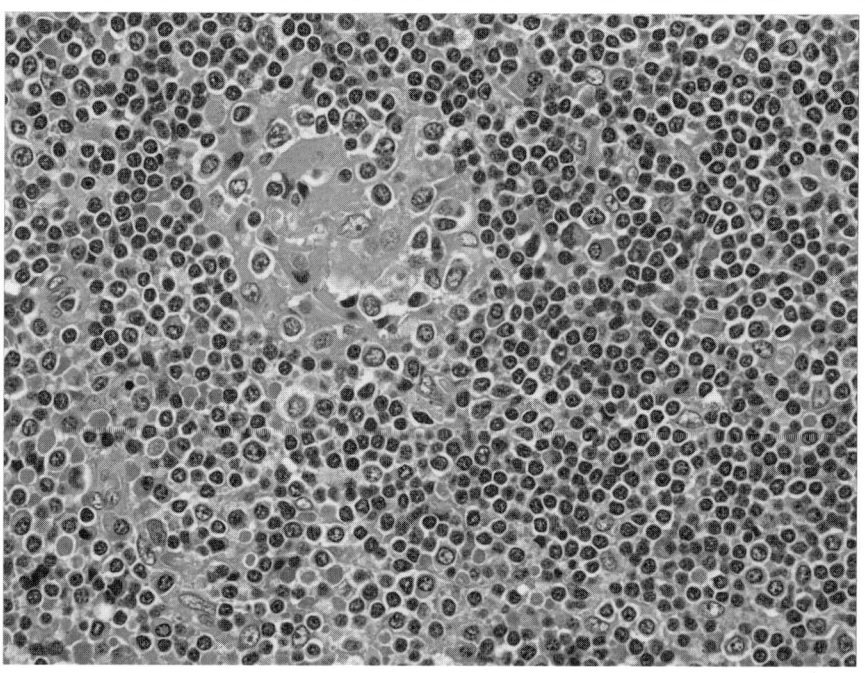

Figure 4. Under higher magnification, the centrocyte-like insinuate between and through the thyroid follicle cells with resultant disruption and destruction of the follicle.

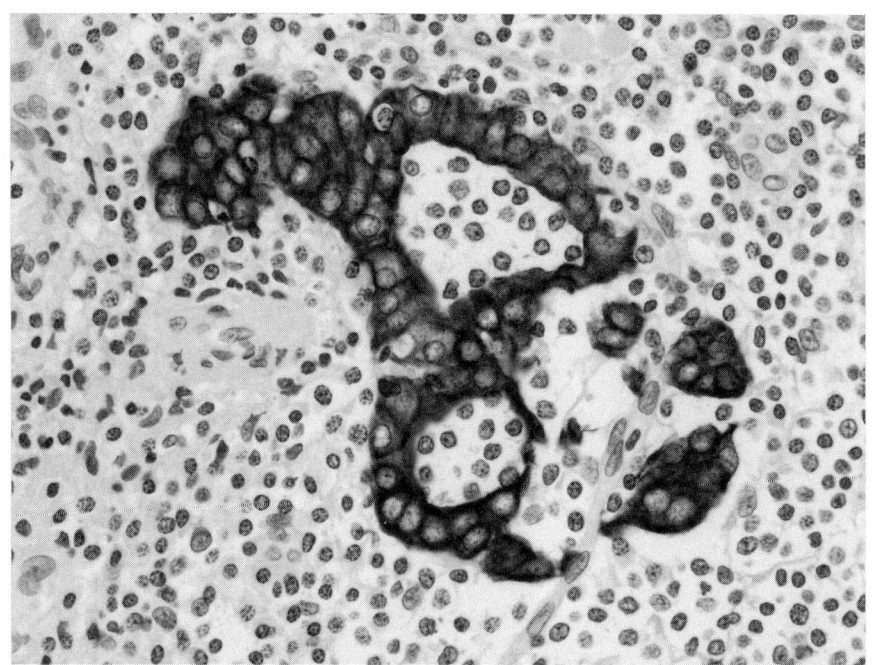

Figure 5. A cytokeratin stain highlights a relatively intact follicle that nonetheless is permeated by centrocyte-like cells, some of which are present within the follicle lumen.

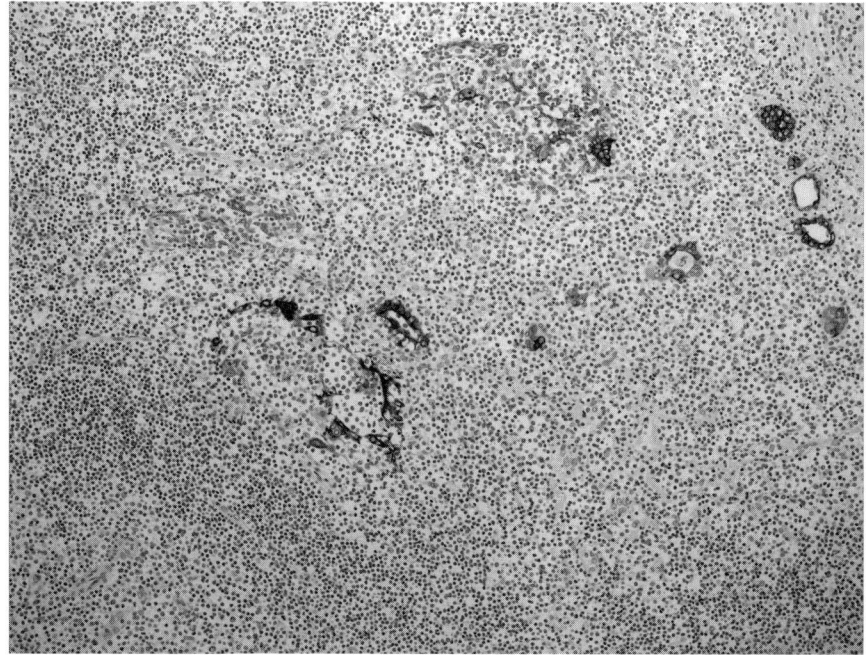

Figure 6. More destructive lymphoepithelial lesions with only remnants of thyroid follicle left. A cytokeratin stain is useful in showing residual epithelial cells within the dense lymphoid infiltrate.

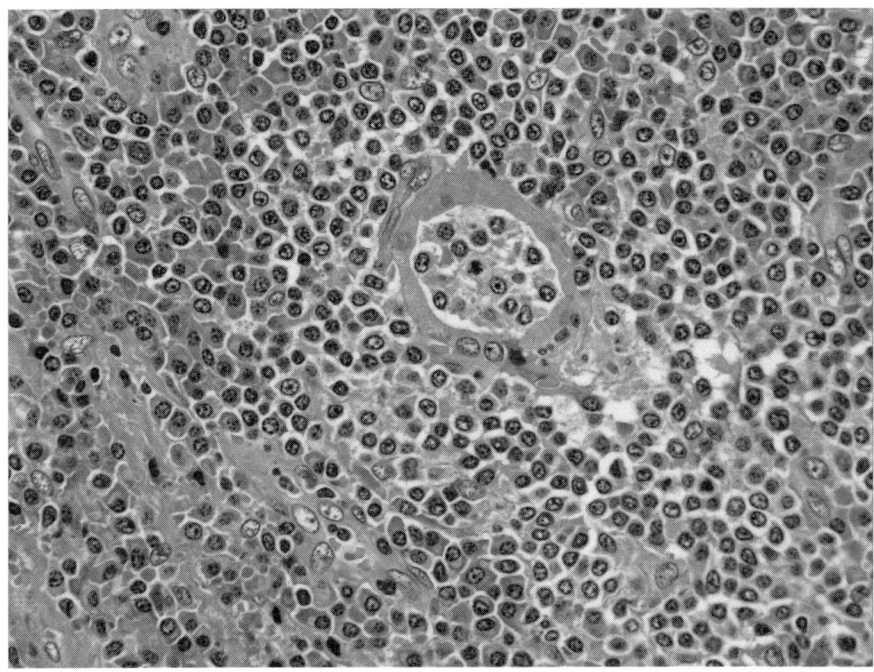

Figure 7. So-called "MALT ball" or "stuffed follicle" where the neoplastic cells reside within the lumen of the thyroid follicle.

truly reactive germinal centers from so-called "follicular colonization". In this phenomenon the centrocyte-like cells home into the germinal centers of lymphoid follicles both in the thyroid gland and draining lymph nodes. The centrocyte-like cells displace the usual cells of the germinal center and this often imparts a nodular or follicular appearance to the neoplastic infiltrate. Morphologically the possibility of follicular lymphoma needs to be separated from a MZBL of MALT type with follicular colonization.

MZBL OF MALT TYPE WITH LARGE CELL TRANSFORMATION (MIXED MZBL AND DIFFUSE LARGE CELL B-CELL LYMPHOMA [DLBCL])

For categorization as MZBL of MALT-type with large cell transformation, areas of typical MZBL of MALT-type, as described above must be histologically evident. This type of primary thyroid lymphoma accounted for just under 50% of all cases in one series (36). The presence of either MZBL of MALT-type with a component of large, blastic lymphoma cells warrants a diagnosis of mixed MZBL and DLBCL. How much large cell or high-grade lymphoma has to be present to make a diagnosis? Whilst this has not been quantified widely, but general principles suggest that confluent clusters, aggregates or sheets of large cells indicate a significant component and hence designation as MZBL of MALT-type with large cell transformation. Usually an obvious cluster

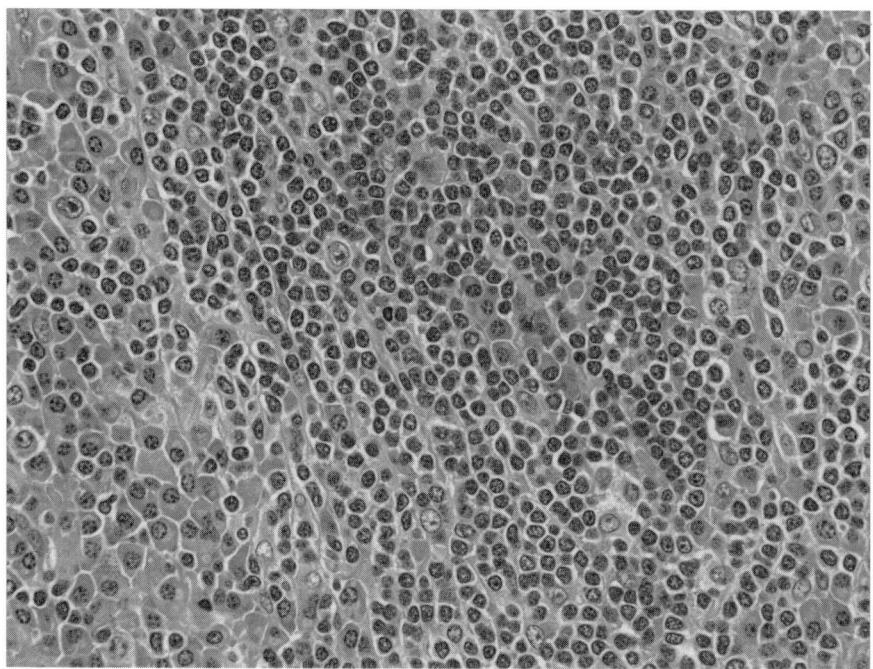

Figure 8. Other cellular components of MALT-lymphoma include plasma cells, larger centroblastic cells and occasional histiocytes. These are admixed with centrocyte-like cells in MZBL of MALT-type.

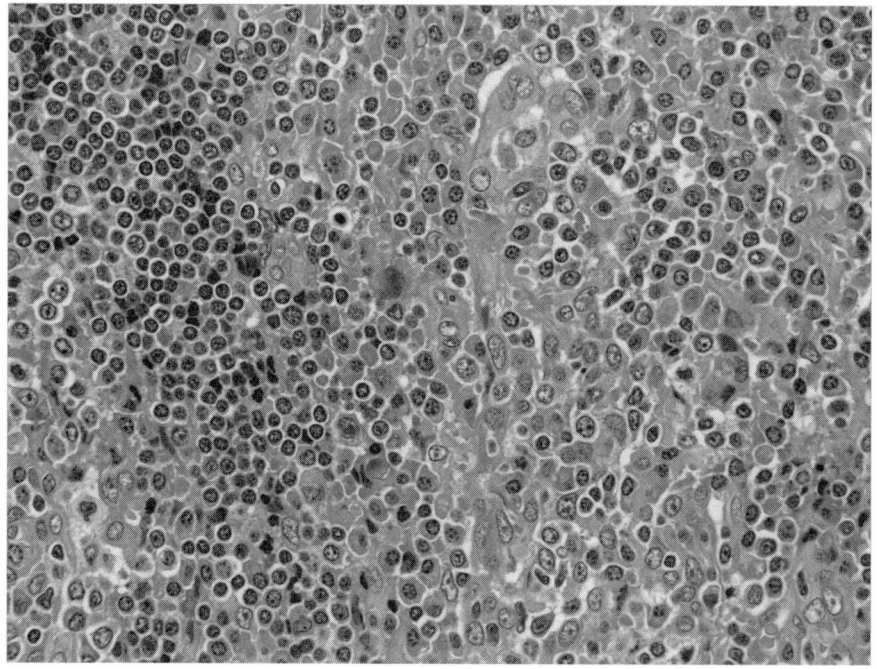

Figure 9. The plasma cell component can be seen to localize around the follicle epithelium: a para-follicular location.

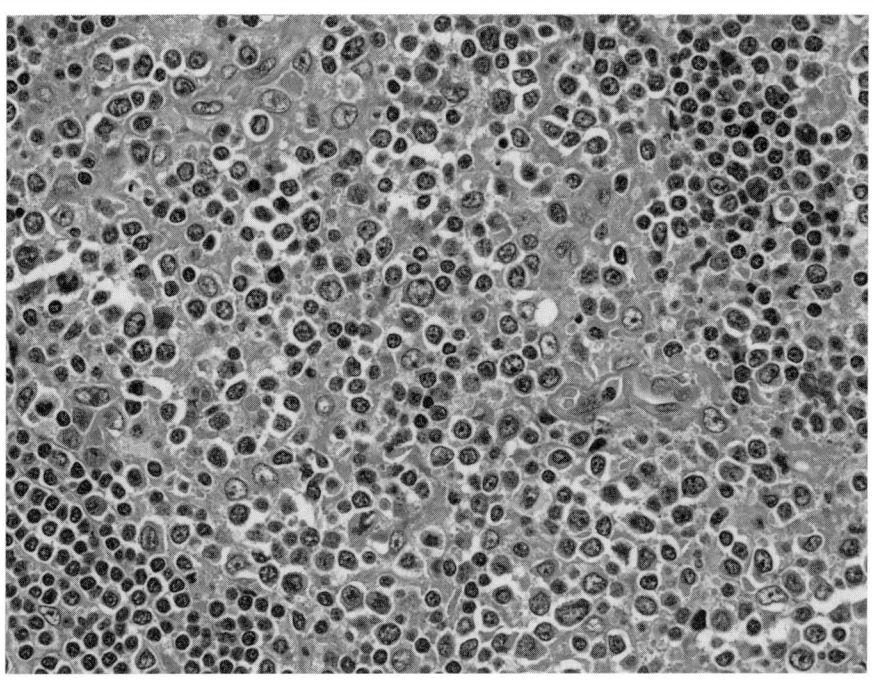

Figure 10. A cluster of centroblastic cells making this a mixed MZBL of MALT-type and DLBCL.

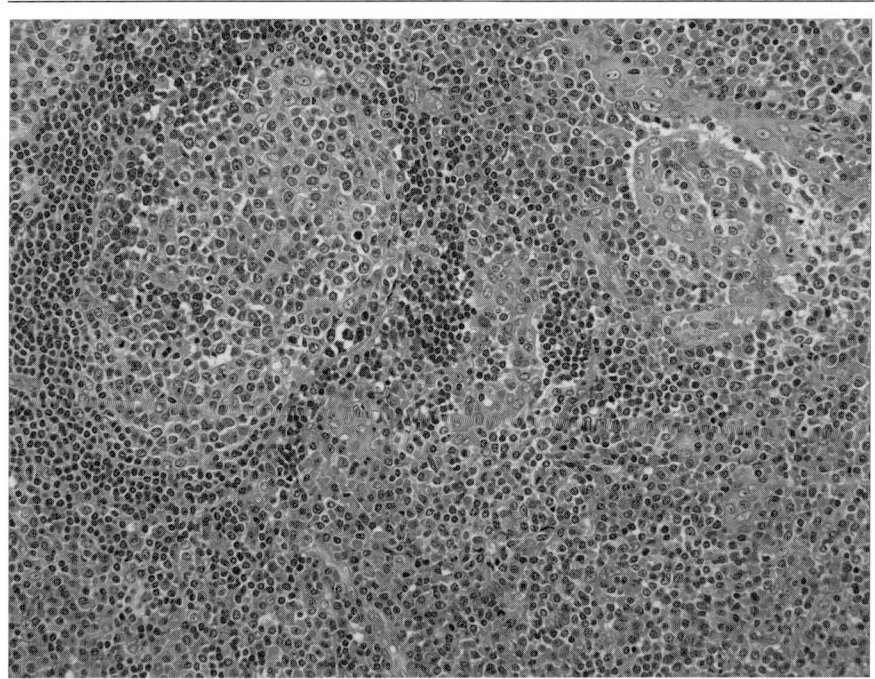

Figure 11. A reactive lymphoid follicle replete with germinal centre and mantle zone, in a MZBL of MALT-type.

or sheet or multiple areas of blast cells are encountered. In the study by Derringer and colleagues the DLBCL component accounted for at least 50% of the lymphoma (36). Thus, it would appear that the large cell component is obvious and easily discerned. The large cells may resemble centroblasts (large cells with vesicular chromatin and a small typically single nucleolus) usually, or even immunoblasts (large cells with vesicular chromatin and a prominent nucleolus) less commonly. In the series reported by Derringer et al, they even noted scattered Reed-Sternberg-like cells and cells reminiscent of the large cells seen in Burkitt's like lymphoma (36). The large cells may permeate diffusely through the thyroid with destruction of thyroid follicular epithelium or may also result in lymphoepithelial lesions (Figure 12). However, a distinct low-grade MZBL component must also be present for this lymphoma to be considered a mixed pattern.

DIFFUSE LARGE B-CELL LYMPHOMA (DLBCL) WITHOUT MZBL OF MALT-TYPE

As the name implies a histologically detectable MZBL of MALT-type as described above is not present. In a study by Skacel and colleagues, they encountered 16 cases of DLBCL without any MZBL but containing lymphoepithelial lesions composed only of large cells. These cases are more appropriately categorized as DLBCL without MZBL of MALT-type because of the absence of the latter component. Even in the absence of a low-grade component, the vast majority (85%) of DLBCL do show some of the morphological features associated with MALT-lymphoma: lymphoepithelial lesions, plasma cells, follicle colonization and monocytoid B-cells are detected although varying in number from case to case (36). In the absence of the MALT-lymphoma morphology, it is impossible to separate primary thyroid DLBCL from secondary involvement of the gland by a nodal primary. Careful examination of several sections may be required to find the morphological features of a MALT-lymphoma in an otherwise pervasive large cell infiltrate of the thyroid. The large cells of DLBCL are identical to the large cells described above.

IMMUNOHISTOCHEMISTRY

The use of immunohistochemistry in thyroid lymphomas is somewhat limited in that there isn't a characteristic or diagnostic immunoprofile. The application of LCA and cytokeratins as a first line investigation usually accomplishes the separation of lymphoma from carcinoma. MZBL of MALT-type, MZBL with blasts and DLBCL are all B-cell lymphomas and will stain positively with traditional B-cell markers (CD20, CD79a). The reactive T-cells decorate with CD3, while light chain restriction in plasma cells, which is seen in about 20% of cases, can be demonstrated with kappa and lambda stains. In some instances light chain restriction (cytoplasmic and membrane staining) can be demonstrated in the neoplastic lymphoid cells too. The neoplastic centrocyte-like cells of MALT origin are usually: CD5, CD10, CD23, cyclin D1 and IgD negative and positive for IgM. This immunophenotype reflects their origin from marginal zone B-cells in sites of chronic organ-specific inflammation caused by autoimmune disease or a specific inflammatory lesion (43–45). The use of bcl-2 immunostaining will also assist in excluding follicular lymphoma from reactive lymphoid follicles. In must be borne in

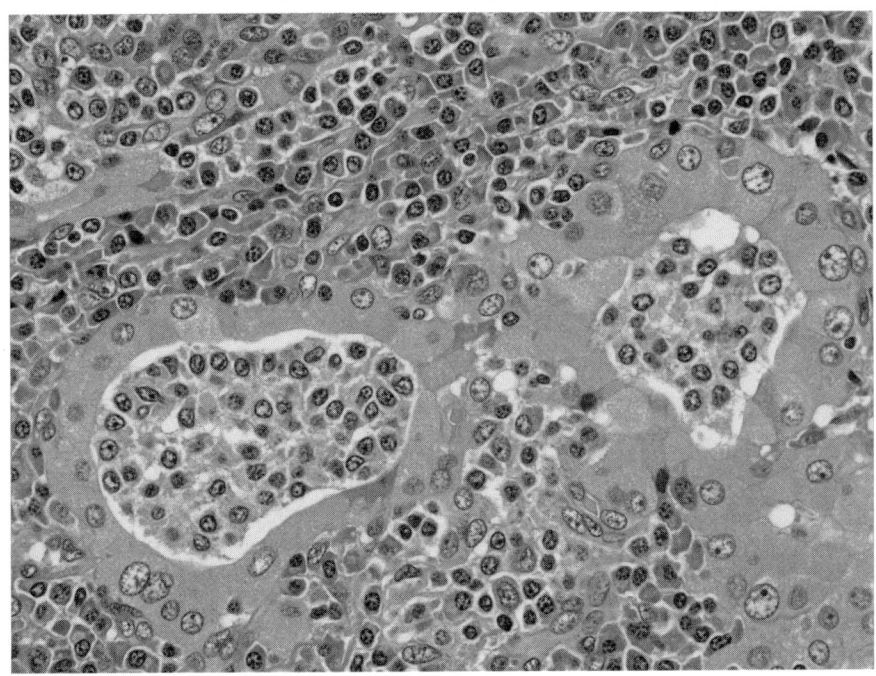

Figure 12. A MZBL of MALT-type with high-grade transformation. Here large cells have formed a lymphoepithelial lesion and occupy a thyroid follicle lumen (MALT-ball).

mind that the centrocyte-like cells in lymphoepithelial lesions and colonized follicles may also express bcl-2 protein (46, 47). Bcl-2 immunoexpression does not separate MZBL of MALT-type from Hashimoto's thyroiditis, as the centrocyte-like cells can be positive in both conditions. However, high-grade lesions lose bcl-2 immunoexpression with an accompanying increase in p53 protein expression (47).

Cytokeratin stains obviously also highlight the thyroid follicle epithelium and the degree of destruction caused by lymphoepithelial lesions. Cytokeratin staining is useful in the DLBCL cases in showing the remnants of epithelium and hence a morphological features of a MALT-lymphoma. Obviously, more directed lymphoid markers could be employed if wanting to exclude or confirm the various other types of lymphoma that may occur primarily in the thyroid gland.

CYTOGENETICS/MOLECULAR BIOLOGY

As with immunohistochemistry, there is no single cytogenetic or molecular aberration that typifies MALT-lymphomas. Within the remit of MALT-lymphomas some similar genetic findings have been noted irrespective of site, however, gastric MALT-lymphomas have been more intensively examined and have chromosomal abnormalities that tend to be commoner at this site than other MALT sites. There are some repetitive abnormalities, however. Trisomy 3 has been identified in approximately 60% of

MALT-lymphomas (48). The t (1;14) translocation involving the *bcl-10* gene, which then undergoes further mutations has been identified in 6–8% of MALT-lymphomas, especially those showing large cell transformation (49). The t (11;18) (q21;q21) translocation, leading to fusion of the *apoptosis inhibitor-2* gene and the MALT lymphoma associated translocation (*MALT1*) gene, has been found in 18–35% of MALT-lymphomas but mainly those occurring in the gastrointestinal tract and are rarely encountered in thyroid MALT-lymphomas (50). Similarly, the t(14;18)(q32;q21) translocation tends not to be present in thyroid MALT-lymphomas (50). It is clear that no single chromosomal abnormality occurs in thyroid MALT-lymphomas and that some translocations within the MALT-lymphoma group are site-specific. It is thought that the various translocations and other cytogenetic abnormalities render the lymphoid tissue unstable and permissive for the process of lymphomagenesis.

RELATIONSHIP BETWEEN LOW- AND HIGH-GRADE MALT-LYMPHOMAS

The coexistence of low- and high-grade MALT-lymphoma suggests either a pathogenetic link between the two components, or that they represent two independent *de novo* clones. The weight of evidence points to a close relationship between the low- and high-grade foci: often there is a transition noted microscopically, both immunohistochemical and molecular studies substantiate commonality and transformation of low-grade to high-grade lymphoma, and the clinical presentation of a sudden and/or rapid increase in size of an already enlarged thyroid gland (51–55). Peng and colleagues performed PCR and mutational analyses to identify clone-specific rearranged immunoglobulin heavy chain gene sequences (55). The PCR products from both the low- and high-grade foci were identical in size and direct sequencing revealed common clone-specific immunoglobulin heavy chain gene rearrangements (55).

DIFFERENTIAL DIAGNOSIS

Anaplastic (small cell) carcinoma

This type of carcinoma is likely to simulate high-grade lymphoma. Attention to the cohesive growth pattern, stromal sclerosis/desmoplasia, absence of MALT-lymphoma morphological features, especially the admixture of plasma cells, should alert one to the possibility of carcinoma. Confirmation is readily achieved by the use of epithelial immunohistochemical markers.

HASHIMOTO'S THYROIDITIS

It is important to note that similar cellular constituents (centrocyte-like and plasma cells) together with lymphoepithelial lesions are encountered in Hashimoto's thyroiditis. Hence, florid cases can be exceptionally difficult to separate from MZBL of MALT-type. It has been suggested that a dense lymphoid infiltrate with fewer intervening reactive lymphoid follicles, broad bands of centrocyte-like or clear cells and large number of lymphoepithelial lesions that diffusely efface the thyroid parenchyma, favour a diagnosis of lymphoma. In the histologically suspicious cases, the demonstration of sheets of B-cells, light chain restriction and heavy chain gene rearrangement are ancillary features that will help in confirming the diagnosis of lymphoma. The clinical picture of sudden or rapid enlargement of the thyroid in a patient previously diagnosed as having Hashimoto's thyroiditis will also be useful. At the end of the day, there are going to be some cases (hopefully a very small number!) that clinical information, light microscopy, immunohistochemistry and molecular techniques will not be able to separate. When unsure, the possibility of lymphoma should be raised and careful follow-up of the patient should be recommended.

PROGNOSTIC FACTORS AND OUTCOME

Several prognostic factors have been advanced as indicators of poor outcome: stage greater than IE, diffuse large cell lymphoma histology, rapid clinical growth, abundant apoptosis, vascular invasion, high mitotic rate, perithyroidal extension and compressive clinical symptoms (36). The most important prognostic factor, however, is stage and this generally is in concert with the histological appearance, with MZBL of MALT-type being a low-grade lesion that is low stage with a very good prognosis and long survival.

Therapy is usually in the form of debulking surgery or combined adjuvant chemotherapy.

REFERENCES

1. Doniach I. The Thyroid Gland. In: Systemic Pathology, volume II. Eds: Wright GP, Symmers WStC. Longmans, Green and Co, London, 1966. Chapter 31, pp. 1095–1122.
2. Brewer DB, Orr JW. Thyroid lymphosarcoma. J Pathol Bacteriol 1953;65:193–5.
3. Compagno J, Oertel JE. Malignant lymphomas and other lymphoproliferative disorders of the thyroid gland. A clinicopathologic study of 245 cases. Am J Clin Pathol 1980;74:1–11.
4. Isaacson P, Wright DH. Malignant lymphoma of mucosa-associated lymphoid tissue. A distinctive type of B-cell lymphoma. Cancer 1983;52:1410–6.
5. Isaacson P, Wright DH. Extranodal malignant lymphoma arising from mucosa-associated lymphoid tissue. Cancer 1984;53:2315–24.
6. Anscombe AM, Wright DH. Primary malignant lymphoma of the thyroid – a tumour of mucosa-associated lymphoid tissue. Review of seventy-six cases. Histopathology 1985;9:81–97.
7. Staunton MD, Greening WP. Clinical diagnosis of thyroid cancer. Br Med J 1973;4:532–5.
8. Gospodarowicz MK, Sutcliffe SB. The extranodal lymphomas. Sem Rad Oncol 1995;5:281–300.
9. Fujimoto Y, Suzuki H, Abe K, Brooks JR. Autoantibodies in malignant lymphoma of the thyroid gland. N Engl J Med 1967;276:380–3.
10. Schwarze EW, Papadimitriou CS. Non-Hodgkin's lymphoma of the thyroid. Pathol Res Pract 1980;167;346–62.
11. Tennvall J, Cavallin-Stahl E, Akerman M. Primary localized non-Hodgkin's lymphoma of the thyroid: A retrospective clinicopathological review. Eur J Surg Oncol 1987;13:297–302.
12. Aozasa K, Tsujimoto M, Sakurai M, et al. Non-Hodgkin's lymphomas in Osaka, Japan. Eur J Cancer Clin Oncol 1985;21:487–92.
13. Freeman C, Berg JW, Cutler SJ. Occurrence and prognosis of extranodal lymphomas. Cancer 1972;29:252–60.
14. Pedersen RK, Pedersen NT. Primary non-Hodgkin's lymphoma of the thyroid gland: a population based study. Histopathology 1996;28:25–32.
15. Aozasa K, Inoue A, Tajima K, et al. Malignant lymphomas of the thyroid gland. Analysis of 79 patients with emphasis on histologic prognostic factors. Cancer 1986;58:100–4.
16. Cox MT. Malignant lymphoma of the thyroid. J Clin Pathol 1964;17:591–601.
17. Grimley RP, Oates GD. The natural history of malignant thyroid lymphoma. Br J Surg 1980;67:475–7.
18. Williams ED. Malignant lymphoma of the thyroid. Clin Endocrinol Metab 1981;10:379–89.

19. Holm LE, Blomgren H, Lowhagen T. cancer risks in patients with chronic lymphocytic thyroiditis. N Engl J Med 1985;312:601–4.
20. Kato I, Tajima K, Suchi T, et al. Chronic thyroiditis as a risk factor of B-cell lymphoma in the thyroid gland. Jpn J Cancer Res 1985;761085–90.
21. Sirota DK, Segal RL. Primary lymphomas of the thyroid gland. J Am Med Ass 1979;242:1743–6.
22. Oertel JE, Heffess CS. Lymphoma of the thyroid and related disorders. Semin Oncol 1987;14:333–42.
23. Garin LA. The diagnostic dilemmas of hyperthyroxinemia and hypothyroxinemia. Adv Intern Med 1988;33:380–3.
24. Jennings AS, Sabiri M. Thyroid lymphoma in a patient with hyperthyroidism. Am J Med 1984;76:551–2.
25. Harris NL, Jaffe ES, Stein H, et al. A revised European-American classification of lymphoid neoplasms: a proposal from the International Lymphoma Study Group. Blood 1994;84:1361–92.
26. Chan JK, Banks PM, Cleary ML, et al. A revised European-American classification of lymphoid neoplasms proposed by the Internation Lymphoma Study Group. A summary version. Am J Clin Pathol 1995;103:543–60.
27. Chan JK, Banks PM, Cleary ML, et al. A proposal for classification of lymphoid neoplasms (by the International Lymphoma Study Group). Histopathology 1994;25:517–36.
28. Harris NL, Jaffe ES, Diebold J, et al. The World Health Organization Classification of Neoplastic Diseases of the Hematopoietic and Lymphoid tissues: Report of the Clinical Advisory Committee Meeting—Airlie House, Virginia, November 1997. J Clin Oncol 1999;17:3835–49.
29. Harris NL, Jaffe ES, Diebold J, et al. The World Health Organization Classification of hematological malignancies report of the Clinical Advisory Committee Meeting – Airlie House, Virginia, November 1997. Mod Pathol 2000;13:193–207.
30. Harris NL, Jaffe ES, Diebold J, et al. The World Health Organization Classification of neoplastic diseases of the hematopoietic and lymphoid tissues. Report of the Clinical Advisory Committee Meeting – Airlie House, Virginia, November 1997. Ann Oncol 1999;10:1419–32.
31. Harris NL, Jaffe ES, Diebold J, et al. The World Health Organization Classification of neoplastic diseases of the hematopoietic and lymphoid tissues: Report of the Clinical Advisory Committee Meeting – Airlie House, Virginia, November 1997. Histopathology 2000;36:69–86.
32. Jaffe ES, Harris NL, Diebold J, Muller-Hermelink HK. WHO classification of lymphomas: a work in progress. Ann Oncol 1998;9:s25–30.
33. Jaffe ES, Harris NL, Diebold J, Muller-Hermelink HK. WHO classification of neoplastic diseases of the hematopoietic and lymphoid tissues. A progress report. Am J Clin Pathol 1999;111:s8–12.
34. Isaacson PG. The current status of lymphoma classification. Br J Haematol 2000;109:258–66.
35. Hardoff R, Bar-Shalom R, Dharan M, Luboshitsky R. Hodgkin's disease presenting as a solitary thyroid nodule. Clin Nucl Med 1995;20:37–41.
36. Derringer GA, Thompson LDR, Frommelt RA, et al. Malignant lymphoma off the thyroid gland. A clinicopathologic study of 108 cases. Am J Surg Pathol 2000;24:623–39.
37. Coltrera MD. Primary T-cell lymphoma of the thyroid. Head Neck 1999;21:160–3.
38. Abdul-Rahman ZH, Gogas HJ, et al. T-cell lymphoma in Hashimoto's thyroiditis. Histopathology 1996;29:455–9.
39. Yamaguchi M, Ohno T, Kita K. Gamma/delta T-cell lymphoma of the thyroid gland. N Engl J Med 1997;336:1391–2.
40. Shanks JH, Harris M, Howat AJ, et al. Angiotropic lymphoma with endocrine involvement. Histopathology 1997;31:161–6.
41. Isaacson PG. Lymphomas of mucosa-associated lymphoid tissue (MALT). Histopathology 1990;16:617–9.
42. Skacel M, Ross CW, Hsi ED. A reassessment of primary thyroid lymphoma: high-grade MALT-type lymphoma as a distinct subtype of diffuse large B-cell lymphoma. Histopathology 2000;37:10–18.
43. Nakamura S, Aoyagi K, Furuse M, et al. B cell monoclonality precedes the development of gastric MALT lymphoma in *Helicobacter pylori*-associated chronic gastritis. Am J Pathol 1998;152:1271–9.
44. Zucca E, Bertoni F, Roggero E, et al. Molecular analysis of the progression from *Helicobacter pylori*-associated chronic gastritis to mucosa-associated lymphoid-tissue lymphoma of the stomach. N Engl J Med 1998;338:804–10.
45. Nardini E, Rizzi S, Menard S, et al. Molecular phenotype distinguishes two subsets of gastric low-grade mucosa-associated lymphoid tissue lymphomas. Lab Invest 2002;82:535–41.
46. Chetty R, Gatter K. bcl-2 immunoexpression in MALT lymphomas. Hum Pathol 1996;27:1246–7.

47. Chetty R, O'Leary JJ, Biddolph SC, Gatter KC. Immunohistochemical detection of p53 and bcl-2 proteins in Hashimoto's thyroiditis and primary thyroid lymphomas. J Clin Pathol 1995;48:239–41.
48. Wotherspoon AC, Finn TM, Isaacson PG. Trisomy 3 in low-grade B-cell lymphomas of mucosa-associated lymphoid tissue. Blood 1995;85:2000–4.
49. Du MQ, Peng H, Liu H, et al. *BCL10* gene mutation in lymphoma. Blood 2000;95:3885–90.
50. Streubel B, Lamprecht A, Dierlamm J, et al. T(14;18)(q32;q21) involving *IGH* and *MALT1* is a frequent chromosomal aberration in MALT lymphoma. Blood 2002;101:2335–9.
51. Chan JK, Ng CS, Isaacson PG. Relationship between high-grade lymphoma and low-grade B-cell mucosa-associated lymphoid tissue lymphoma (MALToma) of the stomach. Am J Pathol 1990;136:1153–64.
52. Du M, Peng H, Singh N, et al. The accumulation of p53 abnormalities is associated with progression of mucosa-associated lymphoid tissue lymphoma. Blood 1995;86:4587–93
53. Hsi ED, Eisbruch A, Greenson JK, et al. Classification of primary gastric lymphomas according to histologic features. Am J Surg Pathol 1998;22:17–27.
54. Peng H, Chen G, Du M, et al. Replication error phenotype and p53 gene mutation in lymphomas of mucosa-associated lymphoid tissue. Am J Pathol 1996;148:643–8.
55. Peng H, Du M, Diss TC, et al. Genetic evidence for a clonal link between low and high-grade components in gastric MALT B-cell lymphoma. Histopathology 1997;30:425–9.

4. MOLECULAR EVENTS IN FOLLICULAR THYROID TUMORS

TODD G. KROLL, M.D., Ph.D.
*Departments of Pathology and Medicine, Endocrinology Division,
University of Chicago Pritzker School of Medicine, Chicago, IL 60637*

INTRODUCTION

The analyses of human thyroid tumor tissues have proven informative in identifying key molecular events in epithelial neoplasia. The thyroid gland gives rise to a variety of epithelial tumors that differ markedly in their biologic patterns. The accessibility of thyroid tumors provides a tractable opportunity to define mechanisms of epithelial cell transformation in a spectrum of related cancers.

Two primary issues must be considered when investigating molecular genetic alterations within human thyroid tumor groups. The first is tumor classification. Thyroid tumors are classified predominantly on the basis of morphologic features interpreted by pathologists. Morphologic features provide initial biologic and clinical information but they have been defined somewhat non-specifically in retrospective series. Thus, thyroid tumor diagnosis can be imprecise [1–4] and can create confusion when correlating molecular genetic alterations with clinical and pathologic features. Mutations that predominate in one thyroid tumor group may be identified in others and the distinction as to whether such tumors are misclassified or contain additional alterations is difficult to ascertain. A second important issue relates to mutation detection. Polymerase chain reaction-based amplification and sequencing of nucleic acids from fresh or fast-frozen tissues are most often employed. Such assays are exquisitely sensitive and prone to cross-contamination, particularly when poorly preserved or archival tissues are used. Polymerase chain reaction can even detect genetic alterations within a minute sub-fraction of tumor cells. The biologic significance of this is often unclear. Tissue

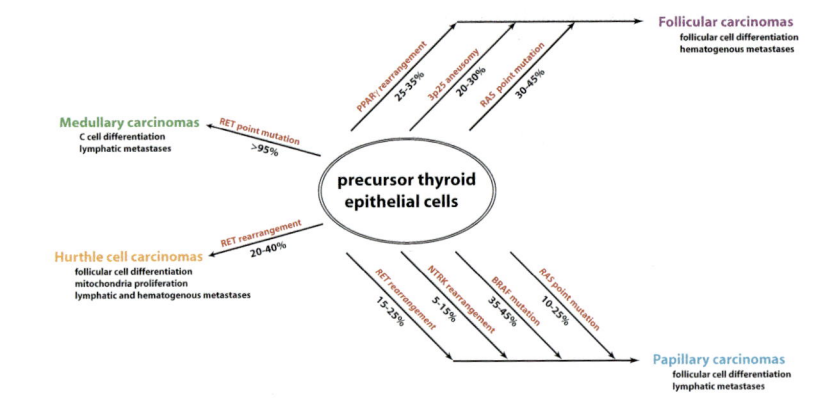

Figure 1. Histologic-Molecular Model of Thyroid Cancer Formation. Four main types of thyroid carcinoma with distinct biologic features are recognized. A subset of each type may progress to poorly differentiated and/or clinically aggressive forms. Genetic alterations that characterize these pathways and sub-pathways are shown.

composition must also be documented rigorously because thyroid tumor resections contain admixtures of tumor, normal thyroid, lymphoid, reactive and stromal elements. All such factors must be considered or erroneous results will be obtained [5–7].

This chapter begins with a histologic-molecular model of thyroid cancer formation and discusses known mutations and emerging biologic and clinical correlates in follicular thyroid tumors. A summary and comparison of thyroid carcinomas with the acute myeloid leukemias follows.

A histologic-molecular model of thyroid cancer

A model that encompasses histologic, molecular, and biologic facets of thyroid cancer formation is shown in Figure 1. At least four sub-types of thyroid cancer with distinct characteristics are recognized. Tumors within each group may progress to poorly differentiated, metastatic, and/or anaplastic forms. The thyroid carcinoma model seems unique relative to other carcinomas in several respects. First, distinct gene mutations define separate pathways of oncogenesis within the thyroid. This is different than a single linear genetic pathway envisioned commonly for other carcinomas such as those arising in the colon [8] and exocrine pancreas [9, 10]. Second, both thyroid specific and non-thyroid specific mutations characterize different thyroid carcinoma subgroups. One particularly interesting class of thyroid-specific mutations is the chromosomal rearrangements that encode gene fusions [11, 12]. Gene fusions been identified infrequently in carcinomas even though they are common in blood cell and soft connective tissue cancers [13]. Third, thyroid cancer mutations correlate with specific biologic properties. For example, *RET* and *PPARγ* rearrangements characterize papillary [14] and follicular [12] thyroid carcinomas that tend to spread via regional lymphatics or blood vessels, respectively. Distinct *RET* germ line point mutations identify different familial medullary thyroid carcinoma patients with propensities for poor outcome and/or concomitant non-thyroid disease [15]. Thus, mutation staus provides predictive biologic information in thyroid cancer and thus may augment our current morphology-based classification and treatment schemes. Even so, it must be kept in mind that a combination of cellular events, not single gene alterations, determines overall thyroid cancer biology. Thyroid tumors with apparently identical single gene mutations but distinct patterns of growth and/or prognoses have been reported [16–21].

PPARγ rearrangements

Somatic rearrangements in the gene encoding the nuclear receptor PPARγ have been identified in thyroid cancers with follicular cell differentiation, frequent encapsulation, vascular invasion and capsular penetration. These are follicular thyroid carcinomas (Figure 1). The discovery of PPARγ rearrangements resulted from mapping [12] of a chromosomal translocation, t(2;3)(q13;p25), which had been identified in follicular thyroid tumors [12, 22–27]. The t(2;3) rearrangement juxtaposes the promoter region and 5′ coding sequence of the PAX8 gene on chromosome 2 with most of the coding sequence of the PPARγ gene on chromosome 3 and results in expression of a chimeric PAX8-PPARγ transcription factor (Figure 2).

PAX8-PPARγ is a thyroid-specific mutation and one member of a family of PPARγ rearrangements in follicular carcinomas. Another follicular carcinoma translocation, t(3;7)(p25;q31) [28], fuses the promoter and 5′ coding sequence of a novel transcription factor gene termed CREB3L2 or BBF2H7 [29] on chromosome 7 with most of the coding sequence of PPARγ (Figure 2). PAX8-PPARγ and CREB3L2-PPARγ (Figure 2) contain identical PPARγ sequences that include wild-type PPARγ DNA binding, ligand binding, RXR dimerization, and transactivation domains [30]. Additional putative PPARγ rearrangements have been detected in other follicular carcinomas [12, 22, 31, 32].

PPARγ rearrangements have been identified in 25–35% of follicular carcinomas based on studies using pathologically well-defined tissues [32–38]. PPARγ rearrangements [32] or RAS gene point mutations but not both [33] are detected early in low stage follicular carcinomas, suggesting the existence of sub-pathways of oncogenesis in follicular carcinoma (Figure 1). Such a model is further supported by distinct patterns of galectin-3 and HBME-1 protein expression in PPARγ rearrangement- versus RAS mutation-positive follicular carcinomas [33] and by an additional genetic subset of follicular carcinomas (25%) that possess 3p25 aneusomy in the absence of PPARγ rearrangement [32].

The mechanisms through which PPARγ rearrangements deregulate thyrocyte growth are being investigated and aberrations in transcription (Figure 3) and other cell functions may be involved. PAX8-PPARγ stimulates proliferation, inhibits apoptosis, and induces anchorage independent growth of human thyroid cells [39], supporting a primary role for PAX8-PPARγ in follicular cell transformation. PAX8-PPARγ also transforms NIH3T3 mouse fibroblasts in colony assays [39], demonstrating that PAX8-PPARγ can alter both thyrocyte and non-thyrocyte growth functions. PAX8-PPARγ has little ability to stimulate transcription from PPARγ response elements *in vitro* and also inhibits transcription mediated by wild-type PPARγ [12, 39], activities that fit

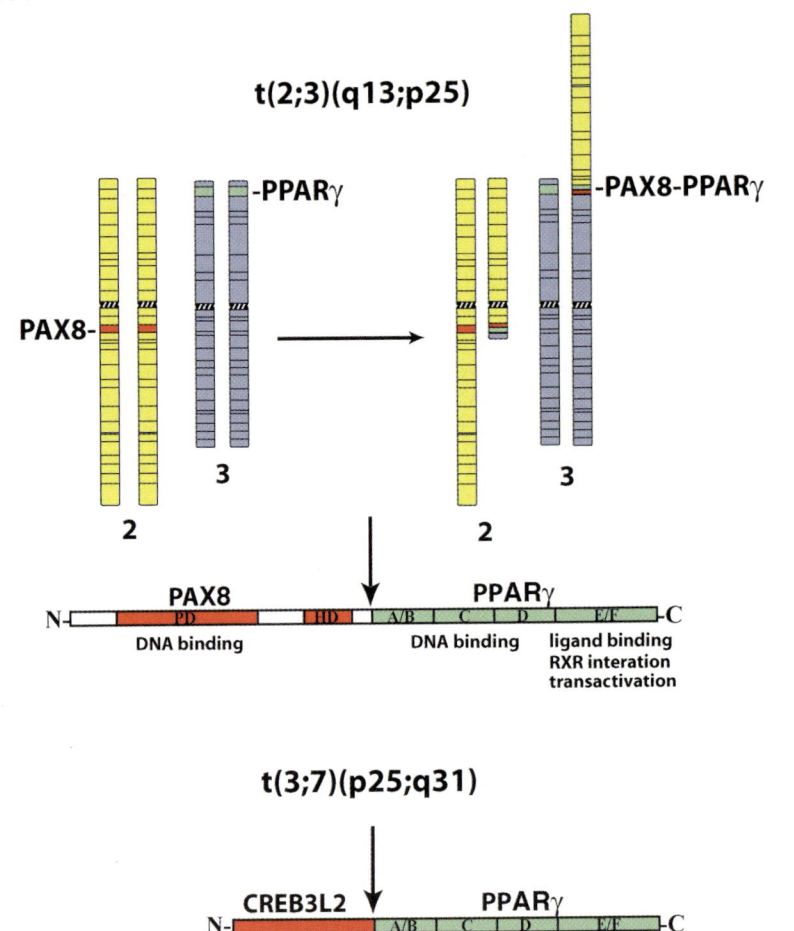

Figure 2. PPARγ Gene Rearrangements in Follicular Thyroid Carcinoma. The breakpoints of two chromosomal rearrangements, t(2;3)(q13;p25) and t(3;7)(p25;q31), have been cloned from human follicular thyroid carcinomas. Each rearrangement encodes a chimeric fusion protein that contains identical domains (A-E) of the PPARγ nuclear receptor.

well with the known tumor suppressor-like effects of wild-type PPARγ in a variety of epithelial cells [40–44]. In general, wild-type PPARγ stimulation inhibits thyroid cell growth [45, 46] and a reduction in PPARγ expression has also been noted in a significant subgroup of thyroid cancers without *PPARγ* rearrangement [32, 38]. The retinoblastoma tumor suppressor protein and cell cycle regulators may be involved [45, 47, 48].

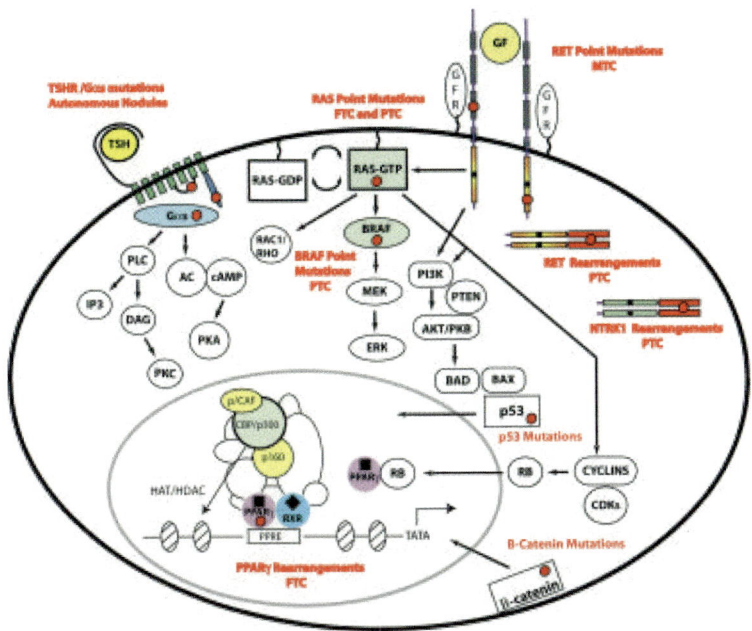

Figure 3. Molecular Pathways in Follicular Thyroid Tumors. Schematic representation of major molecular pathways involved in follicular thyroid tumors. Some, but not all, components and inter-connections of these pathways are indicated. Mutations are note in red and by red dots. Abbreviations: TSHR, thyroid stimulating hormone receptor; Gαs, guanine nucleotide stimulatory factor α; PLC, phospholipase C; IP3, inositol triphosphate; DAG, diacylglycerol; PKC, protein kinase C; AC, adenyl cyclase; cAMP, cyclic adenosine monophosphate; PKA, protein kinase A; RAC1/RHO, rac1/rho GTP binding proteins; GFR, growth factor receptor; GF, growth factor; RET, ret tyrosine receptor kinase; NTK1, ntrk1 tyrosine receptor kinase; GTP, guanine diphosphate; GTP, guanine triphosphate; RAS, ras GTP binding protein; BRAF, braf serine/threonine kinase; MEK, mitogen activated protein kinase kinase; ERK, extracellular signal regulated kinase (mitogen activated protein kinase); PI3K, phosphoinositol-3-kinase; PTEN, pten dual specificity phosphatase; AKT, akt serine/threonine kinase; PKB, protein kinase B; BAD and BAX, proapoptotic bcl-2 family members; p53, p53 tumor suppressor protein; RB, rb retinoblastoma tumor suppressor protein; CDKs, cyclin-dependent kinases; PPARγ, peroxisome proliferator-activated receptor γ; RXR, retinoid X receptor; p/CAF, CBP/p300, p160, nuclear receptor co-activators; HAT, histone acetyl transferase; HDAC, histone deacetylase complex. TATA, tata box.

Although inhibition of wild-type PPARγ by PAX8-PPARγ appears to be functionally important, the CREB3L2-PPARγ fusion protein appears to exhibit little inhibitory activity [30], suggesting that other mechanisms are also critical. PAX and CREB3L2 rearrangements have been noted in other cancers, supporting the idea that contributions of these domains in PAX8-PPARγ and CREB3L2-PPARγ are functionally important. For example, the *PAX3* and *PAX7* genes are rearranged in alveolar rhabdomyosarcoma [49–51] and *CREB3L2* is rearranged in fibromyxoid sarcoma [29]. Wild-type PAX8, a transcription factor required for normal thyroid follicular cell development [52], also possesses transforming activities *in vitro* [53].

Follicular adenomas with *PAX8-PPARγ* rearrangement have been identified at apparent lower frequency than in follicular carcinomas [33, 34, 36] and it seems most reasonable to consider these early (precursor/in situ) follicular carcinomas [32] unless genetic and/or clinical distinctions from the follicular carcinomas can be documented. *PPARγ* rearrangements are expected in at least some follicular adenomas because differential diagnosis of follicular adenomas from carcinomas is not precise. The possibility that *PPARγ* rearrangements mark a subset of follicular carcinomas, some even before histologic evidence of invasiveness is apparent, suggests that molecular analyses of fine needle aspiration biopsies may be useful to detect these follicular cancers [54]. However, the exact diagnostic utility of PPARγ rearrangements in diagnosis will not be clear until the biologic and molecular relatedness of follicular carcinomas and adenomas with *PPARγ* rearrangement is better defined. Papillary (follicular variant) and Hurthle cell carcinomas with *PPARγ* rearrangement have been observed infrequently [32, 34, 55], suggesting that these thyroid cancers arise via alternate transformation pathways (Figure 1).

Clinical and pathological characteristics of follicular carcinoma patients with *PPARγ* rearrangements have been examined. Follicular carcinomas with *PPARγ* rearrangement tend to have well-defined foci of vascular invasion and capsular penetration but not lymph node metastases [32, 33]. They also tend to present at younger patient age than follicular carcinomas without *PPARγ* rearrangement [32, 33] and progress and metastasize in some cases [23, 35]. Even so, few *PPARγ* rearrangements have been detected in anaplastic thyroid carcinomas [34, 35], which are highly aggressive cancers thought to arise from follicular and papillary carcinomas. Further studies are required to define the biologic characteristics and patterns of progression of follicular thyroid tumors with *PPARγ* rearrangement.

RET rearrangements

Somatic rearrangements in the gene encoding the *RET* receptor tyrosine kinase have been identified in a subset of thyroid cancers that exhibit follicular cell differentiation, characteristic papillary and/or nuclear morphologies, and a propensity for lymph node metastases. These are papillary thyroid carcinomas (Figure 1). Interestingly, the *RET* gene plays a fundamental role in multiple thyroid cancers. Whereas rearrangements of *RET* characterize papillary thyroid carcinomas [11, 14], germ-line *RET* point mutations characterize medullary thyroid carcinomas arising in the multiple endocrine neoplasia type 2 [56–59] and family medullary thyroid carcinoma syndromes. Thus, different *RET* mutations (rearrangements or point mutations) arising in different cellular contexts (follicular or C cell lineages) promote formation of different thyroid cancers (Figure 1). The *RET* rearrangements are discussed in detail in Chapter 12.

RET rearrangements in papillary carcinoma are thyroid-specific mutations and most often result from para-centric chromosomal inversions. For example, the *RET* gene at chromosome 10q11 is recombined frequently with other 10q loci such as *H4* in PTC1 [60] and *ELE1* in PTC3 [61, 62]. Several less frequent reciprocal translocations involving *RET* and other chromosomal loci have been described, particularly in papillary carcinoma patients exposed to radiation in the Chernobyl accident [63–65]. All known *RET* rearrangements result in expression of cytoplasmic, chimeric fusion proteins that contain the intracellular tyrosine kinase domain of RET fused to domains of non-RET (termed RET fusion genes or RFG) genes. The extracellular cadherin-like, cysteine-rich, and transmembrane domains of RET are not retained in the RFG-RET fusion proteins.

Experiments expressing RFG-RET fusion proteins in thyroid cell lines support a central role of the RAS-BRAF-MEK-ERK pathway in neoplastic transformation of follicular cells into papillary carcinomas (Figure 3). The RFG-RET fusion proteins stimulate follicular cell proliferation and inhibit differentiation [66–70]. Apoptosis may also be altered [71]. These biologic effects are mediated by ligand-independent dimerization [72, 73], cytoplasmic relocation [73], and constitutive activation of the RET tyrosine kinase. Adaptor molecules such as Shc, Frs2, Enigma, and Grb proteins interact with RET proteins [69, 74–78] and stimulate downstream RAS-BRAF-MAPK-ERK and other signal transduction pathways.

Transgenic mouse lines engineered to express RFG-RET fusion proteins in the thyroid document their ability to promote formation of papillary carcinoma-like tumors *in vivo* [79–82]. However, these transgenic lines do not all develop thyroid tumors with high penetrance or short latency and few, if any, develop tumors that metastasize without co-expression of additional mutations, arguing that multiple alterations are required for expression of the full papillary carcinoma phenotype [66, 67, 83].

RET rearrangements have been detected in 15–25% of papillary carcinomas and have been considered specific based on RTPCR and Southern blot experiments [70, 84–91]. *RET* rearrangements appear to arise early in papillary carcinoma because they are most common in low stage and the occult/micropapillary tumors [89, 92–94]. Papillary carcinomas with *RET* rearrangements may also present at younger patient age than papillary carcinomas without *RET* rearrangements [87, 95, 96], in a manner that resembles *PPARγ* rearrangements in follicular carcinoma. Other strong clinicopathologic correlates of *RET* rearrangement include classic papillary (not follicular variant) morphology [97, 98] and the presence of lymph node spread [86, 87, 96, 98]. The ELE1-RET (PTC3) fusion protein may be more frequent in the aggressive tall cell [17] and solid [16, 20] papillary carcinoma subtypes. A significant fraction of papillary carcinomas with *RET* alterations appear to progress to poorly differentiated thyroid carcinoma [99] but few *RET* rearrangements have been detected in anaplastic thyroid cancers [84, 89].

A few recent reports have noted *RET* rearrangements, somewhat unexpectedly, in benign and malignant Hurthle cell tumors [18, 19] and in thyroid hyalinizing trabecular adenomas [100, 101]. These Hurthle cell carcinomas with *RET* rearrangements appear to have increased tendency for lymphatic spread [102], supporting a biologic connection to papillary carcinoma as well. Thus, one intriguing possibility is that the Hurthle cell tumors with *RET* rearrangement are actually papillary carcinomas with additional morphologic and perhaps biologic features. An alternate possibility that must be excluded is that the *RET* rearrangements are present in a small fraction of the tumor cells because a only combined high cycle RTPCR and nucleotide probe hybridization have so far demonstrated their presence.

NTRK1 rearrangements

Somatic rearrangements in the gene encoding the *NTRK1* receptor tyrosine kinase have been identified in 5–15% of papillary thyroid carcinomas (Figure 1). These are discussed further in Chapter 12. In essence, *NTRK1* rearrangements bear strong resemblance to *RET* rearrangements in several respects. First, both NTRK1 and RET are receptors for neurotrophic ligands [103] and are not normally expressed in follicular epithelial cells. Second, both *NTRK1* and *RET* rearrangements were identified by transfection of papillary carcinoma DNA into NIH3T3 cells [11, 14, 85]. Third, both *NTRK1* and *RET* rearrangements arise frequently from subtle intra-chromosomal inversions. Fourth, both *NTRK1* and *RET* rearrangements lead to expression of fusion proteins with constitutive tyrosine kinase activation. For example, rearrangements at 1q21 often fuse the NTRK1 tyrosine kinase domain to other proteins such as *TPM* and *TPR* [104–106]. Fifth, both *NTRK1* and *RET* rearrangements may be more frequent in younger patients and in patients with lymph node metastases [95, 96, 107]. Last, the NTRK1 and RET fusion proteins activate related signal transduction pathways in thyroid follicular cells [66, 108–111] (Figure 3). Expression of the NTRK1 fusion proteins in the thyroid of transgenic mice leads to follicular hyperplasia- and papillary carcinoma-like proliferations [112].

RAS mutations

Somatic point mutations in *RAS* genes have been detected frequently in both nonthyroid [113] and thyroid (Figure 1) cancers. This contrasts the thyroid-specific gene rearrangements involving *PPARγ*, *RET*, and *NTRK1*. *RAS* mutations are most common in follicular versus papillary and Hurthle cell tumors [33, 91, 114–120] and have been detected in 20–50% of follicular adenomas and carcinomas [33, 91, 119–122]. The presence of *RAS* mutations in both follicular adenomas and carcinomas is consistent with a model in which many *RAS*-initiated follicular carcinomas develop from adenoma (morphologic) precursors. Experimental evidence supports this contention in that mutated RAS is insufficient to induce a fully transformed phenotype *in vitro* [66, 123–126] or follicular carcinoma *in vivo* [127, 128]. *N-RAS* mutations appear to predominate over *K-RAS* and *H-RAS* mutations in follicular thyroid tumors and mutations in codon 61 of *N-RAS* may be the most prevalent [33, 119, 120, 129]. The possibilities that *K-RAS* mutations are more frequent in papillary compared to follicular thyroid tumors [114, 115, 130], radiation-associated carcinomas [114], and/or aggressive thyroid cancers [130] require further investigation, particularly in view of the primary role of *K-RAS* mutations in pancreatic ductal carcinomas [10, 131] that are highly aggressive.

Recent studies have correlated the clinical and pathologic features with *RAS* mutation status. Thyroid carcinoma patients with *RAS* mutations may present at older age and with larger tumors [33] and may more frequently have less differentiated, high stage cancers [130, 132–134]. Careful pathologic evaluation of classic from follicular variant papillary carcinomas has noted another potentially interesting pattern. Follicular variants seem to contain more *N-RAS* (75%) and *H-RAS* (25%) mutations and few if any *RET* rearrangements, whereas classic papillary carcinomas seem to contain more *RET* rearrangements (30–35%) and few if any *RAS* mutations [98]. Follicular variants papillary carcinomas also had statistically lower rates of lymph node metastases and higher rates of tumor encapsulation and vascular invasion (follicular carcinoma-like features) compared to classic papillary carcinomas [98]. Thus, the existence of a morphologic and molecular "hybrid" thyroid cancer with some features of papillary and follicular carcinoma needs to be further explored.

Mouse modeling experiments have documented that *RAS* mutations are important role in tumorigenesis and tumor maintenance[128, 131, 135, 136] and RAS proteins transduce multiple stimuli from the thyroid follicular cell surface (Figure 3) as discussed further in Chapter 7.

BRAF mutations

Somatic point mutations in the *BRAF* gene have been identified recently in thyroid and other cancers [137]. *BRAF* encodes a serine/threonine kinase downstream of RAS and it transduces signals from multiple stimuli (Figure 3). A mutation that alters valine 599 to glutamic acid (V599E) in the BRAF kinase domain has been identified in 35–45% of papillary thyroid carcinomas [70, 90, 91, 120, 138–140] and in some undifferentiated/anaplastic thyroid carcinomas [90, 138]. *BRAF* mutations have been detected in few other benign or malignant thyroid tumors [70, 90, 91] and seem not to co-exist with *RAS* point mutations or *RET* rearrangements [70, 91, 138], thereby defining an additional sub-pathway in papillary carcinoma (Figure 1).

Papillary thyroid carcinoma patients with *BRAF* mutations tend to present at older age [90], at higher stage [90, 138], and with more frequent distant metastases compared to papillary carcinoma patients without *BRAF* mutation. Thus, mutated *BRAF* may define an aggressive papillary carcinoma form. In agreement with this possibility, mutated BRAF exhibits enhanced kinase activity and increased transformation efficiency compared to wild-type BRAF *in vitro* [137].

Thyroid stimulating hormone receptor and G protein mutations

Iodide uptake and thyroid hormone biosynthesis and metabolism are coordinately regulated with proliferation in thyroid follicular epithelial cells. These differentiated thyroid functions are controlled by the thyroid stimulating hormone receptor (TSHR) and its downstream signaling molecules (Figure 3) such as cyclic AMP and phospholipase C [141–143]. Somatic mutations in molecular components of the TSHR pathway have been detected in 60% or more of benign TSH-independent (autonomous/hyperfunctioning) thyroid nodules. The remaining 40% of autonomous nodules are postulated to contain undefined alterations in the same TSHR system [144]. Approximately 90% of mutations involve TSHR, often in the third intracellular loop or transmembrane regions of this seven-spanning membrane receptor [145, 146]. 5–10% of the mutations involve the G protein subunit Gsα/gsp activated by TSHR ligands [147]. Thus, constitutive stimulation of the TSHR pathway underlies most autonomous thyroid tumors [148].

Autonomous thyroid tumors usually exhibit hyperplastic morphology and transgenic mice and other animal models with an activated TSHR-Gsα/gsp-cAMP axis [149, 150] develop follicular hyperplasia and hyper-functioning thyroid tumors, supporting a fundamental role of the TSHR system. Furthermore, nodular hyperthyroidism in nonautoimmune autosomal dominant hyperthyroidism [151] and the McCune-Albright Syndrome [152] have been associated with germ-line mutations in TSHR-Gsα/gsp axis. Although chronic stimulation of the TSHR pathway promotes formation of benign thyroid nodules, this seems to provide little increased risk of thyroid cancer. Additional cellular alterations [153], potentially including the down-regulation of PPARγ[154], are apparently required.

B-catenin and p53 mutations

Stage at presentation is a key prognostic factor in thyroid carcinoma. Mutations in the genes encoding B-*catenin*, a component of the Wnt signaling pathway [155], and *p53*, an important tumor suppressor and a sensor of genome stability, have been identified most often in advanced stage thyroid cancer. Mutations in exon 3 of B-*catenin* have been detected in 25–60% of poorly differentiated and anaplastic thyroid carcinomas [156, 157], and the expression of B-*catenin* protein is often reduced or re-localized from the plasma membrane to the cytoplasm and nucleus in these [156–158] and some follicular and papillary [157–160] thyroid carcinomas. p53 mutations have been identified mostly in poorly differentiated and anaplastic thyroid carcinomas [161–164] and they appear to interfere with differentiated functions in thyroid cells [165, 166] and promote thyroid cancer invasion and metastases in transgenic mouse models [83, 167]. The p53 pathways are discussed in detail in Chapter 8.

Aneuploidy and other chromosomal aberrations

A low level of chromosomal instability is observed in benign thyroid tumors and well-differentiated thyroid cancers such as papillary carcinoma, a moderate level of chromosomal instability is observed in follicular carcinoma, and higher levels of chromosomal instability are observed in Hurthle cell, poorly differentiated/anaplastic, and metastatic carcinomas. Thus, increased chromosomal instability and aneuploidy correlate generally with increased thyroid cancer aggressiveness. On the other hand, microsatellite instability is relatively infrequent in thyroid cancer [168–174]. Exposure to ionizing radiation increases genetic instability and thyroid carcinoma prevalence as discussed in Chapter 11.

Analyses of human thyroid tumors with conventional cytogenetics and fluorescence in situ hybridization have identified additional recurrent chromosomal abnormalities. Hyperplastic nodules from thyroid goiters often contain one or two clonal numerical changes, including trisomies of chromosomes 7, 10, 12, 17, and/or 22, whereas follicular adenomas more frequently contain three or more numerical chromosomal alterations and/or balanced chromosomal rearrangements [25, 175–178]. However, it should be kept in mind that karyotypes frequently present an incomplete picture of chromosomal content because the cultures may frequently appear diploid as the result of contaminating normal cells. All suspected genetic alterations must be verified in primary thyroid tumor tissues.

The chromosomal regions 2p21 and 19q13 are rearranged in approximately 10% and 20%, respectively, of thyroid follicular adenomas with clonal cytogenetic aberrations. Both the 2p21 [26, 175, 179] and 19q13 [24, 175, 180] loci fuse with multiple different partner chromosomes in different follicular adenomas. The 2p21 and 19q13 breakpoints have been mapped using follicular adenoma cell lines that contain t(2;7)(p21;p15), t(2;20;3)(p21;q11;p25), t(5;19)(q13;13), or t(1;19)(p35;q13). The 2p21 breakpoint appears to involve a novel candidate gene termed *THADA* [181, 182] and the 19q13 breakpoint a novel transcription factor gene termed *ZNF331/RITA* [183–185]. It will be informative to define the cell biologic and biochemical mechanisms of these new thyroid rearrangements.

Additional genetic imbalances have been defined in follicular thyroid tumors using loss of heterozygosity studies and comparative genomic hybridization techniques. Genetic gains predominate over losses in follicular adenomas, whereas genetic losses predominate over gains in follicular, Hurthle, and anaplastic thyroid carcinomas. The most consistent losses in follicular cancers involve chromosomes 2p [186–189], 2q [186–188], 3p [169, 174, 187–191], 7q [188, 192, 193], 9 [174, 187, 188, 194, 195], 10q [196–198], 11q [187, 189, 195, 197, 199, 200], 13q [187, 188, 196, 197], 17q [201], 18q [174, 187, 197], and 22q [187, 188, 195, 202, 203] regions. In addition to these losses, Hurthle cell carcinomas harbor deletions at 1q, 8q, 9q, 14q, and 17p [174, 194, 201]. The possibility that at least some of these genomic loci contain genes important in thyroid tumor pathogenesis is reinforced by the fact that three regions (2q13, 3p25 and 7q31) have been shown to be involve follicular carcinoma rearrangements [12, 30]. Thus, functionally important loci may be targeted by multiple genetic mechanisms.

Summary

Knowledge of the molecular events that govern human thyroid tumorigenesis has grown considerably in the past ten years. Key genetic alterations and new oncogenic pathways have been identified. Molecular genetic aberrations in thyroid carcinomas bear noteworthy resemblance to those in acute myelogenous leukemias. Thyroid carcinomas and myeloid leukemias both possess transcription factor gene rearrangements—*PPARγ*-related translocations in thyroid carcinoma and *RARα*-related and *CBF*-related translocations (amongst others) in myeloid leukemia [204]. PPARγ and RARα are closely related members of the same nuclear receptor subfamily, and the PML-RARα and PAX8-PPARγ fusion proteins both function as dominant negative inhibitors of their wild-type parent proteins [12, 205, 206]. Thyroid carcinomas and myeloid leukemias [207–210] also both harbor *NRAS* mutations (15–25% of both cancers) and receptor tyrosine kinase mutations – *RET* mutations in thyroid carcinomas and *FLT3* mutations in myeloid leukemias [211, 212]. The *NRAS* and tyrosine receptor kinase mutations are not observed in the same thyroid carcinoma or leukemia patients [209, 213], suggesting that multiple initiating pathways exist in both. Lastly, thyroid carcinomas [214] and myeloid leukemias [209, 215] possess p53 mutations at relatively low frequency (10–15%) in patients who tend to be older and have more aggressive, therapy resistant disease. Such parallels are unlikely to occur by chance alone and argue that common mechanisms underlie these diverse epithelial and hematologic cancers.

The comparison of thyroid carcinomas and myeloid leukemias may highlight areas of thyroid cancer investigation worthy of further focus. For example, few collaborating mutations have been defined in thyroid carcinomas even though they play a clear role in myeloid leukemias [212, 216], as exemplified by *RARα* rearrangements [217, 218] and *FLT3* mutations [219] that together dictate the promyelocytic leukemia phenotype. Functional interactions between collaborating mutations are possible at multiple levels, and it is tempting to speculate that some thyroid carcinomas might develop through an unique combination or co-activation of RET and RAS and/or RET and PPARγ (and/or other) signaling systems. In fact, the ELE1-RET (PTC3) fusion protein contains the ELE1 nuclear receptor co-activator domain [220, 221] and it appears to physically associate with and inhibit wild-type PPARγ in some papillary carcinomas [222].

The similarities of the fusion proteins in thyroid carcinoma and myeloid leukemia suggest that a more directed search for fusion genes in non-thyroid carcinomas is warranted. In fact, novel fusion genes have been identified recently in aggressive midline [223, 224], secretory breast [225], and renal cell [226–232] carcinomas, although the epithelial nature of the latter is not well-documented. Interestingly, these cancers all tend to present more frequently in adolescence and young adulthood in a manner similar to thyroid and myeloid [233] malignancies that have fusion genes. The analyses of cancers that present earlier in life may enhance fusion gene recognition in other carcinoma types.

Definition and biologic characterization of the precursor cells that give rise to thyroid carcinoma will also be important. Myeloid leukemias are thought to arise from stem/progenitor cells that acquire disturbed self-renewal and differentiation capacities but retain characteristics of the myeloid lineages. Although the presence of comparable stem/progenitor cells in the thyroid are not defined, distinct thyroid cancer lineages and patterns of differentiation exist and candidate stem/progenitor cells such as the p63-immunoreactive solid cell nests [234] are apparent.

A last important area is development of molecular based therapies for thyroid carcinoma patients resistant to standard radio-iodine treatment. Treatments for such cancers are limited and pathways defined by thyroid cancer mutations are prime targets for pharmacologic interventions with molecular inhibitors. Tyrosine kinase inhibitors [235–239] and nuclear receptor ligands [240–242] have proven dramatically effective in some myeloid leukemia patients. Various molecular inhibitors are being investigated now in thyroid cancer models [45, 243–249]. Such developments predict that the thyroid cancer model will continue to provide biologic insights into human carcinoma biology and that improved pathologic diagnosis and treatment for thyroid cancer patients sit on the not too distant horizon.

BIBLIOGRAPHY

1. Tischler, A.S. and R.A. DeLellis, Tumors of thyroid follicular epithelium: where have we been and where are we going? Endocr Pathol, 2002. **13**(4): p. 267–9.
2. Baloch, Z.W. and V.A. Livolsi, Follicular-patterned lesions of the thyroid: the bane of the pathologist. Am J Clin Pathol, 2002. **117**(1): p. 143–50.
3. Saxen, E., et al., Observer variation in histologic classification of thyroid cancer. Acta Pathol Microbiol Scand [A], 1978. **86A**(6): p. 483–6.
4. Hirokawa, M., et al., Observer variation of encapsulated follicular lesions of the thyroid gland. Am J Surg Pathol, 2002. **26**(11): p. 1508–14.
5. O'Sullivan, M.J., et al., Malignant peripheral nerve sheath tumors with t(X;18). A pathologic and molecular genetic study. Mod Pathol, 2000. **13**(12): p. 1336–46.
6. Ladanyi, M., et al., Re: O'Sullivan MJ, Kyriakos M, Zhu X, Wick MR, Swanson PE, Dehner LP, Humphrey PA, Pfeifer JD: malignant peripheral nerve sheath tumors with t(X;18). A pathologic and molecular genetic study. Mod pathol 2000;13:1336–46. Mod Pathol, 2001. **14**(7): p. 733–7.
7. Tamborini, E., et al., Lack of SYT-SSX fusion transcripts in malignant peripheral nerve sheath tumors on RT-PCR analysis of 34 archival cases. Lab Invest, 2002. **82**(5): p. 609–18.
8. Fearon, E.R. and B. Vogelstein, A genetic model for colorectal tumorigenesis. Cell, 1990. **61**(5): p. 759–67.
9. Hruban, R.H., R.E. Wilentz, and S.E. Kern, Genetic progression in the pancreatic ducts. Am J Pathol, 2000. **156**(6): p. 1821–5.
10. Jaffee, E.M., et al., Focus on pancreas cancer. Cancer Cell, 2002. **2**(1): p. 25–8.
11. Fusco, A., et al., A new oncogene in human thyroid papillary carcinomas and their lymph- nodal metastases. Nature, 1987. **328**(6126): p. 170–2.
12. Kroll, T.G., et al., PAX8-PPARγ1 fusion oncogene in human thyroid carcinoma [corrected]. Science, 2000. **289**(5483): p. 1357–60.
13. Mitelman, F., Recurrent chromosome aberrations in cancer. Mutat Res, 2000. **462**(2–3): p. 247–53.
14. Grieco, M., et al., PTC is a novel rearranged form of the ret proto-oncogene and is frequently detected in vivo in human thyroid papillary carcinomas. Cell, 1990. **60**(4): p. 557–63.
15. Yip, L., et al., Multiple endocrine neoplasia type 2: evaluation of the genotype-phenotype relationship. Arch Surg, 2003. **138**(4): p. 409–16; discussion 416.
16. Thomas, G.A., et al., High prevalence of RET/PTC rearrangements in Ukrainian and Belarussian post-Chernobyl thyroid papillary carcinomas: a strong correlation between RET/PTC3 and the solid-follicular variant. J Clin Endocrinol Metab, 1999. **84**(11): p. 4232–8.
17. Basolo, F., et al., Potent Mitogenicity of the RET/PTC3 Oncogene Correlates with Its Prevalence in Tall-Cell Variant of Papillary Thyroid Carcinoma. Am J Pathol, 2002. **160**(1): p. 247–54.
18. Chiappetta, G., et al., The RET/PTC oncogene is frequently activated in oncocytic thyroid tumors (Hurthle cell adenomas and carcinomas), but not in oncocytic hyperplastic lesions. J Clin Endocrinol Metab, 2002. **87**(1): p. 364–9.
19. Cheung, C.C., et al., Molecular basis off hurthle cell papillary thyroid carcinoma. J Clin Endocrinol Metab, 2000. **85**(2): p. 878–82.
20. Nikiforov, Y.E., et al., Distinct pattern of ret oncogene rearrangements in morphological variants of radiation-induced and sporadic thyroid papillary carcinomas in children. Cancer Res, 1997. **57**(9): p. 1690–4.
21. Kroll, T.G., Molecular rearrangements and morphology in thyroid cancer. Am J Pathol, 2002. **160**(6): p. 1941–4.
22. Jenkins, R.B., et al., Frequent occurrence of cytogenetic abnormalities in sporadic nonmedullary thyroid carcinoma. Cancer, 1990. **66**(6): p. 1213–20.
23. Roque, L., et al., Deletion of 3p25->pter in a primary follicular thyroid carcinoma and its metastasis. Genes Chromosomes Cancer, 1993. **8**(3): p. 199–203.
24. Bondeson, L., et al., Chromosome studies in thyroid neoplasia. Cancer, 1989. **64**(3): p. 680–5.
25. Roque, L., et al., Cytogenetic findings in 18 follicular thyroid adenomas. Cancer Genet Cytogenet, 1993. **67**(1): p. 1–6.
26. Teyssier, J.R., et al., Chromosomal changes in thyroid tumors. Relation with DNA content, karyotypic features, and clinical data. Cancer Genet Cytogenet, 1990. **50**(2): p. 249–63.
27. Sozzi, G., et al., A t(2;3)(q12-13;p24-25) in follicular thyroid adenomas. Cancer Genet Cytogenet, 1992. **64**(1): p. 38–41.

28. Lui, W.O., et al., Balanced translocation (3;7)(p25;q34): another mechanism of tumorigenesis in follicular thyroid carcinoma? Cancer Genet Cytogenet, 2000. **119**(2): p. 109–12.
29. Storlazzi, C.T., et al., Fusion of the FUS and BBF2H7 genes in low grade fibromyxoid sarcoma. Hum Mol Genet, 2003. **12**(18): p. 2349–58.
30. Lui, W., et al., unpublished data. 2004.
31. Dwight, T., et al., Involvement of the PAX8/peroxisome proliferator-activated receptor gamma rearrangement in follicular thyroid tumors. J Clin Endocrinol Metab, 2003. **88**(9): p. 4440–5.
32. French, C., et al., Genetic and Biologic Subgroups of Early Stage Follicular Thyroid Cancer. Am J Pathol, in press, 2003.
33. Nikiforova, M., et al., Ras Point Mutations and PAX8-PPARg Rearrangement in Thyroid Tumors: Evidence for Distinct Molecular Pathways in Thyroid Follicular Carcinoma. J Clin Endocrinol Metab, in press, 2003.
34. Nikiforova, M.N., et al., PAX8-PPARgamma rearrangement in thyroid tumors: RT-PCR and immunohistochemical analyses. Am J Surg Pathol, 2002. **26**(8): p. 1016–23.
35. Dwight, T., et al., Involvement of PAX8/PPARγ1 in Follicular Thyroid Tumors. JCEM, in press, 2003.
36. Marques, A.R., et al., Expression of PAX8-PPARgamma1 Rearrangements in Both Follicular Thyroid Carcinomas and Adenomas. J Clin Endocrinol Metab, 2002. **87**(8): p. 3947–52.
37. Cheung, L., et al., Detection of the PAX8-PPAR gamma fusion oncogene in both follicular thyroid carcinomas and adenomas. J Clin Endocrinol Metab, 2003. **88**(1): p. 354–7.
38. Aldred, M.A., et al., Peroxisome proliferator-activated receptor gamma is frequently downregulated in a diversity of sporadic nonmedullary thyroid carcinomas. Oncogene, 2003. **22**(22): p. 3412–6.
39. Powell, J., et al., The PAX8-PPARg fusion oncoprotein transforms immortalized human thyrocytes through a mechanism probably involving wild-type PPARg inhibition. Oncogene, 2003. **in press**.
40. Girnun, G.D., et al., APC-dependent suppression of colon carcinogenesis by PPARgamma. Proc Natl Acad Sci U S A, 2002. **99**(21): p. 13771–6.
41. Sarraf, P., et al., Differentiation and reversal of malignant changes in colon cancer through PPARgamma. Nat Med, 1998. **4**(9): p. 1046–52.
42. Mueller, E., et al., Terminal differentiation of human breast cancer through PPAR gamma. Mol Cell, 1998. **1**(3): p. 465–70.
43. Mueller, E., et al., Effects of ligand activation of peroxisome proliferator-activated receptor gamma in human prostate cancer. Proc Natl Acad Sci USA, 2000. **97**(20): p. 10990–5.
44. Sarraf, P., et al., Loss-of-function mutations in PPAR gamma associated with human colon cancer. Mol Cell, 1999. **3**(6): p. 799–804.
45. Martelli, M.L., et al., Inhibitory effects of peroxisome poliferator-activated receptor gamma on thyroid carcinoma cell growth. J Clin Endocrinol Metab, 2002. **87**(10): p. 4728–35.
46. Ohta, K., et al., Ligands for peroxisome proliferator-activated receptor gamma inhibit growth and induce apoptosis of human papillary thyroid carcinoma cells. J Clin Endocrinol Metab, 2001. **86**(5): p. 2170–7.
47. Fajas, L., et al., PPARgamma controls cell proliferation and apoptosis in an RB-dependent manner. Oncogene, 2003. **22**(27): p. 4186–93.
48. Fajas, L., et al., The retinoblastoma-histone deacetylase 3 complex inhibits PPARgamma and adipocyte differentiation. Dev Cell, 2002. **3**(6): p. 903–10.
49. Galili, N., et al., Fusion of a fork head domain gene to PAX3 in the solid tumour alveolar rhabdomyosarcoma. Nat Genet, 1993. **5**(3): p. 230–5.
50. Barr, F.G., et al., Rearrangement of the PAX3 paired box gene in the paediatric solid tumour alveolar rhabdomyosarcoma. Nat Genet, 1993. **3**(2): p. 113–7.
51. Shapiro, D.N., et al., Fusion of PAX3 to a member of the forkhead family of transcription factors in human alveolar rhabdomyosarcoma. Cancer Res, 1993. **53**(21): p. 5108–12.
52. Mansouri, A., K. Chowdhury, and P. Gruss, Follicular cells of the thyroid gland require Pax8 gene function. Nat Genet, 1998. **19**(1): p. 87–90.
53. Maulbecker, C.C. and P. Gruss, The oncogenic potential of Pax genes. Embo J, 1993. **12**(6): p. 2361–7.
54. French, C., et al., Thyroid cancer with PPARg rearrangement detected by flourescence in situ hybridization in fine needle aspiration biopsies. manuscript submitted, 2004.
55. Roque, L., et al., Karyotypic characterization of papillary thyroid carcinomas. Cancer, 2001. **92**(10): p. 2529–38.
56. Kawai, K., et al., Tissue-specific carcinogenesis in transgenic mice expressing the RET proto-oncogene with a multiple endocrine neoplasia type 2A mutation. Cancer Res, 2000. **60**(18): p. 5254–60.

57. Michiels, F.M., et al., Development of medullary thyroid carcinoma in transgenic mice expressing the RET protooncogene altered by a multiple endocrine neoplasia type 2A mutation. Proc Natl Acad Sci U S A, 1997. **94**(7): p. 3330–5.
58. Donis-Keller, H., et al., Mutations in the RET proto-oncogene are associated with MEN 2A and FMTC. Hum Mol Genet, 1993. **2**(7): p. 851–6.
59. Mulligan, L.M., et al., Germ-line mutations of the RET proto-oncogene in multiple endocrine neoplasia type 2A. Nature, 1993. **363**(6428): p. 458–60.
60. Pierotti, M.A., et al., Characterization of an inversion on the long arm of chromosome 10 juxtaposing D10S170 and RET and creating the oncogenic sequence RET/PTC. Proc Natl Acad Sci USA, 1992. **89**(5): p. 1616–20.
61. Bongarzone, I., et al., Frequent activation of ret protooncogene by fusion with a new activating gene in papillary thyroid carcinomas. Cancer Res, 1994. **54**(11): p. 2979–85.
62. Santoro, M., et al., Molecular characterization of RET/PTC3; a novel rearranged version of the RET proto-oncogene in a human thyroid papillary carcinoma. Oncogene, 1994. **9**(2): p. 509–16.
63. Fugazzola, L., et al., Oncogenic rearrangements of the RET proto-oncogene in papillary thyroid carcinomas from children exposed to the Chernobyl nuclear accident. Cancer Res, 1995. **55**(23): p. 5617–20.
64. Ito, T., et al., Activated RET oncogene in thyroid cancers of children from areas contaminated by Chernobyl accident. Lancet, 1994. **344**(8917): p. 259.
65. Klugbauer, S., et al., High prevalence of RET rearrangement in thyroid tumors of children from Belarus after the Chernobyl reactor accident. Oncogene, 1995. **11**(12): p. 2459–67.
66. Santoro, M., et al., The TRK and RET tyrosine kinase oncogenes cooperate with ras in the neoplastic transformation of a rat thyroid epithelial cell line. Cell Growth Differ, 1993. **4**(2): p. 77–84.
67. Wang, J., et al., Conditional expression of RET/PTC induces a weak oncogenic drive in thyroid PCCL3 cells and inhibits thyrotropin action at multiple levels. Mol Endocrinol, 2003. **17**(7): p. 1425–36.
68. De Vita, G., et al., Expression of the RET/PTC1 oncogene impairs the activity of TTF-1 and Pax-8 thyroid transcription factors. Cell Growth Differ, 1998. **9**(1): p. 97–103.
69. Knauf, J.A., et al., RET/PTC-induced dedifferentiation of thyroid cells is mediated through Y1062 signaling through SHC-RAS-MAP kinase. Oncogene, 2003. **22**(28): p. 4406–12.
70. Kimura, E.T., et al., High prevalence of BRAF mutations in thyroid cancer: genetic evidence for constitutive activation of the RET/PTC-RAS-BRAF signaling pathway in papillary thyroid carcinoma. Cancer Res, 2003. **63**(7): p. 1454–7.
71. Castellone, M.D., et al., Ras-mediated apoptosis of PC CL3 rat thyroid cells induced by RET/PTC oncogenes. Oncogene, 2003. **22**(2): p. 246–55.
72. Tong, Q., S. Xing, and S.M. Jhiang, Leucine zipper-mediated dimerization is essential for the PTC1 oncogenic activity. J Biol Chem, 1997. **272**(14): p. 9043–7.
73. Monaco, C., et al., The RFG oligomerization domain mediates kinase activation and re-localization of the RET/PTC3 oncoprotein to the plasma membrane. Oncogene, 2001. **20**(5): p. 599–608.
74. Pandey, A., et al., The Ret receptor protein tyrosine kinase associates with the SH2- containing adapter protein Grb10. J Biol Chem, 1995. **270**(37): p. 21461–3.
75. Alberti, L., et al., Grb2 binding to the different isoforms of Ret tyrosine kinase. Oncogene, 1998. **17**(9): p. 1079–87.
76. Arighi, E., et al., Identification of Shc docking site on Ret tyrosine kinase. Oncogene, 1997. **14**(7): p. 773–82.
77. Melillo, R.M., et al., Docking protein FRS2 links the protein tyrosine kinase RET and its oncogenic forms with the mitogen-activated protein kinase signaling cascade. Mol Cell Biol, 2001. **21**(13): p. 4177–87.
78. Durick, K., G.N. Gill, and S.S. Taylor, Shc and Enigma are both required for mitogenic signaling by Ret/ptc2. Mol Cell Biol, 1998. **18**(4): p. 2298–308.
79. Santoro, M., et al., Development of thyroid papillary carcinomas secondary to tissue-specific expression of the RET/PTC1 oncogene in transgenic mice. Oncogene, 1996. **12**(8): p. 1821–6.
80. Powell, D.J., Jr., et al., The RET/PTC3 oncogene: metastatic solid-type papillary carcinomas in murine thyroids. Cancer Res, 1998. **58**(23): p. 5523–8.
81. Jhiang, S.M., et al., Targeted expression of the ret/PTC1 oncogene induces papillary thyroid carcinomas. Endocrinology, 1996. **137**(1): p. 375–8.
82. Cho, J.Y., et al., Early cellular abnormalities induced by RET/PTC1 oncogene in thyroid-targeted transgenic mice. Oncogene, 1999. **18**(24): p. 3659–65.

83. Powell Jr, D.J., et al., Altered gene expression in immunogenic poorly differentiated thyroid carcinomas from RET/PTC3p53-/- mice. Oncogene, 2001. **20**(25): p. 3235–46.
84. Santoro, M., et al., Ret oncogene activation in human thyroid neoplasms is restricted to the papillary cancer subtype. J Clin Invest, 1992. **89**(5): p. 1517–22.
85. Bongarzone, I., et al., High frequency of activation of tyrosine kinase oncogenes in human papillary thyroid carcinoma. Oncogene, 1989. **4**(12): p. 1457–62.
86. Jhiang, S.M., et al., Detection of the PTC/retTPC oncogene in human thyroid cancers. Oncogene, 1992. **7**(7): p. 1331–7.
87. Sugg, S.L., et al., ret/PTC-1, -2, and -3 oncogene rearrangements in human thyroid carcinomas: implications for metastatic potential? J Clin Endocrinol Metab, 1996. **81**(9): p. 3360–5.
88. Bounacer, A., et al., High prevalence of activating ret proto-oncogene rearrangements, in thyroid tumors from patients who had received external radiation. Oncogene, 1997. **15**(11): p. 1263–73.
89. Tallini, G., et al., RET/PTC oncogene activation defines a subset of papillary thyroid carcinomas lacking evidence of progression to poorly differentiated or undifferentiated tumor phenotypes. Clin Cancer Res, 1998. **4**(2): p. 287–94.
90. Nikiforova, M.N., et al., BRAF Mutations in Thyroid Tumors Are Restricted to Papillary Carcinomas and Anaplastic or Poorly Differentiated Carcinomas Arising from Papillary Carcinomas. J Clin Endocrinol Metab, 2003. **88**(11): p. 5399–404.
91. Soares, P., et al., BRAF mutations and RET/PTC rearrangements are alternative events in the etiopathogenesis of PTC. Oncogene, 2003. **22**(29): p. 4578–80.
92. Viglietto, G., et al., RET/PTC oncogene activation is an early event in thyroid carcinogenesis. Oncogene, 1995. **11**(6): p. 1207–10.
93. Sugg, S.L., et al., Distinct multiple RET/PTC gene rearrangements in multifocal papillary thyroid neoplasia. J Clin Endocrinol Metab, 1998. **83**(11): p. 4116–22.
94. Corvi, R., et al., Frequent RET rearrangements in thyroid papillary microcarcinoma detected by interphase fluorescence in situ hybridization. Lab Invest, 2001. **81**(12): p. 1639–45.
95. Bongarzone, I., et al., Age-related activation of the tyrosine kinase receptor protooncogenes RET and NTRK1 in papillary thyroid carcinoma. J Clin Endocrinol Metab, 1996. **81**(5): p. 2006–9.
96. Bongarzone, I., et al., RET/NTRK1 rearrangements in thyroid gland tumors of the papillary carcinoma family: correlation with clinicopathological features. Clin Cancer Res, 1998. **4**(1): p. 223–8.
97. Tallini, G. and S.L. Asa, RET oncogene activation in papillary thyroid carcinoma. Adv Anat Pathol, 2001. **8**(6): p. 345–54.
98. Zhu, Z., et al., Molecular profile and clinical-pathologic features of the follicular variant of papillary thyroid carcinoma. An unusually high prevalence of ras mutations. Am J Clin Pathol, 2003. **120**(1): p. 71–7.
99. Santoro, M., et al., RET activation and clinicopathologic features in poorly differentiated thyroid tumors. J Clin Endocrinol Metab, 2002. **87**(1): p. 370–9.
100. Cheung, C.C., et al., Hyalinizing trabecular tumor of the thyroid: a variant of papillary carcinoma proved by molecular genetics. Am J Surg Pathol, 2000. **24**(12): p. 1622–6.
101. Papotti, M., et al., RET/PTC activation in hyalinizing trabecular tumors of the thyroid. Am J Surg Pathol, 2000. **24**(12): p. 1615–21.
102. Belchetz, G., et al., Hurthle cell tumors: using molecular techniques to define a novel classification system. Arch Otolaryngol Head Neck Surg, 2002. **128**(3): p. 237–40.
103. Alberti, L., et al., RET and NTRK1 proto-oncogenes in human diseases. J Cell Physiol, 2003. **195**(2): p. 168–86.
104. Greco, A., et al., TRK-T1 is a novel oncogene formed by the fusion of TPR and TRK genes in human papillary thyroid carcinomas. Oncogene, 1992. **7**(2): p. 237–42.
105. Butti, M.G., et al., A sequence analysis of the genomic regions involved in the rearrangements between TPM3 and NTRK1 genes producing TRK oncogenes in papillary thyroid carcinomas. Genomics, 1995. **28**(1): p. 15–24.
106. Greco, A., et al., Chromosome 1 rearrangements involving the genes TPR and NTRK1 produce structurally different thyroid-specific TRK oncogenes. Genes Chromosomes Cancer, 1997. **19**(2): p. 112–23.
107. Musholt, T.J., et al., Prognostic significance of RET and NTRK1 rearrangements in sporadic papillary thyroid carcinoma. Surgery, 2000. **128**(6): p. 984–93.
108. Roccato, E., et al., Role of TFG sequences outside the coiled-coil domain in TRK-T3 oncogenic activation. Oncogene, 2003. **22**(6): p. 807–18.
109. Roccato, E., et al., Biological activity of the thyroid TRK-T3 oncogene requires signalling through Shc. Br J Cancer, 2002. **87**(6): p. 645–53.

110. Greco, A., et al., Role of the TFG N-terminus and coiled-coil domain in the transforming activity of the thyroid TRK-T3 oncogene. Oncogene, 1998. **16**(6): p. 809–16.
111. Borrello, M.G., et al., The oncogenic versions of the Ret and Trk tyrosine kinases bind Shc and Grb2 adaptor proteins. Oncogene, 1994. **9**(6): p. 1661–8.
112. Russell, J.P., et al., The TRK-T1 fusion protein induces neoplastic transformation of thyroid epithelium. Oncogene, 2000. **19**(50): p. 5729–35.
113. Bos, J.L., ras oncogenes in human cancer: a review. Cancer Res, 1989. **49**(17): p. 4682–9.
114. Wright, P.A., et al., Papillary and follicular thyroid carcinomas show a different pattern of ras oncogene mutation. Br J Cancer, 1989. **60**(4): p. 576–7.
115. Wright, P.A., et al., Radiation-associated and 'spontaneous' human thyroid carcinomas show a different pattern of ras oncogene mutation. Oncogene, 1991. **6**(3): p. 471–3.
116. Shi, Y.F., et al., High rates of ras codon 61 mutation in thyroid tumors in an iodide-deficient area. Cancer Res, 1991. **51**(10): p. 2690–3.
117. Lemoine, N.R., et al., Activated ras oncogenes in human thyroid cancers. Cancer Res, 1988. **48**(16): p. 4459–63.
118. Manenti, G., et al., Selective activation of ras oncogenes in follicular and undifferentiated thyroid carcinomas. Eur J Cancer, 1994. **7**: p. 987–93.
119. Vasko, V., et al., Specific pattern of RAS oncogene mutations in follicular thyroid tumors. J Clin Endocrinol Metab, 2003. **88**(6): p. 2745–52.
120. Fukushima, T., et al., BRAF mutations in papillary carcinomas of the thyroid. Oncogene, 2003. **22**(41): p. 6455–7.
121. Lemoine, N.R., et al., High frequency of ras oncogene activation in all stages of human thyroid tumorigenesis. Oncogene, 1989. **4**(2): p. 159–64.
122. Namba, H., K. Matsuo, and J.A. Fagin, Clonal composition of benign and malignant human thyroid tumors. J Clin Invest, 1990. **86**(1): p. 120–5.
123. Fusco, A., et al., One- and two-step transformations of rat thyroid epithelial cells by retroviral oncogenes. Mol Cell Biol, 1987. **7**(9): p. 3365–70.
124. Gire, V., C.J. Marshall, and D. Wynford-Thomas, Activation of mitogen-activated protein kinase is necessary but not sufficient for proliferation of human thyroid epithelial cells induced by mutant Ras. Oncogene, 1999. **18**(34): p. 4819–32.
125. Gire, V. and D. Wynford-Thomas, RAS oncogene activation induces proliferation in normal human thyroid epithelial cells without loss of differentiation. Oncogene, 2000. **19**(6): p. 737–44.
126. Fagin, J.A., Minireview: branded from the start-distinct oncogenic initiating events may determine tumor fate in the thyroid. Mol Endocrinol, 2002. **16**(5): p. 903–11.
127. Portella, G., et al., The Kirsten murine sarcoma virus induces rat thyroid carcinomas in vivo. Oncogene, 1989. **4**(2): p. 181–8.
128. Santelli, G., et al., Production of transgenic mice expressing the Ki-ras oncogene under the control of a thyroglobulin promoter. Cancer Res, 1993. **53**(22): p. 5523–7.
129. Oyama, T., et al., N-ras mutation of thyroid tumor with special reference to the follicular type. Pathol Int, 1995. **45**(1): p. 45–50.
130. Garcia-Rostan, G., et al., ras mutations are associated with aggressive tumor phenotypes and poor prognosis in thyroid cancer. J Clin Oncol, 2003. **21**(17): p. 3226–35.
131. Aguirre, A.J., et al., Activated Kras and Ink4a/Arf deficiency cooperate to produce metastatic pancreatic ductal adenocarcinoma. Genes Dev, 2003. **17**(24): p. 3112–26.
132. Manenti, G., et al., Selective activation of ras oncogenes in follicular and undifferentiated thyroid carcinomas. Eur J Cancer, 1994. **30A**(7): p. 987–93.
133. Basolo, F., et al., N-ras mutation in poorly differentiated thyroid carcinomas: correlation with bone metastases and inverse correlation to thyroglobulin expression. Thyroid, 2000. **10**(1): p. 19–23.
134. Hara, H., et al., N-ras mutation: an independent prognostic factor for aggressiveness of papillary thyroid carcinoma. Surgery, 1994. **116**(6): p. 1010–6.
135. Rochefort, P., et al., Thyroid pathologies in transgenic mice expressing a human activated Ras gene driven by a thyroglobulin promoter. Oncogene, 1996. **12**(1): p. 111–8.
136. Chin, L., et al., Essential role for oncogenic Ras in tumour maintenance. Nature, 1999. **400**(6743): p. 468–72.
137. Davies, H., et al., Mutations of the BRAF gene in human cancer. Nature, 2002. **417**(6892): p. 949–54.
138. Namba, H., et al., Clinical implication of hot spot BRAF mutation, V599E, in papillary thyroid cancers. J Clin Endocrinol Metab, 2003. **88**(9): p. 4393–7.
139. Cohen, Y., et al., BRAF mutation in papillary thyroid carcinoma. J Natl Cancer Inst, 2003. **95**(8): p. 625–7.

140. Xu, X., et al., High prevalence of BRAF gene mutation in papillary thyroid carcinomas and thyroid tumor cell lines. Cancer Res, 2003. **63**(15): p. 4561–7.
141. Roger, P., et al., Mitogenic effects of thyrotropin and adenosine 3′,5′-monophosphate in differentiated normal human thyroid cells in vitro. J Clin Endocrinol Metab, 1988. **66**(6): p. 1158–65.
142. Corvilain, B., et al., Role of the cyclic adenosine 3′,5′-monophosphate and the phosphatidylinositol-Ca2+ cascades in mediating the effects of thyrotropin and iodide on hormone synthesis and secretion in human thyroid slices. J Clin Endocrinol Metab, 1994. **79**(1): p. 152–9.
143. Nguyen, L.Q., et al., A dominant negative CREB (cAMP response element-binding protein) isoform inhibits thyrocyte growth, thyroid-specific gene expression, differentiation, and function. Mol Endocrinol, 2000. **14**(9): p. 1448–61.
144. Trulzsch, B., et al., Detection of thyroid-stimulating hormone receptor and Gsalpha mutations: in 75 toxic thyroid nodules by denaturing gradient gel electrophoresis. J Mol Med, 2001. **78**(12): p. 684–91.
145. Parma, J., et al., Somatic mutations in the thyrotropin receptor gene cause hyperfunctioning thyroid adenomas. Nature, 1993. **365**(6447): p. 649–51.
146. Russo, D., et al., Thyrotropin receptor gene alterations in thyroid hyperfunctioning adenomas. J Clin Endocrinol Metab, 1996. **81**(4): p. 1548–51.
147. Lyons, J., et al., Two G protein oncogenes in human endocrine tumors. Science, 1990. **249**(4969): p. 655–9.
148. Krohn, K. and R. Paschke, Clinical review 133: Progress in understanding the etiology of thyroid autonomy. J Clin Endocrinol Metab, 2001. **86**(7): p. 3336–45.
149. Michiels, F.M., et al., Oncogenic potential of guanine nucleotide stimulatory factor alpha subunit in thyroid glands of transgenic mice. Proc Natl Acad Sci USA, 1994. **91**(22): p. 10488–92.
150. Zeiger, M.A., et al., Thyroid-specific expression of cholera toxin A1 subunit causes thyroid hyperplasia and hyperthyroidism in transgenic mice. Endocrinology, 1997. **138**(8): p. 3133–40.
151. Duprez, L., et al., Germline mutations in the thyrotropin receptor gene cause non-autoimmune autosomal dominant hyperthyroidism. Nat Genet, 1994. **7**(3): p. 396–401.
152. Weinstein, L.S., et al., Activating mutations of the stimulatory G protein in the McCune-Albright syndrome. N Engl J Med, 1991. **325**(24): p. 1688–95.
153. Suzuki, H., M.C. Willingham, and S.Y. Cheng, Mice with a mutation in the thyroid hormone receptor beta gene spontaneously develop thyroid carcinoma: a mouse model of thyroid carcinogenesis. Thyroid, 2002. **12**(11): p. 963–9.
154. Ying, H., et al., Mutant thyroid hormone receptor beta represses the expression and transcriptional activity of peroxisome proliferator-activated receptor gamma during thyroid carcinogenesis. Cancer Res, 2003. **63**(17): p. 5274–80.
155. Morin, P.J., et al., Activation of beta-catenin-Tcf signaling in colon cancer by mutations in beta-catenin or APC. Science, 1997. **275**(5307): p. 1787–90.
156. Garcia-Rostan, G., et al., Frequent mutation and nuclear localization of beta-catenin in anaplastic thyroid carcinoma. Cancer Res, 1999. **59**(8): p. 1811–5.
157. Garcia-Rostan, G., et al., Beta-catenin dysregulation in thyroid neoplasms: down-regulation, aberrant nuclear expression, and CTNNB1 exon 3 mutations are markers for aggressive tumor phenotypes and poor prognosis. Am J Pathol, 2001. **158**(3): p. 987–96.
158. Cerrato, A., et al., Beta- and gamma-catenin expression in thyroid carcinomas. J Pathol, 1998. **185**(3): p. 267–72.
159. Ishigaki, K., et al., Aberrant localization of beta-catenin correlates with overexpression of its target gene in human papillary thyroid cancer. J Clin Endocrinol Metab, 2002. **87**(7): p. 3433–40.
160. Bohm, J., et al., Expression and prognostic value of alpha-, beta-, and gamma-catenins indifferentiated thyroid carcinoma. J Clin Endocrinol Metab, 2000. **85**(12): p. 4806–11.
161. Sozzi, G., et al., Cytogenetic and molecular genetic characterization of papillary thyroid carcinomas. Genes Chromosomes Cancer, 1992. **5**(3): p. 212–8.
162. Sapi, Z., et al., Contribution of p53 gene alterations to development of metastatic forms of follicular thyroid carcinoma. Diagn Mol Pathol, 1995. **4**(4): p. 256–60.
163. Donghi, R., et al., Gene p53 mutations are restricted to poorly differentiated and undifferentiated carcinomas of the thyroid gland. J Clin Invest, 1993. **91**(4): p. 1753–60.
164. Fagin, J.A., et al., High prevalence of mutations of the p53 gene in poorly differentiated human thyroid carcinomas. J Clin Invest, 1993. **91**(1): p. 179–84.
165. Battista, S., et al., A mutated p53 gene alters thyroid cell differentiation. Oncogene, 1995. **11**(10): p. 2029–37.
166. Fagin, J.A., et al., Reexpression of thyroid peroxidase in a derivative of an undifferentiated thyroid carcinoma cell line by introduction of wild-type p53. Cancer Res, 1996. **56**(4): p. 765–71.

167. La Perle, K.M., S.M. Jhiang, and C.C. Capen, Loss of p53 promotes anaplasia and local invasion in ret/PTC1-induced thyroid carcinomas. Am J Pathol, 2000. **157**(2): p. 671–7.
168. Lazzereschi, D., et al., Microsatellite instability in thyroid tumours and tumour-like lesions. Br J Cancer, 1999. **79**(2): p. 340–5.
169. Rodrigues-Serpa, A., A. Catarino, and J. Soares, Loss of heterozygosity in follicular and papillary thyroid carcinomas. Cancer Genet Cytogenet, 2003. **141**(1): p. 26–31.
170. Soares, P., et al., Benign and malignant thyroid lesions show instability at microsatellite loci. Eur J Cancer, 1997. **33**(2): p. 293–6.
171. Bauer, A.J., et al., Evaluation of adult papillary thyroid carcinomas by comparative genomic hybridization and microsatellite instability analysis. Cancer Genet Cytogenet, 2002. **135**(2): p. 182–6.
172. Vermiglio, F., et al., Absence of microsatellite instability in thyroid carcinomas. Eur J Cancer, 1995. **31A**(1): p. 128.
173. Nikiforov, Y.E., M. Nikiforova, and J.A. Fagin, Prevalence of minisatellite and microsatellite instability in radiation-induced post-Chernobyl pediatric thyroid carcinomas. Oncogene, 1998. **17**(15): p. 1983–8.
174. Segev, D.L., et al., Polymerase chain reaction-based microsatellite polymorphism analysis of follicular and Hurthle cell neoplasms of the thyroid. J Clin Endocrinol Metab, 1998. **83**(6): p. 2036–42.
175. Belge, G., et al., Cytogenetic investigations of 340 thyroid hyperplasias and adenomas revealing correlations between cytogenetic findings and histology. Cancer Genet Cytogenet, 1998. **101**(1): p. 42–8.
176. Roque, L., et al., Significance of trisomy 7 and 12 in thyroid lesions with follicular differentiation: a cytogenetic and in situ hybridization study. Lab Invest, 1999. **79**(4): p. 369–78.
177. Barril, N., A.B. Carvalho-Sales, and E.H. Tajara, Detection of numerical chromosome anomalies in interphase cells of benign and malignant thyroid lesions using fluorescence in situ hybridization. Cancer Genet Cytogenet, 2000. **117**(1): p. 50–6.
178. Antonini, P., et al., Numerical aberrations, including trisomy 22 as the sole anomaly, are recurrent in follicular thyroid adenomas. Genes Chromosomes Cancer, 1993. **8**(1): p. 63–6.
179. Bol, S., et al., Structural abnormalities of chromosome 2 in benign thyroid tumors. Three new cases and review of the literature. Cancer Genet Cytogenet, 1999. **114**(1): p. 75–7.
180. Bartnitzke, S., et al., Cytogenetic findings on eight follicular thyroid adenomas including one with a t(10;19). Cancer Genet Cytogenet, 1989. **39**(1): p. 65–8.
181. Bol, S., et al., Molecular cytogenetic investigations define a subgroup of thyroid adenomas with 2p21 breakpoints clustered to a region of less than 450 kb. Cytogenet Cell Genet, 2001. **95**(3-4): p. 189–91.
182. Rippe, V., et al., Identification of a gene rearranged by 2p21 aberrations in thyroid adenomas. Oncogene, 2003. **22**(38): p. 6111–4.
183. Belge, G., et al., Delineation of a 150-kb breakpoint cluster in benign thyroid tumors with 19q13.4 aberrations. Cytogenet Cell Genet, 2001. **93**(1-2): p. 48–51.
184. Belge, G., et al., Breakpoints of 19q13 translocations of benign thyroid tumors map within a 400 kilobase region. Genes Chromosomes Cancer, 1997. **20**(2): p. 201–3.
185. Rippe, V., et al., A KRAB zinc finger protein gene is the potential target of 19q13 translocation in benign thyroid tumors. Genes Chromosomes Cancer, 1999. **26**(3): p. 229–36.
186. Tung, W.S., et al., Allelotype of follicular thyroid carcinomas reveals genetic instability consistent with frequent nondisjunctional chromosomal loss. Genes Chromosomes Cancer, 1997. **19**(1): p. 43–51.
187. Roque, L., et al., Chromosome imbalances in thyroid follicular neoplasms: a comparison between follicular adenomas and carcinomas. Genes Chromosomes Cancer, 2003. **36**(3): p. 292–302.
188. Kitamura, Y., et al., Allelotyping of follicular thyroid carcinoma: frequent allelic losses in chromosome arms 7q, 11p, and 22q. J Clin Endocrinol Metab, 2001. **86**(9): p. 4268–72.
189. Ward, L.S., et al., Studies of allelic loss in thyroid tumors reveal major differences in chromosomal instability between papillary and follicular carcinomas. J Clin Endocrinol Metab, 1998. **83**(2): p. 525–30.
190. Hunt, J.L., et al., Loss of heterozygosity of the VHL gene identifies malignancy and predicts death in follicular thyroid tumors. Surgery, 2003. **134**(6): p. 1043–7; discussion 1047–8.
191. Herrmann, M.A., et al., Cytogenetic and molecular genetic studies of follicular and papillary thyroid cancers. J Clin Invest, 1991. **88**(5): p. 1596–604.
192. Zhang, J.S., et al., Differential loss of heterozygosity at 7q31.2 in follicular and papillary thyroid tumors. Oncogene, 1998. **17**(6): p. 789–93.
193. Trovato, M., et al., Loss of heterozygosity of the long arm of chromosome 7 in follicular and anaplastic thyroid cancer, but not in papillary thyroid cancer. J Clin Endocrinol Metab, 1999. **84**(9): p. 3235–40.
194. Frisk, T., et al., Low frequency of numerical chromosomal aberrations in follicular thyroid tumors detected by comparative genomic hybridization. Genes Chromosomes Cancer, 1999. **25**(4): p. 349–53.

195. Kitamura, Y., et al., Allelotyping of anaplastic thyroid carcinoma: frequent allelic losses on 1q, 9p, 11, 17, 19p, and 22q. Genes Chromosomes Cancer, 2000. **27**(3): p. 244–51.
196. Zedenius, J., et al., Deletions of the long arm of chromosome 10 in progression of follicular thyroid tumors. Hum Genet, 1996. **97**(3): p. 299–303.
197. Zedenius, J., et al., Allelotyping of follicular thyroid tumors. Hum Genet, 1995. **96**(1): p. 27–32.
198. Yeh, J.J., et al., Fine-structure deletion mapping of 10q22-24 identifies regions of loss of heterozygosity and suggests that sporadic follicular thyroid adenomas and follicular thyroid carcinomas develop along distinct neoplastic pathways. Genes Chromosomes Cancer, 1999. **26**(4): p. 322–8.
199. Nord, B., et al., Sporadic follicular thyroid tumors show loss of a 200-kb region in 11q13 without evidence for mutations in the MEN1 gene. Genes Chromosomes Cancer, 1999. **26**(1): p. 35–9.
200. Matsuo, K., S.H. Tang, and J.A. Fagin, Allelotype of human thyroid tumors: loss of chromosome 11q13 sequences in follicular neoplasms. Mol Endocrinol, 1991. **5**(12): p. 1873–9.
201. Grebe, S.K., et al., Frequent loss of heterozygosity on chromosomes 3p and 17p without VHL or p53 mutations suggests involvement of unidentified tumor suppressor genes in follicular thyroid carcinoma. J Clin Endocrinol Metab, 1997. **82**(11): p. 3684–91.
202. Hemmer, S., et al., DNA copy number changes in thyroid carcinoma. Am J Pathol, 1999. **154**(5): p. 1539–47.
203. Hemmer, S., et al., Comparison of benign and malignant follicular thyroid tumours by comparative genomic hybridization. Br J Cancer, 1998. **78**(8): p. 1012–7.
204. Gilliland, D.G. and M.S. Tallman, Focus on acute leukemias. Cancer Cell, 2002. **1**(5): p. 417–20.
205. Okuda, T., et al., Expression of a knocked-in AML1-ETO leukemia gene inhibits the establishment of normal definitive hematopoiesis and directly generates dysplastic hematopoietic progenitors. Blood, 1998. **91**(9): p. 3134–43.
206. Jansen, J.H., et al., Multimeric complexes of the PML-retinoic acid receptor alpha fusion protein in acute promyelocytic leukemia cells and interference with retinoid and peroxisome-proliferator signaling pathways. Proc Natl Acad Sci USA, 1995. **92**(16): p. 7401–5.
207. Neubauer, A., et al., Prognostic importance of mutations in the ras proto-oncogenes in de novo acute myeloid leukemia. Blood, 1994. **83**(6): p. 1603–11.
208. Radich, J.P., et al., N-ras mutations in adult de novo acute myelogenous leukemia: prevalence and clinical significance. Blood, 1990. **76**(4): p. 801–7.
209. Stirewalt, D.L., et al., FLT3, RAS, and TP53 mutations in elderly patients with acute myeloid leukemia. Blood, 2001. **97**(11): p. 3589–95.
210. Coghlan, D.W., et al., The incidence and prognostic significance of mutations in codon 13 of the N-ras gene in acute myeloid leukemia. Leukemia, 1994. **8**(10): p. 1682–7.
211. Nakao, M., et al., Internal tandem duplication of the flt3 gene found in acute myeloid leukemia. Leukemia, 1996. **10**(12): p. 1911–8.
212. Gilliland, D.G. and J.D. Griffin, The roles of FLT3 in hematopoiesis and leukemia. Blood, 2002. **100**(5): p. 1532–42.
213. Kiyoi, H., et al., Prognostic implication of FLT3 and N-RAS gene mutations in acute myeloid leukemia. Blood, 1999. **93**(9): p. 3074–80.
214. Greenblatt, M.S., et al., Mutations in the p53 tumor suppressor gene: clues to cancer etiology and molecular pathogenesis. Cancer Res, 1994. **54**(18): p. 4855–78.
215. Wattel, E., et al., p53 mutations are associated with resistance to chemotherapy and short survival in hematologic malignancies. Blood, 1994. **84**(9): p. 3148–57.
216. Higuchi, M., et al., Expression of a conditional AML-ETO oncogene bypasses embryonic lethality and establishes a murine model of human t(8;21) acute myeloid leukemia. Cancer Cell, 2002. **1**: p. 63–74.
217. He, L.Z., et al., Two critical hits for promyelocytic leukemia. Mol Cell, 2000. **6**(5): p. 1131–41.
218. Pollock, J.L., et al., A bcr-3 isoform of RARalpha-PML potentiates the development of PML-RARalpha-driven acute promyelocytic leukemia. Proc Natl Acad Sci U S A, 1999. **96**(26): p. 15103–8.
219. Kelly, L.M., et al., PML/RARalpha and FLT3-ITD induce an APL-like disease in a mouse model. Proc Natl Acad Sci U S A, 2002. **99**(12): p. 8283–8.
220. Heinlein, C.A., et al., Identification of ARA70 as a ligand-enhanced coactivator for the peroxisome proliferator-activated receptor gamma. J Biol Chem, 1999. **274**(23): p. 16147–52.
221. Yeh, S. and C. Chang, Cloning and characterization of a specific coactivator, ARA70, for the androgen receptor in human prostate cells. Proc Natl Acad Sci USA, 1996. **93**(11): p. 5517–21.
222. Monaco, C., et al., unpublished data.
223. French, C.A., et al., BRD4 bromodomain gene rearrangement in aggressive carcinoma with translocation t(15;19). Am J Pathol, 2001. **159**(6): p. 1987–92.

224. French, C.A., et al., BRD4-NUT fusion oncogene: a novel mechanism in aggressive carcinoma. Cancer Res, 2003. **63**(2): p. 304–7.
225. Tognon, C., et al., Expression of the ETV6-NTRK3 gene fusion as a primary event in human secretory breast carcinoma. Cancer Cell, 2002. **2**(5): p. 367–76.
226. Argani, P., et al., Primary renal neoplasms with the ASPL-TFE3 gene fusion of alveolar soft part sarcoma: a distinctive tumor entity previously included among renal cell carcinomas of children and adolescents. Am J Pathol, 2001. **159**(1): p. 179–92.
227. Renshaw, A.A., et al., Renal cell carcinomas in children and young adults: increased incidence of papillary architecture and unique subtypes. Am J Surg Pathol, 1999. **23**(7): p. 795–802.
228. Clark, J., et al., Fusion of splicing factor genes PSF and NonO (p54nrb) to the TFE3 gene in papillary renal cell carcinoma. Oncogene, 1997. **15**(18): p. 2233–9.
229. Heimann, P., et al., Fusion of a novel gene, RCC17, to the TFE3 gene in t(X;17)(p11.2;q25.3)-bearing papillary renal cell carcinomas. Cancer Res, 2001. **61**(10): p. 4130–5.
230. Davis, I.J., et al., Cloning of an Alpha-TFEB fusion in renal tumors harboring the t(6;11)(p21;q13) chromosome translocation. Proc Natl Acad Sci U S A, 2003. **100**(10): p. 6051–6.
231. Loewy, J.W., et al., Statistical methods that distinguish between attributes of assessment: prolongation of life versus quality of life. Med Decis Making, 1992. **12**(2): p. 83–92.
232. Hsi, A.C., D.J. Davis, and F.C. Sherman, Neonatal gangrene in the newborn infant of a diabetic mother. J Pediatr Orthop, 1985. **5**(3): p. 358–60.
233. Rowley, J.D., Molecular genetics in acute leukemia. Leukemia, 2000. **14**(3): p. 513–7.
234. Reis-Filho, J.S., et al., p63 expression in solid cell nests of the thyroid: further evidence for a stem cell origin. Mod Pathol, 2003. **16**(1): p. 43–8.
235. Weisberg, E., et al., Inhibition of mutant FLT3 receptors in leukemia cells by the small molecule tyrosine kinase inhibitor PKC412. Cancer Cell, 2002. **1**(5): p. 433–43.
236. Kelly, L.M., et al., CT53518, a novel selective FLT3 antagonist for the treatment of acute myelogenous leukemia (AML). Cancer Cell, 2002. **1**(5): p. 421–32.
237. Spiekermann, K., et al., The protein tyrosine kinase inhibitor SU5614 inhibits FLT3 and induces growth arrest and apoptosis in AML-derived cell lines expressing a constitutively activated FLT3. Blood, 2003. **101**(4): p. 1494–504.
238. Druker, B.J., et al., Activity of a specific inhibitor of the BCR-ABL tyrosine kinase in the blast crisis of chronic myeloid leukemia and acute lymphoblastic leukemia with the Philadelphia chromosome. N Engl J Med, 2001. **344**(14): p. 1038–42.
239. Druker, B.J., et al., Efficacy and safety of a specific inhibitor of the BCR-ABL tyrosine kinase in chronic myeloid leukemia. N Engl J Med, 2001. **344**(14): p. 1031–7.
240. Tallman, M.S., et al., All-trans retinoic acid in acute promyelocytic leukemia: long-term outcome and prognostic factor analysis from the North American Intergroup protocol. Blood, 2002. **100**(13): p. 4298–302.
241. Rego, E.M., et al., Retinoic acid (RA) and As2O3 treatment in transgenic models of acute promyelocytic leukemia (APL) unravel the distinct nature of the leukemogenic process induced by the PML-RARalpha and PLZF-RARalpha oncoproteins. Proc Natl Acad Sci USA, 2000. **97**(18): p. 10173–8.
242. Fenaux, P., et al., A randomized comparison of all transretinoic acid (ATRA) followed by chemotherapy and ATRA plus chemotherapy and the role of maintenance therapy in newly diagnosed acute promyelocytic leukemia. The European APL Group. Blood, 1999. **94**(4): p. 1192–200.
243. Carniti, C., et al., PP1 inhibitor induces degradation of RETMEN2A and RETMEN2B oncoproteins through proteosomal targeting. Cancer Res, 2003. **63**(9): p. 2234–43.
244. Carlomagno, F., et al., The kinase inhibitor PP1 blocks tumorigenesis induced by RET oncogenes. Cancer Res, 2002. **62**(4): p. 1077–82.
245. Carlomagno, F., et al., ZD6474, an orally available inhibitor of KDR tyrosine kinase activity, efficiently blocks oncogenic RET kinases. Cancer Res, 2002. **62**(24): p. 7284–90.
246. Strock, C.J., et al., CEP-701 and CEP-751 inhibit constitutively activated RET tyrosine kinase activity and block medullary thyroid carcinoma cell growth. Cancer Res, 2003. **63**(17): p. 5559–63.
247. Carlomagno, F., et al., Efficient inhibition of RET/papillary thyroid carcinoma oncogenic kinases by 4-amino-5-(4-chloro-phenyl)-7-(t-butyl)pyrazolo[3,4-d]pyrimidine (PP2). J Clin Endocrinol Metab, 2003. **88**(4): p. 1897–902.
248. Podtcheko, A., et al., The selective tyrosine kinase inhibitor, STI571, inhibits growth of anaplastic thyroid cancer cells. J Clin Endocrinol Metab, 2003. **88**(4): p. 1889–96.
249. Lanzi, C., et al., Inhibition of transforming activity of the ret/ptc1 oncoprotein by a 2-indolinone derivative. Int J Cancer, 2000. **85**(3): p. 384–90.

5. MOLECULAR EPIDEMIOLOGY OF THYROID CANCER

MARTIN SCHLUMBERGER

Service de Medecine Nucleaire, Institut Gustave Roussy, 39 rue Camille Desmoulins, 94805 Villejuif, France

INTRODUCTION

Molecular biology studies have greatly enhanced our knowledge of thyroid tumorigenesis, although their impact in clinical practice is still negligible.

Most benign and malignant thyroid tumors have a monoclonal origin, suggesting that genetic events are responsible for their occurrence (34). These may involve the activation of oncogenes or the inactivation of tumor-suppressor genes. Several genetic abnormalities (point mutations or gene rearrangements) have been evidenced in human thyroid tumors (review in 14,40,53). Several *in vitro* and *in vivo* animal models, including transgenic mice that reproduce the human situations, are also available.

ONCOGENES AND THYROID TUMORS

Tyrosine kinase receptors

Growth factors act on the target cell through interaction with specific membrane receptors, some of which belong to the family of tyrosine kinase receptors. The genes encoding these receptors are frequently involved in the pathogenesis of human cancers, including thyroid cancer. Whenever uncontrolled activation of a tyrosine kinase receptor gene occurs, either through overexpression or activating mutations, increased responsiveness to growth factors or ligand-independent gene activation ensues, both of which then activate the signaling pathways downstream. Three tyrosine kinase receptor genes are known to be associated with the pathogenesis of papillary thyroid cancer: the *met* gene through overexpression and the *ret* and *trk* genes through gene rearrangements.

Ret/PTC *oncogene*

MOLECULAR BASIS OF *Ret*/PTC REARRANGEMENTS. The *ret* proto-oncogene is a 21-exon gene located on chromosome 10q11-2 that encodes a membrane tyrosine kinase receptor. The ret receptor together with the glial cell line-derived neurotropic factor (GDNF) receptor (GFRα-1), an extracellular protein tethered to the cell membrane, form a receptor for GDNF. The ret receptor may also combine with other members of the GFRα receptor family, thereby forming receptors for other peptides (artemin, neurturin, persephin). The ret protein is composed of an extra-cellular domain, with a distal cadherin-like domain and a juxta-membrane cystein-rich domain, a transmembrane domain and an intra-cellular domain with tyrosine-kinase activity. The gene is expressed in a variety of neuronal cell lineages including thyroid C cells and adrenal medulla but is not expressed in normal thyroid follicular cells.

Under normal conditions, the ret ligands induce receptor dimerization and tyrosine trans-phosphorylation of the receptor kinase domain, thus activating the pathways downstream. When the gene is mutated, ligand interaction is no longer needed for receptor activation and the downstream pathways are continuously activated: ret/PTC kinase activity promotes interaction with shc, an intermediate in the RAS-RAF-MEK-MAP kinase pathway. Inappropriate activation of this pathway induces abnormal proliferation and differentiation in many human cancers and also induces genomic instability.

Ret activation was first evidenced by transfection experiments and was initially found exclusively in papillary thyroid carcinoma (PTC). The resulting oncogene was thus called *ret*/PTC (16,18,40). All activated forms of the *ret* proto-oncogene are due to chromosomal rearrangements in which the 3' or tyrosine kinase domain of the *ret* gene is fused with the 5' domain of a foreign gene. The foreign gene is constitutively expressed, resulting in permanent expression of the rearranged *ret* gene. These rearranged genes have coiled-coil domains that activate the ret protein through permanent dimerization. They also lack the intracellular juxta-membrane domain that normally exerts a negative regulatory effect on ret tyrosine kinase activity. Finally, the chimeric protein lacks the extracellular and transmembrane domains and is located in the cytosol. Three major forms of the *ret* rearrangements have been identified in epithelial thyroid tumors:

Ret/PTC$_1$, is formed through an intra-chromosomal rearrangement fusing the *ret* tyrosine kinase domain to a gene designated H4, whose function is still unknown.

Ret/PTC$_2$, is formed through an inter-chromosomal rearrangement fusing the *ret* tyrosine kinase domain to a gene located on chromosome 17 that encodes the RIα regulatory subunit of cAMP-dependent protein kinase A.

Ret/PTC$_3$, is formed through an intra-chromosomal rearrangement fusing the *ret* tyrosine kinase domain to a gene designated ELE1, whose function is still unknown.

In the three major *ret* rearrangements *(ret*/PTC$_{1;2;3}$), the breakpoints of the *ret* gene are located in the same intronic region, between exons 11 and 12. Several other ret/PTC rearrangements have been observed that differ because of the location of the breakpoint in the *ret* gene or because of the partner gene.

Recent studies have shown that the unique spatial proximity of *ret* and H4 partner genes in the nuclear matrix of thyroid cells (but not in other cell types) may be a major reason for the development of *ret* rearrangement following exposure to ionizing radiation and may explain why *ret*/PTC are found exclusively in papillary thyroid carcinomas (30).

FREQUENCY OF *ret*/PTC REARRANGEMENTS. The frequency of *ret*/PTC rearrangements in papillary thyroid carcinomas occurring in adult patients who never received neck irradiation during childhood varies between 2.5 and 35% among the different series (3,4,11). *Ret*/PTC1 and *ret*/PTC3 are the most frequent rearrangements in these tumors and *ret*/PTC2 is less frequent. Variations in the frequency and type of rearrangements could be due to differences in the geographical origins of the populations studied or in the sensitivity of the method used to detect the rearrangements. In children with sporadic papillary thyroid carcinoma without a history of radiation exposure, the incidence of *ret*/PTC-positive tumors is similar to that observed in adult patients of the same ethnic background (3,11). *Ret*/PTC rearrangements are more frequently found in papillary thyroid carcinomas occurring after exposure to ionizing radiation during childhood, due to external irradiation or to the Chernobyl accident (see below).

In patients who did not previously receive neck irradiation, rearranged *ret* genes were detected only in papillary thyroid carcinomas. All other tumors studied (thyroidal or non thyroidal) were negative for *ret*/PTC1 (48). In two series, 15–21% of thyroid adenomas were *ret*/PTC positive, but the existence of micropapillary thyroid carcinomas cannot be excluded (20).

That *ret*/PTC rearrangement is found in papillary thyroid microcarcinomas suggests that it is an early event in thyroid carcinogenesis (59). In patients with multifocal disease, diverse *ret*/PTC rearrangements were found in different tumors from the same patient, indicating that these tumors had arisen through distinct initiating events (54).

A high frequency of *ret*/PTC rearrangements has also been found in Hürthle cell papillary thyroid carcinomas (7), and in about 10% of poorly-differentiated thyroid carcinomas, demonstrating that these *ret*-positive tumors derive from papillary thyroid carcinomas (50). On the other hand, *ret*/PTC-positive tumors lack evidence of progression to undifferentiated tumor phenotypes (55).

Transfection of the *ret*/PTC1 gene in normal rat thyroid cells resulted in loss of differentiation and of TSH growth dependency. However, cells were totally transformed only after transfection with *ret*/PTC and mutated *ras* genes, suggesting that simultaneous activation of several genes is necessary for tumor progression. Transgenic mice in which the *ret*/PTC1 gene is expressed in thyroid tissue develop papillary thyroid carcinoma, which is histologically identical to the human cancer (24,49). However, in this model all thyroid cells possess the rearrangement but only a few cells give rise to tumors a few months after birth, suggesting that at least one more mutation is needed to give rise to PTC. The use of the *ret*/PTC3 gene results in a more aggressive histological and clinical behavior. This is consistent with a more aggressive type of human papillary thyroid carcinomas in which *ret*/PTC3 can be evidenced (42,56).

Trk oncogene

The *trk* proto-oncogene is located on chromosome 1. It encodes a membrane tyrosine kinase receptor for the nerve growth factor (NGF). *Trk* expression is restricted to peripheral nerve ganglia.

Activated forms of the *trk* proto-oncogene are the result of chromosomal rearrangements in which the 3' or tyrosine kinase domain of *trk* is fused with the 5' domain of a foreign gene (17,40). The foreign gene is constitutively expressed giving rise to permanent expression of the rearranged *trk* gene. These genes have domains that induce *trk* activation through permanent dimerization. All the breakpoints in these chimeric genes are located in the same *trk* domain.

Several rearrangements have been found in human thyroid tumors:

N-*trk* is formed through an intra-chromosomal rearrangement fusing the *trk* tyrosine kinase domain with the 5' region of the non muscular tropomyosine gene.

Trk-T_1 and *trk*-T_2 are formed through fusion of the *trk* tyrosine kinase domain with the 5' region of the translocated promoter region (*tpr*) gene.

Trk-T_3 is formed through fusion of the *trk* tyrosine kinase domain with the 5' region of a gene called *tag* (*trk* activating gene).

Trk rearrangements have only been found in papillary thyroid carcinomas. Their frequency is lower than that of *ret*/PTC, ranging from 0 to 10% (3,5,42).

Met oncogene

The *met* proto-oncogene encodes a membrane tyrosine kinase receptor. Its ligand is the hepatocyte growth factor (HGF) or scatter factor (SF). HGF-SF is a potent mitogen for epithelial cells and promotes cell motility and invasion.

The *met* proto-oncogene can be activated either as a result of rearrangement with unrelated sequences (this mechanism is not found in thyroid carcinoma) or through overexpression. Overexpression of the *met* oncogene was found in about 50% of papillary thyroid carcinomas and this may be a factor in metastatic spread (9). Negative or low *met* oncogene expression has been found in the other histologic types.

A relationship has been found between *ras* and *ret* activation and *mg* overexpression in human thyroid epithelial cells. This overexpression may in turn sustain their growth through the action of HGF secreted by stromal cells.

Defects in the intracellular signaling pathway: *ras* and *b-raf*

The *ras* genes (*H-ras*, *K-ras* and *N-ras*) encode a 21 kD protein (p21) involved in signal transmission from cell membrane receptors to growth factors to the nucleus. The *ras* gene is activated by point mutations in codon 12 or 61 and sometimes in codon 13 or 59.

Ras mutations were initially found in up to 50% of benign or malignant thyroid tumors and was the most frequent genetic alteration found in these tumors. All three *ras* genes (H, K and N) were found to be activated at a similar frequency (11–15%) in thyroid tumors. No predominance of mutations in critical codons (12,13 or 61) or in base substitution was reported. The frequency of *ras* mutations in papillary thyroid tumors is in general lower than in follicular tumors and varies from 0 to 60% in different series (6,25,35,52,62). In subsequent studies, controversial results were reported and a recent review found that the frequency of ras mutations was lower than initially reported: *ras* oncogene mutations were found more frequently in follicular carcinomas (34%) than in benign adenomas (19%), codon 61 being the most frequently involved; *ras* mutations are more rarely observed in other types of thyroid tumors, being present in 11% of papillary thyroid cancers (58).

The tumorigenic role of the *ras* gene in the thyroid has been studied in normal follicular cells transfected with a mutated *ras* gene. Under such conditions, follicular cell proliferation is increased and the expression of differentiation markers such as thyroglobulin, thyroperoxidase and NIS is reduced or abolished. Transgenic mice, with *ras* gene expression targeted at thyroid cells, develop both thyroid hyperplasia and papillary thyroid cancer (44), and follicular adenoma or carcinoma (47), with a decline in the expression of differentiation markers. Mutated ras proteins stimulate cell division, inhibit cell differentiation and cause genomic instability and facilitate additional mutagenic events.

B-raf gene has been found to be activated by mutation in human cancers, in 66% of malignant melanomas and in less than 15% of colon carcinomas. In melanomas, 98% of the mutations are a missence thymine (T) to adenine (A) transversion at codon 1796, resulting in a valine to glutamate substitution at residue 599 (V599E). This mutation was found in 36% and 69% of papillary thyroid carcinomas but was not found in any of the other types of follicular cell derived tumors (8, 26). Moreover, there was no overlap with *ret*/PTC, *ras* and *b-raf* mutations. Thus, the frequent activation at various points of this pathway may be a key event in the pathogenesis of papillary thyroid carcinoma.

PAX8-PPARγ1 fusion gene

Cytogenetic studies of follicular carcinomas have evidenced abnormalities in chromosomes 2 and 3 (19), and the molecular basis for a chromosomal translocation t(2; 3)(q13; p25) was recently reported. The chromosome 2q13 breakpoint lies within the coding region of the thyroid transcription factor Pax8, and the 3p25 breakpoint within the coding region of PPARγ isoform 1 (27). Pax8 (Paired Box 8) is a transcription factor that plays a role in thyroid ontogenesis and in the expression of several thyroid specific genes. PPARγ (Peroxisome Proliferator-Activated Receptor gamma) is a transcription factor belonging to the hormone nuclear receptor family. Through dimerization with RXRα (Retinoid X Receptor alpha), PPARγ plays a role in the regulation of lipid metabolism, the inflammatory process, differentiation, the cell cycle and tumorigenesis. The fusion protein consists of PAX8 paired and homeobox binding domains, and PPARγ1 DNA binding, ligand binding, dimerization, and transactivation domains. When the PAX8-PPARγ1 fusion gene was transfected to heterologous cells, it did not transactivate promoter constructs containing PPAR response elements, either alone or in the presence of troglitazone, the PPAR ligand agonist. The fusion construct did however prevent wild-type PPARγ1–mediated transactivation, indicating that it may have a dominant negative effect. This negative effect may inhibit terminal differentiation and growth suppression induced by PPARγ agonists.

The PAX8-PPARγ1 translocation was found in 26%–63% of follicular carcinomas and in 8–13% of follicular adenomas. It was not found in normal thyroid tissues, nor in nodular hyperplasia, papillary, Hürthle cell and anaplastic carcinomas (27,30,38,39).

In one series of follicular carcinomas, 86% revealed either ras (58%) or PPARγ1/PAX8 (30%) mutations, and there was no overlap between these two mutations. PPARγ1/PAX8 rearrangement was almost exclusively found in follicular carcinomas that occurred at a younger age, that were small and widely invasive; in contrast, *ras* mutations occurred with a similar frequency in both adenomas and follicular carcinomas; these carcinomas occurred at an older age, were larger and were less invasive. All these data suggest two different pathways in follicular tumorigenesis (39).

The PAX8-PPARγ1 translocation is associated with PPARγ1 protein overexpression. PPARγ1 expression is downregulated in some thyroid carcinomas (1) and is overexpressed in some tumors without a detectable PAX8-PPARγ1 translocation, which suggests that PPARγ may have other translocation partners. Indeed, a novel gene, located at 7q34 and provisionally named FTCF (follicular thyroid carcinoma fusion) was recently detected fused to the 5′ region (exons1–6) of the PPARγ1 gene, leading to expression of a FTCF-PPARγ1 fusion transcript and fusion protein.

Defects in the TSH stimulation pathway: TSH-receptor gene and *gsp* oncogene mutations

TSH stimulates follicular cell proliferation and differentiation by binding to a membrane receptor, the TSH-receptor (TSH-R). The TSH-R belongs to the receptor family with 7 transmembrane domains coupled to G proteins. These are heterotrimeric proteins, composed of three sub-units, α, β and γ. Binding of TSH to its receptor stimulates the enzyme adenylate-cyclase, through interaction with a Gs protein, that in turn increases the intra-cellular concentration of cAMP. This acts as a second messenger stimulating protein kinase A (PKA). Activated PKA phosphorylates different target proteins and particularly, the cAMP-responsive transcription factor (cAMP responsive element binding protein, or CREB) in the nucleus. Other pathways may be involved in the intra-cellular transduction of the message.

Several point mutations activating the TSH-R have been described in toxic adenomas with wide variations in frequency (from 10% to more than 80%) between the different series. Such differences may be explained by geographical variations, patient selection but also because different regions of the TSH-R were studied. Most activating mutations are found within or near the third intra-cellular loop, a region implicated in the interaction with the Gs protein. Transfection experiments have shown that the mutated TSH-R is constitutively activated, but differences exist between different mutations in terms of the extent of the increase in basal cAMP, the activation of signal transmission and response to TSH stimulation (57).

Activating point mutations in one of the 2 critical codons of the α subunit of the Gs protein gene (then called *gsp*) have been found in 7 to 38% of toxic adenomas (46, 57). As a result, mutations were found in these 2 genes in 40–60% of hyperfunctioning adenomas. It may be hypothesized that in negative tumors, alterations in another gene participating in the cAMP pathway may be responsible for the phenotype. Activating mutations of the TSH-R have also been found in the rare hyperfunctioning follicular carcinomas with high radioiodine uptake and thyrotoxicosis (45).

In transgenic mice, gsp and TSH-R activating mutations have been demonstrated to play a role in the development of hyperfunctioning thyroid tissue. The expression of an A2 adenosine receptor gene (equivalent to TSH-R) in thyroid tissue induces diffuse thyroid hyperplasia and early hyperthyroidism (57). The expression of gsp in thyroid tissue induces focal hyperfunctioning, that is equivalent to that of a human hyperfunctioning nodule with late hyperthyroidism (33).

Activating mutations of gsp and TSH-R have also been found in hypofunctioning benign and malignant follicular thyroid tumors but at a low frequency (<10%) (45,51). In follicular thyroid carcinomas they are restricted to a subset of tumors with high basal adenylate cyclase activity. These data suggest that gsp and TSH-R mutations may participate in the tumorigenesis of some hypofunctioning thyroid tumors, by conferring a growth advantage to a cellular clone in which another yet unknown genetic alteration has already abrogated the growth-limiting mechanism, which normally down-regulates the response to cAMP (53).

Tumor suppressor genes and other genetic abnormalities

Tumor suppressor genes code for proteins that normally inhibit or restrict cell division. They become tumorigenic through loss of function and tend to act in a recessive manner. One allele is usually lost as part of a large deletion of chromosomal material, while the other allele is inactivated by a point mutation.

No genomic abnormalities were found in *Rb*, the retinoblastoma gene. However, transgenic mice with thyroid specific expression of a human papilloma virus, type E7, develop nodular goiter and subsequently papillary and follicular thyroid carcinomas (28). This protein can functionally inactivate the Rb protein, suggesting that the latter acts in the negative control of cell proliferation (14,53).

A high frequency of inactivating point mutations (22 to 83%) in the *p53* gene were observed in anaplastic but not in differentiated thyroid carcinomas (10,13,23). These data suggest that inactivation of the *p53* gene may be a key event in progression from differentiated to anaplastic carcinoma and that this alters cell differentiation. Conversely, the bcl2 protein is expressed in differentiated thyroid carcinomas but is absent in anaplastic tumors (41).

Mutations in the adenomatous polyposis colonic (*APC*) gene probably contribute to the development of thyroid cancer seen in familial adenomatous polyposis, but linkage analysis excluded the APC gene as a rare susceptibility gene for familial papillary thyroid carcinoma.

Germline inactivating mutations in the *PTEN* gene are found in 80% of patients with in Cowden's disease (multiple hamartomas, breast and follicular thyroid tumors) (12). If no hamartomas are present, *PTEN* germline mutations are found in only 5% of the families with breast and thyroid tumors. PTEN, the phosphatase and tensin homolog gene is an inhibitor of Akt1, a critical intermediary in several Phosphatidyl Inositol 3 (PI3) kinase signaling transduction pathway. In sporadic follicular thyroid carcinoma, mutations are rare but *PTEN* gene expression is decreased and expression and phosphorylation of Akt are increased and this may be involved in follicular pathogenesis (43).

Linkage studies have permitted chromosomal mapping of at least 3 syndromes with a preponderance of familial PTC (29). A syndrome of familial PTC together with papillary renal neoplasia has been mapped to 1q21. This syndrome is clinically and genetically distinct from other familial tumor syndromes and is not a variant of familial papillary renal carcinoma caused by inherited activating mutations of the *MET* protooncogene. A familial syndrome characterized by PTC alone has been mapped to 2q21. Two different studies reported genetic linkage to 19p13.2 of a large kindred with different clinical features: in one family all thyroid tumors were oxyphilic (TCO) and many were benign; in the other one no oxyphilic changes were found and all tumors were PTC.

There are also a number of familial disorders potentially related to familial PTC, including familial goiter syndromes, one syndrome located at 14q and another at Xp22. Finally, thyroid nodules may be associated with either hypothyroidism or hyperthyroidism when gene mutations are components of pathways of thyroid metabolism or its regulation.

Loss of genetic sequences has been described in the long arm of chromosome 11 (11q13) in sporadic follicular thyroid tumors and, as described above in the short arm of chromosome 3, but only in follicular carcinomas (19,40).

Simian virus 40 (SV40) large T antigen (Tag) sequences have been detected in several human tumors, and are believed to be the result of SV40 infections. The presence of the Tag region of SV40 has been demonstrated in 66% of papillary thyroid cancer and in 100% of anaplastic thyroid cancer, as well as in normal thyroid tissue adjacent to these tumors (60). The high prevalence of SV40 footprints has been interpreted as a possible participation of this oncogenic virus in the onset/progression of specific thyroid carcinomas. Further studies are needed to understand the role of this finding in thyroid tumorigenesis.

RADIATION-ASSOCIATED THYROID TUMORS

The thyroid gland is highly sensitive to radiation during childhood, the excess relative risk per Gray being 7.7, and 88% of thyroid cancers occurring in these subjects being attributable to radiation. The irradiated thyroid gland is thus an adequate model for the study of radiocarcinogenesis

Genetic predisposition

Several epidemiological studies have suggested a familial predisposition to developing a thyroid carcinoma after irradiation. Firstly, approximately 3–5% of patients with thyroid cancer, without previous exposure to radiation, have a familial history of the same disease (29). Secondly, when both individuals in sibling pairs were irradiated, the occurrence of thyroid tumors was concordant more often than would have been expected by chance. Thirdly, patients with one radiation-induced tumor (thyroid, salivary, neural, parathyroid) are more likely to develop another tumor than patients with comparable risk factors but who had never had a tumor. This predisposition may be related to a defect in DNA repair mechanisms, but lifestyle risk factors may also explain some of these epidemiological findings.

Age at exposure

Epidemiological studies have shown that the carcinogenic effects of radiation are maximal during early childhood and then decrease rapidly with increasing age. This has been linked to the growth rate of the thyroid gland. Carcinogenesis is a multi-step process, and after the occurrence of a genetic abnormality, several cell divisions are needed for lesions to accumulate and for clonal expansion.

Indeed, a number of experiments in rats have shown that after thyroid exposure to radiation, the risk of developing a thyroid tumor is increased when cell proliferation is stimulated (administration of goitrogens, high or low iodine diet, partial thyroidectomy, TSH stimulation) and decreased when cell proliferation is decreased (hypophysectomy, administration of L-thyroxine). In a recent study in rats, high and low iodine diet both increase proliferation, and both induced thyroid adenomas but no thyroid malignancies occurred. Thus both a mutagenic event (radiation exposure) and increased proliferation rate are needed for the occurrence of thyroid carcinoma (2).

Ionising radiation is less carcinogenic in adults, in whom growth has already been completed: during adulthood, thyroid cell replication rarely occurs (doubling time: 8 years). In contrast, in children thyroid cells are in the process of active replication and this could allow intracellular accumulation of abnormalities that heighten the likelihood of an emerging abnormal clone of transformed cells.

Genetic abnormalities in radiation-associated thyroid tumors

Irradiation of the thyroid may directly induce *ret*/PTC rearrangements. This was found to be the case when *ret*/PTC rearrangements were induced in a dose-dependent fashion after *in vitro* irradiation of human cell lines of undifferentiated thyroid cancer (22). Chromosomal loci involved in the *ret*/PTC1 rearrangement (i.e. *ret* and H4) are juxtaposed during the interphase in normal human thyroid cells, providing a target for radiation to induce simultaneous double-stranded DNA breaks that lead to erroneous nonhomologous recombination via end-joining (37).

Ret/PTC rearrangements were found in 55–85% of papillary thyroid carcinomas that developed in children who had been exposed to external radiation or contaminated during the Chernobyl accident (4,11,15,21,42,56,61). In both cases, intrachromosomal rearrangements (*ret*/PTC1&3) were predominant. However, in papillary thyroid carcinomas that emerged early after the Chernobyl accident, the *ret*/PTC3 form was more frequently observed and was associated with a solid growth pattern and a more aggressive phenotype (56). In contrast, in papillary thyroid carcinoma occurring either after external irradiation or more than 10 years after the Chernobyl accident, *ret*/PTC1 was the predominant form and was associated with a less aggressive phenotype (classical papillary thyroid carcinoma and diffuse sclerosing variant). *Ret*/PTC rearrangements were also found in 11–45% of thyroid adenomas that occurred after external irradiation during childhood, and in 52% following exposure in Chernobyl (6,11).

Trk rearrangements were found at a similar low frequency in spontaneous and radiation-associated papillary thyroid carcinomas (3,5,42).

Activating mutations in the *ras* genes have been found in thyroid tumors from patients with a history of external irradiation, at a frequency similar to that observed in apparently spontaneous tumors (6). In contrast, in tumors that developed in children after the Chernobyl accident, *ras* point mutations were found in 25% of the follicular tumors but not in papillary thyroid carcinomas (36,61). In spontaneous thyroid tumors, transversions (a base change from purine to pyrimidine or vice-versa) as well as transitions (a base change from purine to purine or pyrimidine to pyrimidine) were detected in the *ras* genes. In radiation-associated tumors, only transversions were present (6). The exact mechanism of these mutations remains to be determined, but it can be postulated that they arise through an ionizing radiation-induced oxidative lesion, producing 8-OXO-dG which can pair with adenosine during DNA replication (6,53).

The frequency of activating point mutations in the Gαs and TSH-R genes is low (<10%) in tumors occurring either after external irradiation during childhood and after the Chernobyl accident (6). *P53* gene mutations have been detected in a few papillary thyroid carcinomas occurring after external irradiation during childhood and after the Chernobyl accident. These mutations may explain the aggressiveness of some of these tumors (36).

From these data, it can be postulated that radiation may directly lead to DNA strand breaks and *ret* activation through gene rearrangements. The precise nature of possible secondary genetic events resulting in further progression is unknown.

CONCLUSION

Several conclusions can be drawn from the study of oncogenes and tumor suppressor genes in human thyroid tumors (Table 1):

Alterations of membrane tyrosine kinase receptors (*ret*/PTC, *trk*, *met*) are observed only in papillary thyroid carcinomas; the higher frequency of *ret*/PTC rearrangements in radiation-associated papillary thyroid carcinoma and also their discovery in radiation-associated follicular adenomas suggest that they may be directly induced by radiation exposure. *Met* overexpression may be a secondary event.

Activating point mutations of the *ras* genes are found in 11% of papillary thyroid carcinomas. *B-raf* mutations were found in 36% and 69%, with no overlap between *ret*/PTC, *ras* and *b-raf* mutations. The activation of this pathway is frequently observed in papillary thyroid carcinomas and may play a determining role in their pathogenesis.

Ras mutations are found in 20% of benign and in 30% of malignant follicular thyroid tumors. *B-raf* mutations were not found in these tumors. Other genetic abnormalities that may be facilitated by genetic instability induced by *ras* mutations are needed for tumor progression and to determine the histological type of the thyroid tumor.

PPARγ1/PAX8 translocations were found in malignant and benign follicular tumors. In one series of follicular carcinomas, 86% revealed either *ras* or PPARγ1/PAX8 mutations. However, there was no overlap between these two mutations and phenotypes associated with each of these mutations were different, suggesting two different pathways in follicular tumorigenesis.

Table 1. Frequencies (%) of genetic alterations in hypofunctioning thyroid tumors, in the absence of previous neck irradiation.

	Papillary carcinoma	Follicular adenoma	Follicular carcinoma	Anaplastic carcinoma
Tyrosine kinase receptors:				
ret/PTC rearrangement	2.5–35	rare	rare	rare
trk rearrangement	0–15	rare	rare	rare
met overexpression	50–70	rare	rare	rare
Intra-cellular signaling pathway:				
ras point mutation	11	19	34	<40
b-raf point mutation	36–69			
PPARγ-PAX8 rearrangement	NR	8–13	26–63	NR
TSH stimulation pathway:				
TSH-R mutation	rare	<10	<10	rare
gsp	rare	<10	<10	rare
p53 mutations	rare	rare	rare	25 – >80

P53 mutations are observed only in poorly-differentiated or anaplastic thyroid cancers; they play a determining role in progression from differentiated to undifferentiated thyroid carcinomas and in the dedifferentiation process.

TSH-R and Gαs activating point mutations are found in about 60% of hyperfunctioning adenomas; their role in the pathogenesis of hypofunctioning thyroid tumors has not been confirmed.

Several growth factors are overexpressed in thyroid tumors. Paracrine factors such as Fibroblast Growth Factor (FGF1 and 2) are mitogens for thyrocytes, and Vascular Endothelial Cell Growth Factor (VEGF) may play a determining role in tumor neovascularisation. Other growth factors may also play a role, such as insulin like growth factor–1 (IGF1), Epidermal Growth Factor or TGFα. Overexpression of these growth factors is believed to be secondary to other oncogenic events.

Other abnormalities may also play a role in thyroid tumorigenesis. DNA methylation is frequently abnormal in thyroid tumors and this may modify gene functions (31). The status of telomerase may be modified: follicular adenomas are telomerase-negative, and about half of papillary and follicular carcinomas are telomerase-positive. Some telomerase-negative cancers maintain telomere length by a mechanism independent of telomerase (32). Other genetic abnormalities may also exist, and deletions have been demonstrated in follicular tumors, possibly indicating the location of yet unknown tumor suppressor genes.

These data may suggest a scheme for epithelial thyroid tumorigenesis. Ongoing studies of the transcriptome and proteome will rapidly increase our knowledge in the field.

REFERENCES

1. Aldred MA, Morrison C, Gimm O, Hoang-Vu C, Krause U, Dralle H, Jhiang S, Eng C. Peroxisome proliferation-activated receptor gamma is frequently downregulated in a diversity of sporadic nonmedullary thyroid carcinomas. Oncogene 2003; 22: 3412–3416.

2. Boltze C, Brabant G, Dralle H, Gerlach R, Roessner A, Hoang-Vu C. Radiation-induced thyroid carcinogenesis as a function of time and dietary iodine supply: an in vivo model of tumorigenesis in the rat. Endocinology 2002; 143: 2584–2592.
3. Bongarzone I, Fugazzola L, Vigneri P, Mariani L, Mondellini P, Pacini F, Basolo F, Pinchera A, Pilotti S, Pierotti MA. Age-related activation of the tyrosine kinase receptor proto-oncogenes ret and ntrk 1 in papillary thyroid carcinoma. J Clin Endocrinol Metab 1996; 81: 2006–2009.
4. Bounacer A, Wicker R, Caillou B, Cailleux AF, Sarasin A, Schlumberger M, Suarez HG. High prevalence of activating ret proto-oncogene rearrangements in thyroid tumors from patients who had received external radiation. Oncogene. 1997; 15: 1263–73.
5. Bounacer A, Schlumberger M, Wicker R, Du Villard JA, Caillou B, Sarasin A, Suarez HG. Search for NTRK1 proto-oncogene rearrangements in human thyroid tumours originated after therapeutic radiation. Br J Cancer. 2000; 82: 308–14.
6. Challeton C, Bounacer A, Duvillard JA, Caillou B, De Vathaire F, Monier R, Schlumberger M, Suarez HG. Pattern of ras and gsp oncogene mutations in radiation-associated human thyroid tumors. Oncogene 1995; 11: 601–603.
7. Cheung CC, Ezzat S, Ramyar L, Freeman JI, Asa SI. Molecular basis of Hürthle cell papillary thyroid carcinoma. J Clin Endocrinol Metab 2000; 85:878–882.
8. Cohen Y, Xing M, Mambo E, Guo Z, Wu G, Trink B, Beller U, Westra WH, Ladenson PW, Sidransky D. BRAF mutation in papillary thyroid carcinoma. J Natl Cancer Inst 2003; 95: 625–627.
9. Di Renzo MF, Olivero M, Ferro S, Prat M, Bongarzone I, Pilotti S, Belfiore A, Constantino A, Vigneri R, Pierotti MA, Comoglio PM. Overexpression of the c-Met/HGF receptor gene in human thyroid carcinomas. Oncogene 1992; 7: 2549–2553.
10. Donghi R, Longoni A, Pilotti S, Michieli P, Della Porta G, Pierotti MA. Gene p53 mutations are restricted to poorly differentiated and undifferentiated carcinomas of the thyroid gland. J Clin Invest 1993; 91: 1753–1760.
11. Elisei R, Romei C, Vorontsova T, Cosci B, Veremeychik V, Kuchinskaya E, Basolo F, Demidchik EP, Miccoli P, Pinchera A, Pacini F. RET/PTC rearrangements in thyroid nodules: studies in irradiated and not irradiated malignant and benign thyroid lesions in children and adults. J Clin Endocrinol Metab 2000; 86: 3211–3216.
12. Eng C. Will the real Cowden syndrome please stand up: revised diagnostic criteria. J Med Genet 2000; 37: 828–830.
13. Fagin JA, Matsuo K, Karmakar A, Chen DI, Tang SH, Koeffler HP. High prevalence of mutations of the p53 gene in poorly differentiated human thyroid carcinoma. J Clin Invest 1993; 91: 179–184.
14. Fagin JA. Molecular genetics of tumors of thyroid follicular cells. In The Thyroid Eighth Edition. Braverman LE, Utiger RD, Eds. Lippincott, Williams and Wilkins, Philadelphia 2000, pp. 886–898.
15. Fugazzola L, Pilotti S, Pinchera A, Vorontsova TV, Mondellini P, Bongarzone I, Greco A, Astakhova L, Butti MG, Demidchik EP, Pacini F, Pierotti MA. Oncogenic rearrangements of the RET proto-oncogene in papillary thyroid carcinomas from children exposed to the Chernobyl nuclear accident. Cancer Res 1995; 55: 5617–5620.
16. Fusco A, Grieco M, Santoro M, Berlingieri MT, Di Fiore PP, Pilotti S, Pierotti MA, Della Porta G, Vecchio G. A new oncogene in human papillary carcinomas and their lymphnodal metastases. Nature 1987; 328: 170–172.
17. Greco A, Pierotti MA, Bongarzone I, Pagliardini S, Lanzi C, Della Porta G. Trk-T1 is a novel oncogene formed by the fusion of tpr and trk genes in human papillary thyroid carcinomas. Oncogene 1992; 7: 237–242.
18. Grieco M, Santoro M, Berlingieri MT, Melillo RM, Donghi R, Bongarzone I, Pierotti MA, Della Porta G, Fusco A, Vecchio G. PTC is a novel rearranged form of the ret proto-oncogene and is frequently detected in vivo in human thyroid papillary carcinoma. Cell 1990; 60: 557–563.
19. Herrmann MA, Hay ID, Bartelt JDH, Ritland SR, Dahl RJ, Grant CS, Jenkins RB. Cytogenetic and molecular genetic studies of follicular and papillary thyroid cancers. J Clin Invest 1991; 88: 1596–1604.
20. Ishizaka Y, Kobayashi S, Ushijima T, Hirohaschi S, Sugimura T, Nagao M. Detection of RET/PTC transcripts in thyroid adenomas and adenomatous goiter by an RT-PCR method. Oncogene 1991; 6: 1667–1672.
21. Ito T, Seyama T, Iwamoto KS, Mizuno T, Tronko ND, Komissarenko IV, Cherstovoy ED, Satow Y, Takeichi N, Dohi K, Akiyama M. Activated RET oncogene in thyroid cancers of children from areas contaminated by Chernobyl accident. Lancet 1994; 344: 259.
22. Ito T, Semaya T, Iwamoto KS, Hayashi T, Mizuno T, Tsuyama N, Dohi K, Nakamura N, Akiyama M. In vitro irradiation is able to cause RET oncogene rearrangement. Cancer Res 1993; 53: 2940–2943.

23. Ito T, Seyama T, Mizuno T, Tsuyama N, Hayashi T, Hayashi Y, Dohi K, Nakamura N, Akiyama M. Unique association of p53 mutations with undifferentiated but not with differentiated carcinomas of the thyroid gland. Cancer Res 1992; 52: 1369–1371.
24. Jhiang SM, Sagartz JE, Tong Q, Parker-Thornburg J, Capen CC, Cho JY, Xing S, Ledent C. Targeted expression of the RET/PTC 1 oncogene induces papillary thyroid carcinomas. Endocrinology 1996; 137: 375–378.
25. Karga H, Lee JK, Vickery AL, Thor A, Gaz RD, Jameson JL. Ras oncogene mutations in benign and malignant thyroid neoplasms. J Clin Endocrinol Metab 1991; 73: 832–836.
26. Kimura ET, Nikiforova MN, Zhu Z, Knauf JA, Nikiforov YE, Fagin JA. High prevalence of BRAF mutations in thyroid cancer: genetic evidence for constitutive activation of the ret/PTC-RAS-BRAF signaling pathway in papillary thyroid carcinoma. Cancer Res 2003; 63: 1454–1457.
27. Kroll TG, Sarraf P, Pecciarini L, Chen CJ, Mueller E, Spiegelman BM, Fletcher JA. PAX8-PPARγ1 fusion oncogene in human thyroid carcinoma. Science 2000; 289: 1357–60.
28. Ledent C, Marcotte A, Dumont JE, Vassart G, Parmentier M. Differentiated carcinomas develop as a consequence of the thyroid specific expression of a thyroglobulin-human papillomavirus type 16 E7 transgene. Oncogene 1995; 10: 1789–1797.
29. Malchoff CD, Malchoff DM. The genetics of hereditary nonmedullary thyroid carcinoma. J Clin Endocrinol Metab 2002; 87: 2455–2459.
30. Marques AR, Espadinha C, Catarino AL, Moniz S, Pereira T, Sobrinho LG, Leite V. Expression of PAX8-PPAR gamma 1 rearrangements in both follicular thyroid carcinomas and adenomas. J Clin Endocrinol Metab 2002; 87: 3947–52.
31. Matsuo K, Tang SH, Zeki K, Gutman RA, Fagin JA. Aberrant DNA methylation in human thyroid tumors. J Clin Endocrinol Metab 1993; 77: 991–995.
32. Matthews P, Jones CJ, Skinner J, Haughton M, de Micco C, Wynford-Thomas D. Telomerase activity and telomere length in thyroid neoplasia: biological and clinical implications. J pathol 2001; 194: 183–193.
33. Michiels FM, Caillou B, Talbot M, Dessarps-Freichey F, Maunoury MT, Schlumberger M, Mercken L, Monier R. Oncogenic potential of guanine nucleotide stimulatory factor alpha subunit in thyroid glands of transgenic mice. Proc Natl Acad Sci USA 1994; 91: 10488–10492.
34. Namba H, Matsuo K, Fagin JA. Clonal composition of benign and malignant human thyroid tumors. J Clin Invest 1990; 86: 120–125.
35. Namba H, Rubin SA, Fagin JA. Point mutations of ras oncogenes are an early event in thyroid tumorigenesis. Mol Endocrinol 1990; 4: 1474–1479.
36. Nikiforov YE, Nikiforova MN, Gnepp DR, Fagin JA. Prevalence of mutations of ras and p53 in benign and malignant thyroid tumors from children exposed to radiation after the Chernobyl nuclear accident. Oncogene 1996; 13: 687–693.
37. Nikiforova MN, Stringer JR, Blough R, Medvedovic M, Fagin JA, Nikiforov YE. Proximity of chromosomal loci that participate in radiation-induced rearrangements in human cells. Science 2000; 290: 138–141.
38. Nikiforova MN, Biddinger PW, Caudill CM, Kroll TG, Nikiforov YE. PAX8-PPAR gamma rearrangement in thyroid tumors: RT-PCR and immunohistochemical analyses. Am J Surg Pathol. 2002; 26 : 1016–23.
39. Nikiforova MN, Lynch RA, Biddinger PW, Alexander EK, Dorn II GW, Tallini G, Kroll TG, Nikiforov YE. Ras point mutation and PAX8-PPARγ rearrangement in thyroid tumors: evidence for distinct molecular pathways in thyroid follicular carcinoma. J Clin Endocrinol Metab 2003; 88: 2318–2326.
40. Pierotti MA, Bongarzone I, Borrello MG, Greco A, Pilotti S, Sozzi G. Cytogenetics and molecular genetics of carcinomas arising from thyroid epithelial follicular cells. Genes Chromosom Cancer 1996;16: 1–14.
41. Pollina L, Pacini F, Fontanini G, Vignati S, Bevilacqua G, Basolo F. Bcl2, p53 and proliferating cell nuclear antigen expression is related to the degree of differentiation in thyroid carcinomas. Br J Cancer 1996; 73: 139–143.
42. Rabes HM, Demidchik EP, Sidorow JD, Lengfelder E, Beimfohr C, Hoelzel D, Klugbauer S. Pattern of radiation-induced RET and NTRK1 rearrangements in 191 post-Chernobyl papillary thyroid carcinomas: biological, phenotypic and clinical implications. Clin Cancer Res 2000; 6: 1093–1103.
43. Ringel MD, Hayre N, Saito J, Saunier B, Schuppert F, Burch H, Bernet V, Burman KD, Kohn LD, Saji M. Overexpression and overactivation of Akt in thyroid carcinoma. Cancer Res 2001;61: 6105–6111.

44. Rochefort P, Caillou B, Michiels FM, Ledent C, Talbot M, Schlumberger M, Lavelle F, Monier R, Feunteun J. Thyroid pathologies in transgenic mice expressing a human activated RAS gene driven by a thyroglobulin promoter. Oncogene 1996; 12: 111–118.
45. Russo D, Arturi F, Schlumberger M, Caillou B, Monier R, Filetti S, Suarez HG. Activating mutations of the TSH receptor in differentiated thyroid carcinomas. Oncogene 1995; 11: 1907–1911.
46. Russo D, Arturi F, Wicker R, Chazenbalck GD, Schlumberger M, Dugas Duvillard JA, Caillou B, Monier R, Rapoport B, Filetti S, Suarez HG. Genetic alterations in thyroid hyperfunctioning adenomas. J Clin Endocrinol Metab 1995; 80: 1347–1351.
47. Santelli G, De Franciscis V, Portella G, Chiappetta G, D'Alessio A, Califano D, Rosati R, Mineo A, Monaco C, Manzo G, Pozzi L, Vecchio G. Production of transgenic mice expressing the Ki-ras oncogene under the control of a thyroglobulin promoter. Cancer Res 1993; 53: 5523–5527.
48. Santoro M, Carlomagno F, Hay ID, Herrmann MA, Grieco M, Melillo R, Pierotti MA, Bongarzone I, Della Porta G, Berger N, Peix JL, Paulin C, Fabien N, Vecchio G, Jenkins RB, Fusco A. Ret oncogene activation in human thyroid neoplasms is restricted to the papillary cancer sub-type. J Clin Invest 1992; 89: 1517–1522.
49. Santoro M, Chiappetta G, Cerrato A, Salvatore D, Zhang L, Manzo G, Picone A, Portella G, Santelli G, Vecchio G, Fusco A. Development of thyroid papillary carcinomas secondary to tissue-specific expression of the RET/PTC 1 oncogene in transgenic mice. Oncogene 1996; 12: 1821–1826.
50. Santoro M, Papotti M, Chiappetta G, Garcia-Rostan G, Volante M, Johnson C, Camp RL, Pentimalli F, Monaco C, Herrero A, Carcangiu ML, Fusco A, Tallini G. RET activation and clinicopathologic features in poorly differentiated thyroid tumors. J Clin Endocrinol Metab 2002; 87: 370–379.
51. Suarez HG, Du Villard JA, Caillou B, Schlumberger M, Parmentier C, Monier R. gsp mutations in human thyroid tumours. Oncogene 1991; 6: 677–679.
52. Suarez HG, Du Villard JA, Severino M, Caillou B, Schlumberger M, Tubiana M, Parmentier C, Monier R. Presence of mutations in all three ras genes in human thyroid tumors. Oncogene 1990; 5: 565–570.
53. Suarez HG. Genetic alterations in human epithelial tumors. Clin Endocrinol 1998; 48: 531–546.
54. Sugg SL, Ezzat S, Rosen IB, Freeman JL, Asa SL. Distinct multiple RET/PTC gene rearrangements in multifocal papillary thyroid neoplasia. J Clin Endocrinol Metab 1998; 83: 4116–4122.
55. Tallini G, Santoro M, Helie M, Carlomogno F, Salvatore G, Chiapetta G, Carcangiu Ml, Fusco A. RET/PTC oncogene activation defines a subset of papillary thyroid carcinomas lacking evidence of progression to poorly differentiated or undifferentiated tumor phenotypes. Clin Cancer Res 1998; 4: 287–294.
56. Thomas GA, Bunnell H, Cook HA, Williams ED, Nerovnya A, Cherstvoy ED, Tronko ND, Bogdanona TI, Chiapetta G, Viglietto G, Pentimalli F, Salvatore G, Fusco A, Santoro M, Vecchio G. High prevalence of RET/PTC rearrangements in Ukrainian and Belarussian post-Chernobyl thyroid papillary carcinomas: a strong correlation between RET/PTC3 and the solid-follicular variant. J Clin Endocrinol Metab 1999; 84: 4232–4238.
57. Van Sande J, Parma J, Tonacchera M, Swillens S, Dumont J, Vassart G. Genetic basis of endocrine disease. Somatic and germline mutations of the TSH receptor gene in thyroid diseases. J Clin Endocrinol Metab 1995; 80: 2577–2585.
58. Vasko V, Ferrand M, Di Cristofaro J, Carayon P, Henry JF, De Micco C. Specific pattern of ras oncogene mutation in follicular thyroid tumors. J Clin Endocrinol Metab 2003, 88:2745–2752.
59. Viglietto G, Chiappetta G, Martinez-Tello FJ, Fukunaga FH, Tallini G, Rigoupoulou D, Visconti R, Mastro A, Santoro M, Fusco A. RET/PTC oncogene activation is an early event in thyroid carcinogenesis. Oncogene 1995; 11: 1207–1210.
60. Vivaldi A, Pacini F, Martini F, Iaccheri L, Pezzetti F, Elisei R, Pinchera A, Faviana P, Basolo F, Tognon M. Simian virus 40-like sequences from early and late regions in human thyroid tumors of different histotypes. J Clin Endocrinol Metab 2003; 88: 892–9.
61. Williams ED. Cancer after nuclear fallout: lessons from the Chernobyl accident. Nature Rev 2002; 2: 543–549.
62. Wright PA, Lemoine NR, Mayall ES, Wyllie FS, Hughes D, Williams ED, Wynford Thomas D. Papillary and follicular thyroid carcinomas show a different pattern of ras oncogene mutation. Br J Cancer 1989; 60: 576–577.

6. GROWTH FACTORS AND THEIR RECEPTORS IN THE GENESIS AND TREATMENT OF THYROID CANCER[1]

SHEREEN EZZAT

Department of Medicine, University of Toronto, and The Freeman Centre for Endocrine Oncology, Mount Sinai Hospital, Toronto, Ontario, Canada M5G-1X5

INTRODUCTION

The oncogenes and/or tumor suppressor genes that are implicated in the transformation and progression of the majority of thyroid neoplasms remain unknown. Mutations that have been identified in other human malignancies are restricted to a relatively small subset of thyroid neoplasms, if they are identified at all. It would appear that novel genetic alterations are implicated including the well-characterized ret/PTC rearrangements. Numerous factors have been shown to govern thyroid cell differentiation and proliferation. Indeed, increasing evidence suggests that many of these growth factors and their receptors can also be implicated in tumor cell progression in genetically transformed thyrocytes. The molecular mechanisms underlying dysregulated thyroid cell growth and their potential role in the tumorigenic pathway will be discussed.

GROWTH FACTORS AND RECEPTORS

Overview

Growth factors are polypeptides of several major families that regulate cell replication and functional differentiation by directly altering the expression of specific genes (1). They are considered to play an important role in the multistep pathway of tumorigenesis. A number of oncogene products are homologous to growth factors, their receptors,

---

[1] This work was supported in part by grants from the Canadian Institutes of Health Research (MT-14404).

or enzymes that participate in the mitogenic process. In several systems, growth factors have been shown to interact with specific membrane receptors in regulating cell growth and gene expression in an autocrine or paracrine manner. Some are known to affect hormone production and some are, in turn, modulated by hormones (2). A few have been identified in the thyroid where they are considered to play a physiological role in endocrine cell regulation (3;4).

Endocrine cells including thyrocytes are the site of both synthesis and action of growth factors. A number of growth factors have been identified in endocrine cells, including insulin-like growth factors-I and -II (IGF-I, IGF-II) (5;6), epidermal growth factor (EGF) (7;8), transforming growth factor-α (TGFα) (9–11), transforming growth factor-TGF-ß, platelet-derived growth factor (12;13) and basic fibroblast growth factor (bFGF; FGF-2) (14). Growing evidence suggests that human thyroid tumor cells produce multiple peptides that regulate their own function in vitro. The relative significance of these different growth factors in human thyroid neoplasia, however, remains to be established.

THE EPIDERMAL GROWTH FACTOR FAMILY

The EGF family of ligands includes EGF, TGF-α, amphiregulin, heparin-binding EGF-like growth factor (HB-EGF), and betacellulin (BTC) (15). An additional family of EGF-related agonists include neuregulins which include glial growth factors (GGFs), neu differentiation factors (NDFs)/heregulins, ligands for erbβ-3 and erbβ-4. It is still not very clear which specific subsets of erbB receptors become activated in response to each of these ligands.

Transforming growth factor-α

Transforming growth factor-α is expressed as a membrane-anchored protein (16) that may alter pituitary production of TSH as well as cell proliferation (17). TGFα is thought to mediate estrogen-induced cell proliferation in several tissues (18–20). Estrogen stimulation has been implicated in thyroid tumorigenesis most aptly in rodents using a number of synthetic estrogenic compounds. Using a two-stage thyroid tumorigenesis model, one week administration of N-bis(2-hydroxypropyl)nitrosamine, gonadectomized F344 rats of both sexes were implanted with fused pellets containing EB for 32 weeks (21). Thyroid gland weights were increased by EB pellet in a dose-dependent and increased the occurrence of thyroid proliferative lesions in male and female animals. These data provide suggestive evidence for the potential significance of this growth factor in thyroid tumorigenesis.

Epidermal growth factor and receptor (EGF; EGF-R)

The common receptor of EGF and TGF-α, EGF-R, is a 170-kD plasma membrane tyrosine kinase product of the protooncogene v-*erbβ*. EGF-R is over-expressed in several types of human cancers that correlate with tumor aggressiveness. In the thyroid, EGF promotes growth but may inhibit some functional parameters. The normal thyroid displays EGF and EGF-R staining that is variable, but largely cytoplasmic, for both EGF and EGF-R (4;8;22). Nuclear positivity for EGF and EGF-R has been described in both follicular adenomas and follicular carcinomas. In marked contrast, nuclear staining has been reported as almost absent in papillary carcinomas. The absence of nuclear EGF and EGF-R in papillary carcinomas would suggest that the role played by EGF in growth control differs between papillary carcinoma and follicular adenomas/carcinomas of the thyroid (23).

Interestingly, the compound ZD6474, a low molecular weight EGF tyrosine kinase inhibitor was recently shown to have enzymatic functions on RET-derived oncoproteins. This agent blocks the *in vivo* phosphorylation and signaling of the RET/PTC3 and RET/MEN2B oncoproteins and of an EGF-R/RET chimeric receptor. This inhibition was associated with morphological reversion and prevented the growth of human PTC cell lines that carry spontaneous RET/PTC1 rearrangements (24).

As mentioned previously, the EGF-R is one of four highly homologous tyrosine kinase receptors that include erbβ2/HER2/neu/p185, erbβ-3 (HER3), and erbβ-4 (HER4). Growing evidence in support of functional cross-talk between the different members of this receptor family is now well recognized (25). Ligand-induced stimulation can result in transphosphorylation of *neu* via EGF-R (25;26). Over-expression of a wild type EGF-R and heterocomplex formation with *neu* dramatically increases receptor autophosphorylation and binding of EGF (25;27).

Erb β-2/neu in thyroid neoplasia

The specific role of the erbβ-2 proto-oncogene in human carcinomas was investigated in human thyroid tumours including nodular hyperplasias, follicular carcinomas and papillary carcinomas (without and with tall-cell features, insular, or anaplastic de-differentiation). There was no evidence of DNA amplification of erbβ-2 gene itself. Furthermore, sequencing of the transmembrane domain revealed no activating point mutations of the of erbβ-2 gene. The level of mRNA expression, however, was variable with nearly a third of papillary carcinomas showing statistically significant elevated mRNA levels compared with corresponding normal thyroid tissue. These findings, however, did not correlate with other indicators of poor prognosis. Moreover, in contrast to the elevated mRNA levels in thyroid tumours, the level of protein staining correlated with the degree of differentiation. Normal and hyperplastic tissue being strongly positive and poorly differentiated tumours showing negative of erbβ-2 immunostaining. Thus, these studies indicate the absence of mutations or amplifications of the erbβ-2 gene in human thyroid tumours. Elevated erbβ-2 mRNA expression in some thyroid tumours was not associated with clinical features of poor prognosis. Nevertheless, the significance of the elevated mRNA levels remains unclear, as it did not result in protein overexpression. Instead, cytoplasmic erbβ-2 protein detection by immunohistochemistry appears to correlate with differentiation of human thyroid tumours and may be a feature of good prognosis. There does not appear to be a positive relationship between erbβ-2 expression and the well-characterized ret/PTC rearrangements indicating that the two events are likely to be mutually exclusive in genesis and action of these two putative thyroid oncogenes (28).

THE TRANSFORMING GROWTH FACTOR-β

Transforming growth factor (TGF)-β has been implicated in the regulation of normal and neoplastic cell function. TGF-β regulates the expression of various proteins, including p27Kip1 (p27), a cell cycle inhibitory protein. Enhancement of tumor cell growth and invasiveness by transforming growth factor-β (TGF-β) requires constitutive activation of the ras/MAPK pathway. How MEK activation by epidermal growth factor (EGF) influences the response of fully differentiated and growth-arrested thyroid epithelial cells in primary culture to TGF-β1 is not clear. The epithelial tightness was maintained after single stimulation with EGF or TGF-β1 for 48 hours. In contrast, co-stimulation abolished the trans-epithelial resistance and increased the paracellular flux of labeled inulin. Reduced levels of the tight junction proteins claudin-1 and occludin accompanied the loss of barrier function. N-cadherin, expressed only in few cells of untreated or single-stimulated cultures is increased and co-localizes with E-cadherin at adherens junctions. TGF-beta1 only partially inhibited EGF-induced Erk phosphorylation. The MEK inhibitor U0126 prevents Erk1/2 phosphorylation and abrogated the synergistic responses to TGF-β1 and EGF. These observations indicate that concomitant growth factor-induced MEK activation is necessary for TGF-β1 to convert normal thyroid epithelial cells to a mesenchymal phenotype providing evidence for the role of these growth factors in thyroid cell transdifferentiation.(29).

VASCULAR ENDOTHELIAL GROWTH FACTOR

Vascular endothelial growth factor (VEGF) also known as vascular permeability factor (VPG) exists in a number of isoforms in human and rodent tissues including VEGF206h/205r, VEGF189h/188r, VEGF165h/164r, VEGF145h/144r and VEGF121 that differ in their molecular masses and biological activities. The VEGF isoforms bind with two tyrosine-kinase receptors, KDR/flk-1 and flt-1. In addition, VEGF165 binds with co-receptor, neuropilin-1, which is expressed in human endothelial cells and several types of non-endothelial cells including solid tumors. Recent studies on the role of estrogen in the regulation of tumor angiogenesis demonstrated that this steroid induces neovascularization in parallel with early induction of VEGF and the VEGFR2- (flk-1/KDR) protein expression in both blood vessels and non-endothelial cells (30). Moreover, estrogen-induced rat pituitary tumors in Fisher 344 rats express higher VEGF164 and neuropilin-1 levels compared to control untreated rats (31). These findings suggest that over-expression of VEGF and its receptor (VEGFR-2) may play an important role in the early phases of estrogen induced tumor angiogenesis in some endocrine tissues.

FIBROBLAST GROWTH FACTORS & RECEPTORS

Fibroblast growth factors (FGFs)

Basic Fibroblast Growth Factor (now known as FGF-2) is one of an ever-expanding family of FGFs several of which possess mitogenic, angiogenic, and hormone regulatory functions (32). FGF-2 immunoreactivity was described originally in the non-hormone producing folliculo-stellate cells of the pituitary (33). In one mouse model, estrogen-induced tumorigenesis was associated with parallel increases in the expression of a pituitary tumor transforming gene (PTTG) as well as FGF-2 (33). In turn, both PTTG and FGF-2 have been shown to be increased in mRNA expression in papillary thyroid cancer that was also associated with lymph nodal invasion and distant metastasis. These findings were upheld even after consideration of other known prognostic factors such as age and gender of the patient and size and type of the tumor (34). Similarly, increased concentrations of FGF-2 in the serum of patients with differentiated papillary thyroid carcinoma has also been reported (35).

Fibroblast growth factor receptors (FGFRs)

There are 4 mammalian FGFR genes encoding a complex family of transmembrane receptor tyrosine kinases (RTKs) (36). Each prototypic receptor is composed of 3 immunoglobulin (Ig)-like extracellular domains, 2 of which are involved in ligand binding, a single transmembrane domain, a split tyrosine kinase, and a COOH-terminal tail with multiple autophosphorylation sites. Multiple forms of cell-bound or secreted receptors are produced by the same gene. Tissue-specific alternative splicing, variable polyadenylation sites and alternative initiation of translation result in truncated receptor forms (37;38). The first two extracellular loops of FGFR1 can be secreted as soluble circulating FGF binding proteins (39) but their physiological importance remains to be established. Different FGFRs can dimerize, so that truncated forms of FGFR1 block signalling through FGFR1, 2, and 3 (40).

Structural alterations of FGFRs may play a role in human tumorigenesis. FGFR1 is highly expressed in the brain (41) but the shorter (2 Ig-domain) form of FGFR1 is more abundant in some CNS glioblastomas (42). Anti-sense targeted interruption of FGFR1 reduces malignant melanoma cell proliferation and differentiation (43). FGFR2 exon switching has been observed to accompany prostate cell transformation (44).

The expression of FGF-2 and one of its receptors FGFR1 was recently compared in differentiated thyroid cancers, normal thyroids, multinodular goiters, and Graves' disease specimens. The investigators noted that FGF-2 was significantly over-expressed in thyroid carcinomas compared with normal thyroid tissue. More interestingly, increased FGF-2 mRNA expression was independently associated with lymph nodal invasion and distant metastasis at tumor presentation (34).

The biological relevance of the FGF signaling system in thyroid cell growth has been further hinted at from genetically altered mice. Mice deficient for FGFRR2-IIIb were generated by placing translational stop codons and an IRES-LacZ cassette into exon IIIb of FgfR2. Expression of the alternatively spliced receptor isoform, FgfR2-IIIc, is not affected in these mice. The FGFR2-IIIb deficient mice, however, show dysgenesis of several non-endocrine as well as endocrine tissues including the thyroid, adrenals, pancreas, and pituitary. These findings are particularly interesting in view of the fact that FGF ligand expression is not altered with normal FGF8, FGF10, Bmp4, and Msx1 in this animal model (45).

In contrast, gain-of-function mutations in the FGFR-3 gene have been described to result in inhibition of cartilaginous cell growth in the growth plate suggesting an important growth inhibitory signal for this receptor. RT-PCR examination confirmed the expression of this growth factor in papillary thyroid carcinomas. Over-expression of FGFR-3 was successful in specific binding of 125I-FGF-2. Growth rates of cells over-expressing FGFR-3, however, were similar to those of control cells (46). Cells over-expressing FGFR3 continued to grow beyond the density of control cells. These interesting findings suggest a role for FGFR3 in thyroid cancer cell adhesion and/or invasiveness.

The nerve growth factor family

NGF is a growth factor that generally results in anti-proliferative and anti-invasive effects in neuroendocrine tumors. NGF inhibits thyrocyte invasion and reverts the effect of retinoic acid in these cells. This effect is likely mediated by an increase in adhesion to the extracellular matrix proteins laminin and collagen IV and the inhibition of cell migration. NGF also induces expression of its receptor p75 NGF receptor. This receptor can be the subject of rearrangements. Indeed, the thyroid TRK oncogenes are generated by chromosomal rearrangements juxtaposing the neurotrophic tyrosine receptor kinase type 1 (NTRK1) tyrosine kinase domain to foreign activating sequences. TRK oncoproteins display a constitutive tyrosine kinase activity in NIH3T3 cells (47). The TRK oncoproteins' signal transduction involves several signal transducers activated by the NGF-stimulated NTRK1 receptor including fibroblast growth factor receptor substrate (FRS) FRS2 and FRS3, two related adapter proteins activated by fibroblast growth factor and NTRK1 receptors, in the signaling of the thyroid TRK-T1 and TRK-T3 oncogenes. FRS2 and FRS3 are recruited and activated by TRK-T1 and TRK-T3. Expression studies show different expression patterns of the FRS adapters in normal and tumor thyroid samples. FRS3 is expressed in both normal and thyroid tumor samples, whereas FRS2 is not expressed in normal thyroid but is differentially expressed in some tumors. These data are consistent with the notion that the FRS2 and FRS3 adapter proteins may have a role in thyroid carcinogenesis triggered by TRK oncogenes and provide the basis for a new dimension of pharmaco-therapeutic possibilities.

CONCLUSIONS

Thyroid tumors are common neoplasms that exhibit a wide range of biologic behavior. Numerous factors have been shown to govern thyrocyte proliferation. In particular, hormones and growth factors likely play a role as promoters of tumor cell growth in genetically transformed cells. In some instances enhanced growth factors and their receptors may serve as survival signals for neoplastic cells. In other instances, however, abnormal forms of growth factor receptors (such as members of the EGF-R/HER2/neu) may also be important in the early stages of cell transformation and chromosomal instability consistent with the clonal composition of thyroid neoplasms. More detailed structure/function studies of growth factor/receptor functional interactions in morphologically characterized thyroid nodules are required. It is anticipated that these studies will identify signaling patterns that will provide the basis for the development of more specific and effective pharmacotherapeutic agents.

REFERENCES

1. Rizzino A. Growth Factors. In: Kovacs K, Asa SL, editors. Functional Endocrine Pathology. Boston: Blackwell Scientific Publications Inc., 1991: 979–989.
2. Ezzat S. The role of hormones, growth factors and their receptors in pituitary tumorigenesis. Brain Pathol 2001; 11(3):356–370.
3. Asa SL, Ezzat S. The pathogenesis of pituitary tumours. Nat Rev Cancer 2002; 2(11):836–849.
4. van der Laan BFAM, Freeman JL, Asa SL. Expression of growth factors and growth factor receptors in normal and tumorous human thyroid tissues. Thyroid 1995; 5:67–73.
5. Minuto F, Barreca A, del Monte P, Cariola G, Torre GC, Giordano G. Immunoreactive insulin-like growth factor I (IGF-I) and IGF-I-binding protein content in human thyroid tissue. J Clin Endocrinol Metab 1989; 68:621–626.
6. Okimura Y, Kitajima N, Uchiyama T et al. Insulin-like growth factor I (IGF-I) production and the presence of IGF-I receptors in rat medullary thyroid carcinoma cell line 6-23 (clone 6). Biochem Biophys Res Commun 1989; 161:589–595.
7. Di Carlo A, Pisano G, Parmeggiani U, Beguinot L, Macchia V. Epidermal growth factor receptor and thyrotropin response in human thyroid tissues. J Endocrinol Invest 1990; 13:293–299.
8. Duh Q-Y, Gum ET, Gerend PL, Raper SE, Clark OH. Epidermal growth factor receptors in normal and neoplastic thyroid tissue. Surgery 1993; 98:1000–1007.
9. Grubeck-Loebenstein B, Buchan G, Sadeghi R et al. Transforming growth factor beta regulates thyroid growth. role in the pathogenesis of nontoxic goiter. J Clin Invest 1989; 83:764–770.
10. Aasland R, Akslen LA, Varhaug JE, Lillehaug JR. Co-expression of the genes encoding transforming growth factor-α and its receptor in papillary carcinomas of the thyroid. Int J Cancer 1990; 46:382–387.
11. Driman DK, Kobrin MS, Kudlow JE, Asa SL. Transforming growth factor-α in normal and neoplastic human endocrine tissues. Hum Pathol 1992; 23:1360–1365.
12. Heldin N-E, Gustavsson B, Claesson-Welsh L et al. Aberrant expression of receptors for platelet-derived growth factor in an anaplastic thyroid carcinoma cell line. Proc Natl Acad Sci USA 1993; 85:9302–9306.
13. Matsuo K, Tang S-H, Sharifi B, Rubin SA, Schreck R, Fagin JA. Growth factor production by human thyroid carcinoma cells: Abundant expression of a platelet-derived growth factor-β-like protein by a human papillary carcinoma cell line. J Clin Endocrinol Metab 1993; 77:996–1004.
14. Logan A, Gonzalez AM, Buscaglia ML, Black EG, Sheppard MC. Basic fibroblast growth factor is an autocrine factor for rat thyroid follicular cells. Ann NY Acad Sci 1991; 638:453–455.
15. Beerli RR, Hynes NE. Epidermal growth factor-related peptides activate distinct subsets of ErbB receptors and differ in their biological activities. J Biol Chem 1996; 271:6071–6076.
16. Ezzat S, Walpola IA, Ramyar L, Smyth HS, Asa SL. Membrane-anchored expression of transforming growth factor-α in human pituitary adenoma cells. J Clin Endocrinol Metab 1995; 80:534–539.
17. Fisher DA, Lakshmanan J. Metabolism and effects of epidermal growth factor and related growth factors in mammals. Endocr Rev 1990; 11:418–442.
18. Bates SE, Davidson NE, Valverius EM et al. Expression of transforming growth factor α and its messenger ribonucleic acid in human breast cancer: Its regulation by estrogen and its possible functional significance. Mol Endocrinol 1988; 2:543–555.
19. Liu SC, Sanfilippo B, Perroteau I, Derynck R, Salomon DS, Kidwell WR. Expression of transforming growth factor α (TGFα) in differentiated rat mammary tumors: estrogen induction of TGFα production. Mol Endocrinol 1987; 1:683–692.
20. Nelson KG, Takahashi T, Lee DC et al. Transforming growth factor-α is a potential medicator of estrogen action in the mouse uterus. Endocrinology 1992; 131:1657–1664.
21. Son HY, Nishikawa A, Kanki K et al. Synergistic interaction between excess caffeine and deficient iodine on the promotion of thyroid carcinogenesis in rats pretreated with N-bis(2-hydroxypropyl)nitrosamine. Cancer Sci 2003; 94(4):334–337.
22. Mäkinen T, Pekonen F, Franssila K, Lamberg B-A. Receptors for epidermal growth factor and thyrotropin in thyroid carcinoma. Acta Endocrinol (Copen) 1988; 117:45–50.

23. Marti U, Ruchti C, Kampf J et al. Nuclear localization of epidermal growth factor and epidermal growth factor receptors in human thyroid tissues. Thyroid 2001; 11(2):137–145.
24. Carlomagno F, Vitagliano D, Guida T et al. ZD6474, an orally available inhibitor of KDR tyrosine kinase activity, efficiently blocks oncogenic RET kinases. Cancer Res 2002; 62(24):7284–7290.
25. Qian X, LeVea CM, Freeman JK, Dougall WC, Greene MI. Heterodimerization of epidermal growth factor receptor and wild-type or kinase-deficient Neu: A mechanism of interreceptor kinase activation and transphosphorylation. Proc Natl Acad Sci USA 1994; 91:1500–1504.
26. Dougall WC, Quan X, Peterson NC, Miller MJ, Samanta A, Greene MI. The *neu*-oncogene: signal transduction pathways, transformation mechanisms and evolving therapies. Oncogene 1994; 9:2109–2123.
27. Goldman R, Levy RB, Peles E, Yarden Y. Heterodimerization of the erbB-1 and erbB-2 receptors in human breast carcinoma cells: A mechanism for receptor transregulation. Biochem J 1990; 29:11024–11028.
28. Sugg SL, Ezzat S, Zheng L, Freeman JL, Rosen IB, Asa SL. Oncogene profile of papillary thyroid carcinoma. Surgery 1999; 125:46-52.
29. Grande M, Franzen A, Karlsson JO, Ericson LE, Heldin NE, Nilsson M. Transforming growth factor-beta and epidermal growth factor synergistically stimulate epithelial to mesenchymal transition (EMT) through a MEK-dependent mechanism in primary cultured pig thyrocytes. J Cell Sci 2002; 115(Pt 22):4227–4236.
30. Banerjee SK, Sarkar DK, Weston AP, De A, Campbell DR. Over expression of vascular endothelial growth factor and its receptor during the development of estrogen-induced rat pituitary tumors may mediate estrogen-initiated tumor angiogenesis. Carcinogenesis 1997; 18(6):1155–1161.
31. Banerjee SK, Zoubine MN, Tran TM, Weston AP, Campbell DR. Overexpression of vascular endothelial growth factor164 and its co- receptor neuropilin-1 in estrogen-induced rat pituitary tumors and GH3 rat pituitary tumor cells. Int J Oncol 2000; 16(2):253–260.
32. Mason IJ. The ins and outs of fibroblast growth factors. Cell 1994; 78:547–552.
33. Gospodarowicz D, Ferrara N, Schweigerer L, Neufeld G. Structural characterization and biological functions of fibroblast growth factor. Endocr Rev 1987; 8:95–114.
34. Boelaert K, McCabe CJ, Tannahill LA et al. Pituitary tumor transforming gene and fibroblast growth factor-2 expression: potential prognostic indicators in differentiated thyroid cancer. J Clin Endocrinol Metab 2003; 88(5):2341–2347.
35. Komorowski J, Pasieka Z, Jankiewicz-Wika J, Stepien H. Matrix metalloproteinases, tissue inhibitors of matrix metalloproteinases and angiogenic cytokines in peripheral blood of patients with thyroid cancer. Thyroid 2002; 12(8):655–662.
36. Givol D, Yayon A. Complexity of FGF receptors: genetic basis for structural diversity and functional specificity. FASEB J 1992; 6(15):3362–3369.
37. Yan G, Wang F, Fukabori Y, Sussman D, Hou J, McKeehan WL. Expression and transformation of a variant of the heparin-binding fibroblast growth factor receptor (*flg*) gene resulting from splicing of the exon at alternate 3'-acceptor site. Biochem Biophys Res Commun 1992; 183:423–430.
38. Peters KG, Werner S, Chen G, Williams LT. Two FGF receptor genes are differentially expressed in epithelial and mesenchymal tissues during limb formation and organogenesis in the mouse. Develop 1992; 114:233–243.
39. Hanneken A, Ying W, Ling N, Baird A. Identification of soluble forms of the fibroblast growth factor receptor in blood. Proc Natl Acad Sci USA 1994; 91:9170 9174.
40. Werner S, Weinberg W, Liao X et al. Targeted expression of a dominant-negative FGF receptor mutant in the epidermis of transgenic mice reveals a role of FGF in keratinocyte organization and differentiation. EMBO J 1993; 12:2635–2643.
41. Gonzalez AM, Logan A, Ying W, Lappi DA, Berry M, Baird A. Fibroblast growth factor in the hypothalamic-pituitary axis: Differential expression of fibroblast growth factor-2 and a high affinity receptor. Endocrinology 1994; 134:2289–2297.
42. Eisemman A, Ahn AJ, Graziani G, Tronick SR, Ron D. Alternative splicing generates at least five different isoforms of the human bFGF receptor. Oncogene 1991; 6:1195–1202.
43. Becker D, Lee PLP, Rodeck U, Herlyn M. Inhibition of the fibroblast growth factor receptor 1 (FGFR-1) gene in human melanocytes and malignant melanomas leads to inhibition of proliferation and signs indicative of differentiation. Oncogene 1992; 7:2303–2313.
44. Yan G, Fukabori Y, McBride G, Nikolaropolous S, McKeehan WL. Exon switching and activation of stromal and embryonic fibroblast growth factor (FGF)-FGF receptor genes in prostate epithelial cells accompany stromal independence and malignancy. Mol Cell Biol 1993; 13:4513–4522.

45. Revest JM, Spencer-Dene B, Kerr K, De Moerlooze L, Rosewell I, Dickson C. Fibroblast growth factor receptor 2-IIIb acts upstream of Shh and Fgf4 and is required for limb bud maintenance but not for the induction of Fgf8, Fgf10, Msx1, or Bmp4. Dev Biol 2001; 231(1):47–62.
46. Onose H, Emoto N, Sugihara H, Shimizu K, Wakabayashi I. Overexpression of fibroblast growth factor receptor 3 in a human thyroid carcinoma cell line results in overgrowth of the confluent cultures. Eur J Endocrinol 1999; 140(2):169–173.
47. Ranzi V, Meakin SO, Miranda C, Mondellini P, Pierotti MA, Greco A. The signaling adapters fibroblast growth factor receptor substrate 2 and 3 are activated by the thyroid TRK oncoproteins. Endocrinology 2003; 144(3):922–928.

7. BIOLOGY OF RAS IN THYROID CELLS

JUDY L. MEINKOTH

Department of Pharmacology, University of Pennsylvania School of Medicine, Philadelphia, PA 19104

INTRODUCTION

Ras is an almost universal component of signaling pathways in vertebrates, invertebrates and yeast where it plays critical roles in development, proliferation, differentiation and survival. In the twenty years since the first identification of mutated Ras genes in human tumors, intensive effort has been devoted to understanding how Ras promotes neoplastic transformation. What has become clear is that Ras promotes transformation in multiple ways. The effects of Ras are diverse due to the significant complexity of Ras-mediated signaling pathways. Mammalian cells express multiple Ras proteins, which localize to discrete membrane microdomains and exhibit differential affinities towards downstream signaling molecules. The existence of a large number of Ras effectors, many of which are members of multi-gene families, together with extensive sites of crosstalk between Ras and other intracellular signaling pathways, further increases the complexity of Ras-mediated signaling.

Mutations in all three cellular Ras genes (H-, K- and N-Ras) have been identified in benign and malignant thyroid tumors. This has generated immense interest in elucidating the cellular consequences of Ras activation in thyroid cells. The recent discovery of B-Raf mutations in thyroid tumors reaffirms the important contribution of Ras-mediated signaling pathways to thyroid cell transformation. Interestingly, the effects of Ras in thyroid cells are unusual in several respects. Unlike primary fibroblasts where expression of activated Ras induces growth arrest, Ras stimulates proliferation in primary human thyrocytes. Recent data suggests that this may be a consequence of cell type specific effects on cell cycle regulatory proteins. Thyroid cells are one of few cellular models where proliferation is positively regulated by cAMP. As discussed below, crosstalk between cAMP and Ras markedly influences the signaling pathways activated by Ras. Indeed, TSH has been shown to modulate the effects of Ras on differentiation, proliferation and survival. The focus of this chapter is on the effects of Ras activation in thyroid cells, including the role of cellular Ras in TSH driven proliferation and the contribution of sustained Ras activity to thyroid cell transformation.

RAS REGULATION AND SIGNALING

Ras proteins are 21kDa GTP-binding proteins that function as molecular switches, cycling between active GTP- and inactive GDP-bound states. Cellular Ras activity is regulated by the opposing action of guanine nucleotide exchange factors (GEFs) that catalyze GDP dissociation, and GTPase activating proteins (GAPs) that stimulate intrinsic GTPase activity. Multiple RasGEFs and RasGAPs co-exist in most cells, increasing the diversity of signals that regulate Ras activity. Ras proteins are localized to the plasma membrane where they are poised to respond to signals initiated by the activation of cell surface receptors. Cellular Ras activity is maintained at very low levels. In response to signals such as those elicited by growth factors and hormones, Ras becomes activated in a transient manner. For cell surface receptors with tyrosine kinase activity, receptor dimerization induces tyrosine phosphorylation, thereby creating docking sites for signaling molecules such as Grb-2 and Shc, adaptor proteins comprised of SH2 and SH3 domains. Grb-2 is associated with the RasGEF SOS in the cytosol. Recruitment of Grb-2 to the activated receptor localizes SOS to the plasma membrane in close proximity to Ras, facilitating its activation. For G protein-coupled receptors, Ras is activated through second messengers such as diacylglycerol, calcium, and possibly cAMP (Busca et al., 2000; Pak et al., 2002), as well as through heterotrimeric G protein β/γ subunit- and src-mediated pathways.

In its active conformation, Ras binds to a variety of effectors. Effectors are defined as proteins that interact selectively with the GTP-bound form of Ras, and become activated as a consequence of this interaction. Three downstream effector pathways have been characterized in the most detail (Figure 1). They include members of the Raf, PI3K and RalGDS families (reviewed in Reuther et al., 2000; Shields et al.,

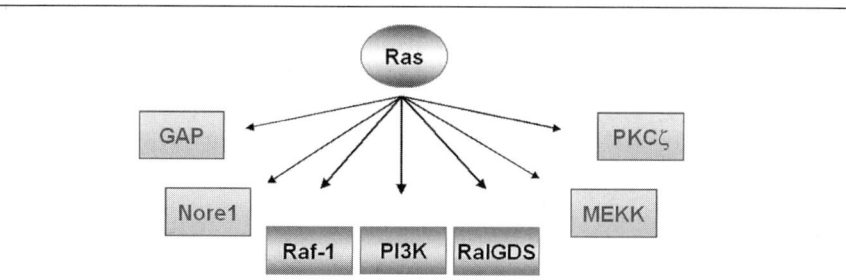

Figure 1. Ras signals through multiple downstream effectors including, but not limited to those illustrated here. In thyroid cells, Ras has been shown to signal through Raf-1, PI3K and RalGDS (shown in bold).

2000). Interaction between GTP-Ras and its first identified target, Raf-1, induces a conformational change that unmasks phosphorylation sites and anchors Raf-1 to the plasma membrane. Once this occurs, Raf-1 activity becomes Ras-independent. Active Raf binds to and phosphorylates MEK1/2 proteins, stimulating their kinase activity. MEK proteins are dual specificity serine/threonine and tyrosine protein kinases that phosphorylate and activate MAPK1/2 (also referred to as ERK1/2), protein kinases that play important roles in many cellular processes including the regulation of gene expression. In a similar fashion, binding of GTP-Ras to the p110 catalytic subunit of PI3K stimulates lipid kinase activity, increasing the production of second messenger phosphoinositide (3,4) P_2 (PIP2) and phosphoinositide (3,4,5) P_3 (PIP3). PIP3 promotes the activation of a kinase cascade that includes PDK-1, Akt (or PKB) and p70 ribosomal S6 protein kinase (p70s6k). These kinases phosphorylate numerous protein substrates with diverse roles in protein synthesis, cell proliferation and cell survival. PI3K also regulates survival through activation of Rac GTPases. Binding of GTP-Ras to RalGDS stimulates GEF activity towards the Ras-related proteins, Ral A and B. Downstream targets of Ral include phospholipase D, Rho, and Rac- and Cdc42-selective GAPs. There are a number of additional putative Ras effectors, including RasGAPs, MEKK, AF6, PKCζ, and Nore1. To date, activated Ras has been shown to signal through MAPK, PI3K and RalGDS in thyroid cells, effects that are markedly influenced by cAMP, an important regulator of thyroid cell function and proliferation (Figure 2).

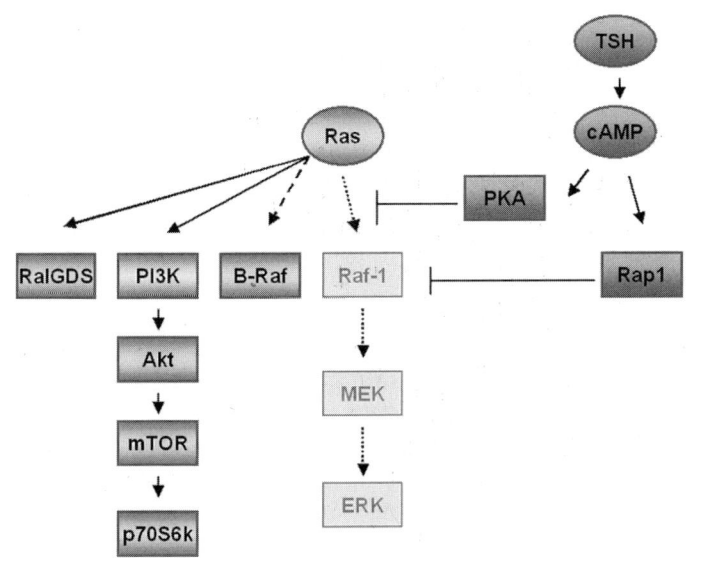

Figure 2. Ras signaling pathways are altered by TSH. TSH elevates cAMP, which activates PKA and Rap1 in thyroid cells. PKA has been reported to disrupt signaling from Ras to Raf-1 by phosphorylating the N-terminus of Raf-1, which decreases the affinity of Raf-1 for Ras. Activated Rap 1 binds to Raf-1, but does not stimulate its activity. It is not yet know whether Ras signals to B-Raf in thyroid cell (dashed line).

RAS MUTATIONS IN THYROID CANCER

A metastatic tumor is the end result of a complex series of steps involving multiple gene products. Work performed over the past decade has identified a number of gene products with putative roles in the initiation and progression of thyroid tumorigenesis. Mutations in Gsα (gsp) and the TSH receptor have been identified in hyperfunctioning adenomas. Ras mutations are prevalent in follicular carcinomas (see below). Mutations in ret, trk and met were identified in papillary carcinomas. Aberrant DNA methylation, leading to loss of expression of the p16 tumor suppressor gene, has been described in both types of cancer. Finally, mutations in p53 appear to play a role in the final dedifferentiation process. The reader is referred to several excellent recent reviews regarding the molecular basis of thyroid cancer (Jhiang, 2000; Gimm, 2001; Puxeddu et al., 2001; Fagin, 2002).

Early reports revealed that Ras mutations were particularly prevalent in benign follicular adenomas and follicular carcinomas, where estimates ranged as high as 50% (Lemoine et al., 1990; Namba et al., 1990; Suarez et al., 1990; Shi et al., 1991; Farid, 1994). The frequency of Ras mutations was initially reported to be similar in benign adenomas and follicular carcinomas, suggesting that Ras played an early role in thyroid transformation. However, more recent studies suggest that Ras mutations are less frequent than was first reported, occurring with an overall frequency of 16–19% (Esapa et al., 1999; Vasko et al., 2003). These studies also revealed a higher frequency of Ras mutations in follicular carcinomas versus adenomas, consistent with a role for Ras in malignant progression. According to recent data, mutations in codon 61 of N-Ras are the most frequent Ras mutation found in thyroid tumors (Nikiforova et al., 2003; Vasko et al., 2003). Besides Ras mutations, a significant proportion of follicular carcinomas exhibit a specific chromosomal translocation that fuses the coding regions for the paired and homeobox binding domains of the Pax-8 transcription factor to the DNA and ligand binding, dimerization and transactivation domains of PPARγ1 (Martelli et al., 2002). Interestingly, follicular carcinomas harboring both Ras mutations and the Pax-8/PPARγ translocation are extremely rare. This indicates either that both changes activate similar signaling pathways or that follicular carcinomas are comprised of at least two distinct tumor types that arise by different mechanisms (Nikiforova et al., 2003).

Although Ras mutations are infrequent in papillary thyroid carcinomas, somatic mutations in B-Raf were recently identified in these tumors (Kimura et al., 2003; Cohen et al., 2003). B-Raf mutations were discovered in a wide range of human tumors only last year (Davies et al., 2002; Rajagopalan et al., 2002). Intriguingly, mutations in B-Raf were found in cancers that typically harbor Ras mutations, such as malignant melanomas, colorectal tumors and ovarian cancers. The most frequent B-raf mutation (V599E) results in the insertion of an acidic residue close to a site of activating phosphorylation in the kinase domain. Recombinant B-RafV559E exhibits increased kinase activity, suggesting constitutive activation of signaling pathways similar to those activated by Ras. Moreover, unlike activated Raf-1 mutants that stimulate transformation through an autocrine mechanism involving Ras, the effects of

B-RafV559E on cell transformation were Ras-independent (Davies et al., 2002). The same B-Raf mutation has now been shown to be the most common genetic change in papillary thyroid carcinomas (Kimura et al., 2003). These results are striking for several reasons. First, there are three mammalian Raf proteins: Raf-1, A-Raf and B-Raf. While Raf-1 is ubiquitously expressed, A- and B-Raf exhibit a more restricted pattern of expression. Intriguingly, B-Raf is expressed in neuronal, neuroendocrine and endocrine cells. Of further interest with regard to thyroid cells, Raf proteins are important sites of integration between signals activated by Ras and cAMP. Cyclic AMP impairs the activation of Raf-1 by serum growth factors and Ras (Figure 2). In contrast, cAMP stimulates B-Raf activity (Erhardt et al., 1995; Vossler et al., 1997; Busca et al., 2000). Therefore, it is perhaps not surprising that melanoma cells harbor B-Raf mutations given their regulation by α-melanocyte stimulating hormone and related proopiomelanocortin-derived peptides that upregulate intracellular cAMP. Similarly, the identification of B-Raf mutations in thyroid tumors is particularly interesting given the growth promoting effects of chronic TSH stimulation. Despite the high frequency of Ras mutations in colorectal cancers, B-Raf mutations were found only in tumors without Ras mutations. In agreement with these results, no overlap was seen between mutations in Ras and B-Raf in papillary thyroid carcinomas (Kimura et al., 2003). These results provide strong support for the notion that B-Raf and Ras mutations are equivalent in their tumorigenic effects. Finally, RET/PTC oncogenes also signal partly through Ras (Barone et al., 2001; Castellone et al., 2003) and possibly through PDK-1 (Kim et al., 2003), a protein kinase that is also activated downstream from Ras. Strikingly, there appears to be no overlap between papillary carcinomas harboring RET/PTC, B-Raf and Ras mutations, which together account for two thirds of all papillary carcinomas. These findings underscore the significant contribution of Ras-mediated signaling pathways to thyroid tumorigenesis. In the following sections, I review what is known regarding the role of endogenous Ras, and the consequences of sustained Ras activity in thyroid cells.

ROLE OF CELLULAR RAS IN THYROID CELLS

TSH regulates the function and proliferation of thyroid follicular cells, highly specialized epithelial cells that synthesize, store and secrete thyroid hormones. Thyroid hormone biosynthesis requires the expression of cell type specific gene products, including the TSH receptor, thyroperoxidase, thyroglobulin and the sodium/iodide symporter (Damante et al., 1994). TSH regulates the expression of these genes in part through effects on thyroid-specific transcription factors such as TTF-1, TTF-2 and Pax-8 (Missero et al., 1998). The proliferation of thyroid cells is TSH-dependent (for recent reviews, see Medina et al., 2000; Kimura et al., 2001). However, for the most part, TSH acts together with insulin or IGF-I and serum to stimulate sustained proliferation. The effects of TSH on function and proliferation are reproduced by cAMP elevating agents and analogs. Positive growth regulation by cAMP is one of the unique features of thyroid cells and stands in marked contrast to the growth inhibitory effects of cAMP in many other cell types (Cook et al., 1993; Sevetson et al., 1993; Wu et al., 1993).

Compared to the effects of ectopic expression of constitutively active Ras, much less is known regarding the roles of endogenous Ras in thyroid cells. TSH-stimulated DNA synthesis was repressed following expression of dominant negative mutant Ras (Ras17N) in Wistar rat thyroid (WRT) (Kupperman et al., 1993) and FRTL-5 cells (Medina et al., 2000; Ciullo et al., 2001). Interference with Rac (Cass et al., 1999) or RhoA (Medina et al., 2002) also impaired TSH-stimulated DNA synthesis and mitogenesis, respectively. RhoA inhibition induced G1 phase cell cycle arrest in FRTL-5 cells (Hirai et al., 1997). Together, these data indicate that Ras family members play an integral role in the proliferation of rat thyroid cells. Whether Ras is required downstream from TSH/cAMP (Medina et al., 2000; Medina et al., 2000; Tsygankova et al., 2000), in addition to functioning downstream from insulin/IGF-I, is controversial (Van Keymeulen et al., 2000).

Although Ras stimulates proliferation through the Raf-1/MAPK cascade in many cells, this effector pathway does not play a major role in TSH signaling. Lamy *et al.* first reported that TSH failed to stimulate MAPK activity in canine thyroid cells (Lamy et al., 1993), in agreement with numerous studies in other cell types where cAMP inhibits growth factor stimulated-MAPK activity. TSH inhibited serum-stimulated MAPK activity in WRT cells (Miller et al., 1997) and treatment with the MEK1 inhibitor PD98059 had no effect on TSH-stimulated DNA synthesis in FRTL-5 cells (Medina et al., 2000). In addition to indicating that TSH does not signal through this cascade, these findings also suggested that Ras is unlikely to signal through the Raf-1/MAPK cascade in the presence of TSH (Figure 2), results that were later confirmed (see below). TSH stimulates p70s6k activity in WRT (Cass et al., 1998) and FRTL-5 cells (Medina et al., 2000), effects that were observed in the absence of insulin. Interference with mTOR, an upstream activator of p70s6k, impaired TSH-stimulated proliferation (Cass et al., 1998; Cass et al., 1999; Coulonval et al., 2000). As p70s6k can be activated downstream from PI3K, the role of PI3K in thyroid cell proliferation was investigated. Treatment with cell permeable PI3K inhibitors, microinjection of a dominant negative PI3K mutant, or injection of a p110-specific antibody inhibited TSH/cAMP stimulated DNA synthesis (Cass et al., 1999). Similarly, expression of dominant negative PI3K induced G1 phase cell cycle arrest in FRTL-5 cells and PI3K inhibitors blocked the stimulatory effects of TSH on cyclin E expression, a molecular marker of G1 phase cell cycle progression (Medina et al., 2000). Wortmannin and LY294002, cell permeable PI3K inhibitors, impaired TSH and insulin-stimulated DNA synthesis in canine thyroid cells (Coulonval et al., 2000) and IGF-I-stimulated proliferation in FRTL-5 cells (Saito et al., 2001). The role of PI3K in thyroid cell proliferation gained further support with the discovery that expression of PTEN, a negative regulator of PI3K, was decreased in a significant proportion of follicular neoplasms (Bruni et al., 2000), and that Akt activity is increased in follicular carcinomas (Ringel et al., 2001).

The acute effects of Ras activation in thyroid cells were first examined following microinjection of purified Ras protein into WRT cells (Kupperman et al., 1993). Microinjection of cellular or activated H-Ras protein was sufficient to stimulate DNA synthesis in quiescent cells. The ability of Ras to stimulate DNA synthesis in starved cells was impaired by co-injection of a Raf-1 antibody or of a dominant negative MEK1 protein (Al-Alawi et al., 1995), invoking a role for the Raf/MAPK cascade in growth stimulation by Ras. When injected into cells that were treated with TSH or 8BrcAMP, however, co-injection of the Raf-1 antibody or of the dominant negative MEK1 protein failed to impair Ras-stimulated DNA synthesis. These results provided the first indication that crosstalk between TSH/cAMP and Ras influences which effector pathways are activated by Ras in thyroid cells (Figure 2). The ability of TSH to influence Ras signaling received additional strong support from Ciullo *et al.* These authors confirmed that Ras and PI3K are required for TSH-stimulated cell cycle progression in FRTL-5 cells (Ciullo et al., 2001). Importantly, they demonstrated that TSH stimulated complex formation between endogenous Ras and PI3K, whereas it impaired association between Ras and Raf-1.

SUSTAINED RAS ACTIVITY AND THYROID CELL PROLIFERATION

The identification of activating Ras mutations in thyroid tumors prompted studies of the consequences of sustained Ras activity in thyroid cells. Early gene transfer studies revealed the oncogenic potential of Ras in thyroid cells *in vitro*. Stable expression of activated H- or K-Ras in FRTL-5 cells was fully transforming. Ras-expressing cells exhibited hormone-independent proliferation, anchorage-independent growth and formed tumors in nude mice (Fusco et al., 1987). In contrast to these results, rat thyroid PC-CL3 cells were only partially transformed by Ras. *In vivo* studies demonstrated that Ras activation was insufficient for tumor formation. When injected into adult Fischer rats, a K-Ras retrovirus induced the formation of differentiated thyroid carcinomas only in goitrogen-treated animals (Portella et al., 1989). Similarly, targeted expression of activated K-Ras to the thyroid gland stimulated hyperplasia and adenoma formation, but only in rare instances tumor formation, which required goitrogen treatment (Santelli et al., 1993). In seeming contrast to these findings, expression of activated H-Ras in the thyroid gland stimulated hyperplasia and papillary thyroid tumors (Rochefort et al., 1996; Feunteun et al., 1997).

The effects of Ras on the proliferation of human thyroid cells are of enormous interest. Using retroviruses, Lemoine *et al.* demonstrated that activated H-Ras stimulates the sustained proliferation of primary human thyroid cells (Lemoine et al., 1990; Bond et al., 1994; Jones et al., 2000). The mitogenic effects of Ras were also seen following acute introduction of activated Ras protein by scrape loading or microinjection (Gire et al., 1999). The ability of Ras to stimulate proliferation in primary thyroid cells is very different from its effects in primary fibroblasts where expression of activated Ras stimulated growth arrest (Serrano et al., 1997; Olson et al., 1998). Ras-expressing human thyroid cells were morphologically transformed and exhibited anchorage-independent growth, but not tumor formation. Strikingly, after 15–25 population doublings, Ras-expressing cells ceased to proliferate and became senescent, results quite similar to the limited growth potential of benign follicular adenomas harboring Ras mutations. These data strongly support the idea that human thyroid cells harbor a cell-intrinsic mechanism that prevents unchecked proliferation, even in the face of sustained expression of activated Ras.

In human cells, Ras-stimulated proliferation was impaired by inhibition of MAPK and PI3K activity. Although both pathways were required, activation of either signaling cascade alone was insufficient to stimulate proliferation (Gire et al., 1999; Gire et al., 2000). These findings are not dissimilar from those observed in rat thyroid cells, where Ras stimulated DNA synthesis through the Raf/MAPK cascade in the absence of TSH (Al-Alawi et al., 1995).

SUSTAINED RAS ACTIVITY AND THYROID DIFFERENTIATION

Ras transformation suppressed differentiated gene expression in rat thyroid cells (Avvedimento et al., 1985; Fusco et al., 1987; Francis-Lang et al., 1992). Intriguingly, H- and K-Ras impaired differentiation in different ways. H-Ras transformation was associated with the loss of Pax-8 and TTF-2 expression, and inactivation of TTF-1 possibly through decreased phosphorylation (Francis-Lang et al., 1992; Velasco et al., 1998). In contrast, TTF-1 expression was abolished in K-Ras transformed cells (Francis-Lang et al., 1992). K-Ras has also been shown to impair the nuclear localization of PKA, thereby preventing PKA-mediated phosphorylation of nuclear transcription factors (Gallo et al., 1995). Ras-transformed human cells retain their differentiated phenotype (Lemoine et al., 1990; Gire et al., 2000), a finding consistent with the occurrence of Ras mutations in differentiated thyroid tumors. It should be noted that de-differentiation is not an obligate response of rat thyroid cells to activated Ras. Using Ras effector domain mutants that signal through discrete downstream effectors (White et al., 1995), Miller *et al.* demonstrated that Ras signaling through the Raf/MAPK cascade impaired thyroglobulin expression in WRT cells, while Ras signaling to RalGDS (Miller et al., 1998) or PI3K did not (Cass et al., 2000). Stable expression of activated MEK-1, a downstream target of Raf, failed to de-differentiate FRTL-5 cells, perhaps due to its relatively modest effects on MAPK activity (Cobellis et al., 1998). Indeed, further studies by the same authors revealed that transient expression of RasS35, the effector domain mutant that signals selectively through Raf-1, or of activated Raf-1 impaired TTF-1 activity (Missero et al., 2000). Furthermore, MEK inhibitors partially blocked the inhibitory effects of Ras on TTF-1 activity. These data indicate that activation of the MAPK cascade impairs differentiated gene expression in rat thyroid cells, and that there are likely to be additional signals through which Ras suppresses thyroid differentiation. Different effects of RhoA on differentiated gene expression have been reported. Stable expression of activated RhoA impaired thyroglobulin and TTF-1 mRNA and protein levels (Medina et al., 2002), however transient expression of activated RhoA failed to repress TTF-1 promoter activity (Missero et al., 2000). Given the inhibitory effects of Ras signaling to MAPK on thyroid differentiation, the ability of TSH to direct Ras signals to alternate effectors such as PI3K and RalGDS would allow TSH to stimulate proliferation through Ras in cells that retain their differentiated character.

RAS AND THYROID CELL SURVIVAL

Although stable expression of activated Ras in thyroid cells confers hormone and anchorage-independent proliferation, it also renders cells more sensitive to apoptosis.

Serum withdrawal induced apoptosis in H- and K-Ras-transformed, but not parental FRTL-5 cells (Di Jeso et al., 1995). H-Ras-transformed WRT cells exhibit an enhanced sensitivity to apoptosis in response to deprivation of adhesion or treatment with MAPK and PI3K inhibitors (Cheng et al., 2001). Inducible expression of activated Ras in PC-CL3 cells stimulated proliferation followed by apoptosis (Shirokawa et al., 2000). Intriguingly, apoptosis was strictly dependent upon TSH or cAMP elevation; in the absence of TSH/cAMP, Ras stimulated proliferation. Although epithelial cells typically perish by anoikis following detachment, Ras stimulated apoptosis in adherent PC-CL3 cells. Interference with either MAPK or JNK impaired apoptosis, invoking a role for these signaling pathways in Ras-mediated apoptosis. Acute infection of WRT, FRTL-5 and PC-CL3 cells with an adenovirus expressing activated H-Ras also stimulated apoptosis, although in this instance cell death occurred in the presence or absence of TSH (Cheng et al., 2003).

The effects of Ras on apoptosis are not limited to rat thyroid cells. Human thyroid cells immortalized by temperature-sensitive SV40 large T antigen underwent rapid cell death following expression of activated Ras at the restrictive temperature (Burns et al., 1993). Exposure to the phorbol ester tumor promoter TPA stimulated apoptosis in human thyroid cells expressing activated H-Ras (Hall-Jackson et al., 1998). Moreover, inhibition of PI3K activity induced apoptosis in H-Ras-expressing human thyroid cells, suggesting that clonal expansion induced by Ras requires PI3K activity to suppress apoptosis (Gire et al., 2000). Together these findings indicate that apoptosis is a conserved response to acute expression of activated Ras in thyroid cells. The relative ease with which rat and human thyroid cells are selected to survive stable expression of activated Ras also indicates that secondary changes that allow for the survival of Ras-expressing thyroid cells are frequent. The elucidation of the factors that dictate whether Ras stimulates transient or sustained proliferation, growth arrest or apoptosis is an exciting area for exploration.

RAS AND GENOMIC INSTABILITY

One of the consequences of Ras mutations in human tumors is destabilization of the karyotype. Expression of activated Ras in a variety of established cell lines and tumor cells induces chromosomal aberrations including an enhanced frequency of gene amplification (Smith et al., 1995), chromosome losses and gains, aberrant chromosome segregation and centrosome amplification (Saavedra et al., 1999). Inducible expression of activated H-Ras in PC-CL3 cells stimulated the formation of micronuclei containing chromosomes and chromosome fragments (Saavedra et al., 2000). Micronuclei with whole chromosomes arise as a consequence of spindle disruption; micronuclei containing chromosome fragments are typically generated by double strand DNA breaks. Although the effects of Ras on micronuclei formation were rapid, they were observed in only a small proportion of cells, perhaps due to the presence of wildtype p53 in these cells. This raises the interesting possibility that Ras predisposes thyroid cells to the acquisition of additional mutations by inducing genomic instability. Over time, cells harboring Ras mutations would acquire additional genetic and epigenetic changes that contribute to their full transformation. In this regard, it is interesting that Ras mutations occur at a higher frequency in follicular versus papillary carcinomas, given the higher degree of aneuploidy observed in follicular carcinomas (Fagin, 2002). It will be interesting to assess whether papillary tumors bearing B-Raf mutations exhibit similar chromosomal aberrations. Whether Ras induces genomic instability in primary human thyroid cells, which exhibit a more stable karyotype than do rodent cells, has not yet been determined.

While chromosomal instability could provide the mechanism for Ras-stimulated apoptosis, the low frequency of micronuclei formation versus the high frequency of apoptosis argues that these events are distinct (Shirokawa et al., 2000). Apoptosis was TSH-dependent, while micronuclei formation was insensitive to cAMP levels. Furthermore, the signaling pathways through which Ras stimulated micronuclei formation and apoptosis were distinct. Therefore, acute expression of activated Ras stimulates multiple signals leading to DNA damage and chromosomal instability in a small proportion of cells and apoptosis in most cells. The changes that occur in the small population of surviving cells that contribute to their survival in the presence of activated Ras remain to be identified.

CELL CYCLE DEREGULATION AND APOPTOSIS

Acute expression of activated Ras stimulated aberrant cell cycle progression followed by apoptosis in WRT cells (Cheng et al., 2003). Infection of quiescent cells with an adenovirus expressing activated H-Ras induced cell cycle progression into S phase. Rather than completing the cell cycle, the majority of Ras-expressing cells exhibited a protracted S phase and ultimately perished by apoptosis. The effects of Ras on cell cycle regulatory proteins were very different from the mitogens, TSH, insulin, and serum. Unlike mitogen treatment, which increased the expression of cyclins D1 and B, Ras rapidly decreased cyclin D1 expression, and failed to increase cyclin B expression. Excessive mitogenic signaling, for example through overexpression of E2F (Nahle et al., 2002), is a potent inducer of apoptosis, as is delayed cell cycle progression (Meikrantz et al., 1995). These findings suggest that the acute effects of Ras on thyroid cell cycle progression are aberrant, and induce an apoptotic response. Similar effects on cell cycle progression and apoptosis have been reported following expression of high mobility group (HMG) proteins in thyroid cells. Impaired expression of HMGA in PC-CL3 cells blocked Ras transformation, suggesting a role for HMGA downstream from Ras (Fedele et al., 2001). When stably overexpressed, HMGA induced aberrant cell cycle progression characterized by premature entry into S phase and delayed transition into G2/M. These aberrant effects on cell cycle progression were accompanied by apoptosis. These data support the idea that conflict between mitogenic pressure and the inability to proceed through the cell cycle generates an apoptotic signal in rat thyroid cells. The high frequency of cell death in Ras-expressing human thyroid cells at the restrictive temperature for SV40 large T (Burns et al., 1993) may reflect a similar mechanism. The deletion of thyroid cells harboring Ras mutations by apoptosis might explain why Ras mutations are not found in a higher proportion of thyroid tumors.

The effects of activated Ras on the expression of p16, p21 and p27, cyclin-dependent kinase inhibitors, in human thyrocytes (Jones et al., 2000) differed from those reported in human fibroblasts (Serrano et al., 1997; Olson et al., 1998). In thyroid cells, acute expression of Ras decreased p27 expression, and failed to increase expression of either p16 or p21. These changes would be expected to increase cyclin-dependent kinase activity, in particular cdk-2 activity, which is potently inhibited by p21 and p27 (reviewed in Sherr et al., 1999). These alterations could contribute to the mitogenic activity of Ras in human thyroid cells. In fibroblasts, Ras stimulated p16 and p21 expression, resulting in G1 phase cell cycle arrest. Cessation of proliferation in human thyroid cells was accompanied by re-expression of p27 and *de novo* expression of p16, changes expected to impair cdk activity (Jones et al., 2000). Interestingly, when HPV E7 was expressed in these cells to inactivate growth suppression by p16 and p27, senescence was bypassed. Although the cells continued to proliferate, proliferation was accompanied by increasing cell death. Therefore, in human and rat thyroid cells, proliferative pressure in the face of signals that impair growth induces apoptosis. This would impose selective pressure for cells in which apoptosis is circumvented, for example through the increased expression of positive regulators of cell cycle progression, decreased expression of growth inhibitors or alterations in cell survival signals. Indeed, unlike acute expression of activated Ras, which abolished the expression of cyclin D1, WRT cells selected to survive constitutive expression of activated Ras exhibited increased levels of cyclin D1 (Cheng et al., 2003). The expression of cyclins D1 (Wang et al., 1998; Muro-Cacho et al., 1999) and E (Lazzereschi et al., 1998; Wang et al., 1998) are frequently increased in thyroid tumors. Decreased expression of p27 in carcinomas versus adenomas has been reported (Erickson et al., 1998; Wang et al., 1998). Methylation of the p16 promoter, resulting in reduced p16 expression, has been reported in many differentiated thyroid tumors (Ivan et al., 1996; Jones et al., 1996). Together these findings suggest that alterations in the expression of cell cycle regulatory proteins may contribute to oncogenic transformation by Ras.

CONCLUSIONS AND PERSPECTIVES

While the frequency of Ras mutations in human tumors is only 20% overall, constitutive signaling through Ras is a conserved feature of a much higher proportion of human tumors. Mutations giving rise to increased production of growth factors or sustained activation of growth factor receptors are frequent events in human tumors. Over the past year, mutations in a Ras effector, B-Raf, have been identified in several types of human cancer (Davies et al., 2002; Rajagopalan et al., 2002). Together, mutations that give rise to constitutive signaling through Ras-mediated pathways comprise a significant proportion of human tumors. The fundamental role of Ras in tumorigenesis is particularly evident in the thyroid gland where mutations in Ras, B-Raf and RET/PTC have now been identified. Expression of activated Ras in thyroid cells *in vitro* elicits morphological transformation, sustained proliferation, apoptosis and genomic instability, hallmarks of human tumor cells (Figure 3). Despite the significant advances that have been made in identifying regulators and targets of Ras, these recent advances highlight how little we know regarding the signaling pathways activated by Ras, as well as the consequences of sustained Ras activity in the thyroid cell.

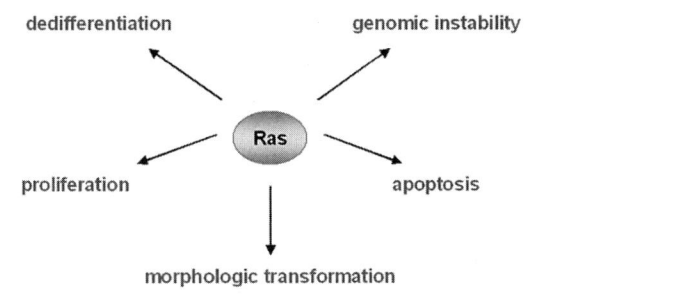

Figure 3. Ras elicits multiple effects in thyroid cells.

Overexpression studies have relied extensively on H- and K- rather than N-Ras, which appears to be a more frequent target for mutation in thyroid cancer. With accumulating evidence that individual Ras proteins localize to different cellular microdomains (Prior et al., 2001; Chiu et al., 2002; Matallanas et al., 2003) and signal in distinct ways (Maher et al., 1995; Villalonga et al., 2001; Walsh et al., 2001), it will be important to assess the specific consequences of N-*ras* activity in thyroid cells. It is interesting that N-Ras provides a survival signal in fibroblasts (Wolfman et al., 2002).

The recent discovery of B-Raf mutations in thyroid tumors paves the way for studies of the contribution of this specific Raf isoform to tumorigenesis. Although cAMP impairs Ras signaling to Raf-1, its effects on B-Raf activity in thyroid cells are largely unknown. Moreover, cAMP itself stimulates several signaling pathways with the potential to regulate B-Raf activity. Thyroid cells are a rich source of Epac, a Rap1-specific GEF (DeRooij et al., 1998; Kawasaki et al., 1998). TSH and cAMP activate endogenous Rap1 in rat (Tsygankova et al., 2001) and canine (Dremier et al., 1997) thyroid cells, effects that are PKA-independent. In other cells, active Rap1 binds to Raf-1 and B-Raf, but with differing consequences. Association between Rap1 and B-Raf stimulates B-Raf activity, whereas Rap-1:Raf-1 complexes are inactive. B-Raf is a substrate for protein kinase A, the other arm of the cAMP signaling pathway. This raises interesting avenues for regulation of B-Raf by cAMP and PKA. The signaling pathways activated by B-Raf in thyroid cells are unknown. While B Raf binds and activates MEK1/2, it remains to be determined whether this pathway is active in TSH-treated cells.

Rap1 has been linked to TSH effects on differentiated gene expression (Tsygankova et al., 2001) and proliferation (Ribeiro-Neto et al., 2002), although the mechanism through which it elicits these effects is not clear. A limited mutational analysis failed to reveal mutations in Rap1 or Epac in follicular adenomas (Vanvooren et al., 2001). Nonetheless, the contribution of Rap1 to thyroid cell biology is important to pursue based on its ability to signal through B-Raf and to affect Ras-mediated signaling. Rap1 was initially isolated as K-rev1, an inhibitor of K-Ras transformation (Kitayama et al., 1989). Although Rap1 clearly functions in Ras-independent pathways, crosstalk between Ras and Rap1 has been shown to modulate the ability of Ras to activate discrete effector pathways. Competition between Rap1 and Ras for downstream signaling molecules may provide a mechanism for balancing the activities of these two signaling molecules and for channeling their effects to discrete effector pathways.

The notion that Ras stimulates genomic instability, predisposing thyroid cells to the acquisition of additional mutations, promises to provide further insight into the molecular mechanisms through which Ras contributes to thyroid cell transformation. Thyroid cancer cell lines and tumors have been shown to exhibit mitotic checkpoint dysfunction, however the genetic and/or epigenetic changes responsible for this have not been identified. A recent analysis failed to reveal mutations in the candidate checkpoint genes, BUB1 or BUBR1 (Ouyang et al., 2002). The relationship between tumors harboring mutations in Ras or B-Raf to DNA damage and effects on p53 deserves further attention given genetic evidence for the acquisition of p53 mutations secondary to mutations in N-Ras in thyroid tumors (Asakawa et al., 2002). In experimental models, stable expression of activated Ras has been shown to induce p53 mutations (Chen et al., 1998). The effects of Ras on cell cycle regulatory proteins needs to be examined in more detail given the unusual effects of Ras on these molecules in human and rat thyroid cells, together with the identification of mutations in cyclins and cyclin-dependent kinase inhibitors in thyroid tumors. It is noteworthy that overexpression of cyclins D1 (Lung et al., 2002) and E (Spruck et al., 1999) has also been linked to genomic instability.

The TSH-dependent nature and relative ease with which rat thyroid cells can be manipulated *in vitro* affords an important cell model for future studies. Transgenic and knock out animal models for discrete Ras and Raf isoforms hold enormous promise for understanding the contributions of these signaling molecules to thyroid tumorigenesis. Whatever is learned from the rodent model systems must be validated in human thyroid cells. With increasing evidence that Ras signals through discrete pathways in rodent versus human cells (Hamad et al., 2002), studies of the signal transduction mechanisms and consequences of Ras and B-Raf activity in human thyroid cells are essential. Finally, while numerous studies have examined the cellular consequences that arise following transient or stable expression of activated Ras, few studies have attempted to model both the primary and secondary adaptive changes that occur in response to sustained Ras activity in the same cells.

REFERENCES

1. Al-Alawi, N., Rose, D. W., Buckmaster, C., Ahn, N., Rapp, U., Meinkoth, J. and Feramisco, J. R., 1995, Thyrotropin-induced mitogenesis is Ras dependent but appears to bypass the Raf-dependent cytoplasmic kinase cascade, *Mol Cell Biol.* **15**: 1162–8.
2. Asakawa, H. and Kobayashi, T., 2002, Multistep carcinogenesis in anaplastic thyroid carcinoma: a case report, *Pathology.* **34**: 94–7.
3. Avvedimento, E. V., Monticelli, A., Tramontano, D., Polistina, C., Nitsch, L. and Di Lauro, R., 1985, Differential expression of thyroglobulin gene in normal and transformed thyroid cells, *Eur J Biochem.* **149**: 467–472.
4. Barone, M. V., Sepe, L., Melillo, R. M., Mineo, A., Santelli, G., Monaco, C., Castellone, M. D., Tramontano, D., Fusco, A. and Santoro, M., 2001, RET/PTC1 oncogene signaling in PC Cl 3 thyroid cells requires the small GTP-binding protein Rho, *Oncogene.* **20**: 6973–82.
5. Bond, J. A., Wyllie, F. S., Rowson, J., Radulescu, A. and Wynford-Thomas, D., 1994, In vitro reconstruction of tumour initiation in a human epithelium, *Oncogene.* **9**: 281–290.

6. Bruni, P., Boccia, A., Baldassarre, G., Trapasso, F., Santoro, M., Chiappetta, G., Fusco, A. and Viglietto, G., 2000, PTEN expression is reduced in a subset of sporadic thyroid carcinomas: evidence that PTEN-growth suppressing activity in thyroid cancer cells is mediated by p27kip1, *Oncogene.* **19:** 3146–3155.
7. Burns, J., Barton, C., Wynford-Thomas, D. and Lemoine, N., 1993, In vitro transformation of epithelial cells by ras oncogenes, *Epithelial Cell Biol.* **2:** 26–43.
8. Busca, R., Abbe, P., Mantoux, F., Aberdam, E., Peyssonnaux, C., Eychene, A., Ortonne, J. P. and Ballotti, R., 2000, Ras mediates the cAMP-dependent activation of extracellular signal-regulated kinases (ERKs) in melanocytes, *EMBO J.* **19:** 2900–10.
9. Cass, L. A. and Meinkoth, J. L., 1998, Differential effects of cyclic adenosine $3'$, $5'$-monophosphate on p70 ribosomal S6 kinase, *Endocrinol.* **139:** 1991–1998.
10. Cass, L. A. and Meinkoth, J. L., 2000, Ras signaling through PI3K confers hormone-independent proliferation that is compatible with differentiation, *Oncogene.* **19:** 924–32.
11. Cass, L. A., Summers, S. A., Prendergast, G. V., Backer, J. M., Birnbaum, M. J. and Meinkoth, J. L., 1999, Protein kinase A-dependent and -independent signaling pathways contribute to cyclic AMP-stimulated proliferation, *Mol Cell Biol.* **19:** 5882–91.
12. Castellone, M. D., Cirafici, A. M., De Vita, G., De Falco, V., Malorni, L., Tallini, G., Fagin, J. A., Fusco, A., Melillo, R. M. and Santoro, M., 2003, Ras-mediated apoptosis of PC CL 3 rat thyroid cells induced by RET/PTC oncogenes, *Oncogene.* **22:** 246–55.
13. Chen, C.-Y., Liou, J., Forman, L. W. and Faller, D. V., 1998, Differential regulation of discrete apoptotic pathways by Ras, *J Biol Chem.* **273:** 16700–16709.
14. Cheng, G., Lewis, A. E. and Meinkoth, J. L., 2003, Ras stimulates aberrant cell cycle progression and apoptosis in rat thyroid cells, *Mol Endocrinol.* **17:** 450–9.
15. Cheng, G. and Meinkoth, J. L., 2001, Enhanced sensitivity to apoptosis in Ras-transformed thyroid cells, *Oncogene.* **20:** 7334–41.
16. Chiu, V. K., Bivona, T., Hach, A., Sajous, J. B., Silletti, J., Wiener, H., Johnson, R. L., 2nd, Cox, A. D. and Philips, M. R., 2002, Ras signalling on the endoplasmic reticulum and the Golgi, *Nat Cell Biol.* **4:** 343–50.
17. Ciullo, I., Diez-Roux, G., Di Domenico, M., Migliaccio, A. and Avvedimento, E. V., 2001, cAMP signaling selectively influences Ras effectors pathways, *Oncogene.* **20:** 1186–92.
18. Cobellis, G., Missero, C. and Di Lauro, R., 1998, Concomitant activation of MEK-1 and Rac-1 increases the proliferative potential of thyroid epithelial cells, without affecting their differentiation, *Oncogene.* **17:** 2047–57.
19. Cohen, Y., Xing, M., Mambo, E., Guo, Z., Wu, G., Trink, B., Beller, U., Westra, W. H., Ladenson, P. W. and Sidransky, D., 2003, BRAF mutation in papillary thyroid carcinoma, *J. Natl. Canc. Inst.* **95:** 625–627.
20. Cook, S. J. and McCormick, F., 1993, Inhibition by cAMP of Ras-dependent activation of Raf, *Science.* **262:** 1059–1062.
21. Coulonval, K., Vandeput, F., Stein, R. C., Kozma, S. C., Lamy, F. and Dumont, J. E., 2000, Phosphatidylinositol 3-kinase, protein kinase B and ribosomal S6 kinases in the stimulation of thyroid epithelial cell proliferation by cAMP and growth factors in the presence of insulin, *Biochem J.* **348:** 351–8.
22. Damante, G. and Di Lauro, R., 1994, Thyroid-specific gene expression, *Biochim Biophys Acta.* **1218:** 255–266.
23. Davies, H., Bignell, G. R., Cox, C., Stephens, P., Edkins, S., Clegg, S., Teague, J., Woffendin, H., Garnett, M. J., Bottomley, W., Davis, N., Dicks, E., Ewing, R., Floyd, Y., Gray, K., Hall, S., Hawes, R., Hughes, J., Kosmidou, V., Menzies, A., Mould, C., Parker, A., Stevens, C., Watt, S., Hooper, S., Wilson, R., Jayatilake, H., Gusterson, B. A., Cooper, C., Shipley, J., Hargrave, D., Pritchard-Jones, K., Maitland, N., Chenevix-Trench, G., Riggins, G. J., Bigner, D. D., Palmieri, G., Cossu, A., Flanagan, A., Nicholson, A., Ho, J. W., Leung, S. Y., Yuen, S. T., Weber, B. L., Seigler, H. F., Darrow, T. L., Paterson, H., Marais, R., Marshall, C. J., Wooster, R., Stratton, M. R. and Futreal, P. A., 2002, Mutations of the BRAF gene in human cancer, *Nature.* **417:** 949–54.
24. DeRooij, J., Zwartkruis, F. J. T., Verheijen, M. H. G., Cool, R. H., Nijman, S. M. B., Wittinghofer, A. and Bos, J. L., 1998, Epac is a Rap1 guanine-nucleotide-exchange factor directly activated by cyclic AMP, *Nature.* **396:** 474–477.
25. Di Jeso, B., Ulianich, L., Racioppi, L., D'Armiento, F., Feliciello, A., Pacifico, F., Consiglio, E. and Formisano, S., 1995, Serum withdrawal induces apoptotic cell death in Ki-ras transformed but not in normal differentiated thyroid cells, *Biochem Biophys Res Commun.* **214:** 819–24.
26. Dremier, S., Pohl, V., Poteet-Smith, C., Roger, P., Corbin, J., Doskeland, S. O., Dumont, J. E. and Maenhaut, C., 1997, Activation of cyclic AMP-dependent protein kinase is required but may not be

sufficient to mimic cyclic AMP-dependent DNA synthesis and thyroglobulin expression in dog thyroid cells, *Mol. Cell. Biol.* **17**: 6717–6726.
27. Erhardt, P., Troppmair, J., Rapp, U. and Cooper, G. M., 1995, Differential regulation of Raf-1 and B-Raf and Ras-dependent activation of mitogen-activated protein kinase by cyclic AMP in PC12 cells, *Mol Cell Biol.* **15**: 5524–5530.
28. Erickson, L. A., Jin, L., Wollan, P. C., Thompson, G. B., van Heerden, J. and Lloyd, R. V., 1998, Expression of p27kip1 and Ki-67 in benign and malignant thyroid tumors, *Mod Pathol.* **11**: 169–74.
29. Esapa, C. T., Johnson, S. J., Kendall-Taylor, P., Lennard, T. W. and Harris, P. E., 1999, Prevalence of Ras mutations in thyroid neoplasia, *Clin Endocrinol* **50**: 529–35.
30. Fagin, J. A., 2002, Minireview: branded from the start-distinct oncogenic initiating events may determine tumor fate in the thyroid, *Mol Endocrinol.* **16**: 903–11.
31. Fagin, J. A., 2002, Perspective: lessons learned from molecular genetic studies of thyroid cancer–insights into pathogenesis and tumor-specific therapeutic targets, *Endocrinology.* **143**: 2025–8.
32. Farid, N. R., Shi, Y., and Zou, M., 1994, Molecular basis of thyroid cancer, *Endocrine Reviews.* **15**: 202–232.
33. Fedele, M., Pierantoni, G. M., Berlingieri, M. T., Battista, S., Baldassarre, G., Munshi, N., Dentice, M., Thanos, D., Santoro, M., Viglietto, G. and Fusco, A., 2001, Overexpression of proteins HMGA1 induces cell cycle deregulation and apoptosis in normal rat thyroid cells, *Cancer Res.* **61**: 4583–90.
34. Feunteun, J., Michiels, F., Rochefort, P., Caillou, B., Talbot, M., Fournes, B., Mercken, L., Schlumberger, M. and Monier, R., 1997, Targeted oncogenesis in the thyroid of transgenic mice, *Horm Res.* **47**: 137–9.
35. Francis-Lang, H., Zannini, M., De Felice, M., Berlingieri, M. T., Fusco, A. and Di Lauro, R., 1992, Multiple mechanisms of interference between transformation and differentiation in thyroid cells, *Mol Cell Biol.* **12**: 5793–800.
36. Fusco, A., Berlingieri, M. T., Di Fiore, P. P., Portella, G., Grieco, M. and Vecchio, G., 1987, One- and two-step transformations of rat thyroid epithelial cells by retroviral oncogenes, *Mol Cell Biol.* **7**: 3365–70.
37. Gallo, A., Feliciello, A., Varrone, A., Cerillo, R., Gottesman, M. E. and Avvedimento, E. V., 1995, Ki-ras oncogene interferes with the expression of cycliin AMP-dependent promoters, *Cell Growth and Difftn.* **6**: 91–95.
38. Gimm, O., 2001, Thyroid cancer, *Cancer Lett.* **163**: 143–56.
39. Gire, V., Marshall, C. and Wynford-Thomas, D., 2000, PI-3-kinase is an essential anti-apoptotic effector in the proliferative response of primary human epithelial cells to mutant RAS, *Oncogene.* **19**: 2269–76.
40. Gire, V., Marshall, C. J. and Wynford-Thomas, D., 1999, Activation of mitogen-activated protein kinase is necessary but not sufficient for proliferation of human thyroid epithelial cells induced by mutant Ras, *Oncogene.* **18**: 4819–32.
41. Gire, V. and Wynford-Thomas, D., 2000, RAS oncogene activation induces proliferation in normal human thyroid epithelial cells without loss of differentiation, *Oncogene.* **19**: 737–44.
42. Hall-Jackson, C. A., Jones, T., Eccles, N. G., Dawson, T. P., Bond, J. A., Gescher, A. and Wynford-Thomas, D., 1998, Induction of cell death by stimulation of protein kinase C in human epithelial cells expressing a mutant ras oncogene: a potential therapeutic target, *Br J Cancer.* **78**: 641–51.
43. Hamad, N. M., Elconin, J. H., Karnoub, A. E., Bai, W., Rich, J. N., Abraham, R. T., Der, C. J. and Counter, C. M., 2002, Distinct requirements for Ras oncogenesis in human versus mouse cells, *Genes Dev.* **16**: 2045–57.
44. Hirai, A., Nakamura, S., Noguchi, Y., Yasuda, T., Kitagawa, M., Tatsuno, I., Oeda, T., Tahara, K., Terano, T., Narumiya, S., Kohn, L. D. and Saito, Y., 1997, Geranylgeranylated rho small GTPase(s) are essential for the degradation of p27Kip1 and facilitate the progression from G1 to S phase in growth-stimulated rat FRTL-5 cells, *J Biol Chem.* **272**: 13–6.
45. Ivan, M., Wynford-Thomas, D. and Jones, C. J., 1996, Abnormalities of the p16INK4a gene in thyroid cancer cell lines, *Eur J. Canc.* **32**: 2369–2370.
46. Jhiang, S. M., 2000, The RET proto-oncogene in human cancers, *Oncogene.* **19**: 5590–7.
47. Jones, C. J., Kipling, D., Morris, M., Hepburn, P., Skinner, J., Bounacer, A., Wyllie, F. S., Ivan, M., Bartek, J., Wynford-Thomas, D. and Bond, J. A., 2000, Evidence for a telomere-independent "clock" limiting RAS oncogene-driven proliferation of human thyroid epithelial cells, *Mol Cell Biol.* **20**: 5690–9.
48. Jones, C. J., Shaw, J. J., Wyllie, F. S., Gaillard, M., Schlumberger, M. and Wynford-Thomas, D., 1996, High frequency deletion of the tumour suppressor gene p16INK4a (MTS1) in human thyroid cancer cell lines, *Mol Cell Endocrinol.* **116**: 115–119.

49. Kawasaki, H., Springett, G. M., Mochizuki, N., Toki, S., Nakaya, M., Matsuda, M., Housman, D. E. and Graybiel, A. M., 1998, A family of cAMP-binding proteins that directly activate Rap1, *Science.* **282:** 2275–2279.
50. Kim, D. W., Hwang, J. H., Suh, J. M., Kim, H., Song, J. H., Hwang, E. S., Hwang, I. Y., Park, K. C., Chung, H. K., Kim, J. M., Park, J., Hemmings, B. A. and Shong, M., 2003, RET/PTC (Rearranged in transformation/papillary thyroid carcinomas) tyrosine kinase phosphorylates and activates phosphoinositide-dependent kinate 1 (PDK1): An alternative phosphatidylinositol 3-kinase-independent pathway to activate PDK1, *Mol Endo* **17:** 1382–1394.
51. Kimura, E. T., Nikiforova, M. N., Zhu, Z., Knauf, J. A., Nikiforov, Y. E. and Fagin, J. A., 2003, High prevalence of BRAF mutations in thyroid cancer: genetic evidence for constitutive activation of the RET/PTC-RAS-BRAF signaling pathway in papillary thyroid carcinoma, *Cancer Res.* **63:** 1454–7.
52. Kimura, T., Van Keymeulen, A., Golstein, J., Fusco, A., Dumont, J. E. and Roger, P. P., 2001, Regulation of thyroid cell proliferation by TSH and other factors: a critical evaluation of in vitro models, *Endocrine Reviews.* **23:** 631–656.
53. Kitayama, H., Sugimoto, Y., Matsuzaki, T., Ikawa, Y. and Noda, M., 1989, A ras-related gene with transformation suppressor activity, *Cell.* **56:** 77–84.
54. Kupperman, E., Wen, W. and Meinkoth, J. L., 1993, Inhibition of thyrotropin-stimulated DNA synthesis by microinjection of inhibitors of cellular Ras and cyclic AMP-dependent protein kinase, *Mol Cell Biol.* **13:** 4477–84.
55. Lamy, F., Wilkin, F., Baptist, M., Posada, J., Roger, P. P. and Dumont, J. E., 1993, Phosphorylation of mitogen-activated protein kinases is involved in the epidermal growth factor and phorbol ester, but not in the thyrotropin/cAMP, thyroid mitogenic pathway, *J Biol Chem.* **268:** 8398–401.
56. Lazzereschi, D., Sambuco, L., Carnovale Scalzo, C., Ranieri, A., Mincione, G., Nardi, F. and Colletta, G., 1998, Cyclin D1 and Cyclin E expression in malignant thyroid cells and in human thyroid carcinomas, *Int J Cancer.* **76:** 806–11.
57. Lemoine, N. R., Staddon, S., Bond, J., Wyllie, F. S., Shaw, J. J. and Wynford-Thomas, D., 1990, Partial transformation of human thyroid epithelial cells by mutant Ha-ras oncogene, *Oncogene.* **5:** 1833–7.
58. Lung, J. C., Chu, J. S., Yu, J. C., Yue, C. T., Lo, Y. L., Shen, C. Y. and Wu, C. W., 2002, Aberrant expression of cell-cycle regulator cyclin D1 in breast cancer is related to chromosomal genomic instability, *Genes Chromosomes Cancer.* **34:** 276–84.
59. Maher, J., Baker, D. A., Manning, M., Dibb, N. J. and Roberts, I. A. G., 1995, Evidence for cell-specific differences in transformation by N-, H- and K-ras, *Oncogene.* **11:** 1639–1647.
60. Martelli, M. L., Juliano, R., LePera, I., Sama, I., Monaco, C., Cammarota, S., Kroll, T., Chiariotti, L., Santoro, M. and Fusco, A., 2002, Inhibitory effects of peroxisome proliferator-activated receptor gamma on thyroid carcinoma cell growth, *J Clin Endocrinol Metab.* **87:** 4728–4735.
61. Matallanas, D., Arozarena, I., Berciano, M. T., Aaronson, D. S., Pellicer, A., Lafarga, M. and Crespo, P., 2003, Differences on the inhibitory specificities of H-Ras, K-Ras and N-Ras (N17) dominant negative mutants are related to their membrane microlocalization, *J Biol Chem.* **278:** 4572–4581.
62. Medina, D. L., Rivas, M., Cruz, P., Barroso, R., Regadera, J. and Santisteban, P., 2002, RhoA activation promotes transformation and loss of thyroid cell differentiation interfering with thyroid transcription factor-1 activity, *Mol Endocrinol.* **16:** 33–44.
63. Medina, D. L. and Santisteban, P., 2000, Thyrotropin-dependent proliferation of in vitro rat thyroid cell systems, *Eur J Endocrinol.* **143:** 161–78.
64. Medina, D. L., Toro, M. J. and Santisteban, P., 2000, Somatostatin interferes with thyrotropin-induced G1-S transition mediated by cAMP-dependent protein kinase and phosphatidylinositol 3-kinase. Involvement of RhoA and cyclin E/cyclin-dependent kinase 2 complexes, *J Biol Chem.* **275:** 15549–56.
65. Meikrantz, W. and Schlegel, R., 1995, Apoptosis and the cell cycle, *J Cell Biochem.* **58:** 160–74.
66. Miller, M. J., Prigent, S., Kupperman, E., Rioux, L., Park, S. H., Feramisco, J. R., White, M. A., Rutkowski, J. L. and Meinkoth, J. L., 1997, RalGDS functions in Ras- and cAMP-mediated growth stimulation, *J Biol Chem.* **272:** 5600–5.
67. Miller, M. J., Rioux, L., Prendergast, G. V., Cannon, S., White, M. A. and Meinkoth, J. L., 1998, Differential effects of protein kinase A on Ras effector pathways, *Mol Cell Biol.* **18:** 3718–26.
68. Missero, C., Cobellis, G., De Felice, M. and Di Lauro, R., 1998, Molecular events involved in differentiation of thyroid follicular cells, *Mol Cell Endocrinol.* **140:** 37–43.
69. Missero, C., Pirro, M. T. and Di Lauro, R., 2000, Multiple ras downstream pathways mediate functional repression of the homeobox gene product TTF-1, *Mol Cell Biol.* **20:** 2783–93.

70. Muro-Cacho, C. A., Holt, T., Klotch, D., Mora, L., Livingston, S. and Futran, N., 1999, Cyclin D1 expression as a prognostic parameter in papillary carcinoma of the thyroid, *Otolaryngol Head Neck Surg.* **120**: 200–7.
71. Nahle, Z., Polakoff, J., Davuluri, R. V., McCurrach, M. E., Jacobson, M. D., Narita, M., Zhang, M. Q., Lazebnik, Y., Bar-Sagi, D. and Lowe, S. W., 2002, Direct coupling of the cell cycle and cell death machinery by E2F, *Nat Cell Biol.* **4**: 859–64.
72. Namba, H., Rubin, S. A. and Fagin, J. A., 1990, Point mutations of Ras oncogenes are an early event in thyroid tumorigenesis, *Mol. Endocrinol.* **4**: 1474–1479.
73. Nikiforova, M. N., Lynch, R. A., Biddinger, P. W., Alexander, E. K., Dorn, G. W., 2nd, Tallini, G., Kroll, T. G. and Nikiforov, Y. E., 2003, RAS point mutations and PAX8-PPAR gamma rearrangement in thyroid tumors: evidence for distinct molecular pathways in thyroid follicular carcinoma, *J Clin Endocrinol Metab.* **88**: 2318–26.
74. Olson, M. F., Paterson, H. F. and Marshall, C. J., 1998, Signals from Ras and Rho GTPases interact to regulate expression of p21Waf1/Cip1, *Nature.* **394**: 220–221.
75. Ouyang, B., Knauf, J. A., Ain, K., Nacev, B. and Fagin, J. A., 2002, Mechanisms of aneuploidy in thyroid cancer cell lines and tissues: evidence for mitotic checkpoint dysfunction without mutations in BUB1 and BUBR1, *Clin Endocrinol* **56**: 341–50.
76. Pak, Y., Pham, N. and Rotin, D., 2002, Direct binding of the B1 adrenergic receptor to the cyclic AMP-dependent guanine nucleotide exchange factor CNrasGEF leads to Ras activation, *Mol Cell Biol.* **22**: 7942–7952.
77. Portella, G., Ferulano, G., Santoro, M., Grieco, M., Fusco, A. and Vecchio, G., 1989, The Kirsten murine sarcoma virus induces rat thyroid carcinomas in vivo, *Oncogene.* **4**: 181–8.
78. Prior, I. A. and Hancock, J. F., 2001, Compartmentalization of Ras proteins, *J. Cell. Sci.* **114**: 1603–1608.
79. Puxeddu, E. and Fagin, J. A., 2001, Genetic markers in thyroid neoplasia, *Endocrinol Metab Clin North Am.* **30**: 493–513.
80. Rajagopalan, H., Bardelli, A., Lengauer, C., Kinzler, K. W., Vogelstein, B. and Velculescu, V. E., 2002, RAF/RAS oncogenes and mismatch-repair status, *Nature.* **418**: 934.
81. Reuther, G. W. and Der, C. J., 2000, The Ras branch of small GTPases: Ras family members don't fall far from the tree, *Curr Opin Cell Biol.* **12**: 157–165.
82. Ribeiro-Neto, F., Urbani, J., Lemee, N., Lou, L. and Altschuler, D. L., 2002, On the mitogenic properties of Rap1b: cAMP-induced G1/S entry requires activated and phosphorylated Rap1b, *Proc. Natl. Acad. Sci. USA.* **99**: 5418–5423.
83. Ringel, M. D., Hayre, N., Saito, J., Saunier, B., Schuppert, F., Burch, H., Bernet, V., Burman, K. D., Kohn, L. D. and Saji, M., 2001, Overexpression and overactivation of Akt in thyroid carcinoma, *Cancer Res.* **61**: 6105–11.
84. Rochefort, P., Caillou, B., Michiels, F. M., Ledent, C., Talbot, M., Schlumberger, M., Lavelle, F., Monier, R. and Feunteun, J., 1996, Thyroid pathologies in transgenic mice expressing a human activated Ras gene driven by a thyroglobulin promoter, *Oncogene.* **12**: 111–8.
85. Saavedra, H. I., Fukasawa, K., Conn, C. W. and Stambrook, P. J., 1999, MAPK mediates RAS-induced chromosome instability, *J Biol Chem.* **274**: 38083–90.
86. Saavedra, H. I., Knauf, J. A., Shirokawa, J. M., Wang, J., Ouyang, B., Elisei, R., Stambrook, P. J. and Fagin, J. A., 2000, The RAS oncogene induces genomic instability in thyroid PCCL3 cells via the MAPK pathway, *Oncogene.* **19**: 3948–54.
87. Saito, J., Kohn, A. D., Roth, R. A., Noguchi, Y., Tatsumo, I., Hirai, A., Suzuki, K., Kohn, L. D., Saji, M. and Ringel, M. D., 2001, Regulation of FRTL-5 thyroid cell growth by phosphatidylinositol (OH) 3 kinase-dependent Akt-mediated signaling, *Thyroid.* **11**: 339–351.
88. Santelli, G., de Franciscis, V., Portella, G., Chiappetta, G., D'Alessio, A., Califano, D., Rosati, R., Mineo, A., Monaco, C., Manzo, G. and et al., 1993, Production of transgenic mice expressing the Ki-ras oncogene under the control of a thyroglobulin promoter, *Cancer Res.* **53**: 5523–7.
89. Serrano, M., Lin, A. W., McCurrach, M. E., Beach, D. and Lowe, S. W., 1997, Oncogenic ras provokes premature cell senescence associated with accumulation of p53 and p16INK4a, *Cell.* **88**: 593–602.
90. Sevetson, B. R., Kong, X. and Lawrence, J. C., 1993, Increasing cAMP attenuates activation of mitogen-activated protein kinase, *Proc. Natl. Acad. Sci. USA.* **90**: 10305–10309.
91. Sherr, C. J. and Roberts, J. M., 1999, CDK inhibitors: positive and negative regulators of G1-phase progression, *Genes Dev.* **13**: 1501–12.
92. Shi, Y.F., Zou, M.J., Schmidt, H., Juhasz, F., Stenzky, V., Robb, D., and Farid, N.R., 1991, *Canc Res* **51**: 2690–2693.

93. Shields, J. M., Pruitt, K., McFall, A., Shaub, A. and Der, C. J., 2000, Understanding Ras: "it ain't over 'till it's over", *Trends in Cell Biol.* **10:** 147–153.
94. Shirokawa, J. M., Elisei, R., Knauf, J. A., Hara, T., Wang, J., Saavedra, H. I. and Fagin, J. A., 2000, Conditional apoptosis induced by oncogenic ras in thyroid cells, *Mol Endocrinol.* **14:** 1725–38.
95. Smith, K. A., Agarwal, K. L., Chernov, M. V., Chernova, O. B., Deguchi, Y., Ishizaka, Y., Patterson, Y. E., Poupon, M. F. and Stark, G. R., 1995, Regulation and mechanisms of gene amplification, *Philos Trans R Soc Lond B Biol Sci.* **347:** 49–56.
96. Spruck, C. H., Won, K. A. and Reed, S. I., 1999, Deregulated cyclin E induces chromosome instability, *Nature.* **401:** 297–300.
97. Suarez, H. G., du Villard, J. A., Severino, M., Cailou, B., Schlumberger, M., M., T., Parmentier, C. and Monier, R., 1990, Presence of mutations in all three ras genes in human thyroid tumors, *Oncogene.* **5:** 565–570.
98. Tsygankova, O. M., Kupperman, E., Wen, W. and Meinkoth, J. L., 2000, Cyclic AMP activates Ras, *Oncogene.* **19:** 3609–15.
99. Tsygankova, O. M., Saavedra, A., Rebhun, J. F., Quilliam, L. A. and Meinkoth, J. L., 2001, Coordinated regulation of Rap1 and thyroid differentiation by cyclic AMP and protein kinase A, *Mol Cell Biol.* **21:** 1921–1929.
100. Van Keymeulen, A., Roger, P. P., Dumont, J. E. and Dremier, S., 2000, TSH and cAMP do not signal mitogenesis through Ras activation, *Biochem Biophys Res Commun.* **273:** 154158.
101. Vanvooren, V., Allgeier, A., Nguyen, M., Massart, C., Parma, J., Dumont, J. E. and Van Sande, J., 2001, Mutation analysis of the Epac–Rap1 signaling pathway in cold thyroid follicular adenomas, *Eur J Endocrinol.* **144:** 605–10.
102. Vasko, V., Ferrand, M., Di Cristofaro, J., Carayon, P., Henry, J. F. and de Micco, C., 2003, Specific pattern of RAS oncogene mutations in follicular thyroid tumors, *J Clin Endocrinol Metab.* **88:** 2745–52.
103. Velasco, J. A., Acebron, A., Zannini, M., Martin-Perez, J., Di Lauro, R. and Santisteban, P., 1998, Ha-ras interference with thyroid cell differentiation is associated with a down-regulation of thyroid transcription factor-1 phosphorylation, *Endocrinology.* **139:** 2796–802.
104. Villalonga, P., Lopez-Alcala, C., Bosch, M., Chiloeches, A., Rocamora, N., Marais, R., Marshall, C. J., Bachs, O. and Agell, N., 2001, Calmodulin binds to K-Ras, but not to H- or N-Ras, and modulates downstream signaling, *Mol. Cell. Biol.* **21:** 7345–7354.
105. Vossler, M. R., Yao, H., York, R. D., Pan, M.-G., Rim, C. S. and Stork, P. J., 1997, cAMP activates MAP kinase and elk-1 through a B-Raf- and Rap1-dependent pathway, *Cell.* **89:** 73–82.
106. Walsh, A. B. and Bar-Sagi, D., 2001, Differential activation of the Rac pathway by Ha-Ras and K-Ras, *J Biol Chem.* **276:** 15609–15615.
107. Wang, S., Wu, J., Savas, L., Patwardhan, N. and Khan, A., 1998, The role of cell cycle regulatory proteins, cyclin D1, cyclin E, and p27 in thyroid carcinogenesis, *Hum Pathol.* **29:** 1304–9.
108. White, M. A., Nicolette, C., Minden, A., Polverino, A., Aelst, L. V., Karin, M. and Wigler, M. H., 1995, Multiple Ras functions can contribute to mammalian cell transformation, *Cell.* **80:** 533–541.
109. Wolfman, J. C., Palmby, T., Der, C. J. and Wolfman, A., 2002, Cellular N-Ras promotes cell survival by downregulation of Jun N-terminal protein kinase and p38, *Mol Cell Biol.* **22:** 1589–1606.
110. Wu, J., Dent, P., Jelinek, T., Wolfman, A., Weber, M. J. and Sturgill, T. A., 1993, Inhibition of EGF-activated MAP kinase signaling pathway by adenosine $3'5'$-monophosphate, *Science.* **262:** 1065–1068.

8. P53 AND OTHER CELL CYCLE REGULATORS

NADIR R. FARID

Osancor Biotech Inc, 31 Woodland Drive, Watford, Herts, U.K., WD17 3BY

INTRODUCTION

Most tumor suppressor genes (whose function in cancer biology was surmised by their inactivation or deletion) turn out to be important in normal cell growth and proliferation. Inactivation of these genes opens the gates to malignant transformation driven by aberrant growth signals. In general, tumor suppressor dysfunction does not initiate genomic instability or aneuploidy, hallmarks of the origin of cancer, but they are at least as susceptible as other genes to the consequences of these destabilizing phenomena. On the other hand, these genes have a predilection to inactivation by epigenetic mechanisms, such as aberrant methylation with the progression of cell transformation.

This chapter focuses on the pathways anchored by the two "big" regulators of the cell cycle: p53 and the retinoblastoma (Rb) genes. Until recently the connections between these two networks was obscure (1). It is now apparent that they regulate and counter-regulate each other in a Ying-Yang fashion. The network centred on p53 is denser and more intricate (2,3), receiving signals from upstream modulators and downstream effectors. In addition to their respective roles at crucial check-points in the cell cycle and DNA repair, the products of both these genes appear to have roles in embryogenesis, cell differentiation and cell fate including senesce(1,4,5).

THE P53 NETWORK

P53 is a transcription factor that transactivates a large number of genes. The abundance of the p53 protein is predominantly regulated through its degradation. Compared to the other features of its biology, our knowledge of the transcriptional regulation is less than complete. The gene is induced by single DNA breaks, radiation, UV light, some chemotherapeutic agents (3) and as demonstrated beautifully recently by interferons α/β (6). P53 tansactivation of its target genes is regulated by posttranslational mechanisms including phosphorylation, acetylation and prolyl isomeration (3,7) or by protein-protein interaction (8). P53 thus modified may select subsets of target promoters by changing its shape and affinity to bind to regulatory DNA sequences that vary among the downstream genes. Little is, however, known about the mechanisms underpinning the selection of the target genes and the divergent cell fates triggered down a given pathway (3,7). In certain situations apparently non-modified P53 can select and activate genes (6).

MDM2 and networks cross-over

P53 is ubiquinated by MDM2, directing it to the proteosomes for degradation. P53/MDM2 makes a finely balanced tandem. Thus, while p53 up-regulates MDM2 gene transcription, the MDM2 protein marks p53 for proteolysis by attaching ubiquitin to its carboxy-terminus (2,3). Furthermore phosphorylation of p53 NH2-terminus (and its activation) influences its binding affinity to MDM2, and thus its degradation (2,3). A deubiquinating enzyme can counteract the degree to which P53 is ubiquinated (9). Moreover, the transcriptional response of P53 may be regulated by the SUMO-1 modification of its carboxy-terminus (10).

And the regulation of MDM2 gets even more complex, in that it is capable of self-ubiquination and is SUMO-1 modified. The latter modification prevents MDM2, s self-ubiquination and therefore, in turn, its ability to ubiquinate P53 (11) The phosphorylation of MDM2 through the phosphatidylinositol 3-kinase (PI3K) pathway (12,13) may also enhances its ability to ubiquinate and thus regulate the cellular level of p53.

Other cues for the p53—anchored pathway also feed through MDM2. Thus growth signals from a number of oncogenes e.g. RAS, induce the ARF gene or stabilize its protein. ARF promotes the accumulation of SUMO-1 modified MDM2 and block the shuffle of MDM2 from the nucleolus to the cytoplasm, thereby stabilizing P53 (14–16).

MDM2 is also the conduit for the regulation of growth factors and allied receptors relevant to proliferation and signaling (17,18)

The influence of ARF on MDM2 function is an important link between the P53 signaling network to that centered on Rb, in that ARF gene transcription is, in turn, regulated by E2F (1). And this influence is far from being unidirectional because MDM2 (which you will recall is transcriptionally regulated by P53) binds to Rb and E2F with resulting increase in E2F gene transcription (19 for review).

Cycle arrest & apoptosis

When the cell is stressed or its function impaired, p53 abundance is increased and the protein activated to arrest cell division until such time as repairs are affected (2,3). P53 mediates the arrest of the cell cycle at the G1/S restriction point and the G2/M phase through the increasing the transcription of p21^{WAF}, an inhibitor of cyclin-dependent kinases. p21 activation is another important node in the cross-communication between p53/Rb networks. p21 activation inhibits the kinases that drive cyclin D and related kinases which phosphorylate RB thus releasing E2F from its grips(1). Other genes regulated by p53 include Reprimo, which arrest the cycle at G2. Interestingly, in epithelial cells 14-3-3σ, by sequestering cyclin 1/CDK1 complexes in the nucleus can affect G2 arrest. Inhibition of 14-3-3σ allows epithelial cells to grow indefinitely (3).

When cellular damage is beyond the capability of the repair mechanisms, apoptosis is orchestrated by p53 (2,3,7). That option is apparently dependent on the abundance of p53 in the cell and is possibly tissue-specific (20). P53 homologs p63 and p73 are not relevant to tumor suppression but they are to apoptosis (21). The transcription of the Bax gene, whose product is pro-apoptotic, is enhanced by p53 apparently through the mediation of another gene (22). Other genes which promote cell death signals and that are induced by p53 include Noxa, p53 A1P1 and PIDD. A1P1 forms complexes with p53 to interact more strongly with the promoters of apoptosis-inducing genes than those involved in cell cycle arrest (8,20). P53 may induce apoptosis through a lysosomal-mitochondrial pathway that is initiated by lysosomal destabilization (23).

Another aspect of the role of p53 as a "guardian of the genome" is its function in maintaining genomic integrity. This is probably achieved by regulating nucleotide excision repair, chromosomal recombination and segregation. That p53 has an important role in DNA repair is supported by its induction of "ribonucleotide reductase" gene following DNA damage (24).

P53 inhibits the formation of new blood vessel in response to trophic factors elaborated (VGEF) by some tumors. Loss of p53 in late progression removes these restraints and allows continued tumor growth and metastases (25).

P53 IN HUMAN CANCERS

P53 is mutated in some 50% of human tumors (see http://perso.curie.fr/Thierry.Soussi, www.iarc.fr/p53/index.html and http://cancergenetics.org/p53.htm, 2,3,7). There are about 18,000 such entries in existing databases, the vast majority of which are missense mutations that apparently disable p53 tumor suppressor function. Table 1 lists the various mechanisms involved in p53 inactivation. While DNA sequence alterations (missense mutations, deletions and insertions, abnormal splicing) are more common in some malignancies compared to others, the other mechanisms shown in Table 1

Table 1. The various ways P53 may be inactivated in malignancies, *modified from (3)*

Mechanism of p53 inactivation	Consequences of inactivation
Missense mutations in the DNA-binding domain	Failure of p53 as a transcription factor
Carboxy-terminus deletions	No p53 tetramers are formed
MDM2 gene amplification	Enhanced p53 proteolysis
ARF deletion	Impaired inhibition of MDM2
Infection by some DNA viruses	Viral products inactivate p53 or increase its degradation
Failure of p53 to localize to the nucleus	p53 does not function

are limited to narrow classes of tumors. Some mechanisms e.g human papilloma virus in cervical cancer, may be related to environmental access of the carcinogen, whereas others may reflect the specific differentiated tissue environment e.g. MDM2 amplification in sarcomas and brain tumors (3). Not all potential mechanisms for inactivation of the p53 pathways have been systematically investigated for the majority of tumors.

Not only do P53 and Rb pathways cross but also the products of some DNA viruses inactivate them both (1–3).

Of the almost 18,000 p53 mutations in human malignancies, 97% are clustered in the core of the DNA-binding domain and 75% represent missense mutations. Until quite recently only a limited number of the tumor-derived missense mutations have been shown to render p53 defective. In order to address this deficiency Kato et al (7) mutated all 393 residues for all possible substitutions, examined the transactivating capacity of the products, after appropriate editing. Overall, 36% of the mutants were functionally inactive and 64% of core domain mutants fell in that category. Except for mutants at the C-terminal tetramerization domain, the functional part of p53 was concentrated between residues 96 and 286. Even within the DNA-binding core, the secondary structures were more susceptible than the connecting loops to functional disruption. By the same token, the conserved regions in closer proximity to DNA were more sensitive to mutations than conserved region not as intimately associated with DNA. At least for some substitutions, there appear to be differential effect on the transactivation of the p53 responsive genes examined (MDM2, BAX, 14-3-3σ, p53A1P1, GADD 45, Noxa, p53R2).

Interestingly, of the 1266 (54.7%) mutants which could be explained by function/mutation notion, 39.1% were inactive for all 8 promoters and have never been reported in tumors, 15.6% were inactive and reported in tumors, 16.1% were reported at least once in tumors but retained wild type transactivating capacity, 1.6% were inactivating mutations but have never been reported in tumors (7) probably because they occur in p53 domains not usually studied for mutations) and finally 27.5% were inactive for only a limited number of promoters. The last category of mutants may well have partial function in tumor suppression but may show pleomorphism in their range of activity against various downstream target genes (7)

P53 mutations in thyroid cancer

The prevalence of p53 mutations (14.3%) in thyroid carcinoma overall is much lower than in common cancers (2,26). Most studies have limited mutation screening to exons 5–8. Apparent mutation hot spots were located at residues 167, 183, 213, 248 and 273, mapping to the DNA-binding core of the p53 protein (2, 26,27). Viewed in the light of recent developments (7), it is apparent that the mutations reported at the caroxby terminal of exon 8 and indeed a few within the DNA-binding core (27), do not influence the transactivating capacity of p53. Such functionally silent mutants may have been accidentally expanded during clonal selection of tumor cells. It cannot, however, be excluded that these apparently functionally silent mutants within the DNA-binding core may have minor disruptive influence on p53's tumor-suppressive function unrelated to its transactivating capacity. In this context, the claim that homozygosity for p53 proline 72 (a polymorphic Arg/Pro site) predisposes to anaplastic carcinoma (28) cannot be sustained. That the silent mutation rate of p53 in thyroid carcinomas was almost 120 fold that expected and 6 times the average rate of p53 silent mutations in the databases, the apparent random distribution of these mutations and distribution of multiple mutations (doublets, triplets) in accordance with Poisson's expectations suggest that p53 is particularly hypermutable in malignant thyroid tumors (2,27).

Almost a third of the mutations in p53 comprise G: C→A: T transitions at CpG dinucleotides and 5 of 6 mutation hotspots (codons 175, 245, 273 and 282) are CpG sites. ^{m}C (5-methylcystosine) is frequently converted to T by spontaneous hydrolytic deamination, forming a basis for an epigenetic mutational mechanism. These epigenetic events occur predominantly in poorly differentiated and anaplastic tumors; with one exception each all transitions at codons 273 and 248 were found in such tumors (2). Although the distribution of C→T/G→A transitions suggest that ^{m}C deamination is as likely to be time-dependent as replication- dependent (29), we speculate that it may occur at the thyroidal stem cell stage.

Even though p53 is only one of many pathways leading to thyroid cancer it appears to have a pivotal role in differentiated thyroid function, in that thyroid –specific differentiation genes are re-expressed on anaplastic thyroid cancer cells harbouring p53 mutant with transfection of wild type p53 (30).

Mutations in radiation related thyroid cancer

The prevalence of p53 mutations thyroid cancers related to radiation is no different from that in the non-irradiated tumor population (2,27). However, the frequency distribution of the mutation spectrum is radically different between two groups (Table 2). Moreover, the radiation—related thyroid tumors show higher G: C→A: T transitions rates and silent mutations than the non-radiation related thyroid tumors. Experimental radiation of thyroid epithelial cells was found to increase the rate of p53 silent mutations (31). The role of radiation in targeting mutation sites is further bolstered by the fact that none of the mutations in radiation related tumors involved CpG dinucleotides as opposed to one-quarter in the non-radiation related tumors.

Table 2. Mutation spectrum in radiation-related compared to non-radiation related thyroid carcinomas

P53 codons	Radiation-related	Non-radiation related
248		8/8
273		9/9
213	6/8	2/8
167	5/5	
183	5/5	
173		3/3
208	2/3	1/3
266		3/3

Only codons with 3 or more mutation events are considered.
χ_2(heterogeneity) = 34.98, p < 0.0005 (df = 7)

The apical pole of thyrocytes copes with significant oxidative stress. The notion that that DNA mutagenesis is induced by oxidation of G (32) and exaggerated by radiation is attractive but is not upheld by the nature (transitions) of p53 mutations actually observed. Other mechanisms of p53 oxireduction by environmental factors (33) cannot be excluded. On the other hand given the abundance of nitrous oxide (NO) synthases in thyroid tissue (34) and documented increased NO in malignant tumors (35), it is conceivable that local NO generation may be responsible for G: C→A:T transitions in poorly differentiated thyroid carcinomas. The scenario for incriminating NO in p53 mutagenesis might, however, be different from that shown in inflammatory bowel disease and rheumatoid arthritis field (36–38).

P53 mutations in different studies

Although the number of samples exhibiting p53 mutations in individual reports in the literature is small, there are enough striking differences between them to warrant comment. Recurrence of the nature and type of mutations in series from individual centers is interesting. Thus in two series from Japan transitions at p53 codon 248 predominated, in a US study mutation were limited to transitions at codon 273, whereas in a third series (from Italy) p53 abnormalities in thyroid tumors were completely limited to frame-shift mutation, uncommon in the database as a whole (see 2 for review). If the possibility of cross-contamination is put aside, one might therefore speculate that local environmental or genetic factors contributing to the differences in mutations from different centers. Given the small numbers of mutations in each series these must remain that—speculations. The differences between radiation-related and spontaneous thyroid tumors considered above are probably on a more secure basis.

The abundance of P53 in thyroid tumors

While mutant p53 have longer half-lives and are thus more abundant in thyroid tumors harboring p53 mutations, p53 abundance may also be regulated by upstream signals in the absence of mutations (2,3,7). Cancer genes involved in malignant thyroid cell transformation mediate some of their effect by repressing cellular p53 levels (13,39). Thus the oncogene RET/PTC was found to reduce the levels of p53 and it is known that the PI3K pathway, normally repressed by the tumor suppressor PTEN, can influence p53 levels by way of phosphorylation of Mdm2 (12,13).

Although there is broad correlation between p53 mutations and immunohistochemical reactivity, documented gene mutation rates are less than estimates based on protein abundance on histology. Aberrant p53 immunoreactivity is detectable in 40–50% of poorly differentiated carcinomas, not significantly more than in anaplastic (50–60%) tumors (40,41). While, however, in undifferentiated cancer p53 expression is widespread, in poorly differentiated carcinoma it is usually observed in a lower proportion of cells and is sometimes confined to specific tumor foci with aggressive/infiltrative growth.

It is likely that a wide range of activities against downstream target genes are necessary for p53 to exert its full tumor suppressive function. This may explain why whereas p53 is frequently mutated, mutations in downstream target genes are rarely found.

MDM2 in thyroid cancer

MDM 2 is upregulated in a small percentage of malignant thyroid tumors. That this occurs, irrespective of the presence of wt p53, suggest that increased MDM2 gene transcription is in response to upstream cues and probably feed upon other targets of MDM2 (42). MDM2 is not amplified nor re-arranged in thyroid tumors. Interestingly, MDM2 transcripts abundance was related to clinical tumor staging (43).

MDM 2 is apparently more likely to be translocated to the nucleus in well-differentiated malignant thyroid tumors than in benign nodular tissue, thus sequestering p53 (44) (or driving the cell cycle via Rb/E2F). An increase in MDM 2 protein by immunocytochemistry is more frequent, found in half the tumors and is related to the expression of the anti-apoptotic protein Bcl-2 (45).

P21 in thyoid cancer

P21 is a downstream transcriptional target of p53 which inhibits Rb phosphorylation in a cyclin-dependent kinase 2-specific but not cyclin-dependent kinase 4-specific sites (46), thus setting up a pathway that uses the cell's normal regulatory machinery involving Rb phosphoryaltion. Interestingly, cyclin D1 involved in the phosphorylation of p21 may influence the cell cycle independent of the cyclin-dependent kinases by sequestering p21 (47). P21 may be induced independent of p53 and plays important roles in differentiation of such tissues as skeletal muscle (48).

P21 protein expression may be reduced in carcinomas with p53 mutations. However, this correlation is far from consistent in that p21 is detected in 1/3 of tumors irrespective of their degree of differentiation and is often co-expressed with p53, suggesting p53 independent induction of p21 in these tumors (49,50). Deletions and mutations of p21 were examined in one study only, comprising 57 thyroid tumors. Exon 2 of the p21 gene was deleted in 12.5% of papillary thyroid carcinomas. The deletion in 3/5 samples was related to a point mutation 16 bps upstream from the splice donor site and result in aberrant RNA splicing. P21codon 31 (Ser→Arg) polymorphism was no more frequent in patients with thyroid cancer compared to controls (51). It was assumed that these mutants were functionally inactive as they mapped in the most evolutionarily conserved part of the gene and as p21 truncated beyond nt 222 were functionally inactive (52). None of the tumors haboring p21 deletion mutant carried p53 or Rb mutations (43,51, see below).

The putative tumor suppressor gene TSG101 is involved in the regulation of the cell cycle by binding to p21 and increasing its stability. The influence of TSG101 on p21 is proliferative-phase and perhaps tissue specific (53,54). TSG 101 transcripts and gene product abundance has been reported to be upregulated in papillary carcinoma (55). Interestingly, TSG101 is encoded in a chromosomal region notorious for its genomic instability and which spans another tumor suppressor gene, *FHIT*, which is frequently deleted in all stages of thyroid tumor formation (56). The notion that frequent abnormal transcripts of TSG101 and *FHIT* reflect genomic instability and are of doubtful biologic significance (57) is likely incorrect.

THE RETINOBLASTOMA GENE NETWORK

Aberrations of the Rb gene is found in ~50% all human tumors (1) and yet it has not been as intensively studied in human cancers as have p53!. Indeed alterations in the Rb signalling pathway, by activation of positive acting components such as G1 cyclins and cyclin-dependent kinases (cdk), by inactivation of negative acting components such as cdk inhibitors and p53, or by mutations in Rb itself has been detected in virtually all human cancers (58).

Rb plays a pivotal role in the G1 checkpoint in the cell cycle, in balancing proliferation and apoptosis and in determining cell fate. It is important for the terminal differentiation of a number of tissues both in the embryonic and extraembryonic tissues (4).

Rb inhibits cell cycle advance when underphosphorylated. Once phosphorylated by two cyclin/cdk complexes Rb releases its control on the cycle. The G1 cyclins upstream of Rb are, in turn, regulated by inhibitors. By controlling the activities of certain transcription factors and thus responding genes Rb permits the cycle to progress from the G1 phase into S phase. The most prominent and important of these transcription factors are members of the E2F family (1). Two classes of cdk inhibitors interpret the responses of the cell to environmental signals: the CIP/KIP and INK4 that silence the cdks.

The G1 phase cyclins are engaged by cdk4 or ckd6 early in G1 and cdk 2 late in G1, to phosphorylate Rb thus releasing E2F to act at their cognate promoters. Early in S phase cyclinA/cdk2 complexes are activated not only to drive the cycle forward but also to terminate the transcriptional influence of E2Fs by phosphorylating them (1,59).

RB in thyroid carcinoma

Rb is deleted not only in retinoblastoma but in a large variety of sporadic tumors including osteosarcoma, carcinomas of the bladder, prostate and small cell lung carcinoma (1). Reports of Rb aberration in thyroid tumors are sparse.

We found in frame deletion of Rb exon 21 in 55% of malignant (but not benign) thyroid tumors (60). Exon 21 is an integral component of the Rb "pocket" that binds E2F and oncogenic DNA virus antigens (1). The Rb deletions were related to defective RNA splicing, although no mutations at the exon/intron junction were found (60). Both copies of the Rb gene were deleted in only one –third of the samples. Immunocytochemical analysis of pRb was, however, reduced or diminished in all positive specimens, suggesting that additional lesions in the promoter or coding sequence of Rb may have inactivated the second allele. It is noteworthy that mice with a single copy of Rb ($Rb^{+/-}$) develop neuroendocrine tumors including medullary thyroid carcinoma (61); it conceivable that a different tissue environment in adult thyroid tissue encourage somatic transformation of epithelial thyroid cells.

For technical and interpretative reasons the loss of Rb immunoreactivity in malignant thyroid tumors was not upheld earlier (see 62 for review). Since then, pRb loss turns out to be a consistent feature of papillary and follicular carcinoma but apparently not that of Hürthel cell or Warthin-like variants of the former (62,63).

The Cyclin-kinase Inhibitors

The CPI/KIP family

P21 is rarely mutated in human neoplasms and has been considered in thyroid carcinoma above under P53.

$P27^{KIP1}$ responds to cellular environmental signals such as growth factors, cell anchorage and contact inhibition. It is also rarely deleted in tumors. $P27^{KIP1}$ protein abundance is regulated post-translationally by way of phosphorylation and proteosome-mediated degradation following ubiquination (1).

$P27^{K1P1}$ protein abundance is reduced in malignant thyroid tumors and is associated with poor clinical outcomes (64,65). Its levels are, however, maintained in a subset of tumors, predominantly those with oncocytic histology including follicular variant of papillary carcinoma (66,67). The cytoplasmic accumulation of $P27^{K1P1}$ is probably related to its sequestration by cyclin D3 (68). This mechanism surmised on my part would need to be directly confirmed. This phenomenon is, however, not without precedent as p21 may be regulated by its being sequestered by cyclin D1(47).

The INK4 family

The two members of the INK4 family, INK4A and INK4B, are closely linked on 9p21, a region of the genome highly mutable in familial melanomas and pancreatic carcinomas. This region thus exhibits a high rate of LOH in tumor tissue. Human tumors contain either mutations in Rb or INK4A, which needs wild type Rb to disrupt the cell cycle. The reading frame of another gene alluded to before in the connection of the p53/Rb networks, ARF, overlaps that of INK4A (1 for review).

Mutations or deletions of INK4A and INK4B are infrequent in primary thyroid carcinomas but are common in thyroid carcinoma cell lines (69–72). Epigenetic silencing of INK4B by hypermethylation may be not an uncommon mechanism for gene silencing in clinical tumor material (72,73). Moreover, LOH at 9p21 may be a more frequent event in thyroid carcinoma than is the recorded inactivation of INK4 family members, suggesting the presence of tumor suppressor genes in the vicinity.

The cyclins

Cyclin D1 is an early G1 cell cycle progression factor (1,2,48). While cyclin D1 regulates Rb activity by way of post-translational modification, Rb enhances the specific transcription of cyclin D1 (74), thus setting up a regulatory feedback loop. Aberrant expression of cyclin D1 through gene amplification or overexpression is a common feature of several cancers. CyclinD1is often amplified only in those tumors that retain wild-type pRb (See 48). We first reported (48,75) the upregulation of cyclin D1 transcripts in $1/3$ of malignant thyroid tumors. Overexpression of cyclin D1, studied in 32 tumors was not related to gene amplification or re-arrangement. Cyclin D1 overexpression was predominantly found in tumors retaining wild type Rb, a fact not emphasized enough in subsequent studies. Our findings have been amply verified at the level of cyclin D1 protein level (43,66,67,76–79) as have our suggestion that gene amplification is not involved in gene product overexpression (64,80). Cyclin D1 (and lack thereof of p27) overexpression has proved to be an important prognostic factor (43,76,78,79) in the prediction of lymph node metastases in papillary thyroid cancer. Moreover cyclin D1 overexpression in papillary microcarcinomas predicted secondaries to the regional lymph nodes (64). Constitutive activation of Ret as a result as of RET/PTC re-arrangement appears to be involved in inducing cyclin D1 over-expression (81). Cyclin D1 may also be upregulated by other oncogenes (82,83).

In well-differentiated papillary thyroid carcinomas cyclin D1 overexpression was related to that of p21 (43,77), which was apparently induced by a p53-independent mechanism (43).

The abundance of the other G1 phase cyclin, cyclin E, appeared to parallel that of cyclin D1 (66,67) and did not appear to be differentially expressed between different tumor types.

E2F

The E2F family of transcription factors is the most important downstream effectors of Rb. They bind to relevant promoters only when heterodimerized with their partner DP. The complexes show specificity for Rb or its homolgos p107 and p130. The E2F family members mediate many of Rb,s effect in embryogenesis, cell differentiation and cell fate as well as apparently functions as a transcription factor independent of Rb (1). E2F is involved in the induction of genes required in initiating and executing DNA replication, DNA repair, cell cycle progression and apoptosis (including Myc and ARF). Beyond the G1/S restriction point E2F regulate genes involved in G2/M checkpoints and mitotic regulation as well as chromosomal dynamics.

The E2F/DP complex is inactivated by cyclinA/cdk2 phosphorylation and its abundance modulated by ubiquitin—mediated degradation.

Although no mutations have been described in E2F in human tumors, it is apparent that its overexpression stimulates cell proliferation and contribute to carcinogenesis. Depending on ambient growth signals it E2F can promote apoptosis in both p53-dependent and—independent manner.

Thyroid carcinomas are reported to overexpress E2F (63,80,84). E2F appeared to be particularly expressed in oxyphilic adenomas and carcinomas (2/3 of samples) (84) compared to non-oxyphilic lesions (1/3 of samples). Anwar developed this theme further by showing that the presence of pRb and E2F can be used to sub-categorize papillary carcinomas: Hürthle and Warthin-like variants which arise within the context of Hashimoto's thyroiditis were Rb and E2F1 positive, whereas papillary carcinoma, including the follicular variant were negative for both (63). Interestingly, metaplastic Hurthle cells associated with thyroid autoimmune disease were only Rb positive. This fascinating observation (63) warrants further follow-up.

Just as with p53, E2F appears to be under negative regulation by TR and the interaction is equally complex in that when bound to E2F promoter the unliganded TR activates transcription, whereas the liganded receptor represses the transcription of S-phase specific DNA polymerase, thymidine kinase and dihydrofolate reductase genes and thus withdrawal of S phase to initiate differentiation (85). A high rate of aberrant TR in thyroid tumors (see the Chapter by Cheng) would release such restraining influence on E2F.

Further afield

It is apparent that the influence of Rb and its downstream interactors extends beyond the S phase of the cell cycle, to G2-M and hence my justification for the discussion the roles in thyroid cancer of cyclins acting later in the cycle and indeed a negative cyclin.

Cyclins A, B1 and cdc2 are factors which regulate the transition from G2 to the M phase of the cycle. Cyclin A and cdc2 were overexpressed in undifferentiated thyroid cancers, as opposed to cyclin B1 which was less frequently overexpressed in this class of tumors (86).

Recently Ito et al (87) found that the expression of cyclin G2 that negatively regulates cell cycle progression could differentiate between papillary and follicular thyroid tumors. Thus, whereas normal thyroid tissues and papillary tumors were negative for cyclin G2, it was expressed in 2/3 follicular adenomas but only 20% of follicular carcinomas.

THYROID HORMONE RECEPTORS & TUMOR SUPPRESSOR NETWORKS

Thyroid hormones have a profound influence on development, growth, energy and intermediary metabolism and, as being recently realized, in carcinognesis (See Chapter 9). Thyroid hormones acting through their receptors (TRs) can be also be modelled as a wide-ranging network with crucial nodes. Not surprisingly the p53-based network overlap that predicated on thyroid hormone action and apparently influence each other. P53 apparently binds to and modulates TRβ activity and depending on cell type and experimental system p53 was reported to repress basal or ligand-mediated activity (88,89). TR can apparently also regulate MDM2 gene transcription independently of p53 (90). The potential for thyroid hormones influencing both tumor suppressor networks discussed above is immediately obvious and is an area where more functional studies would be welcome. Cheng discusses elsewhere in this book the mutation of TR in thyroid carcinoma, I only point out that the frequent silent mutations noted in those studies echo those in p53!

CONCLUSIONS & PRESPECTIVES

Our understanding of the physiologic roles of the many nodes that interconnect within and between the p53 and Rb—based networks is less than complete. However, rapid progress is being made. In thyroid tumors much of the relevant data is predicated on the abundance of specific proteins determined immmuncytochemically. While this approach is rapid, cheap, may relate gene product abundance to histology and even allow the construction of hypotheses on the pathways involved, it gives limited insight into the molecular mechanisms involved.

Studies of the rates and nature of p53 mutation suggest that the gene is highly mutable in thyroid tumors and specifically incriminates a commonly occurring epigenetic event in anaplastic carcinoma, rarely found in well-differentiated tumors. Another common epigenetic mechanism for tumor suppressor inactivation, hypermethylation of regulatory sequences, has been documented in INK4B within the Rb network as well as in genes in independent pathways, involved in cytoskeletal integrity (91). Rb gene is frequently truncated resulting in low levels of Rb protein, a finding that needs to be explored more widely. That p21, which is rarely inactivated in tumors, is also truncated in thyroid carcinomas through aberrant RNA splicing raises suspicions that correct RNA splicing may be impaired in thyroid tumors.

Interestingly, the only two genes within the p53 and Rb networks we found to be differentially regulated in thyroid tumors were A1P1, involved in p53 related apoptosis and cyclin D1 (Puskas L & Farid, NR, unpublished). Cyclin D1, which is important in regulating Rb function and thus cell cylce progression, is upregulated through diverse pathways. Cyclin D1 is also a "cross-over artist" because by sequestering p21 it can extend its proactive influence on to the p53 network. Cyclin D1's abundance is valuable in forecasting the outcome of thyroid carcinoma, even those in the microtumor stage of their evolution (64).

It is apparent that genes entrusted with putting the brakes on the cell cycle, often fail in thyroid tumors. There are many areas of uncertainty or outright ignorance that need to be filled in with systematic studies of genes and gene products within these pathways.

REFERENCES

1. Yamasaki, L Role of the RB tumor suppressor in cancer In DA Franks (Edit) "Signal transduction in cancer", Kluwer Academic Publishers, Boston 2003, pp 208–239.
2. Farid NR 2001 P53 mutations in thyroid carcinoma: Tidings from an old foe *J. Endocrinol. Invest.* 24, 536–545.
3. Vogelstein B, Lane D, Levine AB 2000 Surfing the p53 network *Nature* 408, 307–310.
4. De Bruin A, Wu L, Saavedra HI, Wilson P, Yang Y, Rosol TJ, Weinstein M, Robinson ML, Leone G 2003 Rb function in extraembryonic lineages suppresses apoptosis in the CNS of Rb-deficient mice *Proc Natl Acad Sci USA* 100, 6546–6551.
5. Tyner SD, Venkatachalam S, Choi J, ones S, Ghebranious N, Igelmann H, Lu X, Soron G, Cooper B, Brayton C, Park SH, Thompson T, Harsenty G, Bradely A, Donehower LA 2002 p53 mutants mice that display early ageing-associated phenotypes *Nature* 415, 45–53.
6. Takaoka A, Hayakawa S, Yani H, Stoiber D, Negishsi H, Kikuchi H, Sasaki S, Imai K, Shibue T, Honda K, Taniguchi T 2003 Integration of interferon-α/β signalling to p53 responses in tumour suppression and antiviral defence *Nature (Lon.)* 424, 516–523.
7. Kato S, Han S-Y, Liu W, Otsuka K, Shibata H, Kanamaru R, Ishioka C 2003 Understanding the function-structure and function-mutation relationships of p53 tumor suppressor protein by high-resolution missense mutation analysis Proc. Natl Acad, Sci USA 100, 8424–8429.
8. Samuels-Lev Y, O'Connor DL, Bergamaschi D, Trigiante G, Hsieh JK, Zhong S, Campargue I, Naumovski L, Crook T, Lu X 2001 ASPP proteins specifically stimulate the apoptotic function of p53 Mol.Cell 8, 781–794.
9. Li M, Chen D, Shiloh A, Luo J, Nikolaev A, Qin J, Gu W 2002 Deubiquination of p53 by HAUSP is an important pathway for p53 stabilization *Nature* 416, 648–653.

10. Rodriguez MS, Desterro JM, Lain S, Midgley CA, Lane DP, Hay RT 1999 SUMO-1 modification activates the transcriptional response of p53 *EMBO J* 18, 6455–6461.
11. Buschmann T, Lerner D, Lee CG, Ronai Z 2001The Mdm-2 amino-terminus is required for the MDm2 binding and SUMO-1 modification by E2 SUMO-1 conjugating enzyme ubc9 *J. Biol. Chem.*276, 40389–40395.
12. Yoko O, Shohei K, Toshiyuki O, Yuko I, Toshiaki S, Keiji T, Norihisa M, Yukiko G 2002 Akt enhances mdm2-mediated ubiquination and degradation of p53 *J. Biol. Chem.* 277, 21843–21850.
13. Schon O, Friedler A, Bycroft M, Freund S, Fersht A2002 Molecular mechanisms of the interaction between MDM2 and P53 *J. Mol. Biol.* 323, 491–501.
14. Tao W, Levine AJ 1999 P19^{ARF} stabilizes p53 by blocking nucleo-cytoplasmic shuttling of Mdm2 *Proc. Natl. Acad. Sci.USA* 96, 69378–6941.
15. Kamjo T, Weber JD, Zambetti G, Zindy F, Rouissel, Sherr CJ 1998 Functional and physical interactions at the ARF tumor suppressor with p53 and Mdm2 *Proc. Natl. Acad. Sci.USA* 95, 8292–8297
16. Xirodimas DP, Chisholm J, Desterro JM, Lane DP, Hay RT 2002 P14ARF promotes the accumulation of SUMO-1 conjugated (H) Mdm2 *FEBS Lett.* 528, 207–211.
17. Shenoy SK, McDonald PH, Kohout TA, LefkowitzRJ 2001Regulation of receptor fate by ubiquination ofactivated beta-2 adrenergic receptor and beta-arrestin *Science* 294, 1307–1313.
18. Girnita L, Girnita A, Larsson O 2003 Mdm2-dependent ubiquination and degradation of the insulin-like growth factor 1 receptor *Pro. Natl. Acad. Sci. USA* 100, 8247–8252.
19. Daujat S, Neel H, Piette J 2001 MDM2: life without p53 *TrendsGenet* 17, 459–464.
20. Lane D 2001 How cells choose to die *Nature* 414, 25–27.
21. Flores ER, Tsai KY, Crowley D, Sengupta S, Yang A, McKeon F, Jacks, T 2002 p63 and p73 are required for p53-depedent apoptosis in response to DNA damage *Nature* 416, 560–564.
22. Yu J, wang Z, Kinzler KW, Vogelstein B, Zhang L 2003 *PUMA* mediates the apoptotic response to p53 in colorectal cancer cells *Proc. Natl. Acad. Sci.USA* 100, 1931–1936
23. Yuan X-M, Li W, Dalen H, Lotem J, Kama R, Sachs R, Brunk UT 2002 Lysosomal destabilization in p53-induced apoptosis *Proc. Natl. Acad. Sci.USA* 99, 6286–6291.
24. Tanaka H, Arakawa H, Yamaguchi T, Shiraishi K,Fukuda S, Matusi K, Takei Y, Nakamura Y 2000 A ribonucleotide reductase gene is involved in a p53 cell-cycle checkpoint for DNA damage *Nature* 404, 42–48.
25. Hendrix MJ 2000 De-mystifying the mechanisms(s) of maspin *Nat. Med* 6, 374–376.
26. FaridNR, Shi Y, Zou M 1994 Molecular basis of thyroid cancer *Endocr Rev*.15, 202–232.
27. Shahedian B, Shi Y, Zou M, Farid NR 2001Thyroid carcinoma is characterized by genomic insability: evidence from p53 mutations *Mol. Gene. Metab* 72, 155–163.
28. Boltze C, Roessener A, Landt O, Szibor R, Peters B, Schneider-Stock R 2002 Homozygous praline at codon 72 of p53 as a potential risk factor favoring the development of undifferentiated thyroid carcinoma *In. J. Oncol.* 21, 1151–1154
29. Rodin SI, Rodin AS 1998 Strand asymmetry of CpG transition as indicator of G1 phase –dependent origin of multiple p53 mutations in stem cell *Proc. Natl. Acad. Sci.USA* 95, 11927–11932.
30. Moretti F, Farsetti A, Soddu S, Misiti S, Crescenzi M, Filetti S, Andreoli M, Sacchi A, Ponecorvi A 1997 p53 re-expression inhibits proliferation and restores differentiation of human thyroid anaplastic carcinoma cells *Oncogene* 14, 729–740.
31. Gamble SC, Cook MC, Riches AC, Herceg Z, Bryant PE, Arrand JE 1999 p53 mutations in tumors derived from irradiated human thyroid epithelial cells *Mutat. Res* 425, 231–238
32. Bruner SD, Nor,man DPG, Verdine GL 2000 Structural basis for recognition and repair of the endogenous mutagen 8-oxoguanine in DNA *Nature* 403, 859–866.
33. Asher G, Lotem J, Kama R, Sachs L, Shaul Y 2002 NQ01 stabilizes p53 through a distinct mechanism *Proc. Natl. Acad. Sci. USA* 99, 3099–3104.
34. Colin IM,Nava E, Toussaint D, Maiter DM ,vanDenhove MF, Luscher TF, Ketelslegers JM,Denef JF, Jameson JL1995 Expression of nitric oxide synthase isoforms in the thyroid gland: evidence for a role of nitric oxide in vascular control during goiter formation *Endocrinology* 136, 5283–5290.
35. Patel A, Fenton C, Terrell R, Powers PA, Dinauer C, Tuttle RM, Francis GL 2002 Nitrotyrosine, inducible nitric acid oxide synthase (iNOS), and endothelial nitric oxide synthase (eNOS) are increased in thyroid tumors from children and adolescents *J. Endocrinol. Invest.* 25, 675–683.
36. Kasai K, HattoriY,Nakanishi N,Manaka K, Banba N, Motohashi S, Shimoda S1995 Regulation by inducible nitric oxide production by cytokines in human thyrocytes in culture *Endocrinology* 136, 4261–4270.

37. Hussain SP, Amstad P, Raja K, Ambs S, Nagashima M, Bennett WP, Shields PG, Ham AJ, Swenberg JA, Marrogi AJ, Harris CC 2000 Increased p53 mutation load on non-cancerous colon tissue from ulcerative colitis: a cancer-prone chronic inflammatory disease *Cancer Res.* 60, 3333–3337.
38. Yamanishi Y, Boyle DL, Rosengren S, Green DR, Zvaifler NJ, Firestein GS 2002 Regional analysis of p53 mutations in rheumatoid arthritis synovium *Proc. Natl. Acad. Sci.USA* 99, 10025–10030.
39. Kim DW, Hwang JH, Suh JM, Kim H, Song JH, Hwang ES, Hwang IY, ParkKIC, Chung HK, Kim JM, Park J, Hemmings BA, Shong M 2003 RET/PTC (rearranged in transformation/papillary thyroid carcinoma) tyrosine kinase phosphorylates and activated phosphoinositide-dependent kinase 1(PDK1): an alternative phosphoatidylinositol 3-kinase-indepenedent pathway to activate PDK1 *Mol. Endocrinol.* 17, 1382–1394
40. Dobashi Y, Sugimura H, Sakamoto A, Mernyei M, Mori, M, Oyama T, Machinami R. 1994. Stepwise participation of p53 gene mutation during dedifferentiation of human thyroid carcinoma *Diag Mol Pathol* 3, 9–14.
41. Pilotti S, ColliniP, Del Bo R, Catteretti G, Pierotti MA, Rilke F1994 A novel panel of antibodies that segregates immunocytochemically poorly differentiated carcinoma from undifferentiated carcinoma of the thyroid gland *Am. J. Surg. Pathol* 21, 1466-1473.
42. Zou M, Shi Y, al-Sediary S, Hussian SS, Farid NR 1995 The expression of the MDM2 gene, a p53 binding protein, in thyroid carcinogenesis *Cancer* 76:314–318.
43. Shi Y, Zou M, Varkondi E, Nagy A, Kozma L, Farid NR 2001 Cyclin D1 in thyroid carcinomas *Thyroid* 11, 709–710.
44. Jennings T, Bratslavsky G, Gerasimov G, Troshina K, Bronstein M, Dedov I, Alexandrova G, Figge J 1995 nuclear accumulation of MDM2 protein in well-differentiated papillary thyroid carcinoma *Exp. Mol. Pathol.* 62, 199–206.
45. Park KY, Koh JM, Park HJ, Gong G, Hong SJ, Ahn IM1998 Prevalence of Gs alpha, ras, p53 mutations and ret/PTC rearrangement in differentiated thyroid tumors in a Korean population *Clin.Endocrinol.(Oxf)* 49, 317–323.
46. Brugarolas J, Moberg K, Boyd SD, Taya Y Jacks T, Lees JA 1999 Inhibition of cyclin-dependent kinase 2 by p21 is necessary for retinoblastoma protein –mediated G1 arrest after γ-irradiation *Proc. Natl. Acad. Sci.USA* 96, 1002–1007.
47. Geng Y, Yu Q, Sicinska E, Das M, Bronson RT, Sicinski P 2001 deletion of the $p27^{Kip1}$ gene restores normal development in cyclin D1-defieceint mice *Proc. Natl. Acad. Sci. USA* 98, 194–199
48. Farid NR 1996 Molecular pathogenesis of thyroid carcinoma: the significance of oncogenes, tumor suppressor genes and genomic instability *Exp. Clin. Endocrinol. Diab* 104 (Suppl 4), 1–12.
49. Zedenius J, Larsson C, Wallin G, Backdahl M, Aspenblad U, Hoog A, Borresen AL, Auer G 1996 Alteration of p53 and expression of WAF1/p21 in human thyroid tumors *Thyroid* 6, 1–9.
50. ItoY, Kobyashi T, Takeda T, Komoike Y, Wakasugi E, Tamaki Y, Tsujimoto M, Matsuura N, Monden M 1996 Expression of p21 (WAF1/CIP1) protein in clinical thyroid tissues *Br. J. Cancer* 74, 1269–1274.
51. Shi Y, Zou,M, Farid NR, Al-Sediary ST 1996 Evidence of gene deletion of p21(WAF1/CIP1), a cyclin-dependent protein kinas inhibitor, in thyroid carcinoms *Br. J. Cancer* 74, 1336-1341.
52. El-Diery WS, Tokino T, Velculescu VE, Levy DB, Parsons R, Trent JM, Lin D, Mercer WE, Kinzler KW, Vogelstein B 1993 WAF1 a potential mediator of p53 tumor suppression *Cell* 75, 817–825.
53. Krempler A, Henry MD, Triplett AA, Wagner KU 2002 Targeted deletion of the Tsg 101 gene results in cell cycle arrest at the G1/S and p53-independent cell death *J. Biol. Chem.* 277, 43216-43223.
54. Oh,H, Mammucari C, Nenci A, Cabodi S, Cohen SN, Dotto GP 2002 Negative regulation of cell growth and differentiation by TSG101 through association with p21 (Cip1/WAF1)*Proc. Natl. Acad. Sci. USA* 99, 5430–5435.
55. Liu RT, Huang CC, You HL, Chou FF, Hu CC, Chao P, Chen CM,Cheng JT2002 Overexpression of tumor susceptibility gene TSG 101 in human papillary carcinomas *Oncogene* 21, 4830–4837.
56. Zou M, Shi Y, Farid NR, Al-Sediary ST, Paterson MC 1999 FHIT gene abnormalities in both benign and malignant thyroid tumors *Brit. Cancer J.* 35, 467–472.
57. McIver B,Grebe SK, Wangle, Hay ID ,Yokomizo A, LiuW, Goellner JR, Grant CS ,Smith DI, Eberhardt NL 2000 FHIT and TSG101 in thyroid tumours:aberrant transcripts reflect rare abnormal RNA processing events of uncertain pathogenic or clinical significance *Clin. Endocrinol. (Oxf)* 52:, 49–757.
58. Nevins JR 2001 The Rb/E2F pathway and cancer *Hum. Mol. Genet* 10, 699–703.
59. Lees JA, Weinberg RA1999 Throwing monkey wrenches into the clock: New ways of treating cancer *Proc. Natl. Acad. Sci.USA* 96, 4221–4223.
60. Zou M, Shi Y, Farid NR 1994 Frequent inactivation of the retinoblastoma gene in human thyroid carcinoma *Endocrine J.*2, 193–199.

61. Nikitin AY, Juarez-Perez MI, Li S, Huang L, Lee W-H 1999 *RB*-mediated suppression of spontaneous multiple neuroendocrine neoplasis and lung metastases in $Rb^{+/-}$ mice *Proc. Natl. Acad. Sci.USA* 96, 3916-3921.
62. Anwar F, Emond MJ, Schmidt RA, Hwang HC, Bronner MP 2000 Retinoblastoma expression in thyroid neoplasms *Modern Pathology* 13, 562–569.
63. Anwar F 2003 The phenotype of Huirthle and Warthin-like papillary thyroid carcinoma is distinct from classic papillary carcinoma as to the expression of retinoblastoma protein and E2F1 transcription factor *Appl. Immunohistochem. Mio. Morphol.* 11, 20–27.
64. Khoo M L, Beasley NJ, Ezzat S, Freeman JL, Asa SL 2002 Overexpression of cyclin D1 and underexpression of p27 predict lymph node metastases in papillary thyroid carcinoma *J. Clin. Endocrinol. Metab.* 87, 1814–1818.
65. Resnick MB, SchacterP, Finkelstein Y, Kellner Y, Cohen O Immunohistochemical analysis of p27/kip1 expression in thyroid carcinoma *Mod Pathol* 11, 735–739.
66. Wang S, Wu J, Savas L, Patwardhan N, Khan A 1998 The role of cell cycle regulatory proteins, cyclin D1, cyclin E, and p27 in thyroid carcinogenesis *Hum. Pathol.* 29, 1304–1309.
67. Maynes L, Hutzler MJ, Patwardhan NA, Wang S, Khan A 2000 Cell cycle regulatory protein p27 (kip), cyclins D1 and E and proliferative activity in oncocytic (Hurthle cell) lesions of the thyroid *Endocr. Pathol* 11, 331–340.
68. Baldassarre G, Belletti B, Bruni P, Boccia A, Trapasso F, Pentimalli F, Barone MV,Chiappetta G, VentoMT, Spieza S, Fusco A, Viglietto G 1999 Overexpressed cyclin D3 contributes to retaining the growth inhibitor p27 in the cytoplasm of thyroid tumor cells *J. Clin. Inves.* 104, 865–874.
69. Tung WS, Shevlin DW, Bartsch D, Norton JA, Wells SA Jr Goodfellow PJ 1996 Infrequent CDKN2 mutations in human differentiated thyroid cancers *Mol.Carinog.* 15, 5–10.
70. Jones CJ, Shaw JJ, Wylie FS, Gaillard N, Schlumberger M, Wynford-Thomas D 1996 High frequency deletion of the tumor suppressor gene P16INK4a (MTS1)in human thyroid carcinoma cell lines *Mol.Cell.Endocrinol.* 116, 115–119.
71. Schulte KM, Stuadt S, Niederacher D, Finken-Eigen M, Kohrer K, Goretski PE, Roher HD 1998 Rare loss of heterozigosity of the MTS1 and MTS2 tumor suppressor genes in differentiated human thyroid cancer *Horm. Metab. Res.* 30, 549–554.
72. Elisei R, Shiohara M, Koeffler HP, Fagin JA 1998 Genetic and epigenetic alterations of the cyclin-dependent kinase inhibitors p15INK4b and p16INK4b in human thyroid carcinoma cell lines and primary thyroid carcinomas *Cancer* 83, 2185–2193.
73. Schagdarsurenign U, Gimm O, Hoang-Vu C, Draslle H, Pfiefer GP, Dammann R 2002 Frequent epigenetic silencing of the CpG island promoter of RASSF1A in thyroid carcinoma *Cancer Res.* 62, 3698–3701.
74. Muller H, Lukas J, Schneider A, Warthog P, Barter J, Eilers M, Strauss M 1994 CyclinD1 expression is regulated by the retinoblastoma protein *Proc. Natl. Acad. Sci.USA* 91.2945–2949.
75. Zou M, Shi Y, Farid NR, Al-Sediary ST 1998 Inverse association between cyclinD1overexpression and retinoblastoma gene mutations in thyroid carcinoma *Endocrine* 8,61–64.
76. Khoo ML, Ezzat S, FreemanJL, Asa SL 2002 Cyclin D1 protein overexpression predicts metastatic behaqvior in thyroid papillary microcarcinoma but is not associated with gene amplification *J. Clin. Endocrinol. Metab.* 87,1810–1813.
77. GotoA, SakamotoA, Machinami R 2001 An immunochemical analysis of cyclin D1, p53 and p21 waf1/cip proteinin tumirs originating from the follicular epithelium of the thyroid cell *Pathol. Res. Pract.* 197, 217–222.
78. Basolo F, Caligo MA, Pinchera A, Fedeli F, Baldanzi A, Miccoli P, Iacconi P, Fontanini, G, Pacini F 2000 Cyclin D1 overexpression in thyroid carcinomas: relation With clinco-pathological parameters, retinoblastoma gene product and Ki67labeling index *Thyroid* 10, 741–746.
79. Muro-Cacho CA, Holt T, Klotch D, Mora L, Livingston S, Futran N 1999 Cyclin D1 expression as a prognostic parameter in papillary carcinoma of the thyroid *Otolaryngol. Head Neck Surg.* 120, 200–207.
80. Saiz AD, Olvera M, Rezk S, Florentine BA, McCourty A, Brynes RK 2002 Immunobiolgical expression of cyclin D1, E2F-1 and Ki-67 in benign and malignant thyroid lesions *J. Pathol.* 198, 157–162.
81. HwangJH, Kom DW, Suh, JM, Kim H, SongJH, Hwang ES, Park KC, Chung HK, KimJM, Lee T-H, Yu D-Y, Shong M 2003 Activatiob of signal transducer and activator of transcription 3 by oncogenic RET/PTC (rearranged in transformation/papillary thyroid carcinoma) tyrosine kinase:Roles of specific gene regulation and cellular transformatiom *Mol. Endocrinol.* 17, 1155–1166.

82. Rudolph B, Saffrich R, Zwicker J, Henglein B, Muller R, Ansorge W, Eilers M 1996 Activation of cyclin-dependent kinases by Myc mediates induction of cyclin A, but not apoptosis *EMBO J.* 15, 3065–3067.
83. Rodriguez-Puebla ML. Robles AI, Conti CJ 1999 ras activity and cyclin D1 expression: an essential mechanism of mouse skin tumor development *Mol. Carcinog.* 24, 1–6.
84. Volante M, Croce S, Pecchioni C, Papotti M 2002 E2F transcription factor is over expressed in oxyphilic thyroid tumors *Mod. Pathol* 15, 1038–1043.
85. Nygard M, Wahlsrtom GM, Gustafsson MV, Tokumoto YM, Bondesson M 2003 Hormone-dependent repression of the E2F-1 gene by thyroid hormone receptors *Mol. Endocrinol.* 17, 79–92.
86. Ito Y, Yoshida H, Nakano K, Takamura Y, Kobayashi K, Yokozawa T, Matsuka F, Matsuura N, Kuma K, Miyauchi A 2002 expression of G2-M modulators in thyroid neoplasms: correlation of cyclin A,B1 and cdc2 with differentiation *Pathol. Res. Pract.* 198, 397–402.
87. ItoY, Yoshida H, Uruno T, Nakano K, Takamuar Y, Mia A, Kobayashi K, Yokozawa T, Matsuzuka F, Kuma K, Miyauchi A 2003 Decreased expression of cyclin G2 is significantly linked to the malignant transformation of papillary carcinoma of the thyroid *Anticancer Res.* 23, 2335–2338.
88. Qi J-S, Desai-Yajanik V, Yaun Y Samuels HH 1997 Constitutive activation of gene expression by thyroid hormone receptor results from reversal of p53-mediated suppression *Mol. Cell. Biol.* 17, 7195–7207.
89. Bhat MK, Yu CI, Zhan Q, Hayashi Y, Seth P, Cheng SY 1997 Tumor suppressor p53 is a negative regulator in thyroid hormone receptor signalling pathway *J. Biol. Chem* 272, 28989–28993.
90. Qi J-S, Yaun Y, Desia-Yajanik V, Samuels HH 1997 Regulation of the mdm2 oncogene by thyroid hormone receptor *Mol. Cell. Biol.* 19, 864–872
91. Frisk T, Foukakis t, Dwight T, Lunderg J, Hoog A, Wallis G, Eng C, Zedenius G, Larsson C 2002 Silencing of PTEN tumor-suppressor gene in anaplastic thyroid cancer *Genes Chromosomes Cancer* 35, 74–80.

9. ABNORMALITIES OF NUCLEAR RECEPTORS IN THYROID CANCER

SHEUE-YANN CHENG, PH.D.

Laboratory of Molecular Biology, Center for Cancer Research, National Cancer Institute, National Institutes of Health, Bethesda, MD 20892-4264

INTRODUCTION

Nuclear receptors comprise a large family of ligand-inducible transcription factors that are critically important for growth, differentiation, development, and maintenance of metabolic homeostasis. They regulate the expression of target genes by binding to the specific DNA sequences at the promoters to mediate the biological effects. Many nuclear receptors have multiple isoforms with over-lapping functions or isoform-specific functions (1, 2). The expression of these receptor isoforms is regulated in a tissue- and development-dependent manner. A host of coregulatory proteins that influence the ligand selectivity and DNA binding capacity further modulates the transcriptional activities (3, 4).

Abnormal expression and/or aberrant functions of sex steroid nuclear receptors are known to be involved in the development and progression of such endocrine cancers as breast, ovarian, endometrium, and prostate, but less is known about the role of nuclear receptors in the carcinogenesis of the thyroid. Progress in this area has recently been made as a result of the discoveries of the fusion gene of PAX8 with the peroxisome proliferator-activated receptor γ (PPARγ; PAX8-PPARγ) in follicular thyroid carcinoma and of the spontaneous development of follicular thyroid carcinoma in the homozygous knock-in mutant mice harboring a mutated thyroid hormone β receptor (TRβ). This review will first examine the latest findings on the possible roles of several sex steroid nuclear receptors in thyroid carcinogenesis. It will then discuss the molecular actions of the mutant TRβ in carcinogenesis, particularly in relation to a unique knock-in mouse model of thyroid cancer.

ABNORMAL EXPRESSION OF ESTROGEN AND PROGESTERONE RECEPTORS IN THYROID CANCER

Thyroid carcinoma is more common in women than in men (5). For 2003, the estimate of new cases of thyroid cancer has a female predominance with a 2.9:1 ratio (6). This predominance suggests that estrogens may play a critical role in the development of thyroid carcinoma. In the past two decades, efforts have been made to demonstrate the presence of estrogen receptors (ERs) in thyroid tumors and to correlate tumor malignancy with ER expression. Using a dextran-coated charcoal method and analysis by the method of Scatchard, Miki et al. did not detect ER in the cytosol of normal thyroids, but they found a significantly higher ER in the neoplastic and hyperplastic thyroid tissues (7). Using different biochemical methods, Mizukami et al. (8) and Yane et al. (9) also showed a higher expression of ER in neoplastic thyroid lesions than in normal thyroids or in adjacent normal tissues. Lewy-Trenda examined 72 thyroid glands for the expression of ER by using immunochemical assays with anti-ER antibodies. Positive staining occurred in the nuclei of differentiated thyroid cancer cells (24%), but not in non-neoplastic cells. A small number of oxyphillic (4%) and follicular adenomas (6%) also stained positive for ERs (10).

Consistent with these findings, several studies showed that estrogens stimulate the proliferation of thyroid carcinoma cells (11–13), whereas the antiestrogen, tamoxifen, inhibits the proliferation of a tumor cell line derived from medullary thyroid carcinoma (11). These studies clearly showed that cell proliferation induced by estrogens is mediated by ERs, but little is known about the specific molecular pathways. One study suggested that activation of the mitogen-activated protein kinase by phosphorylation might be one of the key steps in the estrogen-mediated cell proliferation of thyroid cancer cells (13).

The relevance of the increased expression of ERs in thyroid tumorigenesis is not obvious, particularly given that there is no clear correlation in the extent of expression of ER to age, sex, presenting clinical or pathological features, or, in cases of carcinoma, to subsequent metastatic potential (10, 14, 15). Furthermore, the failure of several studies to detect a greater expression of ERs in thyroid tumors than in normal tissues casts further doubt on the significance of expression of ERs in thyroid tumor development and progression (16–19). It is unclear whether the discrepancy among studies is due to the sensitivity of the detection or the intrinsic variability in the expression of ERs in tumor samples. Plainly, more studies are needed to understand whether estrogens and ERs are the major factors that contribute to thyroid cancer's predominance in females.

Fewer studies have investigated the roles of progesterone receptors (PRs) in thyroid carcinogenesis. Because of the interest in understanding thyroid cancer's predominance in females, the expression of PRs in thyroid tumors has been evaluated by means of ligand binding assays, enzyme immunoassays, and/or immunohistochemistry. In a few limited studies, the presence of PR and ER was assessed concurrently in the same samples. In 135 thyroid lesions that included papillary, follicular, medullary, and Hurthle cell carcinomas, van Hoeven detected the presence of PR in 51% of the cases, with the highest abundance in papillary carcinomas, particularly in male patients and women older than 50 years (15). In that same study, ER was found in 46% of the samples. In other studies, however, a higher frequency of ER than PR was found in papillary carcinomas (7, 10, 14). Similar to the findings for ER, no correlations were observed between the expression of PR and age, sex, tumor size, presence of capsular or vascular invasion, or lymph node status (10, 14). Still, how the expression of PR is involved in the development of thyroid cancer has not been assessed.

ALTERED EXPRESSION OF THE RETINOIC ACID RECEPTORS IN THYROID CANCER

Retinoic acids (RAs) are essential for many biological processes including proliferation, development, differentiation, carcinogenesis, and apoptosis. These biological effects are mediated through their receptors (RARs). The retinoids, both the natural and synthetic analogs, have been shown to be effective in preventing several cancers in experimental animals and in reversing pre-neoplastic lesions in humans (20, 21). Whether the retinoids could be effective in re-differentiating thyroid cancer cells to be amenable to radioiodide or TSH-suppressive T4 therapy has prompted several investigators to study the expression of RAR in cancer cell lines and tissues. Using Northern blot analysis, del Senno found that the expression of RARα mRNA was lower in thyroid carcinoma cells than in normal thyroid follicular cells. Moreover, del Senno demonstrated that RA reduces the proliferation and function of thyroid follicular cells (22, 23). These findings were confirmed in a larger study. Using immunohistochemistry and Western blotting, Rochaix et al. compared the expression of RARβ in 40 normal/benign tissues, 16 papillary carcinomas, and two follicular carcinomas. RARβ immunostaining was detected in the nuclei, but was limited to the normal epithelial thyroid tissue. A dramatic decrease in RARβ immunostaining was observed in all 16 papillary carcinomas, but in only one follicular carcinoma (24).

Because the feasibility of retinoid-induced differentiation therapy in thyroid cancer hinges on functional RARs, Schmutzler et al. not only examined the expression of mRNA in several human thyroid carcinoma cell lines and tissues, but also assessed the ligand and DNA binding activities (25). Functional RARs were clearly detectable in the two human thyroid carcinoma cell lines (FTC-133 and FTC-238) and two anaplastic thyroid carcinoma cell lines (HTH74 and C643). Intriguingly, variable levels of mRNA were observed in these cell lines, an observation probably indicative of dysregulation of receptor expression in thyroid cancer (25). These results suggest the heterogeneity in the expression of RARs and the association of the dysregulation of the expression of RAR with thyroid carcinogenesis. However, the available expressed functional RAR seems to be able to respond to RA treatment. In a pilot study, patients with advanced thyroid cancer and without the therapeutic options of operation or radioiodide therapy were treated with 13-cis-retinoic acid (1.5 mg/kg body weight daily for 5 weeks). Overall, tumor regression was observed in 19 patients (38%). However, response to retinoid therapy did not always correlate with increased radioiodine uptake (a re-differentiation marker), and so other direct antiproliferative effects could also be involved (26). These encouraging clinical findings warrant additional studies on the RA-based treatment of thyroid cancer. At present, however, little is known about either the molecular mechanisms by which the expression of RAR is dysregulated during thyroid carcinogenesis or the RA-induced–redifferentiation of follicular cells. Elucidation of these mechanisms should help in the design of an effective treatment of thyroid carcinomas that uses the retinoids.

ABNORMALITIES OF THYROID HORMONE RECEPTORS IN THYROID CANCER

The thyroid hormone receptors (TRs) mediate the pleiotropic activities of the thyroid hormone (T3) in growth, development, and differentiation and in maintaining metabolic homeostasis. The two TR genes, α and β, are located on human chromosomes 17 and 3, respectively. Alternative splicing of the primary transcripts gives rise to five major TR isoforms (α1, α2, β1, β2, and β3). TRα1, TRβ1, TRβ2, and TRβ3 differ in their lengths and amino acid sequences at the amino terminal A/B domain, but they bind T3 with high affinity to mediate gene regulatory activity. By contrast, TRα2, which differs from the other TR isoforms in the C-terminus, does not bind T3, and its precise functions have yet to be elucidated. The expression of TR isoforms is tissue-dependent and developmentally regulated (1, 2).

Early evidence to suggest that mutated TR could be involved in carcinogenesis came from the discovery that TRα1 is the cellular counterpart of the retroviral v-erbA that is involved in the neoplastic transformation leading to acute erythroleukemia and sarcomas (27, 28). The oncogenic role of v-erbA was subsequently demonstrated in mammals in that male transgenic mice overexpressing v-erbA developed hepatocellular carcinoma (29).

In recent years, increasing evidence suggests that aberrant expression and mutation of the TR genes could be associated with human neoplasias. Somatic point mutations of TRα1 and TRβ1 were found in 65% (11/17 tumors) and 76% (13/17 tumors), respectively, of human hepatocellular carcinomas. Many of these mutated TRs have lost T3-binding activity and exhibit aberrant DNA-binding activity (30). Aberrant expression and mutations of TR genes were also found in renal clear cell carcinomas (31). Cloning of TRs from 22 renal clear cell carcinomas and 20 surrounding normal tissues identified somatic mutations in 32% and 14% of cloned TRβ1 and TRα1 cDNAs, respectively (32). Most of the mutations were localized in the hormone-binding domain that leads to loss of T3-binding activity and/or impairment in binding to TREs. Similar to the mutated TRs detected in hepatocellular carcinoma (30, 33), the mutated TRs identified in renal clear cell carcinomas exhibit dominant negative activity (32). These studies suggest that mutated TR plays an important role in the development of these human cancers.

Abnormal expression and somatic mutations of TRs in thyroid cancer

Similar to the expression levels reported for ER, PR, and RAR, an altered expression of TRs was detected in thyroid carcinomas. Comparison of the mRNA expression levels of TR isoforms in normal, hyperplastic, and neoplastic human thyroid tissues indicated that TRβ mRNA is significantly lower in papillary and follicular carcinomas than it is in normal thyroid. No differences, however, were found in the expression levels of TRα1 and TRα2 mRNA (34, 35). These findings suggest an association of the reduced expression of TRβ1 mRNA with the development of thyroid carcinomas.

These studies, however, did not determine whether TRβ1, TRα1, and TRα2 were altered at the protein level.

In addition to the reduced expression of TRβ1 mRNA, a lower expression of TRα1 mRNA was found in 16 papillary thyroid carcinomas from Polish patients. The TRβ1 and TRα1 protein levels, however, were higher in cancerous tissues than in nearby healthy tissues, an indication of the complexity in the regulation of TR expression in these tumors (36). To understand the nature of TRs in these papillary thyroid carcinomas, cDNAs were cloned concurrently from both the tumor lesions and the healthy thyroids as controls. Sequence analyses indicated that 93.8% and 62.5% of papillary thyroid carcinomas had mutations in TRβ1 and TRα1, respectively. In contrast, no mutations were found in healthy thyroid controls, and only 11.1% and 22.2% of thyroid adenomas had mutations in TRβ1 and TRα1, respectively. Functional analysis indicated that these mutated TRs lose their transactivation function and exhibit dominant negative activity (36).

The reduced expression of TRβ1 mRNA in papillary thyroid carcinomas was further confirmed in a more recent study of 16 Japanese patients (37). In contrast to the Polish patients, no amino acid-substitution-mutations were detected in the TRβ1 cDNAs cloned from these papillary thyroid carcinomas. The reasons for the different propensity in the mutations of the TRβ gene in these two groups of patients are not entirely clear. One possibility is that the Polish patients were from the post-Chernobyl population and that radiation exposure is a contributing factor to the high frequency of TR mutations. Indeed, five of the 16 Polish patients with mutated TRs were in their teens when the Chernobyl accident occurred. One of 16 patients received radiation treatment during her childhood because of another disease. The age of other patients ranged from 32–58 years old at the time of the Chernobyl accident (Monika Puzianowska-Kuznicka; personal communication). The validation of this hypothesis would require a cohort study with a larger number of patients and a detailed knowledge of irradiation dose received by the patients.

Another possibility is that the propensity of mutations of TRβ1 in papillary thyroid carcinomas could be affected by the patient's ethnic origin. Genetic variation between different populations occurs frequently. For example, a wide variation in the frequency of RET/PTC rearrangements, a hallmark of papillary thyroid carcinoma, has been reported, ranging from a few percent in Japanese (38) and Saudi Arabian patients (39), to 18.8% in Italian patients (40), to 70% in New Caledonian and 85% in Australian patients (41). The frequency of polymorphisms associated with thyroid diseases also differs in Japanese and Caucasian populations (42). Clarification of the issue of whether genetic background affects the frequency of TRβ1 mutations in papillary thyroid carcinoma awaits additional analyses in patients with different ethnic origins.

Germline mutations of the TRβ gene in thyroid cancer: lessons learned from a unique mouse model of thyroid carcinogenesis

So far, the TR mutants identified in human cancers including thyroid carcinoma are somatic mutations. A knock-in mouse that harbors a germline mutation of the TRβ gene has been created (43). The mutation was targeted to the TRβ gene locus

Table 1. Histologic progression of thyroid neoplasia in 5–14 month-old $TR\beta^{PV/PV}$ mice

Hyperplasia	Capsular invasion	Vascular invasion	Anaplasia	Metastasis
27/27(100%)	23/27(85%)	20/27(74%)	10/27(37%)	7/27(26%)

via homologous recombination and the Cre/loxP system. The mutation is called PV (TRβPV mouse) after a patient with the mutation who suffers from the disease known as resistance to thyroid hormone (RTH) (44, 45). RTH is a syndrome characterized by the elevated levels of circulating thyroid hormone that are associated with non-suppressible TSH. Some of the clinical features include attention-deficit hyperactivity disorder, mental retardation, short stature, decreased weight, tachycardia, and hearing abnormalities (44, 45). PV has a unique mutation in exon 10, a C-insertion at codon 448, which produces a frame shift of the carboxyl-terminal 14 amino acids of TRβ1. *In vitro* studies revealed that PV has completely lost T3-binding activity, lacks transcriptional capacity, and exhibits potent dominant negative activity (46). Extensive characterization of the phenotype indicates that the TRβPV mouse faithfully reproduces the human RTH (43). This TRβPV mouse provides a valuable model for clarifying the role of germline mutations of the TRβ gene in carcinogenesis.

In addition to the phenotypes of RTH, homozygous TRβPV ($TR\beta^{PV/PV}$) mice exhibited the phenotype of age-dependent increased mortality. By the age of about 10 months, 50% had died, and by the age of 14–15 months, all mice were dead. In contrast, the heterozygous ($TR\beta^{PV/+}$) mice did not exhibit such abnormalities. Morphological examinations of the moribund $TR\beta^{PV/PV}$ mice indicate that as these mice aged, they spontaneously developed thyroid carcinoma (47). Histological evaluation of thyroids of 27 moribund $TR\beta^{PV/PV}$ mice showed capsular invasion (85%), vascular invasion (74%), anaplasia (37%), and metastasis to the lung and heart (26%) but not to lymph nodes (Table 1).

Representative examples of the pathological features of capsular invasion (Panel A), vascular invasion (Panel B), anaplasia (Panel C), and metastasis to the lung (Panel D) are shown in Figure 1. The histological features and the metastatic patterns indicate that the thyroid carcinoma developed in $TR\beta^{PV/PV}$ mice is follicular. Thus $TR\beta^{PV/PV}$ mice provide the first animal model for studying the molecular genetics underlying follicular thyroid carcinogenesis.

Using microarrays consisting of 20,000 mouse cDNAs, Ying et al. recently profiled the global alterations in gene expression in the thyroids of $TR\beta^{PV/PV}$ mice at 6 months of age, at which time metastasis had begun (48). They found that 185 genes were up-regulated (2- to 17-fold) and 92 were down-regulated (2- to 20-fold). The majority (∼60%) of these altered genes are unnamed. Functional clustering of named genes with reported functions (100 genes) indicated that ∼39% were tumor-, metastasis/invasion-, and cell cycle-related. Importantly, several tumor-related genes, such as cyclin D1, pituitary tumor transforming gene-1, cathepsin D, and transforming growth factor α, that have been reported to be over-expressed in human thyroid

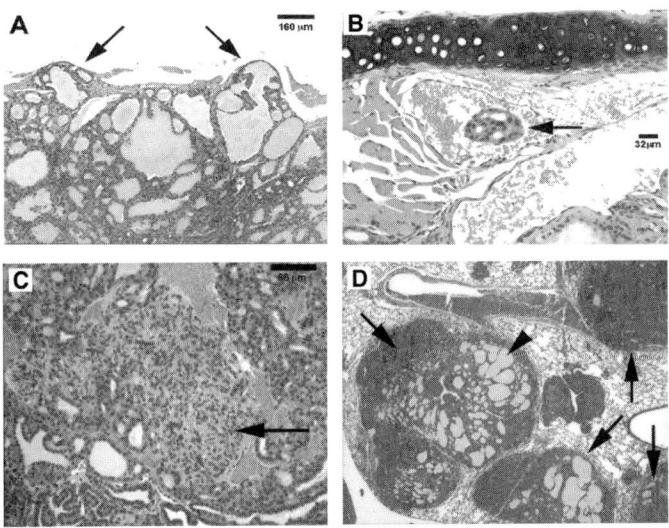

Figure 1. Pathological features in thyroid glands and metastasis in the lung of TRβ$^{PV/PV}$ mice. Histologic sections from tissues of TRβ$^{PV/PV}$ mice showed evidence of capsular invasion in thyroid (A) (arrows), vascular invsion in thyroid (B)(arrows), anaplasia in thyroid (C) and metastatic thyroid carcinoma lesions in lung (arrow).

cancers were found to be activated in the arrays (49–53). Analyses of the gene profiles suggested that the signaling pathways mediated by TSH, peptide growth factors, transforming growth factor-β, tumor necrosis factor-α, and nuclear factor κB were activated, whereas pathways mediated by peroxisome proliferator-activated receptor γ (PPARγ) were repressed (48). These findings suggest that the expression of the TRβ mutant directly and indirectly alters multiple signaling pathways that could contribute to the development of thyroid cancer and that thyroid carcinogenesis is mediated by multiple genetic events.

The frequent occurrence of the somatic mutations in several human cancers (30, 32, 36, 54, 55) and the development of follicular thyroid carcinoma in TRβ$^{PV/PV}$ mice (47) raise the question of whether PV could function to initiate carcinogenesis. On the basis of observations that TRβ$^{PV/PV}$ but not TRβ$^{PV/+}$ mice develop follicular thyroid carcinoma, it is unlikely that PV could act alone to initiate thyroid carcinogenesis. One of the significant differences in phenotypes between TRβ$^{PV/PV}$ and TRβ$^{PV/+}$ mice is that the circulating serum TSH concentration in TRβ$^{PV/PV}$ mice is ~275-fold higher than that in TRβ$^{PV/+}$ mice (43). TSH is the main regulator of thyrocyte differentiation and proliferation, and the possibility that it is an initiator of thyroid carcinogenesis has been intensively studied (56, 57). Recent clinical and biochemical studies, however, do not support the role of TSH as an initiator of follicular carcinoma (58, 57). Additional genetic changes need to occur for the transformation of the hyperproliferative thyroid cells to cancer cells. On the basis of these considerations, it is reasonable to propose that mutation of the two alleles of the TRβ gene could be one of the genetic changes leading to the transformation of the hyperproliferative thyroid cells to cancer cells. This hypothesis needs to be tested in future studies.

ABNORMALITIES OF PEROXISOME PROLIFERATOR-ACTIVATED RECEPTOR γ IN THYROID CANCER

PPARγ is a nuclear receptor that is involved in a wide range of cellular processes including adipogenesis, inflammation, atherosclerosis, cell cycle control, apoptosis, and carcinogenesis (59, 60). PPARγ mRNA is abundantly expressed in adipose tissue, large intestine, and hematopoietic cells, and it is moderately expressed in kidney, liver, and small intestine (61). It was recently found also to express in the thyroid (48). PPARγ inhibits cell growth, and one of the mechanisms in inhibition of cell proliferation is by reducing E2F/DP DNA-binding and transcriptional activity (62). Consistently, activation of PPARγ signaling by its ligands has been shown to block cell proliferation of various malignant cells and, in some cases, to induce differentiation and apoptosis (63–68). Ohta et al. reported that PPARγ mRNA is expressed in human papillary thyroid carcinoma cell lines (69). Significant, but variable expression of PPARγ mRNA was detected in four of the six cell lines studied. Consistent with findings in other cancer cell lines (63–68), cell proliferation was inhibited and apoptosis was induced by treatment with troglitazone. Ohta et al. also found that troglitazone significantly reduced tumor growth and prevented distant metastasis of BHP18–21 tumors in nude mice *in vivo* (69). In a more recent study, Martelli et al. also evaluated whether PPARγ is involved in the growth regulation of normal and tumor thyroid cells (70). No mutations were detected in PPARγ exons 3 and 5 in human thyroid carcinoma cell lines and tissues. The growth of PPARγ-expressing thyroid carcinoma cells was inhibited by treatment with PPARγ agonists, but no growth inhibitory effect was observed in NPA cells by PPARγ agonists that did not express PPARγ. Growth inhibition induced by PPARγ agonists or by overexpression of the PPARγ gene in thyroid carcinoma cells was associated with increased p27 protein levels and apoptotic cell death (70).

TRβ$^{PV/PV}$ mice provide an unprecedented opportunity to study the role of PPARγ in thyroid carcinogenesis *in vivo*. Using quantitative real-time PCR and Northern blotting, Yin et al. found that the expression of PPARγ mRNA was repressed 50%–60% in the thyroids of TRβ$^{PV/PV}$ mice at the ages of 4, 6, and 12 months (71). Immunohistologic analysis demonstrated that the expression of PPARγ protein in the primary lesions of TRβ$^{PV/PV}$ mice was less than that in the thyroids of wild-type mice and was not detectable in the metastasis in the lung (unpublished results), an indication that the expression of PPARγ protein remained low during thyroid carcinogenesis. Moreover, PV was found to abolish ligand (troglitazone)-dependent transcriptional activity of PPARγ in primary cultured thyroid cells from wild-type mice (71). The PV-induced transcriptional repression could be due to PV's competition with PPARγ for binding to the peroxisome proliferator-activated receptor response element (PPRE) present in the PPARγ downstream target genes. Indeed, gel shift assay showed that the *in vitro* translated PV protein could bind to PPRE. This notion is supported by the

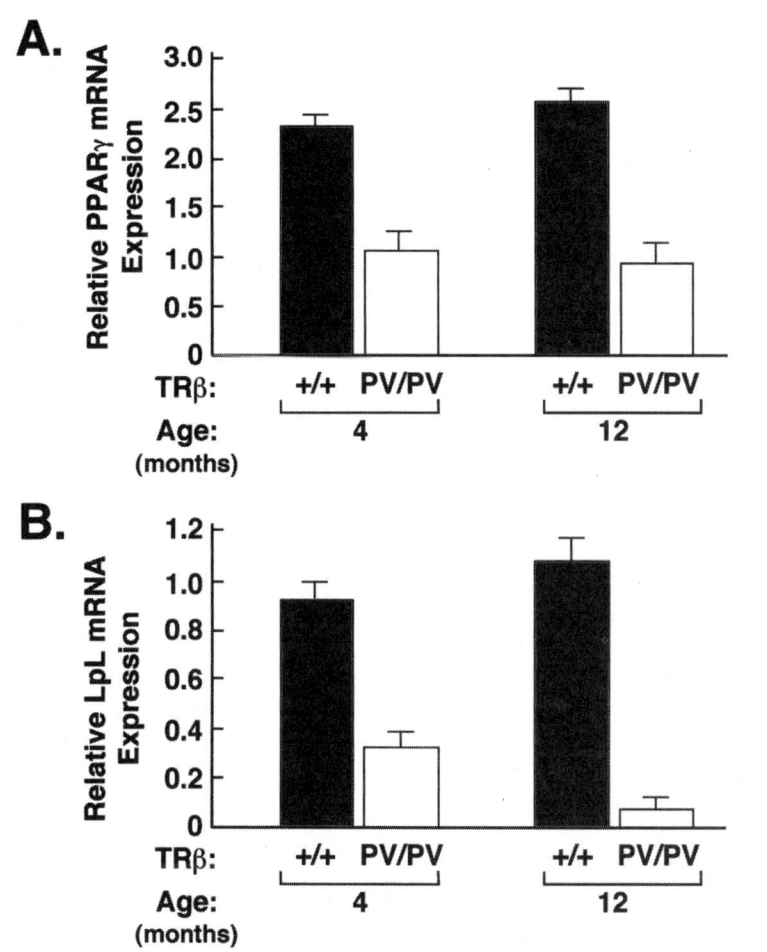

Figure 2. Camparison of the expression of PPARγ and lipoprotein (LpL) mRNA in the thyroids of TRβ$^{PV/PV}$ and wild-type mice at different ages by quantitative real-time PCR. Relative expression levels of PPARγ(A) and LpL(B) mRNA in the thyroid glands were determined using age matched wild-type and mutant mice at the ages of 4 and 12 months as marked. The data are expressed as mean ± SD(n = 4).

finding that the lipoprotein lipase (LpL) gene, a known PPARγ downstream target gene (72), was repressed ~5-fold, as shown by cDNA microarrays (48). Subsequent analyses by quantitative real-time PCR further demonstrated that the expression of the LpL gene was down-regulated (Panel B; Figure 2) concurrently with PPARγ mRNA (Panel A; Figure 2) in the thyroid glands of TRβ$^{PV/PV}$ mice at the ages of 6 and 12 months, thus confirming the repression of PPARγ signal pathways during thyroid carcinogenesis (71). These results indicate that reduced expression of PPARγ mRNA and repression of its transcriptional activity are associated with thyroid carcinogenesis and raise the possibility that PPARγ can be tested as a potential molecular target for prevention and treatment of follicular thyroid carcinoma.

That the attenuation of the PPARγ signaling pathways is associated with the development and progression of follicular thyroid carcinoma is also supported by the findings that the PAX8-PPARγ rearrangement occurs frequently in human follicular thyroid carcinomas, less frequently in adenomas, but not at all in papillary thyroid carcinomas (73–76). Even though the molecular actions of the PAX8-PPARγ rearrangement, particularly in its relation to the thyroid follicular carcinoma, has yet to be clarified, it is known that the fusion of PAX8, a thyroid transcription factor, to the amino terminus of PPARγ results in the loss of the transcriptional activity of PPARγ (73). Moreover, PAX8-PPARγ protein acts to inhibit thiazolidinedione-induced transactivation by PPARγ in a dominant negative manner (73). Taken together, these studies suggest that suppression of PPARγ signaling is closely linked to the development and progression of follicular thyroid carcinoma.

CONCLUDING REMARKS

Studies in the past few decades have clearly established that nuclear receptors play significant roles in the development and progression of several endocrine tumors, such as breast and prostate cancers. Progress in understanding the role of nuclear receptors in thyroid carcinoma lags behind that in breast and prostate cancers. Studies so far indicate that altered expression of ER, PR, RAR, TR, or PPARγ is associated with thyroid carcinomas. More studies are warranted to clarify the functional consequences of altered expressed receptors and to elucidate their signaling pathways in relation to carcinogenesis of the thyroid. These efforts will not only advance our understanding of the molecular genetics of thyroid cancer, but also provide opportunities to develop novel strategies for prevention and treatment.

The discovery that $TR\beta^{PV/PV}$ mice spontaneously develop follicular thyroid carcinoma indicates that, in addition to altered expression of nuclear receptors, mutation of nuclear receptors is another abnormality that could contribute to thyroid carcinogenesis. It is currently unknown whether, in addition to the TRβ gene, mutations of other nuclear receptors could also contribute to the development and progression of thyroid cancer. The finding that the $TR\beta^{PV/PV}$ mouse can be used as an animal model of follicular thyroid carcinoma opens the door to further study of the molecular genetic events underlying carcinogenesis, to identifying signature genes during different stages of tumor progression for clinical diagnosis, and to the testing of drugs and other treatment modalities.

ACKNOWLEDGMENTS

The author thanks all of her colleagues and collaborators who have contributed to the work described in this review.

REFERENCES

1. Cheng, S.-y. Multiple mechanisms for regulation of the transcriptional activity of thyroid hormone receptors. Rev Endocr Metab Disord 1: 9–18, 2000.

2. Yen, P. M. Physiological and molecular basis of thyroid hormone action. Physiol Rev *81*: 1097–1142, 2001.
3. McKenna, N. J., Lanz, R. B., and O'Malley, B. W. Nuclear receptor coregulators: cellular and molecular biology. Endocrinol Rev, *20*: 321–344, 1999.
4. Hermanson, O., Glass, C. K., and Rosenfeld, M. G. Nuclear receptor coregulators: multiple modes of modification. Trends Endocrinol Metab, *13*: 55–60, 2002.
5. Levi, F., Franceschi, S., Gulie, C., Negri, E., and La Vecchia, C. Female thyroid cancer: the role of reproductive and hormonal factors in Switzerland. Oncology, *50*: 309–315, 1993.
6. Jemal, A., Murray, T., Samuels, A., Ghafoor, A., Ward, E., and Thun, M. J. Cancer statistics. CA Cancer J Clin, *53*: 5–26, 2003.
7. Miki, H., Oshimo, K., Inoue, H., Morimoto, T., and Monden, Y. Sex hormone receptors in human thyroid tissues. Cancer, *66*: 1759–1762, 1990.
8. Mizukami, Y., Michigishi, T., Nonomura, A., Hashimoto, T., Noguchi, M., and Matsubara, F. Estrogen and estrogen receptors in thyroid carcinomas. J Surg Oncol, *47*: 165–169, 1991.
9. Yane, K., Kitahori, Y., Konishi, N., Okaichi, K., Ohnishi, T., Miyahara, H., Matsunaga, T., Lin, J. C., and Hiasa, Y. Expression of the estrogen receptor in human thyroid neoplasms. Cancer Lett, *84*: 59–66, 1994.
10. Lewy-Trenda, I. Estrogen and progesterone receptors in neoplastic and non-neoplastic thyroid lesions. Pol J Pathol, *53*: 67–72, 2002.
11. Yang, K., Pearson, C. E., and Samaan, N. A. Estrogen receptor and hormone responsiveness of medullary thyroid carcinoma cells in continuous culture. Cancer Res *48*: 2760–2763, 1988.
12. Banu, K.S., Govindarajulu, P., and Aruldhas, M. M. Testosterone and estradiol have specific differential modulatory effect on the proliferation of human thyroid papillary and follicular carcinoma cell lines independent of TSH action. Endocr Pathol, *12*: 315–327, 2001.
13. Manole, D., Schildknecht, B., Gosnell, B., Adams, E., and Derwahl, M. Estrogen promotes growth of human thyroid tumor cells by different molecular mechanisms. J Clin Endocrinol Metab, *86*: 1072–1077, 2001.
14. Bur, M., Shiraki, W., and Masood, S. Estrogen and progesterone receptor detection in neoplastic and non-neoplastic thyroid tissues. Mod Pathol, *6*: 469–472, 1993.
15. van Hoeven, K. H., Menendez-Botet, C. J., Strong, E. W., and Huvos, A. G. Estrogen and progesterone receptor content in human thyroid disease. Am J Clin Pathol, *99*: 175–181, 1993.
16. Colomer, A., Martinez-Mas, J. V., Matias-Guiu, X., Llorens, A., Cabezas, R., Prat, J., and Garcia-Ameijeiras, A. Sex-steroid hormone receptors in human medullary thyroid carcinoma. Mod Pathol, *9*: 68–72, 1996.
17. Bonacci, R., Pinchera, A., Fierabracci, P., Gigliotti, A., Grasso, L., and Giani, C. Relevance of estrogen and progesterone receptors enzyme immunoassay in malignant, benign and surrounding normal thyroid tissue. J Endocrinol Invest, *19*: 159–164, 1996.
18. Metaye, T., Millet, C., Kraimps, J. L., Aubouin, B., Barbier, J., and Begon, F. Estrogen receptors and cathepsin D in human thyroid tissue. Cancer, *72*: 1991–1996, 1993.
19. Jaklic, B. R., Rushin, J., and Ghosh, B. C. Estrogen and progesterone receptors in thyroid lesions. Ann Surg Oncol, *2*: 429–434, 1995.
20. Verma, A. K. Retinoids in chemoprevention of cancer. J Biol Regul Homeost Agents, *17*: 92–97, 2003.
21. Ralhan, R., and Kaur, J. Retinoids as chemopreventive agents. J Biol Regul Homeost Agents, *17*: 66–91, 2003.
22. del Senno, L., Rossi, R., Gandini, D., Piva, R., Franceschetti, P., and degli Uberti, E. C. Retinoic acid-induced decrease of DNA synthesis and peroxidase mRNA levels in human thyroid cells expressing retinoic acid receptor alpha mRNA. Life Sci, *53*: 1039–1048, 1993.
23. del Senno, L., Rossi, R., Franceschetti, P., delgi Uberti, E. C. Expression of all-trans-retinoic acid receptor RNA in human thyroid cells. Biochem Mol Biol Int, *33*: 1107–1115, 1994.
24. Rochaix, P., Monteil-Onteniente, S., Rochette-Egly, C., Caratero, C., Voigt, J. J., and Jozan, S. Reduced expression of retinoic acid receptor beta protein (RAR beta) in human papillary thyroid carcinoma: immunohistochemical and western blot study. Histopathology, *33*: 337–343, 1998.
25. Schmutzler, C., Brtko, J., Winzer, R., Jakobs, T. C., Meissner-Weigl, J., Simon, D., Goretzki, P. E., and Kohrle, J. Functional retinoid and thyroid hormone receptors in human thyroid-carcinoma cell lines and tissues. Int J Cancer, *76*: 368–376, 1998.
26. Simon, D., Korber, C., Krausch, M., Segering, J., Groth, P., Gorges, R., Grunwald, F., Muller-Gartner, H. W., Schmutzler, C., Kohrle, J., Roher, H. D., and Reiners, C. Clinical impact of retinoids in

redifferentiation therapy of advanced thyroid cancer: final results of a pilot study. Eur J Nucl Med Mol Imaging, 29: 775–782, 2002.
27. Sap, J., Munoz, A., Damm, K., Goldberg, Y., Ghysdael, J., Leutz, A., Beug, H., and Vennstrom, B. The c-erb-A protein is a high-affinity receptor for thyroid hormone. Nature, 324: 635–640, 1986.
28. Thormeyer, D. and Baniahmad, A. The v-erbA oncogene. Int J Mol Med, 4: 351–358, 1999.
29. Barlow, C., Meister, B., Lardelli, M., Lendahl, U., and Vennstrom, B. Thyroid abnormalities and hepatocellular carcinoma in mice transgenic for v-erbA. EMBO J, 13: 4241–4250, 1994.
30. Lin, K. H., Shieh, H. Y., Chen, S. L., and Hsu, H. C. Expression of mutant thyroid hormone nuclear receptors in human hepatocellular carcinoma cells. Mol Carcinog, 26: 53–61, 1999.
31. Puzianowska-Kuznicka, M., Nauman, A., Madej, A., Tanski, Z., Cheng, S., Nauman, J. Expression of thyroid hormone receptors is disturbed in human renal clear cell carcinoma. Cancer Lett, 155: 145–152, 2000.
32. Kamiya, Y., Puzianowska-Kuznicka, M., McPhie, P., Nauman, J., Cheng, S.Y., and Nauman, A. Expression of mutant thyroid hormone nuclear receptors is associated with human renal clear cell carcinoma. Carcinogenesis, 23: 25–33, 2002.
33. Lin, K. H., Zhu, X. G., Shieh, H. Y., Hsu, H. C., Chen, S. T., McPhie, P., and Cheng, S. Y. Identification of naturally occurring dominant negative mutants of thyroid hormone alpha 1 and beta 1 receptors in a human hepatocellular carcinoma cell line. Endocrinology 137: 4073–4081, 1996.
34. Wallin, G., Bronnegard, M., Grimelius, L., McGuire, J., and Torring, O. Expression of the thyroid hormone receptor, the oncogenes c-myc and H-ras, and the 90 kD heat shock protein in normal, hyperplastic, and neoplastic human thyroid tissue. Thyroid, 2: 307–313, 1992.
35. Bronnegard, M., Torring, O., Boos, J., Sylven, C., Marcus, C., and Wallin, G., 1994. Expression of thyrotropin receptor and thyroid hormone receptor messenger ribonucleic acid in normal, hyperplastic, and neoplastic human thyroid tissue. J. Clin Endocrinol Metab, 79: 384–389, 1994.
36. Puzianowska-Kuznick, M., Krystyniak, A., Madej, A., Cheng, S.-y., and Nauman, J. Contribution of functionally impaired thyroid hormone receptor mutants to the tumorigenesis of thyroid papillary cancer. J Clin Endocrinol Metab, 87: 1120–1128, 2002.
37. Takano, T., Miyauchi, A., Yoshida, H., Nakata, Y., Kuma, K., Amino, N. Expression of TRbeta1 mRNAs with functionally impaired mutations is rare in thyroid papillary carcinoma. J Clin Endocrinol Metab 88: 3447–3449, 2003.
38. Namba, H., Yamashita, S., Pei, H. C., Ishikawa, N., Villadolid, M. C., Tominaga, T., Kimura, H., Tsuruta, M., Yokoyama, N., and Izumi, M. Lack of PTC gene (ret proto-oncogene rearrangement) in human thyroid tumors. Endocrinol Jpn, 38: 627–632, 1991.
39. Zou, M., Shi, Y., and Farid, N. R. Low rate of ret proto-oncogene activation (PTC/retTPC) in papillary thyroid carcinomas from Saudi Arabia. Cancer, 73: 176–180, 1994.
40. Cinti, R., Yin, L., Ilc, K., Berger, N., Basolo, F., Cuccato, S., Giannini, R., Torre, G., Miccoli, P., Amati, P., Romeo, G., and Corvi, R. RET rearrangements in papillary thyroid carcinomas and adenomas detected by interphase FISH. Cytogenet Cell Genet, 88: 56–61, 2000.
41. Chua, E. L., Wu, W. M., Tran, K. T., McCarthy, S. W., Lauer, C. S., Dubourdieu, D., Packham, N., O'Brien, C. J., Turtle, J. R., and Dong, Q. Prevalence and distribution of ret/ptc 1, 2, and 3 in papillary thyroid carcinoma in New Caledonia and Australia, J Clin Endocrinol Metab, 85: 2733–2739, 2000.
42. Bednarczuk, T., Hiromatsu, Y., Fukutani, T., Jazdzewski, K., Miskiewicz, P., Osikowska, M., Nauman, J. Association of cytotoxic T-lymphocyte-associated antigen 4 (CTLA 4) gene polymorphism and nongenetic factors with Graves' ophthalmopathy in European and Japanese populations. Eur J Endocrinol, 148: 13–18, 2003.
43. Kaneshige, M., Kaneshige, K., Zhu, X. G., Dace, A., Garrett, L., Carter, T. A., Kazlauskaite, R., Pankratz, D. G., Wynshaw-Boris, A., Refetoff, S., Weintraub, B., Willingham, M. C., Barlow, C., and Cheng, S.-y. Mice with a targeted mutation in the thyroid hormone β receptor gene exhibit impaired growth and resistance to thyroid hormone. Proc Natl Acad Sci USA, 97: 13209–13214, 2000.
44. Yen, P. M. Molecular basis of resistance to thyroid hormone. Trends Endocrinol Metab, 14: 327–333, 2003.
45. Weiss, R. E. and Refetoff, S. Resistance to thyroid hormone. Rev Endocrinol Metab Disord, 1: 97–108, 2000.
46. Meier, C. A., Dickstein, B. M., Ashizawa, K., McClaskey, J. H., Muchmore, P., Ransom, S. C., Merke, J. B., Hao, E. U., Usala, S. J., Bercu, B. B., Cheng, S.-y., and Weintraub, B. D. Variable transcriptional activity and ligand binding of mutant β1 3,3',5-triiodo-L-thyronine receptors from four families with generalized resistance to thyroid hormone. Mol Endocrinol, 6: 248–258, 1992.

47. Suzuki, H., Willingham, M. C., and Cheng, S. Y. Mice with a mutation in the thyroid receptor beta gene spontaneously develop thyroid carcinoma: a mouse model of thyroid carcinogenesis. Thyroid, *12*: 963–969, 2002.
48. Ying, H., Suzuki, H., Furumoto, H., Walker, R., Meltzer, P., Billingham, M. C., and Cheng, S. Y. Alterations in genomic profiles during tumor progression in a mouse model of follicular thyroid carcinoma. Carcinogenesis, *24*: 1467–1479, 2003.
49. Khoo, M. L., Beasley, N. J., Ezzat, S., Freeman, J. L., Asa, S. L. Overexpression of cyclin D1 and underexpression of p27 predict lymph node metastases in papillary thyroid carcinoma. J Clin Endocrinol Metab, *87*: 1814–1818, 2002.
50. Bieche, I., Franc, B., Vidaud, D., Vidaud, M., and Lidereau, R. Analyses of MYC, ERBB2, and CCND1 genes in benign and malignant thyroid follicular cell tumors by real-time polymerase chain reaction. Thyroid, *11*: 147–152, 2001.
51. Heaney, A. P., Nelson, V., Fernando, M., and Horwitz, G., 2001. Transforming events in thyroid tumorigenesis and their association with follicular lesions. J Clin Endocrinol Metab, *86*: 5025–5032, 2001.
52. Ishigaki, K., Namba, H., Nakashima, M., Nakayama, T., Mitsutake, N., Hayashi, T., Maeda, S., Ichinose, M., Kanematsu, T., Yamashita, S. Aberrant localization of beta-catenin correlates with overexpression of its target gene in human papillary thyroid cancer. J Clin Endocrinol Metab, *87*: 433–440, 2002.
53. Holting, T., Goretzki, P. E., and Duh,Q. Y. Follicular thyroid cancer cells: a model of metastatic tumor in vitro. Oncol Rep, *8*: 3–8, 2001.
54. Yen, P. M. and Cheng, S-y. Germline and somatic thyroid hormone receptor mutations in man. J Endocrinolo Invest, *26*: (pages not known), in press, 2003.
55. Lin, K. H., Zhu, X. G., Hsu, H. C., Chen, S. L., Shieh, H. Y., Chen, S. T., McPhie, P., and Cheng, S. Y. Dominant negative activity of mutant thyroid hormone alpha1 receptors from patients with hepatocellular carcinoma. Endocrinology, *138*: 5308–5315, 1997.
56. Kimura, T., Van Keymeulen, A., Golstein, J., Fusco, A., Dumont, J. E., and Roger, P. P. Regulation of thyroid cell proliferation by TSH and other factors: a critical evaluation of in vitro models. Endocr Rev, *22*: 631–656, 2001.
57. Rivas, M. and Santisteban, P. TSH-activated signaling pathways in thyroid carcinogenesis. Molecular Cellular Endo Review (in press), 2003.
58. Fagin, J.A. Branded from the start-distinct oncogenic initiating events may determine tumor fate in the thyroid (minireview). Mol Endocrinol, *16*: 903–911, 2002.
59. Desvergne, B. and Wahli, W. Peroxisome proliferator-activated receptors: nuclear control of metabolism. Endocr Rev, *20*: 649–688, 1999.
60. Fajas, L., Webril, M. B., Auwerx, J. Peroxisome proliferator-activated receptor-gamma: from adipogenesis to carcinogenesis. J Mol Endocrinol, *27*: 1–9, 2001.
61. Fajas, L., Auboeuf, D., Raspe, E., Schoonjans, K., Lefebvre, A. M., Saladin, R., Najib, J., Laville, M., Fruchart, J. C., Deeb, S., Vidal-Puig, A., Flier, J., Briggs, M. R., Staels, B., Vidal, H., and Auwerx, J. The organization, promoter analysis, and expression of the human PPARgamma gene. J Biol Chem, *272*: 18779–18789, 1997.
62. Altiok, S., Xu, M., and Spiegelman, B. M. PPARgamma induces cell cycle withdrawal: inhibition of E2F/DP DNA-binding activity via down-regulation of PP2A. Genes Dev, *11*: 1987–1998, 1997.
63. Tontonoz, P., Singer, S., Forman, B. M., Sarraf, P., Fletcher, J. A., Fletcher, C. D., Brun, R. P., Mueller, E., Altiok, S., Oppenheim, H., Evans, R. M., and Spiegelman, B. M. Terminal differentiation of human liposarcoma cells induced by ligands for peroxisome proliferator-activated receptor gamma and the retinoid X receptor. Proc Natl Acad Sci USA, *94*: 237–241, 1997.
64. Elstner, E., Muller, C., Koshizuka, K., Williamson, E. A., Park, D., Asou, H., Shintaku, P., Said, J. W., Heber, D., and Koeffler, H. P. Ligands for peroxisome proliferator-activated receptor and retinoic acid receptor inhibit growth and induce apoptosis of human breast cancer cells in vitro and in BNX mice. Proc Natl Acad Sci USA, *95*: 8806–8811, 1998.
65. Mueller, E., Sarraf, P., Tontonoz, P., Evans, R. M., Martin, K. J., Zhang, M., Fletcher, C., Singer, S., Spiegelman, B. M. Terminal differentiation of human breast cancer through PPAR. Mol Cell, *1*: 465–470, 1998.
66. Brockman, J. A., Gupta, R. A., and DuBois, R. N. Activation of PPAR leads to inhibition of anchorage-independent growth of human colorectal cancer cells. Gastroenterology, *115*: 1049–1055, 1998.
67. Kuboto, T., Koshizuka, K., Williamson, I. A., Asou, H., Said, J. W., Holden, S., Miyoshi, I., Koeffler, H. P. Ligand for peroxisome proliferator activated receptor (troglitazone) has potent anti-tumor effects against human prostate cancer both in vitro and in vivo. Cancer Res, *58*: 3344–3352, 1998.

68. Sarraf, P., Mueller, E., Jones, D., King, F. J., De Angelo, D. J., Partridge, J. B., Holden, S. A., Chen, L. B., Singer, S., Fletcher, C., and Spiegelman, B. M. Differentiation and reversal of malignant changes in colon cancer through PPAR gamma. Nat Med, *4*: 1046–1052, 1998.
69. Ohta, K., Endo, T., Haraguchi, K., Hershman, J. M., Onaya, T. Ligands for peroxisome proliferator-activated receptor gamma inhibit growth and induce apoptosis of human papillary thyroid carcinoma cells. J Clin Endocrinol Metab *86*: 2170–2177, 2001.
70. Martelli, M. L., Iuliano, R., Le Pera, I., Sama', I., Monaco, C., Cammarota, S., Kroll, T., Chiariotti, L., Santoro, M., Fusco, A. Inhibitory effects of peroxisome poliferator-activated receptor gamma on thyroid carcinoma cell growth. J Clin Endocrinol Metab, *87*: 4728–4735, 2002.
71. Ying, H., Suzuki, H., Zhao, L., Willingham, M. C., Meltzer, P., Cheng, S. Y. Mutant thyroid hormone receptor beta represses the expression and transcriptional activity of peroxisome proliferator-activated receptor gamma during thyroid carcinogenesis. Cancer Res, *63*: 5274–5280, 2003.
72. Schoonjans, K., Peinado-Onsurbe, J., Lefebvre, A. M., Heyman, R. A., Briggs, M., Deeb, S., Staels, B., and Auwerx, J. PPARalpha and PPARgamma activators direct a distinct tissue-specific transcriptional response via a PPRE in the lipoprotein lipase gene. EMBO J., *15*: 5336–5348, 1996.
73. Kroll, T. G., Sarraf, P., Pecciarini, L., Chen, C. J., Mueller, E., Spiegelman, B. M., and Fletcher, J. A. PAX8-PPARgamma1 fusion oncogene in human thyroid carcinoma. Science, *289*: 1357–1360, 2000.
74. Nikiforova, M. N., Biddinger, P. W., Caudill, C. M., Kroll, T. G., and Nikiforov, Y. E. PAX8-PPARgamma rearrangement in thyroid tumors: RT-PCR and immunohistochemical analyses. Am J Surg Pathol, *26*: 1016–1023, 2002.
75. Marques, A. R., Espadinha, C., Catarino, A. L., Moniz, S., Pereira, T., Sobrinho, L. G., Leite, V. Expression of PAX8-PPAR gamma 1 rearrangements in both follicular thyroid carcinomas and adenomas. J Clin Endocrinol Metab, *87*: 3947–3952, 2002.
76. French, C. A., Alexander, E. K., Cibas, E. S., Nose, V., Laguette, J., Faquin, W., Garber, J., Moore, F. Jr., Fletcher, J. A., Larsen, P. R., Kroll, T. G. Genetic and biological subgroups of low-stage follicular thyroid cancers Am J Pathol, *162*: 1053–1060, 2003.

10. MATRIX METALLOPROTEINASES IN THYROID CANCER

YUFEI SHI AND MINJING ZOU

Department of Genetics, King Faisal Specialist Hospital and Research Center, P.O. Box 3354, Riyadh 11211, Saudi Arabia

INTRODUCTION

Cancer is a multistage disorder in which sequential and cumulative genetic aberrations lead to malignant cell transformation (1–2). Approximately 50% of cancer mortality results from invasion and metastasis. Tumor cell invasion and metastasis is a complex multistep process that involves the degradation of extracellular matrix (ECM) proteins by matrix metalloproteinases (MMPs), an important step in the process of cancer invasion and metastasis. Correlation between MMPs overexpression and cancer metastasis have been repeatedly made by numerous studies. Malignant cells rely on these proteinases to disrupt basement membranes, invade surrounding tissues and metastasize to different organs. It is now apparent that not only tumor cells but also non-malignant stromal cells actively participate in the proteolytic degradation of ECM. Tissue inhibitors of metalloproteinases (TIMPs) act as negative regulators of MMPs and it has been shown that they can prevent the spread of cancer in animal models by preserving ECM integrity (3–4).

Matrix metalloproteinases, also called matrixins, constitute a family of zinc-dependent endopeptidases. Twenty-eight members of this family have been identified. Collectively, MMPs play important roles in ECM homeostasis, mediating such normal physiological processes as embryogenesis, organ morphogenesis, reproduction, angiogenesis, and tissue resorption and remodeling (5). The proteolytic activities of MMPs are tightly regulated by endogenous inhibitors, α-macroglobulins, and tissue inhibitors of metalloproteinases (TIMPs) (5). Any disruption of this fine balance can contribute to the pathogenesis of serious diseases such as arthritis, periodontal disease, and cancer metastasis (6).

THE MMP FAMILY AND STRUCTURE

At present, the human MMP family consists of 23 structurally related members (Table1). Historically, the MMPs were divided into subgroups of collagenases, gelatinases, stromelysins, membrane-type MMPs, and other novel MMPs, on the basis of their specificity for ECM components. As the list of MMP substrates has grown and several MMPs can degrade a number of different ECM components, a sequential MMP numbering system has been adapted, and the MMPs are now grouped according to their structure. There are eight distinct structural classes of MMPs: five are secreted and three are membrane-type MMPs (Figure 1) (7).

MMPs are produced and secreted by a number of cell types, including fibroblasts, smooth muscle cells, and endothelial cells. They share several highly conserved domains, including an N-terminal propeptide domain that contains a "cystein switch" sequence that enfolds the zinc atom of the catalytic site to maintain the latency of pro-MMPs, a catalytic domain with a zinc binding site and a conserved methionine, and a C-terminal hemopexin-like domain linked to the catalytic domain by a proline rich hinge region. The catalytic domain contains a zinc binding motif HEXXHXXGXXH, in which the three histidine residues represent the three zinc ligands and the glutamic residue the active site. The hemopexin domain contains a single Cys-Cys bond and plays a role in substrate recognition (for example, it is required for collagenases to cleave triple helical interstitial collagens), interaction with TIMPs, and binding of the enzyme to ECM or cell surface (4–5).

The substrates of MMPs are primarily insoluble proteins of ECM, including interstitial and basement membrane collagens, glycoproteins such as laminin, fibronectin, vitronectin, tenascin and elastin as well as proteoglycans. However, more recent data demonstrate that certain MMPs can degrade proteins other than ECM proteins. Many cell membrane bound precursors of growth factors (TGF-α, TGF-β), growth factor receptors (FGF receptor 1, HER2/neu, HER4) and cell adhesion molecules (CD 44, E-cadherin, αv integrin) have been reported to be MMP substrates. For example, MMP-11 can cleavage of insulin-like growth-factor-binding protein (IGF-BP) to release IGFs (8); MMP 12 can proteolytically process plasminogen to generate angiostatin, an inhibitor of angiogenesis (9); MMP-2 and MMP-9 can proteolytically activate TGF-β and promote tumor invasion and angiogenesis (10); and finally, cleavage of the αv integrin subunit precursor by MMP-14 enhances cancer cell migration (11). Although the significance of these observations is not entirely clear, they reflect the complex nature of MMPs in cancer progression.

REGULATION OF MMP ACTIVITY

The activities of MMPs are regulated at three major levels: transcriptional regulation, activation of latent MMP, and inhibition/deactivation by endogenous inhibitors such as α-macroglobulins and TIMPs.

Table 1. The matrix metalloproteinase (MMP) family

MMP subgroup	MMP	Domain class*	Common name (s)
Collagenase			
Collagenase-1	MMP-1	B	fibroblast collagenase, tissue collagenase, interstitial collagenase
Collagenase-2	MMP-8	B	neutrophil collagenase, granulocyte collagenase, PMN collagenase
Collagenase-3	MMP-13	B	todpole collagenase
Collagenase-4	MMP-18	B	found in Xenopus, no human homologue is known
Stromelysins			
Stromelysin-1	MMP-3	B	transin-1, proteoglycanase, procollagenase-activating protein
Stromelysin-2	MMP-10	B	transin-2
Stromelysin-3	MMP-11	D	
Matrilysins			
Matrilysin	MMP-7	A	matrin, PUMP1, small uterine metalloproteinase
Matrilysin-2	MMP-26	A	endometase
Gelatinases			
Gelatinase A	MMP-2	C	72-kDa gelatinase, 72-kDa type IV collagenase, neutrophil gelatinase
Gelatinase	MMP-9	C	92-kDa gelatinase, 92-kDa type IV collagenase
Membrane-type MMPs			
MT1-MMP	MMP-14	F	MT-MMP1
MT2-MMP	MMP-15	F	MT-MMP2
MT3-MMP	MMP-16	F	MT-MMP3
MT4-MMP	MMP-17	G	MT-MMP4
MT5-MMP	MMP-24	F	MT-MMP5
MT6-MMP	MMP-25	G	MT-MMP6, leukolysin
Other MMPs			
Metalloelastase	MMP-12	B	Macrophage elastase, macrophage metalloelastase
RASI-1	MMP-19	B	
Enamelysin	MMP-20	B	
XMMP	MMP-21	E	homologue of Xenopus XMMP
CMMP	MMP-22	B	found in chicken
Femalysin	MMP-23	H	cysteine array MMP
(no trivial name)	MMP-27	B	
Epilysin	MMP-28	D	
McoI-A	No designation	B	found in mouse
McoI-B	No designation	B	found in mouse
75-kDa gelatinase	No designation	C	found in chichen

*see Figure 1

MMP mRNA levels can be induced by a wide variety of chemical agents (e.g. phorbol esters), growth factors (e.g. epidermal growth factor, EGF), hormones (e.g. thyroid hormone, relaxin) cytokines (e.g. interleukin-1, IL-1 and tumor necrosis factor-α, TNF-α), and physical stress. They may also be down-regulated by suppressive factors such as transforming growth factor-β, retinoic acids and glucocorticoids (5,12). The promoter regions of several MMP genes (MMP-1, MMP-3, MMP-7, MMP-9, MMP-10, MMP-12, and MMP-13) contain some common regulatory DNA

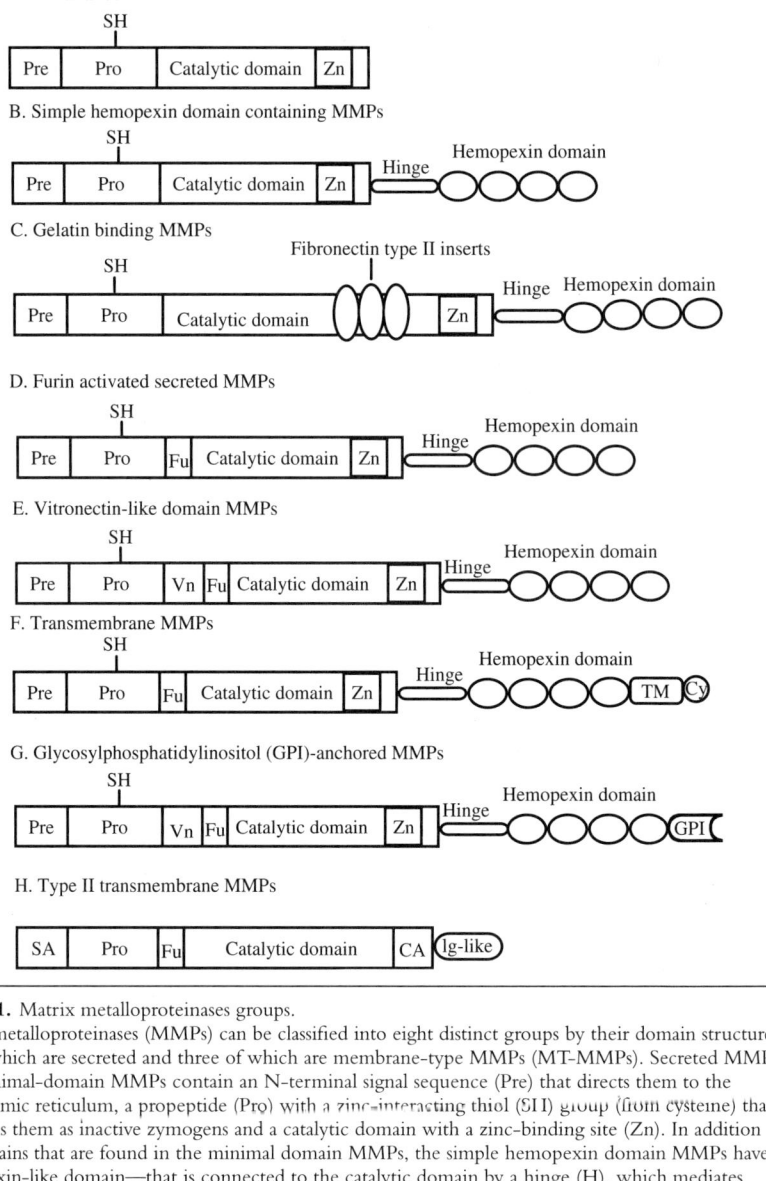

Figure 1. Matrix metalloproteinases groups.
Matrix metalloproteinases (MMPs) can be classified into eight distinct groups by their domain structure, five of which are secreted and three of which are membrane-type MMPs (MT-MMPs). Secreted MMPs: The minimal-domain MMPs contain an N-terminal signal sequence (Pre) that directs them to the endoplasmic reticulum, a propeptide (Pro) with a zinc-interacting thiol (SH) group (from cysteine) that maintains them as inactive zymogens and a catalytic domain with a zinc-binding site (Zn). In addition to the domains that are found in the minimal domain MMPs, the simple hemopexin domain MMPs have a hemopexin-like domain—that is connected to the catalytic domain by a hinge (H), which mediates interactions with tissue inhibitors of metalloproteinases, cell-surface molecules and proteolytic substrates. The first and the last of the four repeats in the hemopexin-like domain are linked by a disulphide bond. The gelatin-binding MMPs contain three inserts that resemble collagen-binding type II repeats of fibronectin (Fi) and is responsible for the specific binding to gelatins and collagens. The furin-activated secreted MMPs contain a recognition motif for intracellular furin-like serine proteinases (Fu) between their propeptide and catalytic domains that allows intracellular activation by these proteinases. This motif is also found in the vitronectin-like insert (Vn) MMPs and the membrane-type MMPs (MT-MMPs). MT-MMPs: MT-MMPs include transmembrane MMPs that have a C-terminal, single-span transmembrane domain (TM) and a very short cytoplasmic domain (Cy), and the glycosylphosphatidylinositol (GPI)-anchored MMPs. MMP-23 represents a third type of membrane-linked MMP. It has an N-terminal signal anchor (SA) that targets it to the cell membrane, and so is a type II transmembrane MMP. MMP-23 is also characterized by its unique cysteine array (CA) and immunoglobulin (Ig)-like domains instead of the hemopexin domain. Adapted from Ref. 7.

sequences. Two important elements for transcriptional regulation are an AP-1 binding site for AP-1 transcription factors which comprise of members of the FOS and JUN family of transcription factors, and a PEA-3 element that binds ETS transcription factors. The AP-1 site, located approximately 70 bp upstream from the transcriptional start site, has been considered to play an important role in the transcriptional activation of the MMP promoters, whereas interaction between AP-1 and PEA-3 site is necessary for basal transcription and trans-activation by cytokines and growth factors. The DNA binding and trans-activation of both AP-1 and ETS transcription factors are regulated by mitogen-activated protein kinases (MAPKs) (12). Interestingly, AP-1 site is not present in the promoter region of MMP-2, a critical metalloproteinase involved in cancer metastasis, and MMP-14, which is involved in the activation of MMP-2 (13). Another transcriptional control of MMP expression is the presence of naturally occurring sequence variation or single nucleotide polymorphisms (SNPs) in the promoters of MMP genes (14). These genetic polymorphisms have been shown to have allele-specific effects on the MMP promoter activities, e.g. an insertion of a guanine at position −1607 in the MMP-1 gene promoter creates the core sequence (5'-GGA-3') of a binding site for the ETS transcription factors. The 2G allele has a higher transcriptional activity in melanoma cells and is associated with more invasive tumors (15).

All MMPs are synthesized as prepro-enzymes. Most MMPs are secreted as inactive, latent pro-MMPs, with the exception of MT-MMPs, which are membrane bound and localize at the cell surface. Since MMP activation occurs after secretion into the extracellular milieu, an important control point for MMP activity is the proteolytic cleavage of pro-MMPs. It has been demonstrated that serine proteases such as trypsin, plasmin, or urokinase initiate activation of MMPs from the zymogen form (16). Some MMPs can also activate other members of the family. A good example is the activation of pro-MMP-2 at the cell surface by MMP-14 and TIMP-2 (17): TIMP-2 binds MMP-14 at its amino terminus and pro-MMP-2 at its carboxyl terminus, which allows an adjacent, non-inhibited MMP-14 to cleave the bound pro-MMP-2. MMP-14 does not fully activate MMP-2 and another already activated MMP-2 is required to remove a residual portion of the MMP-2 propeptide (18). Pro-MMP2 can also be activated by MMP-15 through TIMP-2 independent mechanism (19). Although most MMPs are activated outside the cells by serine proteases or other activated MMPs, MMP-11, MMP-28, and the MT-MMPs can also be activated by intracellular furin-like serine proteases before they reach the cell surface (20).

A final and important control point of MMP activity is the inhibition of activated enzymes by endogenous inhibitors. The main inhibitor of MMPs in tissue fluids is α-macroglobulin, an abundant plasma protein (21). α-Macroglobulin binds to MMPs and the MMP/α-macroglobulin complex then binds to a scavenger receptor and is irreversibly cleared by endocytosis. In a similar way to α-macroglobulin, thrombospondin-2 forms a complex with MMP-2 and facilitates scavenger-receptor-mediated endocytosis and clearance (22). By contrast, thrombospondin-1 binds to pro-MMP-2 and -9 and directly inhibits their activation (23–24). Curiously, thrombospondin-1 has also been reported to increase MMP-2 and -9 activation (25).

Another group of endogenous MMP inhibitors are TIMP family of inhibitors. At present, four structurally related members have been characterized (TIMP-1, TIMP-2, TIMP-3, and TIMP-4) with 40–50% sequence identity at the amino acid levels (26). TIMPs are small, low molecular weight proteins (20–30 kDa). They differ in tissue-specific expression and ability to inhibit various MMPs. They reversibly inhibit active MMPs with relatively low selectivity by occupying the catalytic domain of activated enzymes (27–28). The TIMP/MMP complex is a tight binding, non-covalent complexes with a stoichiometric 1:1 molar ratio. Unlike TIMP-1, TIMP-2, and TIMP-4, which are secreted in soluble form, TIMP-3 has a unique association with ECM. Studies with Timp-2-deficient mice indicate that the dominant physiological function of TIMP-2 is activation of MMP-2 (29). Apart from inhibiting MMPs, TIMP-3 has been shown to promote apoptosis whereas TIMP-1 is active in blocking apoptosis and overexpression of TIMP-2 protect cancer cells from apoptosis (30–32).

MMPs AND TIMPs IN THYROID CANCER PROGRESSION AND METASTASIS

The expression and activity of MMPs are increased in many types of human cancer, and this correlates with advanced tumor stage, increased invasion and metastasis, and shortened survival. Many studies show a negative association between MMPs activity and prognosis (7). MMP-2 and MMP-9 are of particular importance in tumor cell invasion, because they degrade type IV collagen, the main structural component of the basement membrane. Tumor cells expressing high levels of these enzymes are highly metastatic. Cancer cells are not the only source of MMPs. Stromal cells are also participated in the production of MMPs (20). MMPs that are secreted by stomal cells can still be recruited to the cancer cell membrane, e.g. MMP-2 mRNA is expressed by stromal cells of human breast cancers, whereas MMP-2 protein is found on both stromal and cencer cell membranes (33). It has been shown that cancer cells can stimulate tumor stromal cells to produce MMPs in a paracrine fashion through secretion of cytokines, growth factors, and EMMPRIN (extracellular matrix metalloproteinase inducer). EMMPRIN is an intrinsic plasma membrane glycoprotein produced in high amounts by cancer cells, which stimulates local fibroblasts to synthesize MMPs (34). Tumor cell interactions with fibroblasts via EMMPRIN leads to fibroblast-induced local degradation of basement membrane and ECM components, thus facilitating tumor cell invasion. It has been shown that MMP-9 production in tumor infiltrating macrophages play a critical role in angiogenesis and progressive growth of human ovarian tumors in mice (35). Stromal cells and their products have been reported to even cause tumorigenic transformation of adjacent epithelial cells (36).

Earlier studies have shown that invasion by cultured human follicular thyroid carcinoma is correlated with increased production of beta 1 integrins and MMPs (37). Correlation between MMPs and ECM degradation is further demonstrated by the study of plasmin activation system in metastatic follicular thyroid carcinoma cell lines (38). As mentioned earlier, plasmin is a serine protease involved in the activation of MMPs. Plasmin is generated from plasminogen by urokinase-type plasminogen activator (uPA) and tissue-type plasminogen activator (tPA). UPA-mediated plasminogen activation is an important pathway in tumor invasion and can be inactivated by plasminogen activator inhibitors (PAI-1 and –2) (39). Decreased activity of PAI-1 is associated with greater ECM degradation in follicular thyroid carcinoma cell lines (38).

Overexpression of MMP-2, and MMP-9 has been found in thyroid carcinomas and is correlated with large tumor size, high intrathyroid invasion, presence of lymph node metastasis, and advanced disease stage (40). A more comprehensive study of MMPs profile involving seven secreted MMPs (MMP-1, -2, -3, -7, -8, -9, and -13) and three membrane-bound MMPs (MMP-14, -15, and -16) demonstrates that the major MMPs produced in papillary thyroid carcinomas are MMP-2 and MMP-14 (41). The pro-MMP-2 activation and the expression of MMP-14, known to activate pro-MMP-2 at the cell surface, are considerably higher in carcinomas with lymph node metastasis than those without metastasis. MMP-15 expression is confined to 26% of cases. MMP-2, MMP-14, and MMP-15 are immunostained in both carcinoma and stromal cells (41). In a separate study, increased MMP-2 expression is found in follicular and anaplastic thyroid carcinomas, but not in follicular adenomas (42). Interestingly, MMP-2 mRNA expression is restricted to fibroblasts in the stroma adjacent or close to invading tumor cells (42). MMP-1 expression is significantly greater among follicular and papillary thyroid carcinomas compared to benign lesions. However, there is no relationship between MMP-1 expression and invasion, metastasis, or disease recurrence (43). Both carcinoma and stromal cells have been shown to express MMP-1 (43–44). A recent cDNA and tissue microarray study shows that MMP-11 is up-regulated in 67% of papillary thyroid carcinoma tissues (45).

Both TIMP-1 and TIMP-2 expression are increased in thyroid carcinomas, and are correlated with large tumor size and advanced disease stage (40,46), which seem to be contradictory to the role of TIMPs as inhibitors of tumor cell invasion and metastasis. Further study shows stronger TIMP-1 immunostaining in the stromal cells surrounding the tumor, suggesting that the high levels of TIMP-1 transcripts in advanced stage of thyroid carcinoma are likely represent a stroma response to tumor cell invasion. Overexpression of TIMP-1 by gene transfer has resulted in a significant suppression of invasive potential of NPA cells, a poorly differentiated thyroid carcinoma cell line (46). Reduced TIMP-1 expression has been shown in recurrent papillary thyroid carcinoma when compared to non-recurrent carcinomas (43). Apparently, tumor invasion is not dependent on the absolute levels of TIMPs or MMPs. It is the balance between TIMPs and MMPs that determines the potential of thyroid tumor invasion and metastasis. Indeed, the molar ratio of total amounts of MMPs:TIMPs is significantly higher in the thyroid carcinoma samples than in the adenoma and normal samples (41).

Many MMP genes are transcribed at low or undetectable levels in normal thyrocytes. Analysis of MMPs and TIMPs expression *in vitro* demonstrates that MMP-1, -2, -9, -14, and TIMP-1, -2, -3 mRNA are present in normal thyrocytes, malignant thyroid cells and thyroid-derived fibroblasts. The basal levels of MMP-1, -9, and -14 are much lower in thyrocytes than in malignant thyroid cells and thyroid-derived fibroblasts, whereas high basal levels of MMP-2, TIMP-1, -2, and -3 are found in all three cell types without striking difference (47–48). IL-1 can upregulate MMP-1 and MMP-9 mRNA in all the cell types through activating nuclear factor of κB (NF-κB), and has no significant effect on TIMPs, MMP-2, and MMP-14. TNF-α, also acting via

NF-κB passway, can stimulate MMP-9 mRNA expression in malignant thyroid cells and thyroid-derived fibroblasts. EGF, acting via protein tyrosine kinase, can only stimulate MMP-1 expression in malignant cells (49). Phorbol—myristate acetate (PMA, an active phorbol ester) can induce MMP-1, MMP-9 and TIMP-1 mRNA in all the cell types, MMP-14 in malignant thyroid cells and thyroid-derived fibroblasts (47–49). Since PMA, acting via protein kinase C (PKC), can induce *c-jun* and *c-fos* gene expression in human thyroid cells, and their gene products are AP1 transcriptional factors (50), it is likely that PKC is involved in the induction of MMP transcription. Although thyroid-stimulating hormone (TSH) has no significant effect on the basal MMP-1, or TIMP-1 mRNA levels, it can cause a dose-dependent inhibition in PMA or EGF-induced MMP-1 mRNA in malignant cells, and PMA-induced MMP-1 and TIMP-1 mRNA in benign thyroid cells. The repressive action of TSH on MMP-1 mRNA can be mimicked by the forkolin and 8-bromo-cAMP, and can be abrogated by a protein kinase A (PKA) inhibitor, H-89, suggesting that it is PKA-mediated (49). MMP-11, -13, and -18 genes are thyroid hormone responsive genes. Although they have not been shown to be involved in thyroid cancer, they have distinct functions during frog embrogenesis (51).

Several studies have shown that high serum levels of MMP-2, MMP-9, and TIMP-1 are associated with tumor invasion and poor survival in several types of cancer (52–54). Thus, they may be used as prognostic markers in cancer patients. Higher levels of MMP-2 and TIMP-2 are detected by ELISA in peripheral blood of thyroid cancer patients when compared to normal control, and increased blood levels of MMP-3 and MMP-9 appear to be associated with medullary thyroid cancer (55). It remains to be determined whether serum levels of MMPs and TIMPs can be used as diagnostic or prognostic markers for thyroid carcinoma.

MMP INHIBITION IN ANTICANCER THERAPY

Given that MMPs play important role in tumor invasion and metastasis, inhibition of MMPs activity has been the focus of much anticancer research and clinical trials. Pharmaceutical industries have invested considerable effort over the past decade to develop safe and effective MMP inhibitors for use in cancer patient. Three classes of synthetic MMP inhibitors have been developed (Table 2): the collagen peptidomimetics which mimic the collagen amino-acid sequence near the collagenase cleavage site; the collagen non-peptidomimetics which are synthesized based upon the conformation of MMP active site; and the tetracycline derivatives which inhibit the activity of MMPs without antibiotic activity (13, 56–57). Numerous preclinical studies using these MMP inhibitors in cancer models have demonstrated their effectiveness to delay primary tumor growth and inhibit experimental metastasis. Initiation of treatment when tumor burden is minimal has a more profound effect on tumor growth inhibition than at the time of large tumor bulk. Despite of positive preclinical results in the use of MMP inhibitors, most clinical trials have not yielded significant beneficial effects in patients with advanced cancer (57). In the case of BAY12-9566, alarming reports show significantly poorer survival for groups treated with the drug than for placebo-treated group.

Table 2. The matrix metalloproteinase inhibitors for cancer therapy

Inhibitor	Structure	Specificity
Marimastat (BB-2516)	Peptido mimetic	Broad spectrum (2nd generation of BB-94)
Batimastat (BB-94)	Peptido mimetic	Broad spectrum (e.g. MMP-1, 2, 3, 7, 9, 12)
Tanomastat (Bay 12-9566)	Non-peptido mimetic	Broad spectrum (e.g. MMP-2, 9, 11, 13, 14)
Prinomastat (AG3340)	Non-peptido mimetic	Broad spectrum
BMS-275291	Non-peptido mimetic	Broad spectrum
MMI 270 (CGS27023A)	Non-peptido mimetic	Broad spetrum
Metastat (COL-3)	Tetracycline derivative	Gelatinases (MMP-2, 9)

In view of the disappointing results of synthetic MMP inhibitors in clinical trials, we and other investigators have recently explored the potential applications of TIMP gene overexpression for cancer gene therapy (58–60). Antitumor effects have been shown following systemic or local delivery of TIMP-1, TIMP-2, and TIMP-3 genes in animal models (60–63). However, stimulation of mammary tumorigenesis has been reported following systemic TIMP-4 gene delivery. TIMP-4 has been shown to up-regulate Bcl-2 and Bcl-X(L) protein and inhibit apoptosis in human breast cancer cells (64). Given the multifunctional nature of TIMP proteins, further preclinical studies will be needed before initiation of clinical gene therapy trial in patients with cancer.

CONCLUSIONS

As compared with tumors from other organs such as lung, colon, and breast, a limited number of studies have been carried out so far on the involvement of MMPs and TIMPs in thyroid tumorigenesis. Based upon the available data, it is clear that MMPs, especially MMP-2 and MMP-9, and TIMP-1 are involved in thyroid tumor invasion and metastasis. Although TIMP-1 can reduce the invasive potential of thyroid cancer cells *in vitro*, therapeutic intervention *in vivo* has not been attempted yet in animal models to inhibit thyroid tumor growth, invasion, and metastasis, using either synthetic MMP inhibitors or TIMPs gene therapy. Clearly, more studies are needed to fully appreciate the important roles of MMPs and TIMPs in thyroid cancer.

REFERENCES

1. Hanahan, D., and Weinberg, R.A. The hallmarks of cancer. Cell, 100:57–70, 2000.
2. Farid, N.R., Shi, Y., and Zou, M.J. Molecular basis of thyroid cancer. Endocrine Review 15:202–232, 1994.
3. Kohn, E.C., and Liotta, L.A. Molecular insights into cancer invasion: strategies for prevention and intervention. Cancer Res., 55:1856–1862, 1995.
4. DeClerck, Y.A. Interactions between tumor cells and stromal cells and proteolytic modification of the extracellular matrix by metalloproteinases in cancer. European J. Cancer 36:1258–1268, 2000.
5. Nagase, H., and Woessner, J.F. Matrix metalloproteinases. J. Biol. Chem., 274:21491–21494, 1999.
6. Bode, W., Fernandez-Catalan, C., Grams, F., Gomis-Ruth, F.X., Nagase, H., Tschesche, H., and Maskos, K. Insights into MMP-TIMP interactions. Ann. NY Acad. Sci., 878:73–91, 1999.

7. Egeblad, M., and Werb, Z. New functions for the matrix metalloproteinases in cancer progression. Nature Reviews Cancer, 2:163–176, 2002.
8. Manes, S., Mira, E., Barbacid, M.M., Cipres, A., Fernandez-Resa, P., Buesa, J.M., Merida, I., Aracil, M., Marquez, G., and Martinez, A. C. Identification of insulin-like growth factor-binding protein-1 as a potential physiological substrate for human stromelysin-3. J. Biol. Chem., 272:25706–25712, 1997.
9. Cornelius, L.A., Nehring, L.C., Harding, E., Bolanowski, M., Welgus, H.G., Kobayashi, D.K., Pierce, R.A., and Shapiro, S.D. Matrix metalloproteinases generate angiostatin: effects on neovascularization. J. Immunol., 161:6845–6852, 1998.
10. Yu, Q., and Stamenkovic, I. Cell surface-localized matrix metalloproteinase-9 proteolytically activates TGF-beta and promotes tumor invasion and angiogenesis. Genes Dev., 14:163–176, 2000.
11. Kajita, M., Itoh, Y., Chiba, T., Mori, H., Okada, A., Kinoh, H., and Seiki, M. Membrane-type 1 matrix metalloproteinase cleaves CD44 and promotes cell migration. J. Cell Biol., 153:893–904, 2001
12. Fini, M.E., Cook, J.R., Mohan, R., and Brinckerhoft, C.E. in Matrix Metalloproteinases (Parks, W.C. and Mecham, R.P., eds) pp. 299–356, 1998. Academic Press, San Diego.
13. Overall, C.M., and Lopez-Otin, C. Strategies for MMP inhibition in cancer: innovations for the post-trial era. Nature Reviews Cancer, 2:657–672, 2002.
14. Ye, S. Polymorphism in matrix metalloproteinase gene promoters: implication in regulation of gene expression and susceptibility of various diseases. Matrix Biology, 19: 623–629, 2000.
15. Ye, S., Dhillon, S., Turner, S.J., Bateman, A.C., Theaker, J.M., Pickering, R.M., Day, I., and Howell, W.M. Invasiveness of cutaneous malignant melanoma is influenced by matrix metalloproteinase 1 gene polymorphism. Cancer Res., 61: 1296–1298, 2001.
16. Nagase, H. Activational mechanisms of matrix metalloproteinases. Biol. Chem., 378:151–160, 1997.
17. Strongin, A.Y., Collier, I., Bannikov, G., Marmer, B.L., Grant, G.A., Goldberg, G.I. Mechanism of cell surface activation of 72-kDa type IV collagenase. Isolation of the activated form of the membrane metalloprotease. J. Biol. Chem., 270:5331–5338, 1995.
18. Deryugina, E.I., Ratnikov, B., Monosov, E., Postnova, T.I., DiScipio, R., Smith, J.W., Strongin, A.Y. MT1-MMP initiates activation of pro-MMP-2 and integrin alphavbeta3 promotes maturation of MMP-2 in breast carcinoma cells. Exp. Cell Res., 263:209–223, 2001.
19. Morrison, C.J., Butler, G.S., Bigg, H.F., Roberts, C.R., Soloway, P.D., Overall, C.M. Cellular activation of MMP-2 (gelatinase A) by MT2-MMP occurs via a TIMP-2-independent pathway. J. Biol. Chem., 276:47402–47410, 2001.
20. Sternlicht, M.D. and Werb, Z. How matrix metalloproteinases regulate cell behavior. Annu. Rev. Cell Dev. Biol., 17:463–516, 2001.
21. Sottrup-Jensen, L., and Birkedal-Hansen, H. Human fibroblast collagenase-alpha-macroglobulin interactions. Localization of cleavage sites in the bait regions of five mammalian alpha-macroglobulins. J. Biol. Chem., 264:393–401,1989.
22. Yang, Z., Strickland, D.K., and Bornstein P. Extracellular matrix metalloproteinase 2 levels are regulated by the low density lipoprotein-related scavenger receptor and thrombospondin 2. J. Biol. Chem., 276:8403–8408, 2001.
23. Rodriguez-Manzaneque, J.C., Lane, T.F., Ortega, M.A., Hynes, R.O., Lawler, J., and Iruela-Arispe, M.L. Thrombospondin-1 suppresses spontaneous tumor growth and inhibits activation of matrix metalloproteinase-9 and mobilization of vascular endothelial growth factor. Proc. Natl. Acad. Sci. USA, 98:12485–12490, 2001
24. Bein, K., and Simons, M. Thrombospondin type 1 repeats interact with matrix metalloproteinase 2. Regulation of metalloproteinase activity. J. Biol. Chem., 275:32167–32173, 2000.
25. Taraboletti, G., Morbidelli,. L, Donnini, S., Parenti, A., Granger, H.J., Giavazzi, R., and Ziche, M. The heparin binding 25 kDa fragment of thrombospondin-1 promotes angiogenesis and modulates gelatinase and TIMP-2 production in endothelial cells. FASEB J., 14:1674–1676, 2000.
26. Greene, J., Wang, M., Liu, Y.E., Raymond, L.A., Rosen, C., Shi, Y.E. Molecular cloning and characterization of human tissue inhibitor of metalloproteinase 4. J. Biol. Chem., 271:30375–80, 1996.
27. Gomis-Ruth, F.X., Maskos, K., Betz, M., Bergner, A., Huber, R., Suzuki, K., Yoshida, N., Nagase, H., Brew, K., Bourenkov, G.P., Bartunik, H., Bode, W. Mechanism of inhibition of the human matrix metalloproteinase stromelysin-1 by TIMP-1. Nature, 389:77–81, 1997.
28. Edwards, D. R. in *Matrix Metalloproteinase Inhibitors in Cancer Therapy* (eds Clendeninn, N. J. & Appelt, K.) 67–84 (Humana Press, Totowa, New Jersey, 2001).
29. Wang, Z., Juttermann, R., and Soloway, P. D. TIMP-2 is required for efficient activation of proMMP-2 *in vivo*. J. Biol. Chem., 275, 26411–26415, 2000.

30. Baker, A.H., George, S.J., Zaltsman, A.B., Murphy, G., and Newby, A.G. Inhibition of invasion and induction of apoptotic cell death of cancer cell lines by overexpression of TIMP-3. British J. Cancer. 79:1347–11355, 1999.
31. Li, G., and Fridman, R., and Kim, H.R. Tissue inhibitor of metalloproteinase-1 inhibits apoptosis of human breast epithelial cells. Cancer Res., 59:6267–6275, 1999.
32. Valente, P., Fassina, G., Melchiori, A., Masiello, L., Cilli, M., Vacca, A., Onisto, M., Santi, L., Stetler-Stevenson, W.G. and Albini, A. TIMP-2 over-expression reduces invasion and angiogenesis and protects B16F10 melanoma cells from apotosis. Int. J. Cancer, 75:246–253, 1998.
33. Polette, M., Gilbert, N., Stas, I., Nawrocki, B., Noel, A., Remacle, A., Stetler-Stevenson, W.G., Birembaut, P., and Foidart, M. Gelatinase A expression and localization in human breast cancers. An in situ hybridization study and immunohistochemical detection using confocal microscopy. Virchows Arch., 424:641–645, 1994.
34. Huang, S., van Arsdall, M., Tedjarati, S., McCarty, M., Wu, W., Langley, R., and Fidler, I.J. Contributions of stromal metalloproteinase-9 to angiogenesis and growth of human ovarian carcinoma in mice. J. Natl. Cancer Inst., 94:1134–1142, 2002.
35. Guo, H., Zucker, S., Gordon, M.K., Toole, B.P., and Biswas, C. Stimulation of matrix metalloproteinase production by recombinant extracellular matrix metalloproteinase inducer from transfected Chinese hamster ovary cells. J. Biol. Chem., 272:24–27, 1997.
36. Skobe, M., and Fusenig N.E. Tumorigenic conversion of immortal human keratinocytes through stromal cell activation. Proc. Natl. Acad. Sci. USA, 95:1050–1055, 1998.
37. Demeure, M.J., Damsky, C.H., Elfman, F., Goretzki, P.E., Wong, M.G., and Clark, O.H. Invasion by cultured human follicular thyroid cancer correlates with increased beta 1 integrins and production of proteases. World J. Surg., 16:770–776, 1992.
38. Smit, J.W.A., van der Pluijm, G., Romijn, H.A., Lowik, C.W.G.M, Morreau, H., and Gosling, B.M. Degradation of extracellular matrix by metastatic follicular thyroid carcinoma cell lines: role of te plasmin activation system. Thyroid, 9:913–919, 1999.
39. Andreasen, P.A., Kjoller, L., Christensen, L., and Duffy, M.J. The urokinase-type plasminogen activator system in cancer metastasis: a review. Int. J. Cancer, 72:1–22, 1997.
40. Maeta, H., Ohgi, S., and Terada, T. Protein expression of matrix metalloproteinases 2 and 9 and tissue inhibitors of metalloproteinase 1 and 2 in papillary thyroid carcinomas. Virchows Archiv., 438:121–128, 2001.
41. Nakamura, H., Ueno, H., Yamashita, K., Shimada, T., Yamamoto, E., Noguchi, M., Fujimoto, N., Sato, H., Seiki, M., and Okada, Y. Enhanced production and activation of progelatinase A mediated by membrane-type 1 matrix metalloproteinase in human papillary thyroid carcinomas. Cancer Res., 59:467–473, 1999.
42. Zedenius, J., Stahle-Backdahl, M., Enberg, U., Grimelius, L., Larsson, C., Wallin, G., and Backdahl, M. Stromal fibroblasts adjacent to invasive thyroid tumors: expression of gelatinase A but not stromelysin 3 mRNA. World J. Surg., 20:101–106, 1996.
43. Patel, A., Straight, A.M., Mann, H., Duffy, E., Fenton, C., Dinauer, C., Tuttle, R.M., and Francis, G.L. Matrix metalloproteinase (MMP) expression by differentiated thyroid carcinoma of children and adolescents. J. Endocrinol. Investigation, 25:403–408, 2002.
44. Kameyama, K. Expression of MMP-1 in the capsule of thyroid cancer-relationship with invasiveness. Pathol. Res. Pract., 192:20–26, 1996.
45. Wasenius, V.-M., Hemmer, S., Kettunen, E., Knuutila, S., Franssila, K., and Joensuu, H. Hepatocyte growth factor receptor, matrix metalloproteinase-11, tissue inhibitor of metalloproteinase-1, and fibronectin is up-regulated in papillary thyroid carcinoma: a cDNA and tissue microarray study. Clin. Cancer Res., 9:68–75, 2003.
46. Shi, Y., Parhar, R.S., Zou, M., Hammami, M.M., Akhtar, M., Lum, Z.P., Farid, N.R., Al-Sedairy, S.T., Paterson, M.C. Tissue inhibitor of metalloproteinases-1 (TIMP-1) mRNA is elevated in advanced stages of thyroid carcinoma. British J. Cancer. 79:1234–1239, 1999.
47. Aust, G., Hofmann, A., Laue, S., Rost, A., Kohler, T., and Scherbaum, W.A. Human thyroid carcinoma cell lines and normal thyrocytes: expression and regulation of matrix metalloproteinase-1 and tissue matrix metalloproteinase inhibitor-1 messenger-RNA and protein. Thyroid, 7:713–724, 1997.
48. Hofmann, A., Laue, S., Rost, A.-K., Kohler, T., and Scherbaum, W.A., and Aust, G. mRNA levels of membrane-type 1 matrix metalloproteinase (MT1-MMP), MMP-2, and MMP-9 and of their inhibitors TIMP-2 and TIMP-3 in normal thyrocytes and thyroid carcinoma cell lines. Thyroid, 8:203–214, 1998.

49. Korem, S., Resnick, M.B., and Kraiem, Z. Similar and divergent patterns in the regulation of matrix metalloproteinase-1 (MMP-1) and tissue inhibitor of MMP-1 gene expression in benign and malignant human thyroid cells. J. Clin. Endocrinol. Metab., 84:3322–3327, 1999.
50. Heinrich, R., and Kraiem, Z. The protein kinase A pathway inhibits c-jun and c-fos protooncogene expression induced by the protein kinase C and tyrosine kinase pathways in cultured human thyroid follicles. J. Clin. Endocrinol. Metab., 82:1839–1844, 1997.
51. Damjanovski, S., Puzianowska-kuznicka, M., Ishuzuya-Oka, A., and Shi, Y-B. Differential regulation of three thyroid hormone-responsive matrix metalloproteinase genes implicates distinct functions during frog embryogenesis. FASEB J., 14:503–510, 2000.
52. Gohji, K., Fujimoto, N., Hara, I., Fujii, A., Gotoh, A., Okada, H., Arakawa, S., Kitazawa, S., Miyake, H., Kamidono, S., and Nakajima, M. Serum matrix metalloproteinase-2 and its density in men with prostate cancer as a new predictor of disease extension. Int. J. Cancer. 79:96–101, 1998.
53. Pellegrini, P., Contasta, I., Berghella, A.M., Gargano, E., Mammarella, C., and Adorno, D. Simultaneous measurement of soluble carcinoembryonic antigen and the tissue inhibitor of metalloproteinase TIMP1 serum levels for use as markers of pre-invasive to invasive colorectal cancer. Cancer Immunology & Immunotherapy. 49:388–94, 2000.
54. Laack, E., Kohler, A., Kugler, C., Dierlamm, T., Knuffmann, C., Vohwinkel, G., Niestroy, A., Dahlmann, N., Peters, A., Berger, J., Fiedler, W., and Hossfeld, D.K. Pretreatment serum levels of matrix metalloproteinase-9 and vascular endothelial growth factor in non-small-cell lung cancer. Annals of Oncology. 13:1550–7, 2002.
55. Komorowski, J., Pasieka, Z., Jankiewicz-Wika, J., and Stepien, H. Matrix metalloproteinases, tissue inhibitors of matrix metalloproteinases and angiogenic cytokines in peripheral blood of patients with thyroid cancer. Thyroid, 12:655–662, 2002.
56. Zucker, S., Cao, J., and Chen, W.-T. Critical appraisal of the use of matrix metalloproteinase inhibitors in cancer treatment. Oncogene, 19:6642–6650, 2000.
57. Coussens, L.M., Fingleton, B., and Matrisian, L.M. Matrix metalloproteinase inhibitors and cancer: trials and tribulations. Science, 295:2387–2392, 2002.
58. Brand, K. Cancer gene therapy with tissue inhibitors of metalloproteinases (TIMPs). Current Gene Therapy. 2:255–71, 2002.
59. Baker, A.H. Ahonen, M., and Kahari, V.M. Potential applications of tissue inhibitor of metalloproteinase (TIMP) overexpression for cancer gene therapy. Advances in Experimental Medicine & Biology. 465:469–83, 2000.
60. Shi, Y., Parhar, R.S., Zou, M., Al-Mohanna, F.A., and Paterson, M.C. Gene therapy of melanoma pulmonary metastasis by intramuscular injection of plasmid DNA encoding tissue inhibitor of metalloproteinases-1. Cancer Gene Therapy, 9:126–32, 2002.
61. Rigg, A.S. and Lemoine, N.R. Adenoviral delivery of TIMP1 or TIMP2 can modify the invasive behavior of pancreatic cancer and can have a significant antitumor effect in vivo. Cancer Gene Therapy. 8:869–78, 2001.
62. Ahonen, M., Ala-Aho, R., Baker, A.H., George, S.J., Grenman, R., Saarialho-Kere, U., and Kahari, V.M. Antitumor activity and bystander effect of adenovirally delivered tissue inhibitor of metalloproteinases-3. Molecular Therapy: the Journal of the American Society of Gene Therapy, 5:705–15, 2002.
63. Li, H., Lindenmeyer, F., Grenet, C., Opolon, P., Menashi, S., Soria, C., Yeh, P., Perricaudet, M., and Lu, H. AdTIMP-2 inhibits tumor growth, angiogenesis, and metastasis, and prolongs survival in mice. Human Gene Therapy, 12:515–526, 2001.
64. Jiang, Y., Wang, M., Celiker, M.Y., Liu, Y.E., Sang, Q.X., Goldberg, I.D., and Shi, Y.E. Stimulation of mammary tumorigenesis by systemic tissue inhibitor of matrix metalloproteinase 4 gene delivery. Cancer Res., 61:2365–2370, 2001.

11. THE MOLECULAR PATHWAYS INDUCED BY RADIATION AND LEADING TO THYROID CARCINOGENESIS

YURI E. NIKIFOROV, M.D., Ph.D.
Department of Pathology, University of Cincinnati, USA

INTRODUCTION

The association between ionizing radiation and thyroid cancer is well established. It was first proposed in 1950 in children who received X-ray therapy in infancy for an enlarged thymus (1). During the following decades, numerous reports have documented an increased incidence of thyroid neoplasms in children after external radiation for different benign conditions of the head, neck and thorax (2). Since the early 1960s, when the use of radiotherapy for benign conditions was abandoned, the incidence of radiation-associated thyroid malignancy in children gradually decreased (3). Currently, radiation therapy for malignancy continues to be a source of radiation-associated thyroid cancer (4). An increased risk of thyroid cancer has also been linked to environmental irradiation. This was documented in survivors of atomic bomb explosions in Japan in 1945(5), and in residents of the Marshall Islands exposed to fallout after detonation of a thermonuclear device on the Bikini atoll in 1954 (6). In the U.S., exposure to radioiodines from atmospheric nuclear tests in Nevada in the 1950s has been suggested to lead to an excess of thyroid neoplasms (7, 8). In April 1986, an accident at the Chernobyl Nuclear Power Station in the former USSR produced the most serious environmental disasters ever recorded and led to a dramatic increase in the frequency of childhood thyroid cancer in contaminated areas of Belarus, Ukraine, and western Russia (9, 10). This tragic disaster has created one of the most striking paradigms of radiation-induced thyroid tumors and allowed significant progress in the understanding of the molecular pathways induced by radiation. In this chapter, I review the genetic events and molecular mechanisms underlying radiation carcinogenesis in the thyroid gland.

RET/PTC REARRANGEMENTS

Over the last decade, rearrangements of the RET proto-oncogene have been identified as the most common genetic event in thyroid tumors associated with radiation exposure.

The RET proto-oncogene is located on chromosome 10q11.2 and encodes a cell membrane receptor tyrosine kinase (11, 12). The receptor consists of three functional domains: an extracellular domain containing a ligand-binding site, a transmembrane domain, and an intracellular domain that includes a region with protein tyrosine kinase activity. The ligands for RET receptor are neurotrophic factors of the glial cell-line derived neurotrophic factor (GDNF) family, including GDNF, neurtulin, artemin, and persephin (13). Binding of a ligand causes the receptors to dimerize, leading to autophosphorylation of the protein on tyrosine residues and initiation of intracellular signaling cascade. Wild-type RET is expressed in neuronal and neural-crest derived tissues including thyroid parafollicular C-cells, but not in thyroid follicular cells. In thyroid follicular cells, RET can be activated by fusion to different constitutively expressed genes. The product of this rearrangement is a chimeric oncogene named RET/PTC (PTC for papillary thyroid carcinoma).

Structure of RET/PTC oncogenes

Since the original report on RET activation by rearrangement in papillary thyroid carcinomas (14), three major types of the rearrangement have been identified: RET/PTC1, RET/PTC2, and RET/PTC3 (Figure 1). All of them are formed by

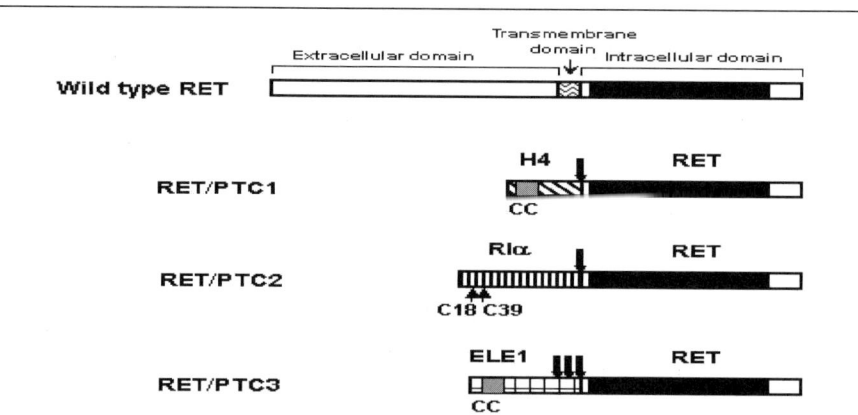

Figure 1. Schematic representation of the wild type RET gene and three major types of RET/PTC rearrangement. The 3' portion of RET participating in the fusion encodes the tyrosine kinase domain (black box) but lacks the transmembrane and extracellular domains. The genes fused with RET encode dimerization domains, either coiled-coil domain (CC) or cysteine residues forming disulfide bonds during dimerization (C18, C39), allowing ligand-independent dimerization and activation of the truncated RET receptor. Block arrows indicate breakpoints.

fusion of the tyrosine kinase domain of RET to the 5' portion of different genes. In RET/PTC1, RET is fused to the H4 (also known as D10S170) gene (14) and in RET/PTC3 to the ELE1 (RFG or ARA70) gene (15, 16). RET/PTC1 and RET/PTC3 are paracentric inversions since both genes participating in the rearrangement are located on chromosome 10q (17, 18). In contrast, RET/PTC2 is formed by reciprocal translocation between chromosomes 10 and 17, resulting in RET fusion to the 5' terminal sequence of the regulatory subunit RIα of the cyclic AMP-dependent protein kinase A (Figure 1).

Recently, several novel types of RET/PTC have been described, most of them in papillary carcinomas from patients with the history of radiation exposure. Five novel types (RET/PTC5, RET/PTC6, RET/PTC7, RET/KTN1, RET/RFG8) were found in post-Chernobyl tumors (20–23), and two other in tumors from patients subjected to therapeutic external radiation (RET/PCM-1, RET/ ΔRFP) (24, 25). All novel types of RET/PTC are translocations and resulted from the fusion of the intracellular domain of RET to heterologous genes located on different chromosomes (Figure 2).

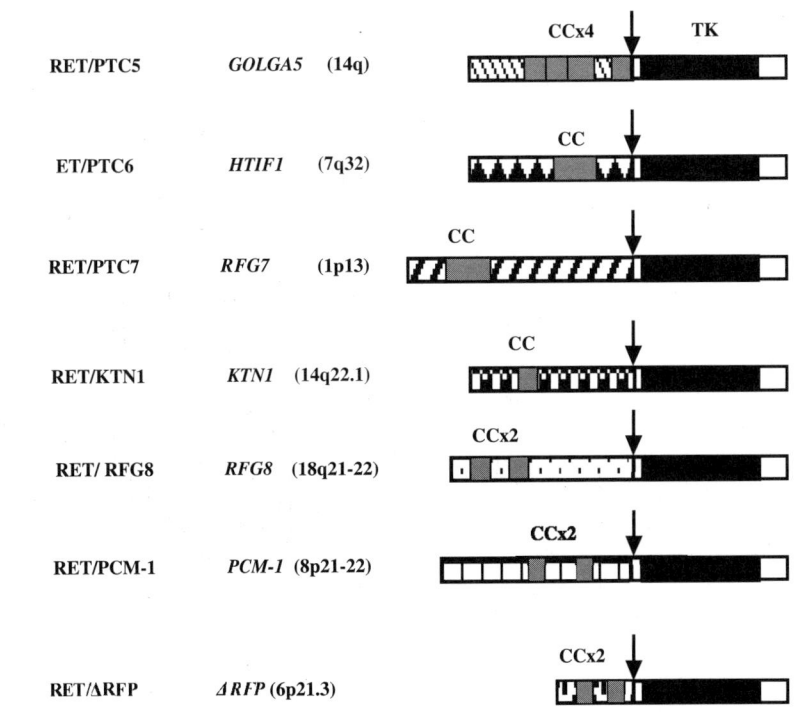

Figure 2. Schematic representation of the novel RET/PTC types found in papillary carcinomas associated with radiation exposure. Each fusion involves the tyrosine kinase (TK) domain of RET and the 5' portion of different genes that encode one or more putative coiled-coil domains (CC) essential for dimerization and RET TK activation. Chromosomal location of the RET fusion partners is shown in brackets. Arrows indicate breakpoints.

The genes fused with RET are constitutively expressed in thyroid follicular cells and drive the expression of the chimeric RET/PTC oncogene. In addition, these partners provide a dimerization domain essential for ligand-independent activation of the RET tyrosine kinase (26, 27). It allows ligand-independent dimerization of the chimeric protein and autophosphorylation of the truncated RET receptor. Indeed, it has been demonstrated that tyrosines 1015 and 1062, which are autophosphorylated in the wild-type RET only upon ligand binding, are constitutively phosphorylated in the RET/PTC chimeric protein (28). The ligand-independent activation of the RET tyrosine kinase is considered essential for the transformation of thyroid cells (29).

Another important role of the genes fused with RET is in determining a subcellular localization of the chimeric protein which lacks the transmembrane domain and cannot be anchored to the cell membrane. In RET/PTC3 protein, for instance, the N-terminal coiled-coil domain of ELE1 (RFG) not only mediates oligomerization of the receptor and chronic kinase activation, but is also responsible for the compartmentalization of the chimeric protein at plasma membrane level, where most of the normal ELE1 (RFG) protein is distributed (30). Thus, different types of RET/PTC chimeric proteins, which have a similar RET tyrosine kinase portion but different N-terminal domains, may be distributed in varies cytoplasmic compartments, allowing them to interact with distinct sets of signaling proteins. This may provide an explanation for some variations in biological properties recently found between different RET/PTC types (reviewed in (31).

RET/PTC prevalence in sporadic and radiation-associated tumors

The prevalence of RET/PTC in papillary carcinomas varies significantly in different studies and geographic regions. In the U.S., the five largest series of adult papillary carcinomas showed the frequency ranging from 11% to 43% (32–36), with the cumulative incidence of 35%. A comparable rate of 30–40% have been found in series from Canada (37)) and Italy (34, 38, 39). In other regions, a wide variation in frequency of RET/PTC has been reported, ranging from 3% in Saudi Arabia (40) to 85% in Australia (41). A higher overall prevalence of RET/PTC has been noted in papillary carcinomas from children and young adults (38, 42–44). Among sporadic tumors of all age groups, RET/PTC1 is the most common type, comprising up to 60–70% of all rearrangements, whereas RET/PTC3 accounts for 20–30% of positive cases and RET/PTC2 for less than 10% (32, 36, 39).

An unusually high incidence of RET/PTC rearrangements has been documented in papillary carcinomas from patients with the history of radiation exposure, including those subjected to either accidental or therapeutic irradiation (Table 1).

In children affected by the Chernobyl nuclear accident, 67–87% of papillary carcinomas removed 5–8 years after exposure and 49–65% of tumors removed 7–11 years after the accident harbored RET/PTC (42, 45–48). Remarkably, in tumors developed less than 10 years after the accident, RET/PTC3 was the most common type, whereas those developed after the longer latency had predominantly RET/PTC1 (Table 2). In patients subjected to therapeutic X-ray irradiation for benign or malignant conditions, the prevalence of RET/PTC was also significantly higher than in the general

Table 1. Prevalence of RET/PTC rearrangements in radiation-induced thyroid cancer

	Total RET/PTC	RET/PTC1	RET/PTC2	RET/PTC3
Environmental Radiation (post Chernobyl)				
Klugbauer et al. (46)	8/12 (67%)	17%	0	50%
Fugazzola et al. (45)	4/6 (67%)	0	17%	50%
Nikiforov et al. (42)	33/39 (87%)	16%	3%	58%
Smida et al. (47)	32/51 (63%)	24%	0	26%
Rabes et al. (48)	94/191 (49%)	25%	0	20%
Therapeutic Radiation				
Bounacer et al. (49)	16/19 (84%)	74%	0	21%

Table 2. RET/PTC prevalence after chernobyl: correlation with the latency period*

Latency period	Total rearrangement positive	RET/PTC1	RET/PTC3	Novel RET/PTC types
≤10years	40/61 (66%)	23%	60%	13%
>10 years	60/130 (46%)	65%	23%	5%

* Modified from Rabes et al. (2000) (48) with permission.

population, being reported at 52–87% (49–51). Exposure to ionizing radiation not only results in a higher prevalence in RET/PTC, but also promotes the fusion of RET to the unusual rearrangement partners, since seven out of eight novel RET/PTC types have been detected in tumors associated with radiation exposure. The novel types comprised up to 13% of all rearrangements found in post-Chernobyl tumors (48) (Table 2).

The fact that post-Chernobyl tumors arising shortly after exposure had mostly RET/PTC3 and those after a longer latent period harbored predominantly RET/PTC1 suggests at least two possibilities. First, radiation may be more effective in inducing RET/PTC3, whereas other factors (still unknown), responsible for the majority of thyroid cancers that are not associated with radiation exposure, lead mostly to RET/PTC1. Second, it is conceivable that radiation is equally efficient in generation of both types, but tumors initiated by RET/PTC3 have a higher growth rate and manifest several years earlier. The latter possibility is supported by the animal experiments demonstrating that RET/PTC3 transgenic mice develop more malignant phenotype and metastatic disease as compared to RET/PTC1 animals (52, 53), and by recent *in-vitro* functional studies showing that RET/PTC3 is a more potent activator of MAPK signaling pathway and more efficient in promoting proliferation of cultured thyroid cells than RET/PTC1 (54).

The occurrence of RET/PTC has been observed after high-dose irradiation of human undifferentiated thyroid carcinoma cells (55) and of fetal human thyroid tissues transplanted into SCID mice (56, 57). In both studies, the rearrangements were detected by RT-PCR as soon as 2 days after exposure. In addition, fetal thyroid cells revealed both RET/PTC1 and RET/PTC3 7 days after irradiation, while only RET/PTC1 persisted and was detectable 2 months later (57). The effective dose of radiation in both studies was high (50 Gy) and lethal for dividing cells, and the cells irradiated in the study by Ito and colleagues (55) were already highly transformed and hence more susceptible to develop secondary genetic defects. Nevertheless, these observations suggest that radiation exposure may lead to the generation of RET/PTC rearrangements in thyroid cells.

Potential mechanisms of RET/PTC generation after radiation exposure

The high prevalence of RET/PTC in post-Chernobyl children and in populations affected by other types of environmental and therapeutic exposures as well as the *in-vitro* studies provide strong evidence for the association between ionizing radiation and RET/PTC rearrangement. The role of radiation appears particularly important for the RET/PTC3 type, since its high prevalence was uniquely associated with papillary carcinomas developed shortly after the Chernobyl accident. The mechanisms of RET/PTC generation in thyroid cells after radiation have been a subject of extensive study over the last years.

Analysis of the breakpoint sites revealed no long-sequence homology between the DNA regions involved in RET/PTC1 fusion in sporadic tumors (58) and in RET/PTC3 in post-Chernobyl carcinomas (59, 60), establishing that these rearrangements result from illegitimate rather than homologous recombination. When the breakpoint sites within the RET and ELE1 genes were mapped and analyzed in 12 post-Chernobyl tumors with RET/PTC3, it appeared that in each tumor the relative position of a breakpoint in the RET gene corresponded to the location of a breakpoint in the ELE1 gene (60). Specifically, after aligning the genes in opposite orientations, the breakpoints were located just across from each other in 5 (42%) tumors (Figure 3, A), while in other tumors they could be aligned by sliding one gene with respect to another (Figure 3, B, C). Similar pattern could be deducted from another study where the breakpoints in 22 post-Chernobyl tumors with RET/PTC3 were characterized (61). Such predilection for the breakpoint site in one gene to correspond to the breakpoint site located within the certain region of the other gene suggests the presence of a stable spatial relationship between these two chromosomal loci within the nucleus (Figure 3).

If the interaction between these loci exists, it should involve folding of chromosome 10 where both RET and ELE1 genes reside separated by a linear distance of ~18 Mb. This is conceivable since one of the levels of DNA packaging involves chromatin arrangement into loops of different size attached to a chromosomal backbone (62). Therefore, although two chromosomal loci are located at a considerable linear distance from each other, they may be closely spaced in the interphase nucleus because of their location at specific areas of chromosomal loop(s).

Indeed, it has been recently demonstrated that chromosomal regions containing the RET and H4 genes are non-randomly positioned with respect to each other in the interphase nuclei of normal thyroid follicular cells (63). Utilizing fluorescence in situ hybridization, two-dimensional distances between RET and H4 were measured in

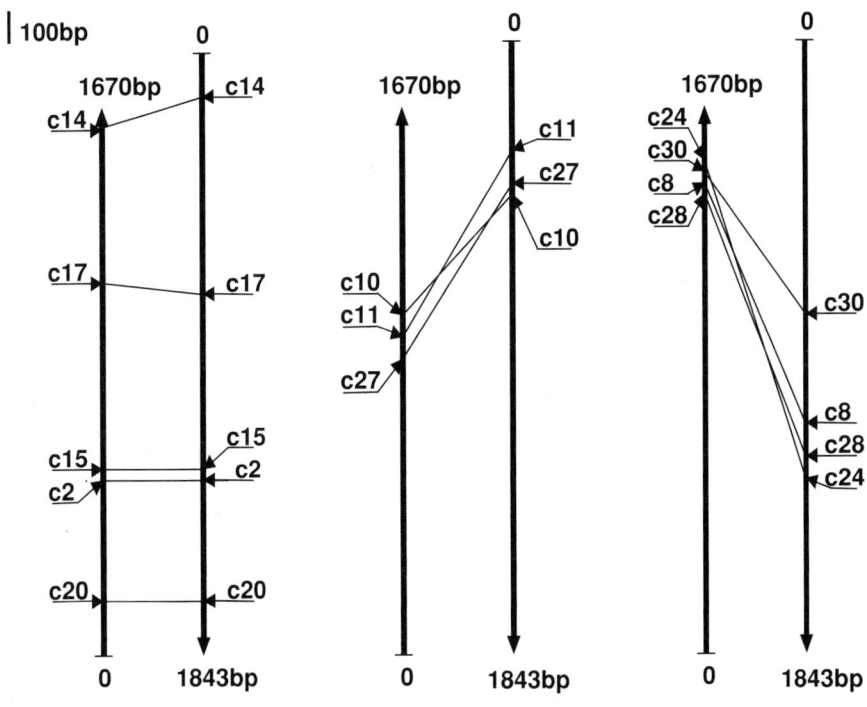

Figure 3. Alignment of the breakpoint sites involved in *RET*/PTC3 in post-Chernobyl tumors demonstrating three patterns of correspondence between the position of breakpoints in each tumor (A, B, C). Modified from Nikiforov et al. (1999) (60) with permission.

the interphase cells and compared with a theoretical Rayleigh model that describes a distribution of distances between two points of linear polymers that fold in a random manner. Previous studies have shown that interphase distances between random loci on the same chromosome conform to the Rayleigh distribution (62, 64). Indeed, in the control experiment, distances between the RET and D10S539 loci, the latter located on chromosome 10q between RET and H4 and is not known to participate in the rearrangement, were found to follow the Rayleigh distribution (Figure 4) (63). As for the RET and H4 distances, they showed a strong deviation from the Rayleigh model, primarily due to the loci either juxtaposed or closer than expected, indicating a non-random manner of RET and H4 interaction. In addition, as many as 35% of primary cultured thyroid cells had at least one pair of RET and H4 genes juxtaposed. These data suggest that generation of RET/PTC rearrangements in thyroid cells may be in part due to the structural organization of chromosome 10, resulting in non-random interaction and spatial approximation of these potentially recombinogenic DNA loci (Figure 4).

It remains unclear, however, whether RET/PTC is a direct consequence of DNA breaks induced by ionizing radiation, or it forms indirectly, after DNA damage has

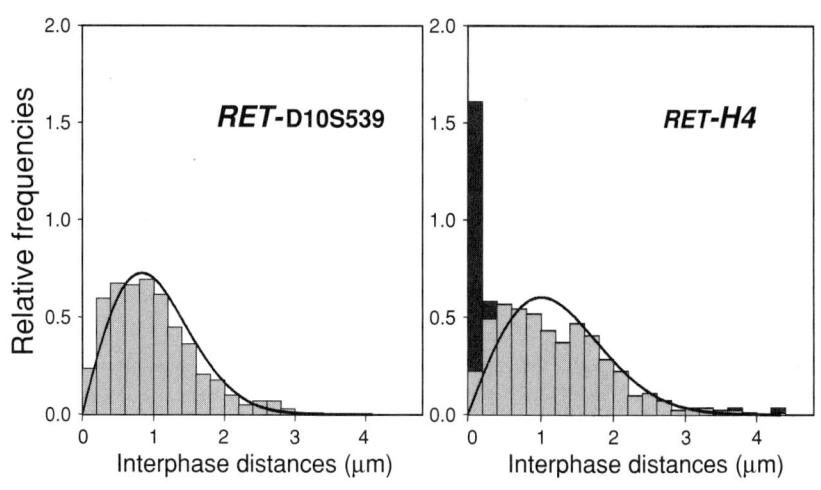

Figure 4. Distribution of interphase distances between RET and D10S539 (A) and RET and H4 (B) in cultured normal thyroid cells as compared with the theoretical Rayleigh distribution (solid line). Dark bars indicate the RET – H4 distances that were in excess over the number expected based on the Rayleigh distribution. From Nikiforova et al. (2000) (63).

been repaired. Important information in this respect can be obtained by mapping and characterization the breakpoint sites involved in the fusion. Thus, if the rearrangement occurred indirectly (as a result of activation or disruption of the recombination machinery), the breakpoints are expected be located within recombinase signal sequences at both participating loci, have similarity in nucleotide composition, or cluster at certain specific hypersensitive DNA regions. However, as it had been convincingly demonstrated in post-Chernobyl tumors with RET/PTC3, the breakpoints within and surrounding ELE1 intron 5 and RET intron 11 were distributed randomly, with no breakpoints occurring at exactly the same base or within an identical sequence in any of 41 tumors reported in three different series (59–61). The breakpoints exhibited no particular nucleotide sequence or composition. In one study, no evidence of AT-rich regions, fragile sites, recombination-specific signal elements, or other target DNA sites (i.e. chi-like motifs, heptamer/nonamer signal sequences) implicated in illegitimate recombination in mammalian cells was found (60). These results favor the direct induction of RET/PTC as a result of random double-strand DNA breaks, rather than disruption of the recombination machinery. However, another study proposed an alternative mechanisms and found at least one topoisomerase I site exactly at or in close proximity to all breakpoints, suggesting the role of DNA breaks induced by this enzyme in the generation of RET/PTC3 (61).

PAX8-PPARfl REARRANGEMENT

Recently, a PAX8-PPARγ fusion has been identified in follicular thyroid carcinomas with cytogenetically detectable translocation t(2;3)(q13;p25) (65). This rearrangement leads to an in-frame fusion of the PAX8 gene, which encodes a paired domain transcription factor, with the peroxisome proliferator-activated receptor (PPAR) γ gene. The structure and biological properties of the fusion gene are discussed in Chapter 4. In the original report, PAX8-PPARγ was detected in 5 out of 8 (63%) follicular carcinomas (65), whereas in the larger follow-up series, the prevalence was 26–35% (66, 67). However, when this alteration was studied separately in follicular carcinomas from patients without a history of radiation and in those exposed to radiation, PAX8-PPARγ fusion was found in 5 out of 12 (42%) sporadic tumors and in all three (100%) tumors associated with radiation (68). Despite the small number of follicular carcinomas in the latter group, this finding points towards the possible association between radiation exposure and PAX8-PPARγ rearrangement. Although papillary carcinoma is by far the most common type of thyroid tumors associated with radiation, an increased risk of follicular carcinoma development has also been documented in these populations (69). Therefore, it is likely that radiation exposure may promote the development of follicular tumors through the generation of PAX8-PPARγ rearrangement in a similar way it involves in the initiation of papillary thyroid carcinogenesis via RET/PTC rearrangement.

RAS MUTATIONS

Point mutations of the three RAS genes, N-RAS, H-RAS, and K-RAS, have been found with various prevalence in thyroid follicular and papillary tumors. The initial reports have suggested that K-RAS mutations in follicular carcinomas may be associated with radiation exposure, since they constituted 3 out of 4 (75%) RAS mutations in patients subjected to radiation, in contrast to 6 out of 25 (25%) RAS mutations in sporadic tumors (70). However, the subsequent studies have not confirmed such an association (Table 3). Indeed, RAS mutations were found in 30% of thyroid tumors from patients with a history of external irradiation and in 42% of sporadic tumors, and similar prevalence of the K-RAS gene mutations was observed in the two groups (71). In a series of post-Chernobyl tumors, no RAS mutations was detected in 33 papillary carcinomas; whereas 3 follicular adenomas and 1 follicular carcinoma harbored N-RAS codon 61 mutation (72). Similar findings were observed in another series of 31 post-Chernobyl papillary carcinomas (73). Two RAS mutations detected in 44

Table 3. Prevalence of RAS mutations in radiation-induced thyroid tumors

Therapeutic Radiation	
Wright et al. (70)	4/12 (33%) after radiation, 3/4 K-RAS (75%) in follicular carcinomas
	25/68 (37%) in non-radiation group, 6/25 (25%) K-RAS
Challeton et al. (71)	10/33 (30%) after radiation
	36/86 (42%) sporadic, similar prevalence of K-RAS mutations
Environmental Radiation (Post-Chernobyl)	
Nikiforov et al. (72)	0/33 in papillary carcinomas
	3/7 in follicular adenomas
	1/1 in follicular carcinoma
Suchy et al. (74)	2/44 in papillary carcinomas (none in codons 12, 13, or 61)
Santoro et al. (73)	0/23 in papillary carcinomas

Table 4. Prevalence of p53 mutations in radiation-induced papillary thyroid cancer

Therapeutic radiation	
Fogelfeld et al. (75)	4/22 (18%) after radiation
	0/18 in control group
Environmental Radiation (post-Chernobyl)	
Hillebrandt et al. (76)	6/26 (23%)
Nikiforov et al. (72)	2/33 (6%)
Smida et al. (77)	5/31 (16%)
Santoro et al. (73)	0/35
Total post-Chernobyl	13/125 (10%)

post-Chernobyl papillary carcinomas in another study were not in critical codons 12, 13, or 61 of the gene (74). These data indicate that activating mutations of the RAS genes do not play a significant role in radiation-induced papillary carcinomas. Similar conclusion can be made for thyroid follicular tumors, the prevalence of RAS mutation in which shows no correlation with the history of radiation.

P53 MUTATIONS

Missense point mutations in exons 5–8 of the p53 tumor suppressor gene have been detected in 4 out of 22 (18%) papillary carcinomas developed in the patients with a history of childhood irradiation to the head and neck area (75). Several studies have reported the prevalence of p53 mutations in post-Chernobyl tumors. In one series, PCR-SSCP analysis revealed two (6%) somatic mutations, both in exon 5, in a series of 33 papillary carcinomas (72). One of those mutations was a missense mutation and another was a silent mutation, as detected by nucleotide sequencing. Other studies reported a 0–23% prevalence of mutations in the critical exons of the p53 gene in pediatric post-Chernobyl papillary carcinomas (Table 4) (73, 76, 77). Despite some variation in the results between these observations, the overall prevalence of p53 mutations in this post-Chernobyl population appears approximately 10%. This indicates that inactivation of the p53 tumor suppressor gene has only a limited role in radiation-induced thyroid carcinogenesis.

OTHER GENETIC EVENTS

A number of other genetic events have been explored as the possible mediators of radiation-induced carcinogenesis in the thyroid gland. Mutations of the GSP and TSH receptor genes were found to play either no role or rarely present in tumors associated with external radiation (71) and in post-Chernobyl tumors (73, 78). It has been recently suggested that mutations in mitochondrial DNA, particularly large-scale deletions, were significantly more frequent in radiation-induced post-Chernobyl tumors in comparison to sporadic neoplasms, and the frequency of these alterations correlated with the levels of radioiodine contamination in the areas of patients' residency (79). Recently, point mutation at nucleotide 1796 of the BRAF gene has been identified as the most common genetic alteration in papillary carcinomas from the general population (80). However, our preliminary data suggest that this mutation is rare in post-Chernobyl papillary carcinomas (Nikiforova et al., manuscript in preparation).

Several types of genomic instability have also been studied in radiation-associated thyroid tumors. These studies were important in the light of the reports of a higher rate of germline mutations at minisatellite loci in children born from parents exposed to radiation after Chernobyl (81, 82). However, post-Chernobyl thyroid carcinomas revealed either no significant minisatellite or microsatellite instability (83), or low rate of microsatellite mutations (84).

CONCLUDING REMARKS

A large volume of information on the genetic alterations in thyroid tumors, generated over the last decade, points towards a significant difference in the molecular pathways involved in the sporadic and radiation-induced carcinogenesis in the thyroid gland. Thus, it appears that the molecular landscape of sporadic papillary and follicular carcinomas is dominated by point mutations, such as those of the BRAF and RAS genes, whereas large-scale chromosomal abnormalities, such as RET/PTC and PAX8-PPARγ rearrangements, are the most common abnormality in radiation-induced tumors. Since ionizing radiation is known to produce single strand and double strand DNA brakes, it is likely that radiation-induced DNA damage plays a direct role in promoting carcinogenesis through the generation of these chromosomal abnormalities.

Significant progress has been achieved in the understanding of why, despite a random distribution of radiation-induced DNA damage, some common cancer-associated chromosomal rearrangements are very specific. It is likely that spatial proximity of potentially recombinogenic chromosomal loci in the nuclei of normal human cells predisposes to these recurrent genetic alterations. It remains unclear, however, whether rearrangements occur directly by mis-rejoining of radiation-induced DNA breaks or they are stimulated by radiation exposure in an indirect way. Some data exist in support of both mechanisms, and further studies are required to explore this important question in more detail. This is crucial for better understanding of the mechanisms of radiation-induced carcinogenesis in humans, and thyroid cancer represents a unique model to address it.

REFERENCES

1. Duffy, B. J., Jr. and Fitzgerald, P. J. Cancer of the thyroid in children: a report of 28 cases. *J Clin Endocrinol Metab*, 31: 1296–1308, 1950.
2. Winship, T. and Rosvoll, R. V. Cancer of the thyroid in children. *Proc Natl Cancer Conf*, 6: 677–681, 1970.
3. Mehta, M. P., Goetowski, P. G., and Kinsella, T. J. Radiation induced thyroid neoplasms 1920 to 1987: a vanishing problem? *Int J Radiat Oncol Biol Phys*, 16: 1471–1475, 1989.
4. Acharya, S., Sarafoglou, K., LaQuaglia, M., Lindsley, S., Gerald, W., Wollner, N., Tan, C., and Sklar, C. Thyroid neoplasms after therapeutic radiation for malignancies during childhood or adolescence. *Cancer*, 97: 2397–2403, 2003.

5. Thompson, D. E., Mabuchi, K., Ron, E., Soda, M., Tokunaga, M., Ochikubo, S., Sugimoto, S., Ikeda, T., Terasaki, M., Izumi, S., and et al. Cancer incidence in atomic bomb survivors. Part II: Solid tumors, 1958–1987. *Radiat Res*, 137: S17–67, 1994.
6. Cronkite, E. P., Bond, V. P., and Conard, R. A. Medical effects of exposure of human beings to fallout radiation from a thermonuclear explosion. *Stem Cells*, 13 Suppl 1: 49–57, 1995.
7. Kerber, R. A., Till, J. E., Simon, S. L., Lyon, J. L., Thomas, D. C., Preston-Martin, S., Rallison, M. L., Lloyd, R. D., and Stevens, W. A cohort study of thyroid disease in relation to fallout from nuclear weapons testing. *Jama*, 270: 2076–2082, 1993.
8. Gilbert, E. S., Tarone, R., Bouville, A., and Ron, E. Thyroid cancer rates and 131I doses from Nevada atmospheric nuclear bomb tests. *J Natl Cancer Inst*, 90: 1654–1660, 1998.
9. Kazakov, V. S., Demidchik, E. P., and Astakhova, L. N. Thyroid cancer after Chernobyl. *Nature*, 359: 21, 1992.
10. Stsjazhko, V. A., Tsyb, A. F., Tronko, N. D., Souchkevitch, G., and Baverstock, K. F. Childhood thyroid cancer since accident at Chernobyl. *Bmj*, 310: 801, 1995.
11. Takahashi, M., Ritz, J., and Cooper, G. M. Activation of a novel human transforming gene, ret, by DNA rearrangement. *Cell*, 42: 581–588, 1985.
12. Takahashi, M. Structure and expression of the ret transforming gene. *IARC Sci Publ* 189–197, 1988.
13. Airaksinen, M. S., Titievsky, A., and Saarma, M. GDNF family neurotrophic factor signaling: four masters, one servant? *Mol Cell Neurosci*, 13: 313–325, 1999.
14. Grieco, M., Santoro, M., Berlingieri, M. T., Melillo, R. M., Donghi, R., Bongarzone, I., Pierotti, M. A., Della Porta, G., Fusco, A., and Vecchio, G. PTC is a novel rearranged form of the ret proto-oncogene and is frequently detected in vivo in human thyroid papillary carcinomas. *Cell*, 60: 557–563, 1990.
15. Santoro, M., Dathan, N. A., Berlingieri, M. T., Bongarzone, I., Paulin, C., Grieco, M., Pierotti, M. A., Vecchio, G., and Fusco, A. Molecular characterization of RET/PTC3; a novel rearranged version of the RETproto-oncogene in a human thyroid papillary carcinoma. *Oncogene*, 9: 509–516, 1994.
16. Bongarzone, I., Butti, M. G., Coronelli, S., Borrello, M. G., Santoro, M., Mondellini, P., Pilotti, S., Fusco, A., Della Porta, G., and Pierotti, M. A. Frequent activation of ret protooncogene by fusion with a new activating gene in papillary thyroid carcinomas. *Cancer Res*, 54: 2979–2985, 1994.
17. Pierotti, M. A., Santoro, M., Jenkins, R. B., Sozzi, G., Bongarzone, I., Grieco, M., Monzini, N., Miozzo, M., Herrmann, M. A., Fusco, A., and et al. Characterization of an inversion on the long arm of chromosome 10 juxtaposing D10S170 and RET and creating the oncogenic sequence RET/PTC. *Proc Natl Acad Sci U S A*, 89: 1616–1620, 1992.
18. Minoletti, F., Butti, M. G., Coronelli, S., Miozzo, M., Sozzi, G., Pilotti, S., Tunnacliffe, A., Pierotti, M. A., and Bongarzone, I. The two genes generating RET/PTC3 are localized in chromosomal band 10q11.2. *Genes Chromosomes Cancer*, 11: 51–57, 1994.
19. Bongarzone, I., Monzini, N., Borrello, M. G., Carcano, C., Ferraresi, G., Arighi, E., Mondellini, P., Della Porta, G., and Pierotti, M. A. Molecular characterization of a thyroid tumor-specific transforming sequence formed by the fusion of ret tyrosine kinase and the regulatory subunit RI alpha of cyclic AMP-dependent protein kinase A. *Mol Cell Biol*, 13: 358–366, 1993.
20. Klugbauer, S., Demidchik, E. P., Lengfelder, E., and Rabes, H. M. Detection of a novel type of RET rearrangement (PTC5) in thyroid carcinomas after Chernobyl and analysis of the involved RET-fused gene RFG5. *Cancer Res*, 58: 198–203, 1998.
21. Klugbauer, S. and Rabes, H. M. The transcription coactivator HTIF1 and a related protein are fused to the RET receptor tyrosine kinase in childhood papillary thyroid carcinomas. *Oncogene*, 18: 4388–4393, 1999.
22. Klugbauer, S., Jauch, A., Lengfelder, E., Demidchik, E., and Rabes, H. M. A novel type of RET rearrangement (PTC8) in childhood papillary thyroid carcinomas and characterization of the involved gene (RFG8). *Cancer Res*, 60: 7028–7032, 2000.
23. Salassidis, K., Bruch, J., Zitzelsberger, H., Lengfelder, E., Kellerer, A. M., and Bauchinger, M. Translocation t(10;14)(q11.2:q22.1) fusing the kinetin to the RET gene creates a novel rearranged form (PTC8) of the RET proto-oncogene in radiation-induced childhood papillary thyroid carcinoma. *Cancer Res*, 60: 2786–2789, 2000.
24. Corvi, R., Berger, N., Balczon, R., and Romeo, G. RET/PCM-1: a novel fusion gene in papillary thyroid carcinoma. *Oncogene*, 19: 4236–4242, 2000.
25. Saenko, V., Rogounovitch, T., Shimizu-Yoshida, Y., Abrosimov, A., Lushnikov, E., Roumiantsev, P., Matsumoto, N., Nakashima, M., Meirmanov, S., Ohtsuru, A., Namba, H., Tsyb, A., and Yamashita,

S. Novel tumorigenic rearrangement, Delta rfp/ret, in a papillary thyroid carcinoma from externally irradiated patient. *Mutat Res*, 527: 81–90, 2003.
26. Tong, Q., Xing, S., and Jhiang, S. M. Leucine zipper-mediated dimerization is essential for the PTC1 oncogenic activity. *J Biol Chem*, 272: 9043–9047, 1997.
27. Jhiang, S. M. The RET proto-oncogene in human cancers. *Oncogene*, 19: 5590–5597, 2000.
28. Salvatore, D., Barone, M. V., Salvatore, G., Melillo, R. M., Chiappetta, G., Mineo, A., Fenzi, G., Vecchio, G., Fusco, A., and Santoro, M. Tyrosines 1015 and 1062 are in vivo autophosphorylation sites in ret and ret-derived oncoproteins. *J Clin Endocrinol Metab*, 85: 3898–3907, 2000.
29. Pierotti, M. A., Bongarzone, I., Borello, M. G., Greco, A., Pilotti, S., and Sozzi, G. Cytogenetics and molecular genetics of carcinomas arising from thyroid epithelial follicular cells. *Genes Chromosomes Cancer*, 16: 1–14, 1996.
30. Monaco, C., Visconti, R., Barone, M. V., Pierantoni, G. M., Berlingieri, M. T., De Lorenzo, C., Mineo, A., Vecchio, G., Fusco, A., and Santoro, M. The RFG oligomerization domain mediates kinase activation and re-localization of the RET/PTC3 oncoprotein to the plasma membrane. *Oncogene*, 20: 599–608, 2001.
31. Nikiforov, Y. E. RET/PTC Rearrangement in Thyroid Tumors. *Endocr Pathol*, 13: 3–16, 2002.
32. Tallini, G., Santoro, M., Helie, M., Carlomagno, F., Salvatore, G., Chiappetta, G., Carcangiu, M. L., and Fusco, A. RET/PTC oncogene activation defines a subset of papillary thyroid carcinomas lacking evidence of progression to poorly differentiated or undifferentiated tumor phenotypes. *Clin Cancer Res*, 4: 287–294, 1998.
33. Jhiang, S. M., Caruso, D. R., Gilmore, E., Ishizaka, Y., Tahira, T., Nagao, M., Chiu, I. M., and Mazzaferri, E. L. Detection of the PTC/retTPC oncogene in human thyroid cancers. *Oncogene*, 7: 1331–1337, 1992.
34. Santoro, M., Carlomagno, F., Hay, I. D., Herrmann, M. A., Grieco, M., Melillo, R., Pierotti, M. A., Bongarzone, I., Della Porta, G., Berger, N., and et al. Ret oncogene activation in human thyroid neoplasms is restricted to the papillary cancer subtype. *J Clin Invest*, 89: 1517–1522, 1992.
35. Lam, A. K., Montone, K. T., Nolan, K. A., and Livolsi, V. A. Ret oncogene activation in papillary thyroid carcinoma: prevalence and implication on the histological parameters. *Hum Pathol*, 29: 565–568, 1998.
36. Nikiforova, M. N., Caudill, C. M., Biddinger, P., and Nikiforov, Y. E. Prevalence of RET/PTC Rearrangements in Hashimoto's Thyroiditis and Papillary Thyroid Carcinomas. *Int J Surg Pathol*, 10: 15–22, 2002.
37. Sugg, S. L., Ezzat, S., Zheng, L., Freeman, J. L., Rosen, I. B., and Asa, S. L. Oncogene profile of papillary thyroid carcinoma. *Surgery*, 125: 46–52, 1999.
38. Bongarzone, I., Fugazzola, L., Vigneri, P., Mariani, L., Mondellini, P., Pacini, F., Basolo, F., Pinchera, A., Pilotti, S., and Pierotti, M. A. Age-related activation of the tyrosine kinase receptor protooncogenes RET and NTRK1 in papillary thyroid carcinoma. *J Clin Endocrinol Metab*, 81: 2006–2009, 1996.
39. Bongarzone, I., Vigneri, P., Mariani, L., Collini, P., Pilotti, S., and Pierotti, M. A. RET/NTRK1 rearrangements in thyroid gland tumors of the papillary carcinoma family: correlation with clinicopathological features. *Clin Cancer Res*, 4: 223–228, 1998.
40. Zou, M., Shi, Y., and Farid, N. R. Low rate of ret proto-oncogene activation (PTC/retTPC) in papillary thyroid carcinomas from Saudi Arabia. *Cancer*, 73: 176–180, 1994.
41. Chua, E. L., Wu, W. M., Tran, K. T., McCarthy, S. W., Lauer, C. S., Dubourdieu, D., Packham, N., O'Brien, C. J., Turtle, J. R., and Dong, Q. Prevalence and distribution of ret/ptc 1, 2, and 3 in papillary thyroid carcinoma in New Caledonia and Australia. *J Clin Endocrinol Metab*, 85: 2733–2739, 2000.
42. Nikiforov, Y. E., Rowland, J. M., Bove, K. E., Monforte-Munoz, H., and Fagin, J. A. Distinct pattern of ret oncogene rearrangements in morphological variants of radiation-induced and sporadic thyroid papillary carcinomas in children. *Cancer Res*, 57: 1690–1694, 1997.
43. Fenton, C. L., Lukes, Y., Nicholson, D., Dinauer, C. A., Francis, G. L., and Tuttle, R. M. The ret/PTC mutations are common in sporadic papillary thyroid carcinoma of children and young adults. *J Clin Endocrinol Metab*, 85: 1170–1175, 2000.
44. Soares, P., Fonseca, E., Wynford-Thomas, D., and Sobrinho-Simoes, M. Sporadic ret-rearranged papillary carcinoma of the thyroid: a subset of slow growing, less aggressive thyroid neoplasms? *J Pathol*, 185: 71–78, 1998.
45. Fugazzola, L., Pilotti, S., Pinchera, A., Vorontsova, T. V., Mondellini, P., Bongarzone, I., Greco, A., Astakhova, L., Butti, M. G., Demidchik, E. P., and et al. Oncogenic rearrangements of the RET

proto-oncogene in papillary thyroid carcinomas from children exposed to the Chernobyl nuclear accident. *Cancer Res*, 55: 5617–5620, 1995.
46. Klugbauer, S., Lengfelder, E., Demidchik, E. P., and Rabes, H. M. High prevalence of RET rearrangement in thyroid tumors of children from Belarus after the Chernobyl reactor accident. *Oncogene*, 11: 2459–2467, 1995.
47. Smida, J., Salassidis, K., Hieber, L., Zitzelsberger, H., Kellerer, A. M., Demidchik, E. P., Negele, T., Spelsberg, F., Lengfelder, E., Werner, M., and Bauchinger, M. Distinct frequency of ret rearrangements in papillary thyroid carcinomas of children and adults from Belarus. *Int J Cancer*, 80: 32–38, 1999.
48. Rabes, H. M., Demidchik, E. P., Sidorow, J. D., Lengfelder, E., Beimfohr, C., Hoelzel, D., and Klugbauer, S. Pattern of radiation-induced RET and NTRK1 rearrangements in 191 post-chernobyl papillary thyroid carcinomas: biological, phenotypic, and clinical implications. *Clin Cancer Res*, 6: 1093–1103, 2000.
49. Bounacer, A., Wicker, R., Caillou, B., Cailleux, A. F., Sarasin, A., Schlumberger, M., and Suarez, H. G. High prevalence of activating ret proto-oncogene rearrangements, in thyroid tumors from patients who had received external radiation. *Oncogene*, 15: 1263–1273, 1997.
50. Elisei, R., Romei, C., Vorontsova, T., Cosci, B., Veremeychik, V., Kuchinskaya, E., Basolo, F., Demidchik, E. P., Miccoli, P., Pinchera, A., and Pacini, F. RET/PTC rearrangements in thyroid nodules: studies in irradiated and not irradiated, malignant and benign thyroid lesions in children and adults. *J Clin Endocrinol Metab*, 86: 3211–3216, 2001.
51. Collins, B. J., Chiappetta, G., Schneider, A. B., Santoro, M., Pentimalli, F., Fogelfeld, L., Gierlowski, T., Shore-Freedman, E., Jaffe, G., and Fusco, A. RET expression in papillary thyroid cancer from patients irradiated in childhood for benign conditions. *J Clin Endocrinol Metab*, 87: 3941–3946, 2002.
52. Powell, D. J., Jr., Russell, J., Nibu, K., Li, G., Rhee, E., Liao, M., Goldstein, M., Keane, W. M., Santoro, M., Fusco, A., and Rothstein, J. L. The RET/PTC3 oncogene: metastatic solid-type papillary carcinomas in murine thyroids. *Cancer Res*, 58: 5523–5528, 1998.
53. Jhiang, S. M., Sagartz, J. E., Tong, Q., Parker-Thornburg, J., Capen, C. C., Cho, J. Y., Xing, S., and Ledent, C. Targeted expression of the ret/PTC1 oncogene induces papillary thyroid carcinomas. *Endocrinology*, 137: 375–378, 1996.
54. Basolo, F., Giannini, R., Monaco, C., Melillo, R. M., Carlomagno, F., Pancrazi, M., Salvatore, G., Chiappetta, G., Pacini, F., Elisei, R., Miccoli, P., Pinchera, A., Fusco, A., and Santoro, M. Potent mitogenicity of the RET/PTC3 oncogene correlates with its prevalence in tall-cell variant of papillary thyroid carcinoma. *Am J Pathol*, 160: 247–254, 2002.
55. Ito, T., Seyama, T., Iwamoto, K. S., Hayashi, T., Mizuno, T., Tsuyama, N., Dohi, K., Nakamura, N., and Akiyama, M. In vitro irradiation is able to cause RET oncogene rearrangement. *Cancer Res*, 53: 2940–2943, 1993.
56. Mizuno, T., Kyoizumi, S., Suzuki, T., Iwamoto, K. S., and Seyama, T. Continued expression of a tissue specific activated oncogene in the early steps of radiation-induced human thyroid carcinogenesis. *Oncogene*, 15: 1455–1460, 1997.
57. Mizuno, T., Iwamoto, K. S., Kyoizumi, S., Nagamura, H., Shinohara, T., Koyama, K., Seyama, T., and Hamatani, K. Preferential induction of RET/PTC1 rearrangement by X-ray irradiation. *Oncogene*, 19: 438–443, 2000.
58. Smanik, P. A., Furminger, T. L., Mazzaferri, E. L., and Jhiang, S. M. Breakpoint characterization of the ret/PTC oncogene in human papillary thyroid carcinoma. *Hum Mol Genet*, 4: 2313–2318, 1995.
59. Bongarzone, I., Butti, M. G., Fugazzola, L., Pacini, F., Pinchera, A., Vorontsova, T. V., Demidchik, E. P., and Pierotti, M. A. Comparison of the breakpoint regions of ELE1 and RET genes involved in the generation of RET/PTC3 oncogene in sporadic and in radiation-associated papillary thyroid carcinomas. *Genomics*, 42: 252–259, 1997.
60. Nikiforov, Y. E., Koshoffer, A., Nikiforova, M., Stringer, J., and Fagin, J. A. Chromosomal breakpoint positions suggest a direct role for radiation in inducing illegitimate recombination between the ELE1 and RET genes in radiation-induced thyroid carcinomas. *Oncogene*, 18: 6330–6334, 1999.
61. Klugbauer, S., Pfeiffer, P., Gassenhuber, H., Beimfohr, C., and Rabes, H. M. RET rearrangements in radiation-induced papillary thyroid carcinomas: high prevalence of topoisomerase I sites at breakpoints and microhomology-mediated end joining in ELE1 and RET chimeric genes. *Genomics*, 73: 149–160, 2001.
62. Yokota, H., van den Engh, G., Hearst, J. E., Sachs, R. K., and Trask, B. J. Evidence for the organization of chromatin in megabase pair-sized loops arranged along a random walk path in the human G0/G1 interphase nucleus. *J Cell Biol*, 130: 1239–1249, 1995.

63. Nikiforova, M. N., Stringer, J. R., Blough, R., Medvedovic, M., Fagin, J. A., and Nikiforov, Y. E. Proximity of chromosomal loci that participate in radiation-induced rearrangements in human cells. *Science*, 290: 138–141, 2000.
64. van den Engh, G., Sachs, R., and Trask, B. J. Estimating genomic distance from DNA sequence location in cell nuclei by a random walk model. *Science*, 257: 1410–1412, 1992.
65. Kroll, T. G., Sarraf, P., Pecciarini, L., Chen, C. J., Mueller, E., Spiegelman, B. M., and Fletcher, J. A. PAX8–PPARgamma1 fusion oncogene in human thyroid carcinoma [corrected]. *Science*, 289: 1357–1360, 2000.
66. French, C. A., Alexander, E. K., Cibas, E. S., Nose, V., Laguette, J., Faquin, W., Garber, J., Moore, F., Jr., Fletcher, J. A., Larsen, P. R., and Kroll, T. G. Genetic and biological subgroups of low-stage follicular thyroid cancer. *Am J Pathol*, 162: 1053–1060, 2003.
67. Cheung, L., Messina, M., Gill, A., Clarkson, A., Learoyd, D., Delbridge, L., Wentworth, J., Philips, J., Clifton-Bligh, R., and Robinson, B. G. Detection of the PAX8–PPAR gamma fusion oncogene in both follicular thyroid carcinomas and adenomas. *J Clin Endocrinol Metab*, 88: 354–357, 2003.
68. Nikiforova, M. N., Biddinger, P. W., Caudill, C. M., Kroll, T. G., and Nikiforov, Y. E. PAX8–PPARgamma rearrangement in thyroid tumors: RT-PCR and immunohistochemical analyses. *Am J Surg Pathol*, 26: 1016–1023, 2002.
69. Shore, R. E. Issues and epidemiological evidence regarding radiation-induced thyroid cancer. *Radiat Res*, 131: 98–111, 1992.
70. Wright, P. A., Williams, E. D., Lemoine, N. R., and Wynford-Thomas, D. Radiation-associated and 'spontaneous' human thyroid carcinomas show a different pattern of ras oncogene mutation. *Oncogene*, 6: 471–473, 1991.
71. Challeton, C., Bounacer, A., Du Villard, J. A., Caillou, B., De Vathaire, F., Monier, R., Schlumberger, M., and Suarez, H. G. Pattern of ras and gsp oncogene mutations in radiation-associated human thyroid tumors. *Oncogene*, 11: 601–603, 1995.
72. Nikiforov, Y. E., Nikiforova, M. N., Gnepp, D. R., and Fagin, J. A. Prevalence of mutations of ras and p53 in benign and malignant thyroid tumors from children exposed to radiation after the Chernobyl nuclear accident. *Oncogene*, 13: 687–693, 1996.
73. Santoro, M., Thomas, G. A., Vecchio, G., Williams, G. H., Fusco, A., Chiappetta, G., Pozcharskaya, V., Bogdanova, T. I., Demidchik, E. P., Cherstvoy, E. D., Voscoboinik, L., Tronko, N. D., Carss, A., Bunnell, H., Tonnachera, M., Parma, J., Dumont, J. E., Keller, G., Hofler, H., and Williams, E. D. Gene rearrangement and Chernobyl related thyroid cancers. *Br J Cancer*, 82: 315–322, 2000.
74. Suchy, B., Waldmann, V., Klugbauer, S., and Rabes, H. M. Absence of RAS and p53 mutations in thyroid carcinomas of children after Chernobyl in contrast to adult thyroid tumours. *Br J Cancer*, 77: 952–955, 1998.
75. Fogelfeld, L., Bauer, T. K., Schneider, A. B., Swartz, J. E., and Zitman, R. p53 gene mutations in radiation-induced thyroid cancer. *J Clin Endocrinol Metab*, 81: 3039–3044, 1996.
76. Hillebrandt, S., Streffer, C., Reiners, C., and Demidchik, E. Mutations in the p53 tumour suppressor gene in thyroid tumours of children from areas contaminated by the Chernobyl accident. *Int J Radiat Biol*, 69: 39–45, 1996.
77. Smida, J., Zitzelsberger, H., Kellerer, A. M., Lehmann, L., Minkus, G., Negele, T., Spelsberg, F., Hieber, L., Demidchik, E. P., Lengfelder, E., and Bauchinger, M. p53 mutations in childhood thyroid tumours from Belarus and in thyroid tumours without radiation history. *Int J Cancer*, 73: 802–807, 1997.
78. Waldmann, V. and Rabes, H. M. Absence of G(s)alpha gene mutations in childhood thyroid tumors after Chernobyl in contrast to sporadic adult thyroid neoplasia. *Cancer Res*, 57: 2358–2361, 1997.
79. Rogounovitch, T. I., Saenko, V. A., Shimizu-Yoshida, Y., Abrosimov, A. Y., Lushnikov, E. F., Roumiantsev, P. O., Ohtsuru, A., Namba, H., Tsyb, A. F., and Yamashita, S. Large deletions in mitochondrial DNA in radiation-associated human thyroid tumors. *Cancer Res*, 62: 7031–7041, 2002.
80. Kimura, E. T., Nikiforova, M. N., Zhu, Z., Knauf, J. A., Nikiforov, Y. E., and Fagin, J. A. High prevalence of BRAF mutations in thyroid cancer: genetic evidence for constitutive activation of the RET/PTC-RAS-BRAF signaling pathway in papillary thyroid carcinoma. *Cancer Res*, 63: 1454–1457, 2003.
81. Dubrova, Y. E., Nesterov, V. N., Krouchinsky, N. G., Ostapenko, V. A., Neumann, R., Neil, D. L., and Jeffreys, A. J. Human minisatellite mutation rate after the Chernobyl accident. *Nature*, 380: 683–686, 1996.
82. Dubrova, Y. E., Grant, G., Chumak, A. A., Stezhka, V. A., and Karakasian, A. N. Elevated minisatellite mutation rate in the post-chernobyl families from ukraine. *Am J Hum Genet*, 71: 801–809, 2002.

83. Nikiforov, Y. E., Nikiforova, M., and Fagin, J. A. Prevalence of minisatellite and microsatellite instability in radiation-induced post-Chernobyl pediatric thyroid carcinomas. *Oncogene*, 17: 1983–1988, 1998.
84. Richter, H. E., Lohrer, H. D., Hieber, L., Kellerer, A. M., Lengfelder, E., and Bauchinger, M. Microsatellite instability and loss of heterozygosity in radiation-associated thyroid carcinomas of Belarussian children and adults. *Carcinogenesis*, 20: 2247–2252, 1999.

12. TRK ONCOGENES IN PAPILLARY THYROID CARCINOMA

ANGELA GRECO, EMANUELA ROCCATO AND MARCO A. PIEROTTI
Istituto Nazionale Tumori, Department of Experimental Oncology Operative Unit #3
Via G. Venezian, 1 20133 Milan Italy

INTRODUCTION

The NTRK1 gene encodes the high affinity receptor for Nerve Growth Factor, and its action regulates neural development and differentiation. Deregulation of NTRK1 activity is associated with several human disorders. Loss of function mutations cause the genetic disease Congenital Insensitivity to Pain with Anhidrosis (CIPA). Constitutive activation of NTRK1 has been detected in several tumor types. An autocrine loop involving NTRK1 and NGF is responsible for tumor progression in prostate carcinoma and in breast cancer. Somatic rearrangements of NTRK1, producing chimeric oncogenes with constitutive tyrosine kinase activity, have been detected in a consistent fraction of papillary thyroid tumors.

The topic of this review is the thyroid TRK oncogenes; the modalities of activation, the mechanism of action, and the contribution of activating sequences will be discussed.

NTRK1 proto-oncogene

NTRK1 (also known as TRKA) is the prototype of a family of genes which also includes NTRK2 (TRKB) and NTRK3 (TRKC), encoding tyrosine kinase receptors for the neurotrophins of the Nerve Growth Factor (NGF) family. NGF is the preferred ligand for NTRK1, brain-derived neurotrophic factor and NT4/5 are ligands for NTRK2, and NT3 is the ligand for NTRK3. Interestingly, NT3 is also capable of binding to NTRK1 and NTRK2, although with low affinity (Barbacid, M., 1995).

All the neurotrophins bind also the p75 low affinity receptor, which belongs to the TNF receptor family, and is devoid of kinase activity (Kaplan, D. R. et al., 2000).

Neurotrophins are responsible for the survival, differentiation and maintenance of specific population of neurons in the developing and adult nervous system (Davies, A. M., 1994). In particular, the NGF/NTRK1 signaling supports survival and differentiation of sympathetic and sensory neurons responsive to temperature and pain. In addition to its neurotrophic functions, NGF also stimulates proliferation of a number of cell types such as lymphocytes, keratinocytes and prostate cells (Otten, U., et al., 1989; Di Marco, E. et al., 1993; Djakiew, D. et al., 1991).

NTRK1 was originally isolated from a human colon carcinoma as a transforming oncogene activated by a somatic rearrangement that fused a non-muscle tropomyosin gene to a novel tyrosine kinase receptor (Martin-Zanca, D. et al., 1986). Cloning of the full length gene (Martin-Zanca, D. et al., 1989) and identification of the NGF as a ligand occurred few years later (Kaplan, D. R. et al., 1991).

The NTRK1 gene is located on chromosome 1q21–22 (Weier, H.-U. G. et al., 1995) and consists of 17 exons distributed within a 25 kb region (Greco, A. et al., 1996). The NTRK1 receptor is a glycosylated protein of 140 kDa, comprising an extracellular portion, including Ig-like and Leucine rich domains for ligand binding, a single transmembrane region, a juxta-membrane domain, a tyrosine kinase domain and a C-terminal tail. Following NGF binding, NTRK1 undergoes dimerization and autophosphorylation of five tyrosine residues (Y490, Y670, Y674, Y675, and Y785). Activated receptor initiates several signal transduction cascades, including the Mitogen Activated Protein Kinase (MAPK), the phosphatidylinositol 3-kinase (PI3K) and the PLC-γ pathways. These signaling cascades culminate in the activation of transcription factors that alter gene expression (Kaplan, D. R. et al., 2000).

NTRK1 in human diseases

Deregulation of NTRK1 activity is associated with several human diseases. Mutations affecting different NTRK1 domains are associated with CIPA (Congenital Insensitivity to Pain with Anhidrosis), a rare recessive genetic disease characterized by loss of pain and temperature sensation, defects in thermal regulation and occasionally mental retardation (Indo, Y. et al., 1996). CIPA is the consequence of a genetic defect in the differentiation and migration of neural crest elements. By studying the effects of different CIPA mutations on NTRK1 biochemical and biological properties, the molecular mechanisms responsible for the disease have been unveiled. CIPA mutations cause inactivation of the NTRK1 receptor by at least three different mechanisms, such as complete inactivation, protein processing alteration, and reduction of receptor activity (Greco, A. et al., 1999; Greco, A. et al., 2000; Miranda, C. et al., 2002a; Miranda, C. et al., 2002b).

NTRK1 gain of function mutations have been described in some human tumors. Activation through genomic rearrangements producing chimeric oncogenes has been detected in a consistent fraction of human papillary thyroid carcinoma, and it will be described later. A 75 amino acids deletion in the extracellular domain of the NTRK1 receptor, resulting in a mutated protein with in vitro transforming activity, has been detected in a patient with acute myeloid leukaemia, indicating that constitutive activation of the NTRK1 receptor may contribute to leukemogenesis (Reuther, G. W. et al., 2000). In human neuroblastoma, expression of NTRK1 is a good prognostic marker, suggesting that lack of NTRK1 expression contributes to malignancy, presumably because it results in the loss of signaling pathways important for growth arrest and/or differentiation of the neural crest derived cells from which these tumors originate (Brodeur, G. M. et al., 1997). In prostatic carcinoma an autocrine loop involving NGF and NTRK1 is responsible for tumor progression (Djakiew, D. et al., 1991), and tumor growth can be blocked by NTRK1 kinase inhibitors (Weeraratna, A. T. et al., 2001). Recently, an autocrine NGF/NTRK1 loop has been demonstrated in breast cancer cells, suggesting that it could represent a potential therapeutic target (Descamps, S. et al., 2001). It is interesting to outline that, at variance with other RTKs such as Met, FGFR, Kit and RET, no oncogenic activation of NTRK1 by point mutations have been found in human cancer. Moreover, the introduction of missense mutations releasing the oncogenic potential of different RTKs showed a distinct effect on NTRK1 receptor. This suggests that, despite the high degree of conservation of certain amino acid residues, the NTRK1 receptor diverges from other RTKs in terms of tridimensional structure and have a distinct auto-inhibitory mechanism (Miranda, C. et al., 2002c).

Thyroid TRK oncogenes

Papillary thyroid carcinoma (PTC) is the most frequent neoplasia originating from the thyroid epithelium, and accounts for about 80% of all thyroid cancers (Hedinger, C. et al., 1988). A consistent fraction (50%) of PTC harbors chromosomal alterations causing somatic rearrangements, and consequent oncogenic activation, of two RTK genes, namely RET and NTRK1 (Pierotti, M. A. et al., 1996). For a long time RET and NTRK1 rearrangements represented the only known genetic alterations in PTC. Recently, mutations of BRAF, alternative to RTK rearrangements, have been reported by different groups, and they represent the most frequent alteration in PTC (Kimura, E. T. et al., 2003; Cohen, Y. et al., 2003; Soares, P. et al., 2003).

Both RET and TRK oncogenes have been discovered in our laboratory by DNA transfection/focus formation assay in NIH3T3 cells, starting from papillary thyroid tumor DNA. Transforming activity correlated with the presence of human RET and TRK sequences in the mouse transfectants DNA (Bongarzone, I. et al., 1989); this provided the basis for the isolation and characterization of the chimeric oncogenes, containing the receptor tyrosine kinase domain preceded by activating sequences from different genes.

Several TRK oncogenes have been isolated from thyroid tumors, differing in the activating genes (Figure 1). The TRK oncogene, identical to that first isolated from colon carcinoma, and containing sequences from the TPM3 gene on chromosome 1q22–23 (Wilton, S. D. et al, 1995), has been frequently found in thyroid tumors (Butti, M. G. et al., 1995). TRK-T1 and TRK-T2 derive both from rearrangement between NTRK1 and TPR gene on chromosome 1q25 (Miranda, C. et al, 1994); however, they display different structure, especially for the different TPR portion

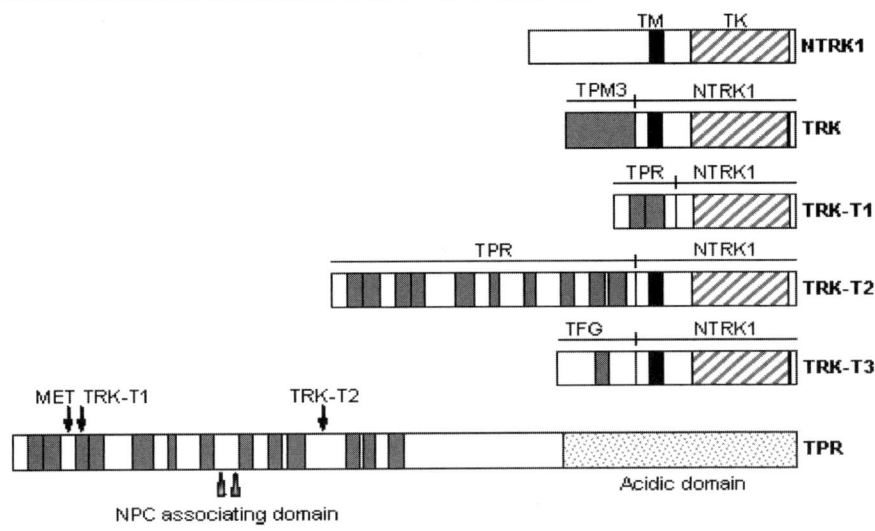

Figure 1. Schematic representation of NTRK1, TRKs and TPR proteins. In the oncoproteins the portions contributed by NTRK1 and activating sequences are indicated. The gray portions represent coiled-coil domains. On TPR the break sites of Met, TRK-T1 and TRK-T2 oncoproteins are indicated by arrows. TM: transmembrane domain, TK: tyrosine kinase domain, NPC: nuclear pore complex.

(Greco, A. et al., 1997; Greco, A. et al., 1992). TRK-T3 is activated by TFG, a novel gene on chromosome 3q11-12 (Greco, A. et al, 1995). All TRK oncogenes but TRK-T1 retain the NTRK1 transmembrane domain. TRK oncogenes display constitutive, ligand-independent tyrosine kinase activity.

In experimental models TRK oncogenes recapitulate the biological effects of the NTRK1 receptor upon NGF stimulation. In fact, they induce morphological transformation of NIH3T3 mouse fibroblasts, and neuronal-like differentiation of PC12 cells (Greco, A. et al., 1993b). The mechanisms by which TRK oncogenes mediate their effects have been in part elucidated (Figure 2). TRK oncoproteins interact to and activate PLCγ Shc, FRS2, FRS3, IRS1 and IRS2. All these molecules, except PLCγ, are recruited by the same tyrosine residue, corresponding to Tyr490 of NTRK1, most likely in a competitive fashion. Such interaction site is crucial for oncogenic activity, in so far its mutation to phenylalanine completely abrogate TRK oncogene biological activity. Moreover, by using a Shc dominant-negative mutant unable to recruit GRB2, we showed a crucial role of Shc adaptor in TRK-T3 biological activity. Conversely, mutation of the PLCγ interaction site did not affect the oncogenic activity. It is worth noting that our studies on TRK oncogenes allowed the identification of novel proteins interacting with NTRK1 kinase, such as IRS1, IRS2 and FRS3 (Miranda, C. et al., 2001; Roccato, E. et al., 2002; Ranzi, V. et al., 2003).

The capability of TPM3, TPR and TFG to activate chimeric tyrosine kinase oncogenes is not restricted to NTRK1; in fact, they have been found fused to other kinase genes. TPM3 and TFG were reported to fuse to ALK in anaplastic large cell lymphoma

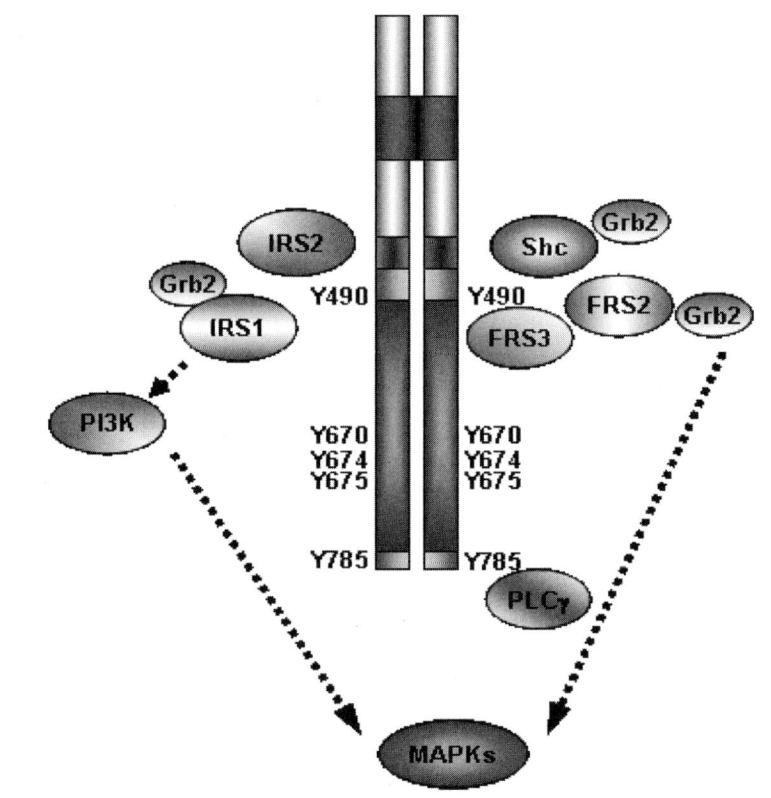

Figure 2. TRK oncogenes signaling pathways. Tyrosine residues are indicated with the number of the corresponding aminoacids of NTRK1.

(Hernandez, L. et al., 2002; Lamant, L. et al., 1999). TPR was first identified as part of the MET oncogene in HOS cells, fused to the TK domain of the hepatocyte growth factor receptor (Park, M. et al., 1986); subsequently it was detected fused to the raf oncogene during the transfection of a rat hepatocarcinoma (Ishikawa, F. et al., 1987). Interestingly, TPR and TFG were first identified in rearranged, oncogenic versions. TPM3 gene encodes a non-muscle tropomyosin isoform. TPR gene encodes a large protein of the nuclear pore complex; recent studies have shown that TPR is a phosphorylated protein involved in mRNA export, through the formation of complexes with different interacting proteins (Shibata, S. et al., 2002; Green, D. M. et al., 2003). TFG encodes a protein of still unknown function.

Role of activating sequences in TRK oncogenic activation

Despite the diversity in structure and function, all the NTRK1 activating proteins contain coiled-coil domains that promote protein dimerization/multimerization. Coiled-coil domains are characterized by heptad repeats with the occurrence of apolar residues

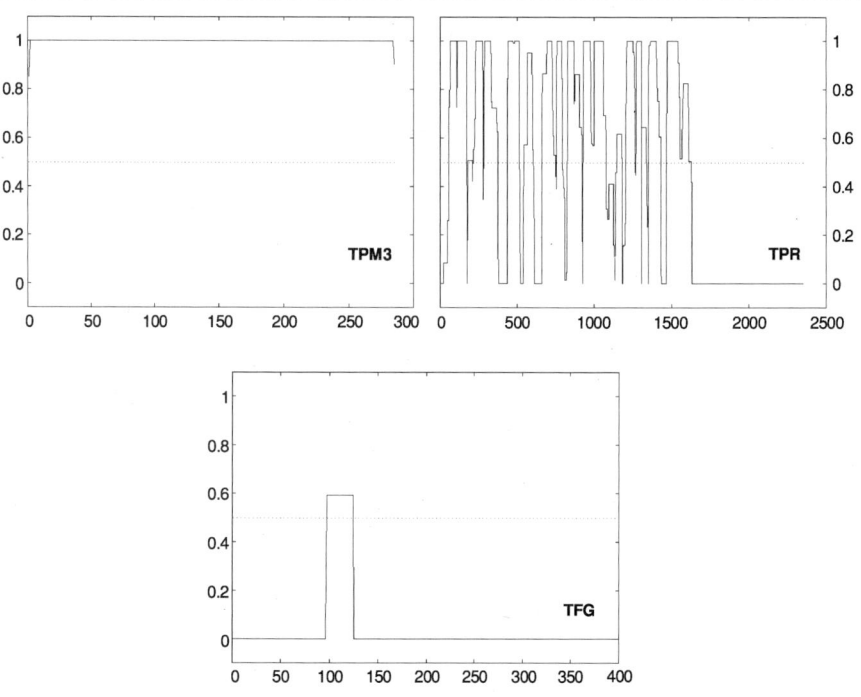

Figure 3. Prediction of coiled-coil domains in TPM3, TPR and TFG with the use of Paircoil program (Berger B., PNAS vol 92, 1995. pag. 8259–8263). The vertical scale represents relative coiled-coil probability; the horizontal scale represents amino acids number.

preferentially in the first (a) and fourth (d) positions (Lupas, A., 1996; Lupas, A. et al., 1991). This confers to the proteins the capability to fold into α-helices that are wound into a superhelix. In Figure 3 the coiled-coil domains detected in TRK activating sequences by sequence analysis with the COIL program are shown.

TPM3 contains numerous, overlapping coiled-coil domains. Several coiled-coil domains are present in TPR, and two of them fall in the region contained in MET and TRK-T1 oncogenes. It has been reported that mutations within the first coiled-coil domain drastically reduces MET transforming activity (Rodrigues, G. A. et al., 1993). TFG contains a single coiled-coil domain, of approximately three heptads, shorter than typical coiled-coil domains (Figures 3 and 4). However, the presence of a hydrophobic residue in position a, would increase the strength of association, despite the short length (Greco, A. et al., 1995). The contribution of TFG coiled-coil domain to TRK-T3 oncogenic activation has been elucidated by studies employing mutants where the domain was either deleted or mutated at leucine residues in position d of each heptad. We have demonstrated that coiled-coil domain plays a crucial role in TRK-T3 oncogenic activation by mediating oncoprotein complexes formation, an essential step for tyrosine kinase activation. Our studies support the model by which coiled-coil domains mediate protein oligomerization of RTK oncogenes leading to constitutive, ligand-independent tyrosine kinase activity (Greco, A. et al., 1998). The TFG coiled-coil domain is predicted to fold into trimers. By size-exclusion chromatography we have demonstrated that the wild type TRK-T3 protein is part of high molecular weight complexes, compatible with the assembly of six oncoproteins molecules, or including other proteins. However, the precise composition of TRK-T3 complexes remains to be determined (Roccato, E. et al., 2003).

Studies on receptor and non receptor tyrosine kinase chimeric oncogenes have demonstrated that the importance of activating genes is related to the coiled-coil domains which mediate the activation above reported. However, an attractive hypothesis is the possibility that activating sequences may contribute with other functions, apart from dimerization. In addition, since the oncogenic rearrangements disabled one allele of the activating gene, the reduced activity of the corresponding protein could play a role in thyroid carcinogenesis. In this respect the thyroid TRK-T3 oncogene represents an attractive model for at least three reasons: 1) the activating portion is provided by TFG, a gene coding for a novel protein whose function remains to be unveiled; 2) the TFG portion contained in TRK-T3 display a single, short coiled-coil domain, corresponding to 14% of the aminoacid residues; 3) TFG might interact with other proteins (see later).

After our initial isolation as part of the TRK-T3 oncogene, the normal TFG counterpart was cloned and characterized (Figure 4).

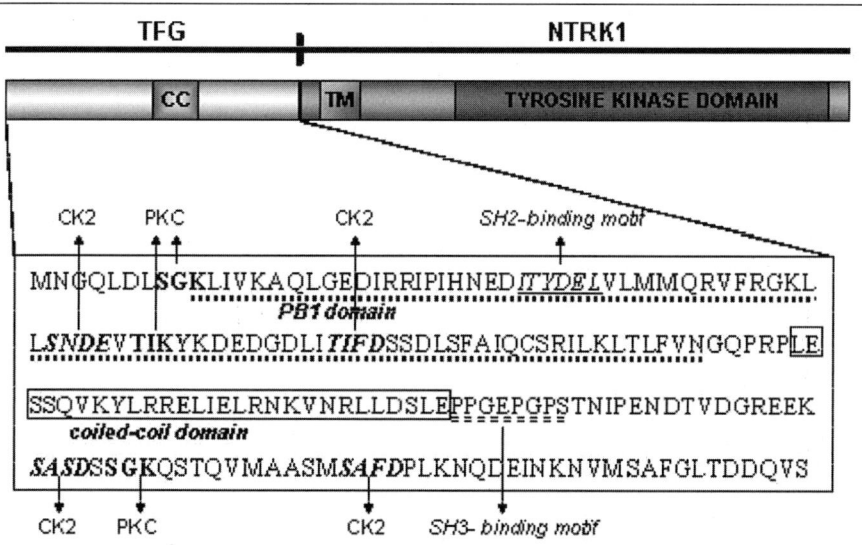

Figure 4. Schematic representation of the TRK-T3 oncogene. The portions contributed by TFG and NTRK1 are indicated. In the box the TFG aminoacidic sequence is reported; specific domains and consensus sites are indicated. CC: coiled-coil domain; TM: transmembrane domain; CK2: putative phosphorylation site for CK2; PKC: putative phosphorylation site for PKC.

TFG gene is ubiquitously expressed in human adult tissues and it is conserved among several species, including C. elegans. In addition to the coiled-coil domain, the TFG protein also contains putative phosphorylation sites for PKC and CK2, glycosilation sites, as well SH2- and SH3-binding sites (Mencinger, M. et al., 1997). Several of these sites are identical in TFG proteins from different species, indicating that the protein might be involved in basic cell processes (Mencinger, M. et al., 1999). We have recently identified a PB1 domain, which encompasses almost entirely the TFG N-terminal portion (Roccato, E. et al., 2003). PB1 is a novel protein module mediating protein oligomerization: in fact it is capable of binding to target proteins containing PC motifs and, as recently discovered, other PB1 domains (Terasawa, H. et al., 2001; Nakamura, K. et al., 2003). Based on the peculiarity of TFG, we have recently focused our interest on the role of sequences outside the coiled-coil domain in TRK-T3 oncogenic activation. On the whole our studies demonstrate that the regions outside the coiled-coil domain give a great contribution to TRK-T3 activation. When deleted, complexes formation is unaffected; however transforming activity is reduced to different extent. More detailed information was provided by studies employing point mutants: transforming activity was significantly reduced by mutating a putative SH2-binding motif, whereas it was abrogated by the mutation of the conserved Lys residue within the PB1 domain. These evidences strongly support the notion that proteins interacting with TFG might play a role in TRK-T3 oncogenic activity (Roccato, E. et al., 2003). The identification of such proteins will give an important contribution to the definition of the modalities by which TRK-T3 triggers thyroid carcinogenesis, as well as to the discovery of TFG normal function.

Genomic features of NTRK1 oncogenic rearrangements

The NTRK1 genomic rearrangements present in the tumor DNA have been cloned and characterized (Figure 5) (Greco, A. et al., 1997; Greco, A. et al., 1995, Butti, M.G. et al, 1995). All the breakpoints fall within a NTRK1 region of 2.9 Kb, showing a GC content of 58.8% (Greco, A. et al., 1993a). The NTRK1 rearrangements are balanced; in fact, in addition to the oncogenic rearrangement containing the 3' moiety of the receptor, the reciprocal product of the rearrangement, containing the 5' portion of NTRK1 fused to the 3' portion of the activating genes, was present in tumor DNA.

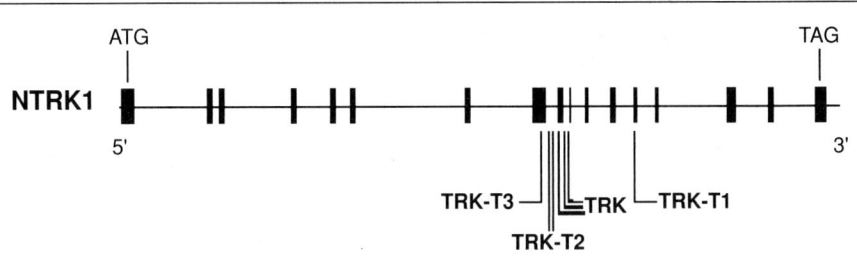

Figure 5. Genomic structure of the NTRK1 gene. The break sites of the different TRK oncogenes are indicated.

Sequencing of the breakpoint regions showed no homologies between the joined extremities. This suggests that the Non Homologous End Joining (NHEJ) mechanism, which requires little or not sequence homology, could be involved in the generation of TRK oncogenes. The NHEJ pathway is activated by ionizing radiations, and this is consistent with the association of PTC with therapeutic or accidental radiation exposure. Analysis of the breakpoint regions in different tumors demonstrated that all the rearrangements are conservative, involving deletion, insertion or duplication of only few nucleotides. In a tumor carrying the TRK-T2 oncogene a peculiar rearrangement was found, with the 5' end of NTRK1 joined to sequences from chromosome 17; however, such additional rearrangement does not contribute to oncogenic activation (Greco, A. et al., 1997).

No cytogenetic studies are available for tumors carrying NTRK1 rearrangements; therefore the type of chromosomal rearrangement generating TRK oncogenes is not documented. A t(1;3) translocation is most likely responsible for the generation of TRK-T3 oncogene (TFG/NTRK1 rearrangement). For TRK, TRK-T1 and TRK-T2, produced by rearrangements with genes located on the q arm of chromosome 1, similarly to NTRK1, three mechanisms of rearrangement can be postulated: deletion, inversion, and reciprocal translocation between the two chromosome 1 homologues. The presence in the tumor DNA of the reciprocal products of the rearrangement allowed us to exclude the deletion. Sequence data recently available in public databases unveiled that NTRK1 has transcriptional orientation opposite to that of TPM3 and TPR. Therefore, intrachromosomal inversion is the only mechanism capable to produce TRK, TRK-T1 and TRK-T2 oncogenes (Figure 6).

The thyroid epithelium is very prone to chromosomal rearrangements. These include the RET and NTRK1 oncogenes in PTC, and the PAX8/PPARγ fusion gene associated with follicular thyroid tumors. This predisposition to gene rearrangements is a peculiarity of thyroid epithelium, at variance with other epithelia, and the understanding of the molecular basis underlying such predisposition represents a fascinating topic. Recently, Nikiforova et al (2000) have shown that, in thyroid interphase nuclei, RET and H4 loci display a distance reduced with respect to other cell type, and suggested that this spatial contiguity may provide the structural basis for the generation of the thyroid RET/H4 (PTC1) oncogene. It is very important to assess whether or not this attractive model also apply to NTRK1 and its partners, rearranging genes. Another possibility is that the high frequency of chromosomal rearrangements in thyroid tumors might reflect the thyrocyte intrinsic capability to repair DNA DSBs, either spontaneous or induced. Yang et al (1999) showed that human thyrocytes exposed in vitro to ionizing radiations failed to induce apoptosis; instead, they showed a significant increase of DNA end-joining activity. In this respect the analysis of the DNA repair kinetics and the status of the enzymes involved in DNA repair in human thyrocytes deserve to be investigated.

CONCLUSIONS

Rearrangements of RET and NTRK1 are frequently detected in human papillary thyroid carcinoma. TRK oncogenes involve different activating genes containing

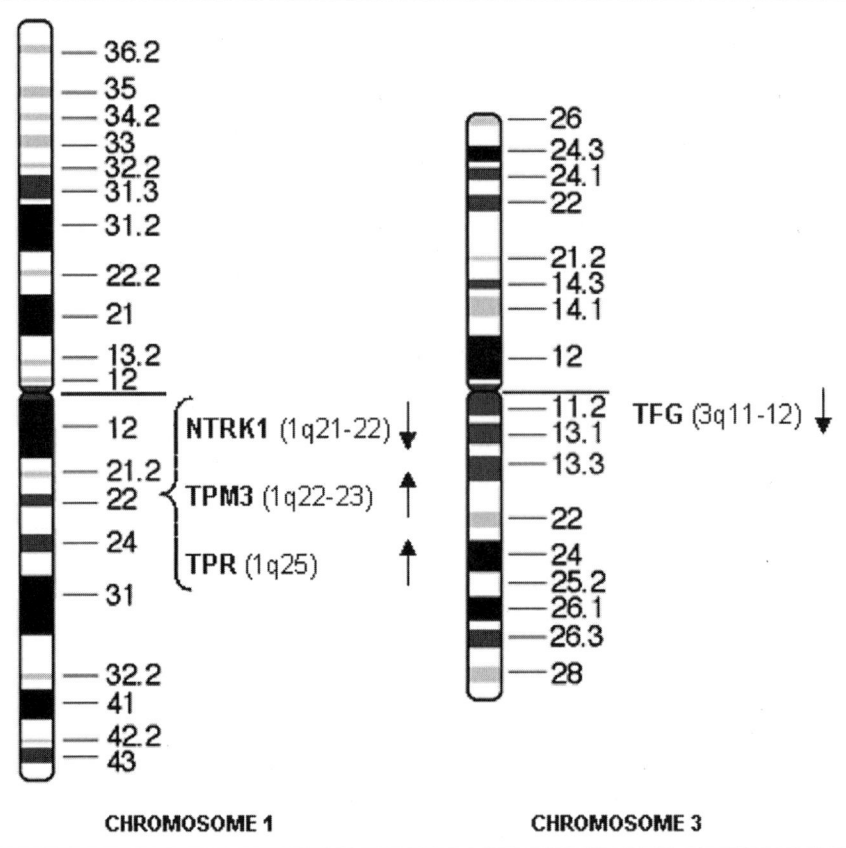

Figure 6. Ideogram of chromosomes 1 and 3 showing the localization of NTRK1, TPM3, TPR and TFG genes. The arrows indicate the transcriptional orientation.

coiled-coil domains that mediate protein dimerization and consequent tyrosine kinase activation. However, also regions outside the coiled-coil domain contribute to oncogenic activation, with modalities presently under investigation. The high proneness of thyroid epithelium to chromosomal rearrangements might reflect structural and enzymatic properties of thyrocytes with respect to DNA repair. The identification and study of such properties will elucidate the mechanisms responsible for the generation of thyroid oncogenes.

REFERENCES

1. Barbacid M. Neurotrophic factors and their receptors. Curr Opin Cell Biol 1995; 7:148–155.
2. Bongarzone I., Pierotti M.A., Monzini N., Mondellini P., Manenti G., Donghi R., Pilotti S., Grieco M., Santoro M., Fusco A., Vecchio G., Della Porta G. High frequency of activation of tyrosine kinase oncogenes in human papillary thyroid carcinoma. Oncogene 1989; 4:1457–1462.
3. Brodeur G.M., Maris J.M., Yamashiro D.J., Hogarty M.D., White P.S. Biology and genetics of human neuroblastomas. J Pediatr Hematol Oncol 1997; 19:93–101.

4. Butti M.G., Bongarzone I., Ferraresi G., Mondellini P., Borrello M.G., Pierotti M.A. A sequence analysis of the genomic regions involved in the rearrangements between TPM3 and NTRK1 genes producing TRK oncogenes in papillary thyroid carcinomas. Genomics 1995; 28:15–24.
5. Cohen Y., Xing M., Mambo E., Guo Z., Wu G., Trink B., Beller U., Westra W.H., Ladenson P.W., Sidransky D. BRAF mutation in papillary thyroid carcinoma. J Natl Cancer Inst 2003; 95:625–627.
6. Davies A.M. The role of neurotrophins in the developing nervous system. J Neurobiol 1994; 25:1334–1348.
7. Descamps S., Toillon R.A., Adriaenssens E., Pawlowski V., Cool S.M., Nurcombe V., Le B., X, Boilly B., Peyrat J.P., Hondermarck H. Nerve growth factor stimulates proliferation and survival of human breast cancer cells through two distinct signaling pathways. J Biol Chem 2001; 276:17864–17870.
8. Di Marco E., Mathor M., Bondanza S., Cutuli N., Marchisio P.C., Cancedda R., De Luca M. Nerve growth factor binds to normal human keratinocytes through high and low affinity receptors and stimulates their growth by a novel autocrine loop. J Biol Chem 1993; 268:22838–22846.
9. Djakiew D., Delsite R., Plufg B., Wrathall J., Lynch J.H., Onoda M. Regulation of growth by a nerve growth factor-like protein which modulates paracrine interactions between a neoplastic epithelial cell line and stromal cells of the human prostate. Cancer Res 1991; 51:3304–3310.
10. Greco A., Fusetti L., Miranda C., Villa R., Zanotti S., Pagliardini S., Pierotti M.A. Role of the TFG N-terminus and coiled-coil domain in the transforming activity of the thyroid TRK-T3 oncogene. Oncogene 1998; 16:809–816.
11. Greco A., Mariani C., Miranda C., Lupas A., Pagliardini S., Pomati M., Pierotti M.A. The DNA rearrangement that generates the TRK-T3 oncogene involves a novel gene on chromosome 3 whose product has a potential coiled-coil domain. Mol Cell Biol 1995; 15:6118–6127.
12. Greco A., Mariani C., Miranda C., Pagliardini S., Pierotti M.A. Characterization of the NTRK1 genomic region involved in chromosomal rearrangements generating TRK oncogenes. Genomics 1993a; 18:397–400.
13. Greco A., Miranda C., Pagliardini S., Fusetti L., Bongarzone I., Pierotti M.A. Chromosome 1 rearrangements involving the genes TPR and NTRK1 produce structurally different thyroid-specific TRK oncogenes. Genes Chrom Cancer 1997; 19:112–123.
14. Greco A., Orlandi R., Mariani C., Miranda C., Borrello M.G., Cattaneo A., Pagliardini S., Pierotti M.A. Expression of TRK-T1 oncogene induces differentiation of PC12 cells. Cell Growth Diff 1993b; 4:539–546.
15. Greco A., Pierotti M.A., Bongarzone I., Pagliardini S., Lanzi C., Della Porta G. TRK-T1 is a novel oncogene formed by the fusion of TPR and TRK genes in human papillary thyroid carcinomas. Oncogene 1992; 7:237–242.
16. Greco A., Villa R., Fusetti L., Orlandi R., Pierotti M.A. The Gly571Arg mutation, associated with the autonomic and sensory disorder CIPA, causes the inactivation of the NTRK1/NGF receptor. J Cell Physiol 2000; 182:127–133.
17. Greco A., Villa R., Pierotti M.A. Genomic organization of the human NTRK1 gene. Oncogene 1996; 13:2463–2466.
18. Greco A., Villa R., Tubino B., Romano L., Penso D., Pierotti M.A. A novel NTRK1 mutation associated with congenital insensitivity to pain anhidrosis. Am J Hum Genet 1999; 64:1207–1210.
19. Green D.M., Johnson C.P., Hagan H., Corbett A.H. The C-terminal domain of myosin-like protein 1 (Mlp1p) is a docking site for heterogeneous nuclear ribonucleoproteins that are required for mRNA export. Proc Natl Acad Sci U S A 2003; 100:1010–1015.
20. Hedinger C, Williams ED, Sobin LH. Histological typing of thyroid tumours. Berlin, Heidelberg: WHO Second Edition, Springer-Verlag, 1988..
21. Hernandez L., Bea S., Bellosillo B., Pinyol M., Falini B., Carbone A., Ott G., Rosenwald A., Fernandez A., Pulford K., Mason D., Morris S.W., Santos E., Campo E. Diversity of genomic breakpoints in TFG-ALK translocations in anaplastic large cell lymphomas: identification of a new TFG-ALK(XL) chimeric gene with transforming activity. Am J Pathol 2002; 160:1487–1494.
22. Indo Y., Tsuruta M., Hayashida Y., Karim M.A., Otha K., Kawano T., Mitsubuchi H., Tonoki H., Awaya Y., Matsuda I. Mutations in TRKA/NGF receptor gene in patients with congenital insensitivity to pain with anhidrosis. Nature Genet 1996; 13:485.
23. Ishikawa F., Takaku F., Nagao M., Sugimura T. Rat c-raf oncogene activation by a rearrangement that produces a fused protein. Mol Cell Biol 1987; 7:1226–1232.
24. Kaplan D.R., Martin-Zanca D., Parada L.F. Tyrosine phosphorylation and tyrosine kinase activity of the trk proto-oncogene product induced by NGF. Nature 1991; 350:158–160.
25. Kaplan D.R., Miller F.D. Neurotrophin signal transduction in the nervous system. Curr Opin Neurobiol 2000; 10:381–391.

26. Kimura E.T., Nikiforova M.N., Zhu Z., Knauf J.A., Nikiforov Y.E., Fagin J.A. High prevalence of BRAF mutations in thyroid cance: gene evidence for constitutive activation of RET/PTC-RAS-BRAF signaling pathway in papillary thyroid carcinoma. Cancer Res 2003; 63:1454–1457.
27. Lamant L., Dastugue N., Pulford K., Delsol G., Mariame B. A new fusion gene TPM3-ALK in anaplastic large cell lymphoma created by a (1;2)(q25;p23) translocation. Blood 1999; 93:3088–3095.
28. Lupas A. Coiled coils: new structures and new functions. Trends Biochem Sci 1996; 21:375–382.
29. Lupas A., Van Dyke M., Stock J. Predicting coiled coilts from protein sequences. Science 1991; 252:1162–1164.
30. Martin-Zanca D., Hughes S.H., Barbacid M. A human oncogene formed by the fusion of truncated tropomyosin and protein tyrosine kinase sequences. Nature 1986; 319:743–748.
31. Martin-Zanca D., Oskam R., Mitra G., Copeland T., Barbacid M. Molecular and Biochemical characterization of the human trk proto-oncogene. Mol Cell Biol 1989; 9:24–33.
32. Mencinger M., Aman P. Characterization of TFG in mus musculus and Caenorhabditis elegans. Biochem Biophys Res Comm 1999; 257:67–73.
33. Mencinger M., Panagopoulos I., Andreasson P., Lassen C., Mitelman F., Aman P. Characterization and chromosomal mapping of the human *TFG* gene involved in thyroid carcinoma. Genomics 1997; 41:372–331.
34. Miranda C., Minoletti F., Greco A., Sozzi G., Pierotti M.A. Refined localization of the human TPR gene to chromosome 1q25 by *in situ* hybridization. Genomics 1994; 23:714–715.
35. Miranda C., Di Virgilio M., Selleri S., Zanotti G., Pagliardini S., Pierotti M.A., Greco A. Novel pathogenic mechanisms of congenital insensitivity to pain with anhidrosis genetic disorder unveiled by functional analysis of neurotrophic tyrosine receptor kinase type1/nervw growth factor receptor mutations. J Biol Chem 2002a; 277:6455–6462.
36. Miranda C., Greco A., Miele C., Pierotti M.A., Van Obberghen E. IRS-1 and IRS-2 are recruited by TrkA receptor and oncogenic TRK-T1. J Cell Physiol 2001; 186:35–46.
37. Miranda C., Selleri S., Pierotti M.A., Greco A. The M581V mutation, associated with a mid form of Congenital Insensitivity to Pain with Anhidrosis, causes partial inactivation of the NTRK1 receptor. J Invest Dermatol 2002b; 119:976–979.
38. Miranda C., Zanotti G., Pagliardini S., Ponzetto C., Pierotti M.A., Greco A. Gain of function mutations of RTK conserved residues display differential effects on NTRK1 kinase activity. Oncogene 2002c; 21:8334–8339.
39. Nakamura K., Johnson G.L. PB1 domains of MEKK2 and MEKK3 interact with the MEK5 PB1 domain for activation of the ERK5 pathway. J Biol Chem 2003; 278:36989–36992.
40. Nikiforova M.N., Stringer J.R., Blough R., Medvedovic M., Fagin J.A., Nikiforov Y.E. Proximity of chromosomal loci that participate in radiation-induced rearrangements in human cells. Science 2000; 290:138–141.
41. Otten U., Ehrhard P., Peck R. Nerve growth factor induces growth and differentiation of human B lymphocytes. Proc Natl Acad Sci USA 1989; 86:10059–10063.
42. Park M., Dean M., Cooper C.S., Schmidt M., O'Brien S.J., Blair D.G., Vande Woude G.F. Mechanism of met oncogene activation. Cell 1986; 45:895–904.
43. Pierotti M.A., Bongarzone I., Borrello M.G., Greco A., Pilotti S., Sozzi G. Cytogenetics and molecular genetics of the carcinomas arising from the thyroid epithelial follicular cells. Genes Chrom Cancer 1996; 16:1–14.
44. Ranzi V., Meakin S.O., Mondellini P., Pierotti M.A., Greco A. The signaling adapters FRS2 and FRS3 are substrates of the thyroid TRK oncoproteins. Endocrinology 2003; 144:922–928.
45. Reuther G.W., Lambert Q.T., Caligiuri M.A., Der C.J. Identification and characterization of an activating TrkA deletion mutation in acute myeloid leukemia. Mol Biol Cell 2000; 20:8655–8666.
46. Roccato E., Miranda C., Ranzi V., Gishizky M.L., Pierotti M.A., Greco A. Biological activity of the thyroid TRK-T3 oncogene requires signaling through Shc. Br J Cancer 2002; 87:645–653.
47. Roccato E., Pagliardini S., Cleris L., Canevari S., Formelli F., Pierotti M.A., Greco A. Role of TFG sequences outside the coiled-coil domain in TRK-T3 oncogenic activation. Oncogene 2003; 22:807–818.
48. Rodrigues G.A., Park M. Dimerization mediated through a leucine zipper activates the oncogenic potential of the *met* receptor tyrosine kinase. Mol Cell Biol 1993; 13:6711–6722.
49. Shibata S., Matsuoka Y., Yoneda Y. Nucleocytoplasmic transport of proteins and poly(A)+ RNA in reconstituted Tpr-less nuclei in living mammalian cells. Genes Cells 2002; 7:421–434.
50. Soares P., Trovisco V., Rocha A.S., Lima J., Castro P., Preto A., Maximo V., Botelho T., Seruca R., Sobrinho-Simoes M. BRAF mutations and RET/PTC rearrangements are alternative events in the etiopathogenesis of PTC. Oncogene 2003; 22:4578–4580.

51. Terasawa H., Noda Y., Ito T., Hatanaka H., Ichikawa S., Ogura K., Sumimoto H., Inagaki F. Structure and ligand recognition of the PB1 domain: a novel protein module binding to the PC motif. EMBO J 2001; 20:3947–3956.
52. Weeraratna A.T., Dalrymple S.L., Lamb J.C., Denmeade S.R., Miknyoczki S.J., Dionne C.A., Isaacs J.T. Pan-trk inhibition decreases metastasis and enhances host survival in experimental models as a result of its selective induction of apoptosis of prostate cancer cells. Clin Cancer Res 2001; 7:2237–2245.
53. Weier H.-U.G., Rhein A.P., Shadravan F., Collins C., Polikoff D. Rapid physical mapping of the human *trk* protooncogene (NTRK1) to human chromosome 1q21–q22 by P1 clone selection, fluorescence *in situ* hybridization (FISH), and computer-assisted microscopy. Genomics 1995; 26:390–393.
54. Wilton S.D., Eyre H., Akkari P.A., Watkins H.C., MacRae C., Laing N.G., Callen, DC. Assignment of the human a-tropomyosin gene TPM3 to 1q22–>q23 by fluorescence in situ hybridisation. Cytogenet Cell Genet 1995; 68:122–124.
55. Yang T.T., Namba H., Hara T., Takmura N., Nagayama Y., Fukata S., Ishikawa N., Kuma K., Ito K., Yamashita S. p53 induced by ionizing radiation mediates DNA end-jointing activity, but not apoptosis of thyroid cells. Oncogene 1997; 14:1511–1519.

13. THYROIDAL IODIDE TRANSPORT AND THYROID CANCER

ORSOLYA DOHÁN AND NANCY CARRASCO

Department of Molecular Pharmacology Albert Einstein College of Medicine Bronx, NY 10461, USA

INTRODUCTION

The current treatment for metastatic papillary and follicular thyroid carcinomas, consists of total thyroidectomy followed by administration of radioiodide for the ablation of any remaining thyroid cancer cells or metastases (1). Radioiodide treatment of thyroid cancer has been employed for over 60 years (2), and this is the most effective targeted and curative radiotherapeutic modality available for any cancer. Radioiodide also destroys any remaining normal thyroid tissue, thus increasing the sensitivity of subsequent ^{131}I scanning and serum Tg measurements for the detection of recurrent or metastatizing disease. This is because, if normal thyroid cells remained after thyroidectomy, they would tend to prevent cancerous cells from being detected by either method. The success rate of this treatment is impressive: the mortality of patients with metastatic thyroid cancer who are treated with ^{131}I is just 3%, as opposed to 12% for those who are not treated (3). Side-effects resulting from this therapy, such as mild sialadenitis, are minimal (3); in most instances they resolve within a few weeks of termination of the treatment.

Two key characteristics of the thyroid contribute to the success of this approach. First, thyrocytes, both normal and cancerous, exhibit a remarkable ability to actively transport iodide (I$^-$). Thus, when radioiodide is administered, it is actively taken up almost exclusively by thyrocytes without affecting other cells. This makes radioiodide therapy a distinctively specific targeted method that delivers radiation from within the cancerous cells themselves. Even though I$^-$ transport activity is significantly lower in the majority of cancerous thyrocytes than in normal ones, the activity remains high enough for accumulated radioiodide to destroy cancerous thyrocytes as well. The decreased ability of cancerous thyrocytes results in the presence of "cold nodules" at tumor sites on thyroid scintigraphic scans. Second, although the thyroid is physiologically crucial, its function can be fully restored after thyroidectomy by thyroid hormone substitutive therapy, thus keeping patients in a euthyroid state.

It has long been well known that active I^- transport is a key attribute of differentiated thyrocytes, as I^- is essential for thyroid hormone biosynthesis. The Na^+/I^- symporter (NIS) is the plasma membrane glycoprotein that mediates active I^- transport from the bloodstream into the cytoplasm of thyrocytes. Using expression cloning in *Xenopus laevis* oocytes, our group isolated the cDNA encoding NIS from rat-thyroid-derived FRTL-5 cells (4). On the basis of a high degree of homology with the rat NIS cDNA, the human, mouse, and pig NIS cDNAs were subsequently cloned (5, 6, 7). NIS-mediated active I^- transport has also been documented in a few other tissues, including salivary glands, gastric mucosa, and lactating (but not non-lactating) mammary gland (8, 9). These findings and the generation of high affinity anti-NIS Abs have led to a thorough molecular characterization of NIS (10) (11) and to the analysis of both thyroidal and extrathyroidal I^- transport in health and disease (9, 12–14).

FUNCTION AND STRUCTURE OF NIS

NIS couples the inward translocation of Na^+ down its electrochemical gradient to the simultaneous inward "uphill" translocation of I^- against its electrochemical gradient. NIS activity is inhibited by the "classic" competitive inhibitors perchlorate and thiocyanate (9, 15–18). Two Na^+ are transported per each I^- (19). The Na^+ gradient that provides the driving force for I^- uptake is maintained by the Na^+/K^+ ATPase. In the thyroid, both NIS and the Na^+/K^+ ATPase are located on the basolateral side of the thyroid follicular cells, facing the blood supply (20). Rat NIS (rNIS) is a 618-amino acid protein (relative molecular mass 65,196) (4); both human and pig NIS, which contain 643 amino acids each, are highly homologous (75.9% and 74.2%, respectively) to rNIS (6, 7). Based on extensive experimental testing, we have proposed a NIS secondary structure model with 13 transmembrane segments (Figure 1) (12). The amino and carboxy termini face extra- and intracellularly, respectively (10). NIS is a glycoprotein; three of its Asp residues (225, 485, 497) are glycosylated in the endoplasmic reticulum (21). However, glycosylation is not essential for proper NIS function, as indicated by the observation that a non-glycosylated NIS protein is properly targeted to the plasma membrane and displays I^- transport activity with an identical K_m value (~20–30 μM) to that of wild-type (WT) NIS (21). The ca 70-amino acid hydrophilic carboxy terminus is the main phosphorylated region of the protein (22). Freeze-fracture electron microscopy studies of NIS-expressing *Xenopus laevis* oocytes revealed the appearance of 9-nm intramembrane particles corresponding to NIS (19). The size of these particles suggested that NIS may function as a multimeric protein. Recent co-immunoprecipitation experiments indicate that NIS is indeed an oligomer (23). A putative leucine zipper motif constituted by leucines at positions 199, 206, 213 and 220 may be the structural basis for NIS oligomerization (4).

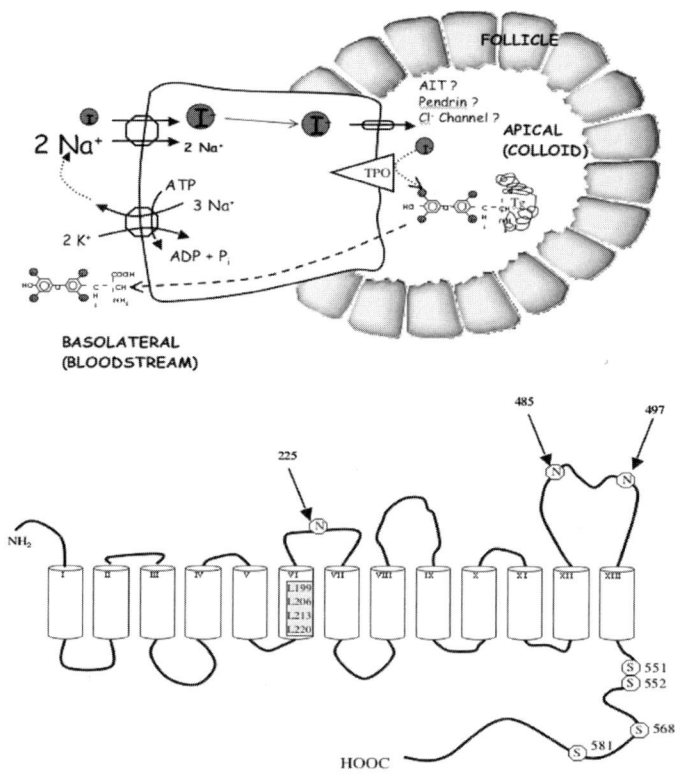

Figure 1. Iodide transport and biosynthetic pathway of thyroid hormones T_3 and T_4 in the thyroid follicular cell. Thyroid follicles are comprised of a layer of epithelial cells surrounding the colloid. The basolateral surface of the cell is shown on the left side of the figure, and the apical surface on the right. Active accumulation of I^-, mediated by the Na^+/I^- symporter (NIS) [top circle], driven by the Na^+ gradient generated by the Na^+/K^+ ATPase [bottom circle]; once I^- effluxes towards the colloid [cylinder], (TPO) [triangle] catalyzes the organification of I^- on the thyroglobulin (Tg) molecule. Dotted line pointing from the apical to the basolateral surface indicates endocytosis of iodinated Tg, followed by its phagolysosomal hydrolysis and secretion of thyroid hormones.
Secondary structure model of NIS. Transmembrane segments are numbered with Roman numerals I-XIII. The N-terminus faces the extracellular milieu and the C-terminus the cytosol. N-glycosylation sites are indicated by arrows and the leucine zipper motif in the VI transmembrane segment is shaded gray. Serines on the C-terminus are indicated.

NIS EXPRESSION IN THYROID CANCER

Given that most thyroid cancers exhibit decreased or absent radioiodide accumulation, the prevailing expectation for a long time was that NIS expression would be found to be decreased or absent in cancerous thyrocytes. The first investigations addressing this issue, carried out using RT-PCR and showing lower mRNA levels in cancerous than in normal thyrocytes, seemed to confirm these expectations (24–28). RT-PCR is an easy-to-perform and very effective technique to detect mRNA expression even in very small tissue samples. However, determinations of mRNA levels by either RT-PCR or

Northern blot analysis provide no information on RNA stability. In addition, mRNA levels of proteins like NIS, with long half-lives and complex posttranscriptional regulation, do not necessarily correlate with actual protein expression (29). Immunoblot analyses to directly assess protein expression would address this limitation; however, this requires significantly larger tissue samples, which are not often available from human specimens.

Immunoblot analyses may provide satisfactory quantitative and qualitative information on NIS protein expression and some posttranslational modifications, but not on subcellular distribution. The subcellular localization of NIS is particularly significant because, as pointed out earlier, NIS is functional *only* when it is properly targeted to the plasma membrane. Hence, immunohistochemical analysis of NIS expression in thyroid cancer was carried out (20, 30, 31). In addition to revealing the subcellular distribution of NIS, immunohistochemistry offers the advantage that NIS protein expression in the carcinomatous tissue can be compared to the surrounding normal tissue in the same thyroid gland. Surprisingly, immunohistochemical studies of NIS protein expression in thyroid cancer have shown that as many as 70% of thyroid cancers actually exhibit NIS protein overexpression (Figure 2B), as compared to the surrounding normal tissue, although in these cancerous cells NIS is mainly located in intracellular membrane compartments rather than in the plasma membrane. NIS was absent only in about 30% of the cases (20, 31). Thus far, no NIS mutations resulting in impaired protein expression or altered plasma membrane trafficking have been identified in thyroid cancer (32). These findings have had a significant impact on research approaches aiming to improve the effectiveness of radioiodide therapy, since they emphasize the importance of stimulating NIS targeting to and/or retention at the plasma membrane rather than stimulating NIS expression at the transcriptional level.

UNDERSTANDING NIS REGULATION IN HEALTH AND DISEASE MAY IMPROVE THE EFFECTIVENESS OF RADIOIODIDE TREATMENT

TSH and I^- are the two main factors that regulate NIS expression: TSH stimulates and I^- decreases it. Hence, TSH stimulation and I^- depletion of residual thyroid carcinoma tissue are the two most important modulators routinely used to optimize radioiodide treatment. To achieve maximum therapeutic effect, thyroidectomized patients must have TSH levels above 30 mU/l and must have been on a low I^- diet for two weeks prior to initiation of radioiodide treatment (1).

TSH has long been known to be a key regulator not only of NIS expression but also of thyroidal I^- uptake (i.e., NIS activity). No thyroidal NIS expression is observed in hypophysectomized rats (because of the lack of TSH), but thyroidal NIS expression is restored as early as 24 h after treatment with TSH. In intact (i.e., non-hypophysectomized) rats, treatment with the I^- organification inhibitor propylthiouracil causes elevated TSH levels, which in turn lead to higher NIS expression than in control animals (10). TSH regulates NIS expression at both the transcriptional and posttranscriptional levels. Several groups have demonstrated that TSH upregulates I^- transport by a cAMP-mediated increase in NIS transcription, while withdrawing TSH causes decreased cAMP levels and diminished NIS transcription (33).

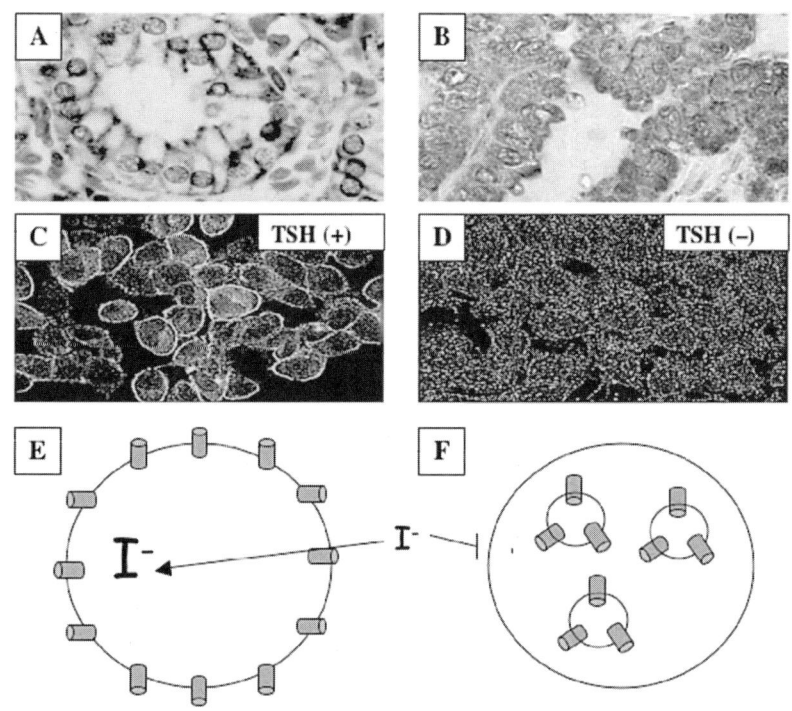

Figure 2. A: NIS immunohistochemistry in Graves' disease. NIS is localized in the basolateral plasmamembrane **B**: NIS immunohistochemistry in follicular carcinoma shows the intracellular localization of the significantly overexpressed NIS protein **C**: Indirect immunofluorescence analysis of NIS localized in the plasma membrane of FRTL-5 cells kept in the presence of TSH, **D**: intracellular NIS localization in TSH deprived FRTL-5 cells **E**: schematic representation of NIS plasma membrane localization and iodide transport in FRTL-5 cells kept in the presence of TSH **F**: schematic representation of NIS localized in the intracellular membrane compartments in TSH deprived FRTL-5 cells, resulting in lack of iodide transport.

The detailed analysis of the rat and human NIS promoters has confirmed the significant role of Pax8 in NIS expression (34–36). In rat, the proximal NIS promoter was found to contain a TTF1 binding site and a TSH-responsive element where a putative transcription factor NTF-1 (NIS TSH-responsive factor 1) interacts (39). NIS upstream enhancer (NUE-2495 to -2260) contains two Pax-8 binding sites and a degenerate CRE (cAMP-responsive element sequence), which are essential for full TSH cAMP-dependent transcription of NIS (34). Interestingly, during chronic TSH stimulation when the catalytic subunit of PKA is downregulated, cAMP is still able to stimulate NIS transcription, indicating the existence of both PKA-dependent and independent mechanisms (34). Recently, a thyroid-specific far-upstream (−9847 to −8968) enhancer in the human NIS gene – highly homologous to the rat NUE – has been reported. It contains putative Pax-8 and TTF-1 binding sites and a CRE-like sequence. The TTF-1 binding site is not required for full activity (35, 36).

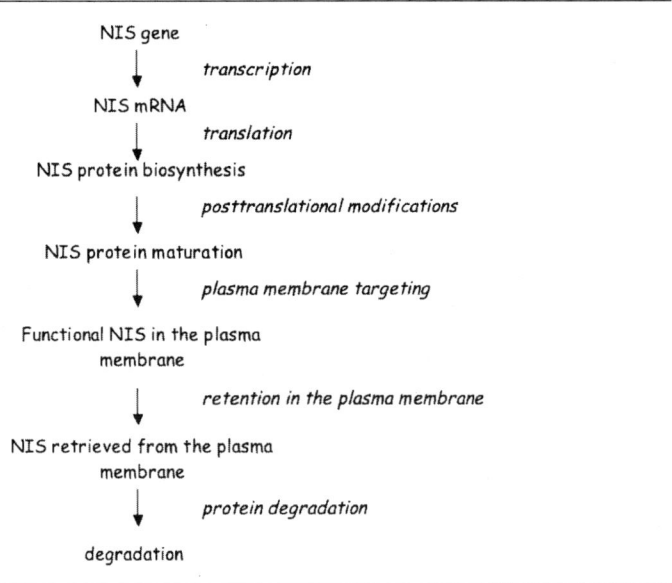

Figure 3. Multiple levels of NIS regulation.

FRTL-5 cells are rat-thyroid-derived, well-differentiated normal thyroid epithelial cells that grow in media supplemented with TSH. These cells are frequently used as an *in vitro* model system to study TSH regulation. In FRTL-5 cells, NIS expression is TSH dependent. Kaminsky *et al.* (37) observed that, in the absence of TSH in the medium, intact FRTL-5 cells did not transport I$^-$, whereas membrane vesicles prepared from the same TSH-deprived cells surprisingly maintained their I$^-$ transporting ability. This suggested that mechanisms other than transcriptional might also operate in regulating NIS activity in response to TSH. Riedel *et al.* (22) investigated this phenomenon in detail. They observed that in the absence of TSH, there was no *de novo* NIS synthesis in FRTL-5 cells, while previously synthesized NIS was redistributed from the plasma membrane to intracellular membrane compartments. (Figure 2 C,D,E,F) These authors also demonstrated that NIS has a long half-life: 5 days in the presence and 3 days in the absence of TSH. Considering the TSH regulation of NIS expression and the long half-life of NIS, it is clear that NIS mRNA levels alone are not a good indicator of actual NIS protein levels. Instead, NIS protein levels must be assessed directly with anti-NIS Abs. In addition, it is also essential to keep in mind that NIS protein expression, in turn, does not necessarily correlate with NIS activity, because such factors as subcellular distribution of NIS to the plasma membrane play a key role in NIS function; hence, it is crucial to quantitate NIS activity (Figure 3).

TSH modulates NIS phosphorylation

The mechanism by which TSH regulates the subcellular distribution of NIS is unknown. Phosphorylation has been shown to be implicated in the activation and subcellular distribution of several transporters (38–40). NIS has several consensus sites for kinases, including those for cAMP-dependent protein kinase, protein kinase C, and casein kinase-2 (9, 22). Furthermore, TSH actions in the thyroid are mainly mediated by cAMP. All these points raised the possibility that phosphorylation might be involved in the regulation of NIS subcellular distribution. When FRTL-5 cells were labeled with ^{32}Pi, lysed, and immunoprecipitated with anti-NIS Ab, it was observed in the autoradiogram that NIS was phosphorylated, independently of the presence of TSH in the culture medium (22). The phosphopeptide map obtained after NIS digestion with trypsin was markedly different when TSH was present from that when TSH was absent (22).

The predominant phosphorylated region of NIS was determined by treatment of the immunoprecipitated symporter with CNBr. CNBr cleaves polypeptides at methionine residues. The anti-NIS Ab generated against the last 16 amino acids of NIS recognized an 11-kDa polypeptide observed also by autoradiography. The densitometric quantitation of the autoradiogram indicated that the major phosphorylation region of NIS is the carboxy terminus (22). Moreover, TSH increased the phosphorylation level of the COOH terminus of NIS ~16-fold. For the identification of which of the serine residues within the COOH terminus are phosphorylated, S551, S552, S568, and S581 (Fig. 1) were replaced individually and simultaneously with alanine. Significantly, the replacement of the four serines of the COOH terminus promoted phosphorylation of threonines in NIS, suggesting that there is an important biological pressure to preserve phosphorylation of NIS at the COOH terminus (22). Future experiments should elucidate whether NIS phosphorylation is involved in trafficking and/or retention of NIS at the plasma membrane.

Regulation of NIS expression by I$^-$

As indicated above, I$^-$ itself, the substrate of NIS, also regulates NIS expression, but the mechanism of this regulation is less clear than that of TSH. For over 60 years, it has been known that I$^-$ organification and, consequently, thyroid hormone biosynthesis, are blocked when the intracellular concentration of I$^-$ rises to a certain threshold. This phenomenon (i.e., the inhibition of I$^-$ organification by a high concentration of I$^-$) is called the Wolff-Chaikoff effect, and it has been used to block thyroid function in hyperthyroid patients (41, 42). I$^-$ also suppresses I$^-$ transport in a time- and dose-dependent manner, an effect that has been investigated by several groups both *in vitro* and *in vivo* (43–45). As I$^-$ transport decreases, the intrathyroidal I$^-$ concentration falls, the inhibition of organification is relieved, and thyroid hormone synthesis resumes; thus, by downregulating its own I$^-$ transport, the thyroid "escapes" from the inhibitory effect of I$^-$ overload. Grollmann *et al* (45) investigated the effect of I$^-$ preincubation on I$^-$ uptake in FRTL-5 cells, and found that I$^-$ preincubation of these cells suppresses I$^-$ uptake in a dose- and time-dependent manner. These authors observed decreased I$^-$ transport after a 2-h incubation with 100 μM of NaI (45)

With the availability of the NIS cDNA and anti-NIS Abs, the inhibitory effect of I$^-$ on its own transport in the thyroid has been partially reinvestigated by several groups. In dog, Uytterspot *et al* (46) found that I$^-$ inhibited both TPO and NIS mRNA expression, but no protein levels were measured. In FRTL-5 cells, Spitzweg et al (47) and Eng et al (48) published somewhat contradictory results. Spitzweg et al (47) reported a 50% decrease in I^- uptake. However, in these uptake studies, the specific activity of the radioactive I^- used in the transport measurements was diluted out by preincubation with unlabeled I^-, which results in its intracellular accumulation. Without taking this factor into account, the interpretation of these findings is uncertain. These authors also reported a decrease in NIS mRNA levels, but did not determine NIS protein. In contrast, Eng et al. (48) did not find decreased NIS mRNA levels after I^- preincubation. Instead, they found that both the levels and the half-life of the NIS protein were significantly decreased. Hence, Eng et al. (48) concluded that I^- regulates its own transport in FRTL-5 cells mostly by posttranscriptional mechanisms. Surprisingly, the same authors found that both NIS mRNA and protein levels were decreased *in vivo* in response to the administration of I^- (49). Evidently, a thorough molecular examination of the regulatory effect of I^- on I^- transport simultaneously assessing NIS expression, subcellular localization, and kinetic properties is required to understand the intriguing role of I^- in its own transport.

Effect of spatial organization of thyroid cells

It is clear from earlier studies that the spatial organization and apical-basolateral polarization of thyroid epithelial cells significantly influence their functions, including I^- transport, I^- organification, and protein expression. Roger et al (50) isolated human thyroid epithelial cells from normal subjects and grew the cells in the presence or absence of serum. They observed that, whereas cells grown in the presence of serum formed monolayers, in the absence of serum the cells formed aggregates. Following TSH stimulation, cells in aggregates exhibited more avid I^- transport than cells in monolayers. Interestingly, this TSH stimulatory effect was abolished by the addition of serum to the medium. Takasu et al (51) showed that, in porcine thyroid cells, polarity is important for I^- uptake, and a follicular structure is required for I^- organification. Kogai et al (52) have recently reinvestigated the effect of spatial organization of thyrocytes on NIS expression and function. They showed that TSH upregulates both NIS mRNA and protein levels in 2- and 3-dimensional human thyrocyte primary cultures, but a significant increase in I^- uptake occurs only in 3-dimensional structures.

SPECIFIC CONSIDERATIONS RELATED TO RADIOIODIDE TREATMENT

A prerequisite for the success of radioiodide treatment is the retention of the radioisotope for a sufficiently long time so the necessary dose is delivered to destroy the malignant tissue. The retention time of radioiodide in thyrocytes is determined by I^- uptake and I^- efflux. At steady-state conditions, I^- accumulation reflects the equilibrium between the rates of influx and efflux (Figure 4).

In the healthy thyroid gland, NIS mediates the active accumulation of I^-, whereas the mechanisms involved in I^- efflux are poorly understood (see "I^- efflux: pendrin and AIT" below). I^- organification – i.e., the TPO-mediated iodination of the tyrosine residues on the thyroglobulin molecule – occurs on the colloidal surface of the apical membrane. Iodinated thyroglobulin molecules remain in the colloid, surrounded

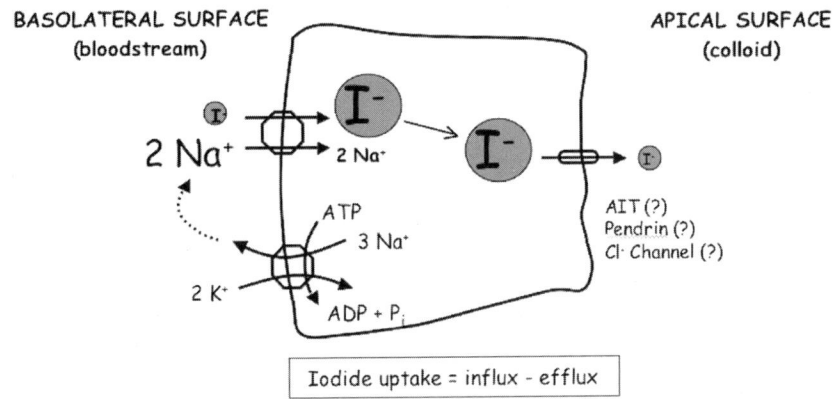

Figure 4. Determinants of iodide accumulation.

by the thyroid epithelial cells, thus increasing the radioiodide retention time in the thyroid gland. In contrast, in thyroid cancer, the typical follicular architecture of normal thyroid tissue is not conserved, as the malignantly transformed epithelial cells lose their polarity (53). Hence, these cells display no well-defined colloidal space, and as a result, thyroglobulin leaks out into the extracellular space and the bloodstream. Most differentiated thyroid cancers exhibit TPO protein expression, but at levels lower than those considered normal (54–56); TPO gene mutations have also been reported in some differentiated thyroid carcinomas (57). Furthermore, earlier studies in humans showed impaired or absent I^- organification in thyroid cancer (58), underscoring the loss or reduction of organification in thyroid cancer.

More recently, the organification effect in radioiodide retention time has been assessed *in vivo* in non-NIS-expressing tumors into which both rat and human NIS have been introduced under the control of tissue-specific promoters. Since these tumors do not express TPO, they do not organify I^-. Cho et al (59) reported radioiodide retention time greater than 24 h in hNIS-expressing xenografted human glioma cells in rats, and observed a longer survival in animals with NIS-expressing tumors versus control animals with non-NIS-expressing tumors. Spitzweg et al (60) introduced NIS in a recombinant adenovirus into a human prostate carcinoma cell line under the regulation of the prostate specific antigen (PSA) promoter. They reported a retention time of 5.6+/−1.4 h in NIS-expressing prostate carcinoma xenografts in nude mice and a remarkable decrease (over 80%) of the size of these xenografts after a single ip injection of 3 mCi ^{131}I. Dingli and colleges (61), for their part, expressed NIS in a myeloma cell line using a transcriptionally targeted lentiviral vector, where the therapeutic or reporter gene is under the control of minimal immunoglobulin promoter and enhancer elements (immunoglobulin κ-light chain enhancer elements). These authors also investigated the so-called bystander effect. β-particles emitted during the decay of ^{131}I can travel a distance of 0.2–2.4 mm. Therefore, the isotope is capable of destroying "bystanding" non-NIS-expressing cells. Dingli et al. (61) also treated myeloma xenografts containing variable numbers of radioiodide-transporting, NIS- and non-NIS-transduced tumor cells. The result was striking: all tumors in which 50–100% of the cells expressed NIS had completely regressed two weeks after a single dose of 1 mCi ^{131}I.

The above results provide strong evidence against the widely held notion that radioiodide therapy is likely to be ineffective in non-thyroidal cells that, while functionally expressing NIS (whether endogenously or by targeted transfection), lack the ability to organify I$^-$. The reasoning was that the absence of organification resulted in the isotope not being retained in the cells for a sufficiently long time. Yet, in the mentioned studies (59, 61, 62), radioiodide treatment was effective even in the *absence* of I$^-$ organification.

If organification is not essential for radioiodide therapy to be effective, sufficient iodide uptake mediated by NIS and slow I$^-$ efflux are the requirements for successful radioiodide therapy.

I$^-$ efflux: pendrin and AIT

Several groups have tried to identify the mediator of apical I$^-$ efflux in thyroid epithelial cells. Two recently cloned molecules are the main candidates: pendrin and the apical iodide transporter (AIT) (Figure 1).

In 1997, a gene defective in Pendred syndrome (PDS) was identified by positional cloning (63). Pendred syndrome is characterized by sensorineural (most often prelingual) deafness and goiter with defective organification. In PDS, goiter can develop at any age or may be absent, whereas deafness is generally present (63). Pendrin has been localized on the apical membrane of the thyroid epithelial cells by immunohistochemistry (64). In heterologous expression systems, pendrin has been shown to transport iodide, chloride, formate, and nitrate (65).

The organification defect characteristic of Pendred syndrome was attributed to defective pendrin-mediated apical I$^-$ transport into the colloid, where organification occurs (Figure 1). Surprisingly, although the recently generated Pds knockout mice are completely deaf, they do not exhibit a pathologic thyroidal phenotype (66); therefore, pendrin's function as the apical I$^-$ transporter remains to be further investigated.

By means of a PCR cloning strategy based on NIS-sequence homologies, a 610-amino-acid protein-coding gene was recently cloned from a human kidney cDNA library. The newly identified protein shares both a strikingly high identity (46%) and similarity (70%) to hNIS (67). This protein, called the human apical iodide transporter (hAIT), has been localized to the apical membrane of thyroid epithelial cells; however, a thorough molecular and kinetic characterization is required to unequivocally establish whether hAIT mediates "downhill" movements of I$^-$ from the cytosol to the colloid.

AIT (SLC5A8) expression in thyroid carcinomas has not yet been investigated. Interestingly, Li et al (68) found, while screening hypermethylated sequences in colon carcinoma cell lines and human colon carcinoma tissues, that the hAIT gene is heavily methylated and hAIT mRNA expression is decreased or absent. Reintroducing AIT into colon cancer cell lines harboring methylated endogenous AIT suppressed their ability to form colonies in soft agar and xenograft tumors in athymic mice. Based on their observations, the authors suggested that AIT could play a role as a tumor suppressor in colon cancer (68).

STUNNING

Stunning is the decrease in radioiodide uptake in thyroid tissue caused by previous exposure of the tissue to a tracer dose of the radioisotope for dosimetry. Stunning was first described almost 50 years ago (69), and since then, several clinical studies have been carried out to investigate its deleterious effect on radioiodide therapy. Before treatment with radioiodide, patients usually undergo diagnostic and dosimetric studies. After administering a tracer dose of radioiodide, the percentage of radioiodide uptake in the tumor tissue is determined and used as a basis to calculate the appropriate therapeutic dose. However, stunning is often observed, so that the percentage of radioiodide uptake measured upon administration of the therapeutic dose is significantly lower than that when the tracer dose was first administered for dosimetry. It is hypothesized that stunning is caused by radiation damage to the cells from the previously administered tracer dose. When stunning occurs, the delivered radioiodide therapeutic dose is insufficient for successful ablation of the malignant tissue (70). While most studies have investigated stunning *in vivo* during the treatment of patients (71), Postgard et al (72) recently reported an *in vitro* study revealing more about the possible mechanism of ^{131}I stunning. These investigators used porcine thyroid cell primary cultures grown on a filter in a bicameral chamber. The apical and basolateral media were separated by the cells assembled into a monolayer. Thyroid cells kept in TSH- and methimazole-supplemented medium were exposed to different amounts of ^{131}I. Stable iodide (10 nM) was administered to control cells. Transepithelial ^{125}I transport (from the basal to the apical membrane) was evaluated after a 3-day washout period. Iodide transport decreased 50% with a 3-Gy absorbed dose, and it was almost completely inhibited with an 80-Gy dose. The transepithelial electrical resistance of the cell monolayer was unchanged, showing that the integrity of the epithelial monolayer remained intact. The presence of perchlorate – the competitive inhibitor of I^- transport – during ^{131}I incubation, partially prevented the reduction of ^{125}I transport. Considering that there was no cell damage from radiation exposure and that the same amount of stable iodide had no effect on transport, these authors concluded that decreased I^- transport after ^{131}I exposure was most probably the result of a direct effect of radiation on thyroid function.

IMPROVING I^- TRANSPORT IN THYROID CANCER

To achieve an optimal therapeutic effect with maximum radioiodide uptake in thyroid carcinoma metastases, TSH has to be above 30 mU/l in thyroidectomized patients, who must be on a low iodide diet for two weeks prior to treatment (1, 73).

Radioiodide uptake in thyroid cancer could be increased by stimulation of NIS activity. Experimental therapies aiming at restoring NIS function in thyroid cancer have concentrated only on increasing NIS transcription. However, as mentioned earlier, TSH and I$^-$ are the main regulators of NIS expression and plasma membrane targeting; therefore, high TSH and low I$^-$ levels are optimal for upregulating NIS expression and cell surface targeting. Clearly, elucidation of the mechanisms involved in NIS targeting to and retention at the plasma membrane may result in novel therapies for thyroid cancer treatment, since NIS is overexpressed in 70% of thyroid cancers but not properly targeted to the plasma membrane (20).

Several groups have attempted to induce NIS transcription in non-NIS-expressing thyroid carcinoma cell lines. Transcriptionally inactive promoter regions often contain hypermethylated CpG rich regions (5-methylcytidine immediately followed by guanidine). These methylated sites of the DNA were found to bind specifically to histone-deacetylase complexes. The N-terminal lysines of unacetylated histones are positively charged and interact with DNA phosphates preventing the binding of transcription factors. When the positive charge of the N-terminus is neutralized via acetylation of the lysines, their electrostatic interaction with the DNA is disrupted, making the binding of transcription factors to the DNA possible. Therefore, inhibiting histone deacetylase activity and/or demethylating CpG-rich promoter regions would initiate transcriptional activity.

As the hNIS promoter has CpG-rich regions, Venkataraman et al. (74) hypothesized that hypermethylation of the hNIS promoter resulting in transcriptional failure could be responsible for decreased or absent NIS expression. These authors were able to restore hNIS mRNA expression in 4 out of 7 cell lines using 5-azacytidine and sodium butyrate treatment. The increase in NIS mRNA transcritpion correlated with demethylation of the untranslated region in the first exon of the hNIS gene. They also investigated NIS mRNA expression by Northern blot and methylation status of the hNIS promoter in proximity to the TATA box in human thyroid tumors. NIS mRNA expression was observed in 16 out of 22 carcinomas, including papillary, follicular, and anaplastic subtypes. These findings suggest that, in these cases, posttranscriptional mechanisms are probably responsible for decreased I$^-$ uptake. In the six non-NIS-mRNA-expressing papillary carcinomas, the hNIS promoter was strongly methylated.

Kitazono et al. (75) reported increased NIS mRNA expression detected by Northern blot and quantitative RT-PCR in four human thyroid carcinoma cell lines (two follicular and two anaplastic) *in vitro* after treatment with depsipeptide, a histone deacetylase inhibitor. This increase in NIS mRNA expression was accompanied by an increase in I$^-$ uptake.

Zarnegar et al. (76) used another histone-deacetylase inhibitor, trichostatin, in papillary, Hurthle, and follicular carcinoma-derived cell lines, and found increased NIS mRNA expression by quantitative PCR. NIS protein levels and I$^-$ uptake activity were not determined.

Other investigators have tried to achieve redifferentiation of thyroid cancer cells with *trans*-retinoic acid (tRa) treatment in thyroid carcinomas to restore radioiodide uptake. Schmutzler et al (77) were able to upregulate NIS mRNA expression by growing follicular thyroid carcinoma-derived cell lines in media supplemented with 1 μM tRa for one week, but no effect was observed on either protein expression or I$^-$ uptake ability. Surprisingly, the same treatment decreased I$^-$ uptake activity in the highly differentiated FRTL-5 cell line (78).

CONCLUDING REMARKS

The role of thyroidal I$^-$ transport in the treatment of thyroid cancer is difficult to overestimate. For over 60 years, the administration of radioiodide to thyroid cancer patients after thyroidectomy has been the most effective internal targeted anticancer radiotherapy available, on account of the unique specificity of NIS. Radioiodide therapy is not only effective and specific, it is also remarkably free of severe side effects. This article shows how, upon isolation of the NIS cDNA and the characterization of the NIS molecule, considerable strides have been made in our understanding of NIS regulation at all levels, including biosynthesis, biogenesis, half-life, targeting, and subcellular localization. These advances considerably increase our potential ability to manipulate the system to optimize the effectiveness of radioiodide treatment. In addition, the discovery that NIS is expressed endogenously in breast cancer has raised, for the first time, the realistic prospect of effectively applying radioiodide therapy in extrathyroidal cancers that express NIS endogenously. Finally, recent studies on the transfer of the NIS gene to cancers that otherwise lack endogenous NIS expression, have opened the door to the possible use of radioiodide therapy in these cancers as well.

ACKNOWLEDGMENTS

Research in our laboratory is supported by the National Institutes of Health: grants R01-DK41544 and R01-CA098390.

REFERENCES

1. Mazzaferri EL 2000 Thyroid diseases: tumors. Radioiodine and other treatment and outcomes. In: Braverman LE, Utiger, R.D. (ed) Werner & Ingbar's The Thyroid, Eight Edition, 2000 ed. Lipincott Williams & Wilkins, pp 904–930.
2. Seidlin SM, Marinelli, L.D., Oshry, E. 1946 Radioactive iodine thearpy. Journal of the American Medical Association Dec 7, 1946.
3. Mazzaferri EL, Jhiang SM 1994 Long-term impact of initial surgical and medical therapy on papillary and follicular thyroid cancer. Am J Med 97:418–28.
4. Dai G, Levy O, Carrasco N 1996 Cloning and characterization of the thyroid iodide transporter. Nature 379:458–60.
5. Smanik PA, Liu Q, Furminger TL, et al. 1996 Cloning of the human sodium Iodide symporter. Biochem Biophys Res Commun 226:339–45.
6. Selmi-Ruby S, Watrin C, Trouttet-Masson S, et al. 2003 The porcine sodium/iodide symporter gene exhibits an uncommon expression pattern related to the use of alternative splice sites not present in the human or murine species. Endocrinology 144:1074–85.
7. Pinke LA, Dean DS, Bergert ER, Spitzweg C, Dutton CM, Morris JC 2001 Cloning of the mouse sodium iodide symporter. Thyroid 11:935–9.
8. Tazebay UH, Wapnir IL, Levy O, et al. 2000 The mammary gland iodide transporter is expressed during lactation and in breast cancer. Nat Med 6:871–8.
9. Dohan O, De la Vieja A, Paroder V, et al. 2003 The sodium/iodide Symporter (NIS): characterization, regulation, and medical significance. Endocr Rev 24:48–77.

10. Levy O, Dai G, Riedel C, et al. 1997 Characterization of the thyroid Na+/I- symporter with an anti-COOH terminus antibody. Proc Natl Acad Sci U S A 94:5568–73.
11. Paire A, Bernier-Valentin F, Selmi-Ruby S, Rousset B 1997 Characterization of the rat thyroid iodide transporter using anti-peptide antibodies. Relationship between its expression and activity. J Biol Chem 272:18245–9.
12. De La Vieja A, Dohan O, Levy O, Carrasco N 2000 Molecular analysis of the sodium/iodide symporter: impact on thyroid and extrathyroid pathophysiology. Physiol Rev 80:1083–105.
13. Riedel C, Dohan O, De la Vieja A, Ginter CS, Carrasco N 2001 Journey of the iodide transporter NIS: from its molecular identification to its clinical role in cancer. Trends Biochem Sci 26:490–6.
14. Spitzweg C, Harrington KJ, Pinke LA, Vile RG, Morris JC 2001 Clinical review 132: The sodium iodide symporter and its potential role in cancer therapy. J Clin Endocrinol Metab 86:3327–35.
15. Carrasco N 1993 Iodide transport in the thyroid gland. Biochim Biophys Acta 1154:65–82.
16. Wolff J 1998 Perchlorate and the thyroid gland. Pharmacol Rev 50:89–105.
17. Yoshida A, Sasaki N, Mori A, et al. 1997 Different electrophysiological character of I-, ClO4-, and SCN- in the transport by Na+/I- symporter. Biochem Biophys Res Commun 231:731–4.
18. Yoshida A, Sasaki N, Mori A, et al. 1998 Differences in the electrophysiological response to I- and the inhibitory anions SCN- and ClO-4, studied in FRTL-5 cells. Biochim Biophys Acta 1414:231–7.
19. Eskandari S, Loo DD, Dai G, Levy O, Wright EM, Carrasco N 1997 Thyroid Na+/I- symporter. Mechanism, stoichiometry, and specificity. J Biol Chem 272:27230–8.
20. Dohan O, Baloch Z, Banrevi Z, Livolsi V, Carrasco N 2001 Rapid communication: predominant intracellular overexpression of the Na(+)/I(-) symporter (NIS) in a large sampling of thyroid cancer cases. J Clin Endocrinol Metab 86:2697–700.
21. Levy O, De la Vieja A, Ginter CS, Riedel C, Dai G, Carrasco N 1998 N-linked glycosylation of the thyroid Na+/I- symporter (NIS). Implications for its secondary structure model. J Biol Chem 273:22657–63.
22. Riedel C, Levy O, Carrasco N 2001 Post-transcriptional regulation of the sodium/iodide symporter by thyrotropin. J Biol Chem 276:21458–63.
23. Dohan O, Ginter, Ch., Carrasco, N. Oligonerization of the Na^+/I^- symporter. In preparation.
24. Lin JD, Chan EC, Chao TC, et al. 2000 Expression of sodium iodide symporter in metastatic and follicular human thyroid tissues. Ann Oncol 11:625–9.
25. Ringel MD, Anderson J, Souza SL, et al. 2001 Expression of the sodium iodide symporter and thyroglobulin genes are reduced in papillary thyroid cancer. Mod Pathol 14:289–96.
26. Lin JD, Hsueh C, Chao TC, Weng HF 2001 Expression of sodium iodide symporter in benign and malignant human thyroid tissues. Endocr Pathol 12:15–21.
27. Arturi F, Russo D, Schlumberger M, et al. 1998 Iodide symporter gene expression in human thyroid tumors. J Clin Endocrinol Metab 83:2493–6.
28. Lazar V, Bidart JM, Caillou B, et al. 1999 Expression of the Na+/I- symporter gene in human thyroid tumors: a comparison study with other thyroid-specific genes. J Clin Endocrinol Metab 84:3228–34.
29. Cazzola M, Skoda RC 2000 Translational pathophysiology: a novel molecular mechanism of human disease. Blood 95:3280–8.
30. Saito T, Endo T, Kawaguchi A, et al. 1998 Increased expression of the sodium/iodide symporter in papillary thyroid carcinomas. J Clin Invest 101:1296–300.
31. Wapnir IL, van de Rijn M, Nowels K, et al. 2003 Immunohistochemical profile of the sodium/iodide symporter in thyroid, breast, and other carcinomas using high density tissue microarrays and conventional sections. J Clin Endocrinol Metab 88:1880–8.
32. Russo D, Manole D, Arturi F, et al. 2001 Absence of sodium/iodide symporter gene mutations in differentiated human thyroid carcinomas. Thyroid 11:37–9.
33. Kogai T, Endo T, Saito T, Miyazaki A, Kawaguchi A, Onaya T 1997 Regulation by thyroid-stimulating hormone of sodium/iodide symporter gene expression and protein levels in FRTL-5 cells. Endocrinology 138:2227–32.
34. Ohno M, Zannini M, Levy O, Carrasco N, di Lauro R 1999 The paired-domain transcription factor Pax8 binds to the upstream enhancer of the rat sodium/iodide symporter gene and participates in both thyroid-specific and cyclic-AMP-dependent transcription. Mol Cell Biol 19:2051–60.
35. Taki K, Kogai T, Kanamoto Y, Hershman JM, Brent GA 2002 A thyroid-specific far-upstream enhancer in the human sodium/iodide symporter gene requires Pax-8 binding and cyclic adenosine $3',5'$-monophosphate response element-like sequence binding proteins for full activity and is differentially regulated in normal and thyroid cancer cells. Mol Endocrinol 16:2266–82.

36. Schmitt TL, Espinoza CR, Loos U 2002 Characterization of a thyroid-specific and cyclic adenosine monophosphate-responsive enhancer far upstream from the human sodium iodide symporter gene. Thyroid 12:273–9.
37. Kaminsky SM, Levy O, Salvador C, Dai G, Carrasco N 1994 Na(+)-I- symport activity is present in membrane vesicles from thyrotropin-deprived non-I(-)-transporting cultured thyroid cells. Proc Natl Acad Sci U S A 91:3789–93.
38. Glavy JS, Wu SM, Wang PJ, Orr GA, Wolkoff AW 2000 Down-regulation by extracellular ATP of rat hepatocyte organic anion transport is mediated by serine phosphorylation of oatp1. J Biol Chem 275:1479–84.
39. Krantz DE, Waites C, Oorschot V, et al. 2000 A phosphorylation site regulates sorting of the vesicular acetylcholine transporter to dense core vesicles. J Cell Biol 149:379–96.
40. Ramamoorthy S, Blakely RD 1999 Phosphorylation and sequestration of serotonin transporters differentially modulated by psychostimulants. Science 285:763–6.
41. Plummer H, S. 1923 Results of administering iodine to patients having exophthalmic goiter. JAMA 80:1955.
42. Wolff J, Chaikoff, I.,L. 1948 Plasma inorganic iodide as a homeostatic regulator of thyroid function. Journal of Biological Chemistry 174:555–564.
43. Braverman LE, Ingbar, S.H. 1963 Changes in thyroidal function during adaptation to large doses of iodide. Journal of Clinical Investigations 42:1216–1231.
44. Panneels V, Van Sande J, Van den Bergen H, et al. 1994 Inhibition of human thyroid adenylyl cyclase by 2-iodoaldehydes. Mol Cell Endocrinol 106:41–50.
45. Grollman EF, Smolar A, Ommaya A, Tombaccini D, Santisteban P 1986 Iodine suppression of iodide uptake in FRTL-5 thyroid cells. Endocrinology 118:2477–82.
46. Uyttersprot N, Pelgrims N, Carrasco N, et al. 1997 Moderate doses of iodide in vivo inhibit cell proliferation and the expression of thyroperoxidase and Na+/I- symporter mRNAs in dog thyroid. Mol Cell Endocrinol 131:195–203.
47. Spitzweg C, Joba W, Morris JC, Heufelder AE 1999 Regulation of sodium iodide symporter gene expression in FRTL-5 rat thyroid cells. Thyroid 9:821–30.
48. Eng PH, Cardona GR, Previti MC, Chin WW, Braverman LE 2001 Regulation of the sodium iodide symporter by iodide in FRTL-5 cells. Eur J Endocrinol 144:139–44.
49. Eng PH, Cardona GR, Fang SL, et al. 1999 Escape from the acute Wolff-Chaikoff effect is associated with a decrease in thyroid sodium/iodide symporter messenger ribonucleic acid and protein. Endocrinology 140:3404–10
50. Roger P, Taton M, Van Sande J, Dumont JE 1988 Mitogenic effects of thyrotropin and adenosine 3′,5′-monophosphate in differentiated normal human thyroid cells in vitro. J Clin Endocrinol Metab 66:1158–65.
51. Takasu N, Ohno S, Komiya I, Yamada T 1992 Requirements of follicle structure for thyroid hormone synthesis; cytoskeletons and iodine metabolism in polarized monolayer cells on collagen gel and in double layered, follicle-forming cells. Endocrinology 131:1143–8.
52. Kogai T, Curcio F, Hyman S, Cornford EM, Brent GA, Hershman JM 2000 Induction of follicle formation in long-term cultured normal human thyroid cells treated with thyrotropin stimulates iodide uptake but not sodium/iodide symporter messenger RNA and protein expression. J Endocrinol 167:125–35.
53. Fitzgerald PJ, Foote, F.W. 1949 The function of of various types of thyroid carcinoma as revealed by the radioautographic demonstration of of radioactive iodine. J. Clin. Endocrinol. 9:1153–1170.
54. De Micco C, Kopp F, Vassko V, Grino M 2000 In situ hybridization and immunohistochemistry study of thyroid peroxidase expression in thyroid tumors. Thyroid 10:109–15.
55. Czarnocka B, Pastuszko D, Janota-Bzowski M, et al. 2001 Is there loss or qualitative changes in the expression of thyroid peroxidase protein in thyroid epithelial cancer? Br J Cancer 85:875–80.
56. Christensen L, Blichert-Toft M, Brandt M, et al. 2000 Thyroperoxidase (TPO) immunostaining of the solitary cold thyroid nodule. Clin Endocrinol (Oxf) 53:161–9.
57. Smanik PA, Fithian LJ, Jhiang SM 1994 Thyroid peroxidase expression and DNA polymorphisms in thyroid cancer. Biochem Biophys Res Commun 198:948–54.
58. Valenta L 1966 Metastatic thyroid carcinoma in man concentrating iodine without organification. J Clin Endocrinol Metab 26:1317–24.
59. Cho JY 2002 A transporter gene (sodium iodide symporter) for dual purposes in gene therapy: imaging and therapy. Curr Gene Ther 2:393–402.

60. Spitzweg C, O'Connor MK, Bergert ER, Tindall DJ, Young CY, Morris JC 2000 Treatment of prostate cancer by radioiodine therapy after tissue-specific expression of the sodium iodide symporter. Cancer Res 60:6526–30.
61. Dingli D, Diaz RM, Bergert ER, O'Connor MK, Morris JC, Russell SJ 2003 Genetically targeted radiotherapy for multiple myeloma. Blood 102:489–96.
62. Spitzweg C, Dietz AB, O'Connor MK, et al. 2001 In vivo sodium iodide symporter gene therapy of prostate cancer. Gene Ther 8:1524–31.
63. Everett LA, Glaser B, Beck JC, et al. 1997 Pendred syndrome is caused by mutations in a putative sulphate transporter gene (PDS). Nat Genet 17:411–22.
64. Mian C, Lacroix L, Alzieu L, et al. 2001 Sodium iodide symporter and pendrin expression in human thyroid tissues. Thyroid 11:825–30.
65. Scott DA, Wang R, Kreman TM, et al. 2000 Functional differences of the PDS gene product are associated with phenotypic variation in patients with Pendred syndrome and non-syndromic hearing loss (DFNB4). Hum Mol Genet 9:1709–15.
66. Everett LA, Belyantseva IA, Noben-Trauth K, et al. 2001 Targeted disruption of mouse Pds provides insight about the inner-ear defects encountered in Pendred syndrome. Hum Mol Genet 10:153–61.
67. Rodriguez AM, Perron B, Lacroix L, et al. 2002 Identification and characterization of a putative human iodide transporter located at the apical membrane of thyrocytes. J Clin Endocrinol Metab 87:3500–3.
68. Li H, Myeroff L, Smiraglia D, et al. 2003 SLC5A8, a sodium transporter, is a tumor suppressor gene silenced by methylation in human colon aberrant crypt foci and cancers. Proc Natl Acad Sci USA 100:8412–7.
69. Rawson RW 1965 Physiological considerations in the management of thyroid cancer. Nucl Med (Stuttg):Suppl 2:319+.
70. Koch W, Knesewitsch P, Tatsch K, Hahn K 2003 [Stunning effects in radioiodine therapy of thyroid carcinoma: existence, clinical effects and ways out]. Nuklearmedizin 42:10–4.
71. Yeung HW, Humm JL, Larson SM 2000 Radioiodine uptake in thyroid remnants during therapy after tracer dosimetry. J Nucl Med 41:1082–5.
72. Postgard P, Himmelman J, Lindencrona U, et al. 2002 Stunning of iodide transport by (131)I irradiation in cultured thyroid epithelial cells. J Nucl Med 43:828–34.
73. Robbins RJ, Tuttle RM, Sonenberg M, et al. 2001 Radioiodine ablation of thyroid remnants after preparation with recombinant human thyrotropin. Thyroid 11:865–9.
74. Venkataraman GM, Yatin M, Marcinek R, Ain KB 1999 Restoration of iodide uptake in dedifferentiated thyroid carcinoma: relationship to human Na+/I-symporter gene methylation status. J Clin Endocrinol Metab 84:2449–57.
75. Kitazono M, Robey R, Zhan Z, et al. 2001 Low concentrations of the histone deacetylase inhibitor, depsipeptide (FR901228), increase expression of the Na(+)/I(-) symporter and iodine accumulation in poorly differentiated thyroid carcinoma cells. J Clin Endocrinol Metab 86:3430–5.
76. Zarnegar R, Brunaud L, Kanauchi H, et al. 2002 Increasing the effectiveness of radioactive iodine therapy in the treatment of thyroid cancer using Trichostatin A, a histone deacetylase inhibitor. Surgery 132:984–90; discussion 990.
77. Schmutzler C, Winzer R, Meissner-Weigl J, Kohrle J 1997 Retinoic acid increases sodium/iodide symporter mRNA levels in human thyroid cancer cell lines and suppresses expression of functional symporter in nontransformed FRTL-5 rat thyroid cells. Biochem Biophys Res Commun 240:832–8.
78. Schmutzler C, Kohrle J 2000 Retinoic acid redifferentiation therapy for thyroid cancer. Thyroid 10:393–406.

14. MOLECULAR SIGNALING IN THYROID CANCER

NICHOLAS J. SARLIS* AND SALVATORE BENVENGA**

*Department of Endocrine Neoplasia & Hormonal Disorders, The University of Texas – M. D. Anderson Cancer Center, Houston, Texas 77082, USA
**Sezione di Endocrinologia, Dipartimento Clinico Sperimentale di Medicina e Farmacologia
& Programma di Endocrinologia Molecolare Clinica, University of Messina, Messina, I-98151, Italy

INTRODUCTION

Molecular signaling – or signal transduction – is central to our understanding of the core biological processes in any type of cancer. Defining the responses of cancerous cells to environmental and endogenous signals, and comparing them to those exhibited by their counterpart normal parental cells can provide valuable insight into the intimate mechanisms underlying malignancy formation, progression, invasion and spread to distant sites (metastasis). Further, detailed knowledge of cancer cell signaling allows us to envisage molecular strategies, upon which novel anticancer therapies will be founded. Ideally, within the context of a particular cancer, our understanding of where and how signal transduction pathways become deranged should enable us to design therapies targeted to the "diseased" elements of the relevant pathway(s). Moreover, the delineation of the evolution of such molecular derangements at each step along the oncogenic transformation process could provide us with the opportunity to intervene at early or intermediate stages of cancer development, i.e., prior to the emergence of irreversible genomic instability, which usually accompanies the transition of a microscopic (or *in situ*) malignancy to the phenotypes of invasive macroscopic carcinoma and metastatic disease (1). In many cases, alterations in molecular signaling in cancer cells are etiologically linked to the oncogenic process. Undoubtedly, the oncogenic potential of a molecule along a signaling pathway can be released through multiple genetic mechanisms (e.g., point mutation or over-/underexpression), ultimately leading to tumor formation. However, it is also true that a number of (qualitative or quantitative) changes in signaling pathway molecular elements could merely represent an epiphenomenon of the oncogenic process, and, hence, the potential significance of the existing descriptive data on such changes needs to be scrutinized carefully and with due circumspection.

All the above notions are highly relevant to thyroid cancer (TC). Indeed, during the past decade, a rapidly evolving body of knowledge has been accumulated on signaling pathways in TC, and their significance in its pathogenesis and progression. An excellent example of the complexity and interconnectedness of such pathways is the thyrotropin (TSH)-dependent signaling system. Although most of the elements of molecular signaling in TC cells are shared with those existing in normal thyrocytes, some are certainly unique to TC cells, such as protein products of fusion genes (*RET/PTC* and *Pax-8/PPARγ*, as presented in the Chapters 4 & 7 respectively. Additionally, other shared elements that are expressed in both normal and malignant thyroid tissues may be altered in specific ways (e.g., overexpressed or mutated) in malignant thyrocytes, a sound example being protein products of mutationally activated *ras* or *b-raf* genes, expanded upon in Chapter 7. Of note, as the thyroid follicular cell is an endocrine cell, it possesses a wide variety of "identity-specific" signaling systems, which are pertinent to the multitude of its endocrine functions and are correlated with its status of differentiation. Specific alterations in these endocrine function-related systems can accompany malignant transformation (e.g., loss of thyroglobulin [Tg] or sodium-iodide symporter [NIS] expression), and usually coexist with derangements in signaling pathways unrelated to the endocrine character of the cell, as commented upon in the contributions in Chapters 13 & 17.

In this chapter, we make an effort to present the currently accumulated knowledge in this important field by appropriately categorizing the various pathways studied to-date, and summarizing the molecular (known or suspected) derangements along these pathways. We will focus our contribution on carcinomas arising from the follicular epithelial cells (thyrocytes), i.e. papillary, follicular and anaplastic TC's (PTC's, FTC's and ATC's, respectively). Further, we will restrict our review to membrane receptor-associated signaling systems. Intracellular (including nuclear) receptor signaling is also an integral part of cell regulation, as recently highlighted by the role of the Pax-8/PPARγ oncoprotein in FTC's (see Chapter 4) and the presence of functional estrogen and thyroid hormone receptors in PTC's and FTC's (refer to Chapter 9), but we will not comment on this subject as it is exhaustively dealt with by other contributors.

In broad terms, signaling essentially begins with the signal molecule/ligand-sensing receptors, and is based on modulation of the activity of "downstream" pathways (or cascades) that are dependent upon the activation of the aforementioned receptors. In order to place some degree of conceptual order in an unwieldy body of data, we have attempted to categorize signaling in TC cells that occurs via activation of plasma membrane receptors and their downstram effector systems, i.e., (i) G-protein coupled receptors (GPCR's) and associated proteins and (ii) enzyme-coupled receptors and downstream pathway elements. Of note, although ion channels and various symporters (e.g., NIS) are expressed in TC, to-date, the only definitive demonstration of a functional ion channel-coupled membrane receptor signaling system pertains to the presence of muscarinic acetylcholine (calcium channel-coupled) receptors in immortalized, yet not truly malignant, thyroid cell lines (2, 3). Moreover, signal sensing and propagation in TC cells also occur through miscellaneous, not yet fully elucidated mechanisms, for example, those responsible for responses of thyrocytes to generic environmental cellular insults, such as hypoxia (4) or hydrogen peroxide/reactive oxygen species (5); additionally, it is believed that thyroglobulin (6, 7) or inorganic iodide (8) can initiate specific cellular effects. In this chapter, we will not comment on these mechanisms, the details of which remain unknown as of yet.

The major signaling systems operative in TC cells and their interrelationship with other important elements controlling thyrocyte growth, apoptosis, and differentiation are summarized schematically in Figure 1, shown at the end of the chapter.

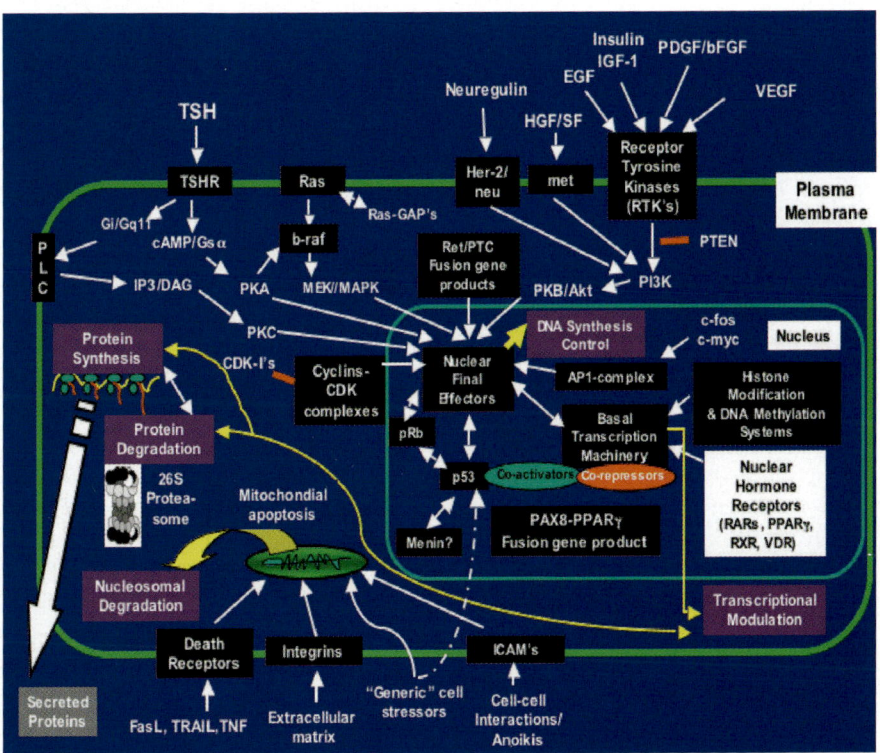

Figure 1. Membrane receptor-dependent signaling pathways involved in the regulation of thyrocyte growth, function, and differentiation. Cross-interacting circuits have been omitted for clarity purposes. Changes in specific elements of the above pathways are intimately associated with TC development, propagation, "aggressiveness", morphologic phenotype, and acquisition of metastatic potential. For more details, refer to the text. All abbreviations are defined in the text, as well as in the List of Abbreviations. Boxes of different colors designate functional categories of the various molecules or pathways.

ELEMENTS AND PATHWAYS OF MOLECULAR SIGNALING VIA PLASMA MEMBRANE RECEPTORS IN TC

G-protein coupled receptors (GPCR's) systems, associated proteins, and downstream effectors

TSH receptor (TSHR) and G-proteins

The *par excellence* thyroid-specific GPCR is the TSHR. It is a typical member of the GPCR family containing seven-transmembrane (TM) domain receptors, and transduces the signal of ambient TSH to the thyrocyte (9). Its ligand, TSH, upon binding onto TSHR activates thyroid function, proliferation and differentiation via activation of both G-protein- and inositol triphosphate (IP3)/phospholipase C (PLC)-dependent pathways.

The trophic role of the TSHR system is considered highly significant; in fact, suppression of endogenous pituitary TSH production by thyroid hormone treatment in patients with TC following thyroidectomy is considered standard therapy in this malignancy, leading to decreased morbidity and mortality, at least for well-differentiated TC's (as reviewed in [10]). TSH also possesses a lesser, inhibitory effect on TSHR signaling, as chronic stimulation of this system leads to down-regulation of TSHR expression (11). Additionally, TSH exposure can also desensitize TSHR-dependent signaling by activating a G-protein-coupled kinase (GRK), which phosphorylates TSHR (12). The phosphorylated TSHR then attracts arrestins, which are proteins inhibiting the G-protein dependent signaling cascade (see below) (13, 14). Of note, TSHR expression may be lost (or at least severely diminished) in some TC's; consequently, the growth of these tumors is not expected to be modulated by ambient TSH, i.e., in the clinical context, to respond to TSH-suppressive therapy with exogenous thyroid hormone (15). Although activating TSHR mutations represent the molecular basis of several autonomously functioning benign thyroid adenomas (reviewed in [16] and [17]), such mutations have only very rarely been reported in TC (18–20). Indeed, most authorities believe that TSHR-activating mutations play a minimal role in the development of TC (21, 22). Transfection of TSHR in cell lines derived from ATC's -and consequently transplanted in nude mice- has led to decreased growth rate and tumor formation *vs.* wild type (non-transfected) cells (23), suggesting highly complex interactions of the TSHR signaling system with other pathways gorverning cell growth, apoptosis and differentiation in TC.

The TSHR is associated with submembranic proteins, the G-proteins, which are responsible for the downstream delivery of its signal. Each G-protein consists of an α–subunit and a $\beta\gamma$–subunit dimer. The predominant type of the α-subunit in thyrocytes is the $G_s\alpha$ variant. In the resting state, G-proteins bind guanosine diphosphate (GDP) via their α-subunit, while their three subunits α, β and γ are tightly bound in a trimer configuration. Upon binding of TSH on TSHR, GDP is dissociated from the α-subunit and replaced by GTP, thus leading to dissociation of the subunit from the β– and γ– subunits, and the formation of an active α–subunit. The latter binds to "downstream" effectors and modulates their action, primarily activating adenylyl cyclase (AC), leading to cyclic adenosine $3',5'$-monophosphate (cyclic AMP or cAMP) production (see below). The subunit possesses intrinsic GTPase activity, hydrolyzing bound GTP to GDP, thus, rendering itself inactive. In that state, the α–subunit is able to re-associate with the β– and γ–subunits, rendering the conformation of the αβγ complex to its "baseline" inactive state, and, thus, terminating the action of the ligand (TSH) (24). Other submembranic moieties, such as the RGS proteins (Regulators of G-protein Signaling), are capable of accelerating the hydrolysis of GTP to GDP, also enhancing the kinetics of termination of the hormone signal (25). Hyperactivity of $G_s\alpha$ can ensue from mutations at either of two "hot spots", i.e. residues Arg201 or Gln227. In a functional sense, these are inactivating mutations, as they abrogate the enzymatic GTPase function or alter the affinity for GTP/GDP, the final result being "locking" the G-protein in its GTP-bound active conformation. At this point, G_s becomes an oncogene or *gsp* (*G-s*timulatory *p*rotein).

$G_s\alpha$ mutations have been described in some autonomously functioning thyroid benign adenomas (26), but seem to be extremely rare in TC (27). The above observations are corroborated by the fact that the thyroid manifestations of McCune-Albright syndrome, a sporadic genetic disease caused by a post-zygotic activating mutation of the $G_s\alpha$ gene (28), classically have included benign thyroid neoplasms (mainly follicular adenomas), and not TC (29). Interestingly, however, clear-cell TC has been recently described in a single case of a patient with McCune-Albright syndrome. In this patient's tumor, malignant thyrocytes enriched for the mutant allele for $G_s\alpha$ (30, 31). Furthermore, in transgenic mouse models, sustained activation of the TSHR/G_s pathway generated by expression of mutant $G_s\alpha$ (32), cholera toxin (33), or a G_s-coupled A2 adenosine receptor (34) caused thyrocyte hyperplasia and hyperfunction, but not cancer, suggesting that this pathway alone is not sufficient to cause malignant transformation.

In addition to stimulation of $G_s\alpha$, TSHR activation also induces stimulation of G_i, as demonstrated by TSH-dependent inhibition of AC in certain *in vitro* systems. This inhibition partially opposes the stimulation of AC through $G_s\alpha$, and can be relieved by pertussis toxin (35). Activation of the G_i/G_0 system via stimulation of the P2-purinergic receptor by extracellular adenosine triphosphate (ATP) in thyroid FRTL-5 cells induces activation of phospholipase A_2 (PLA_2) (36). PLA_2 hydrolyzes the *sn*-2 ester bond of cellular phospholipids, producing a free fatty acid and a lysophospholipid, both of which are lipid signaling molecules. The activation of this signaling pathway is a point of "cross-talk" with pathways activated by mitogens and growth factors (see below). The free fatty acid produced is frequently arachidonic acid (AA, i.e., 5,8,11,14-eicosatetraenoic acid), the precursor of the eicosanoid family that includes prostaglandins, thromboxanes, leukotrienes and lipoxins (reviewed in [37]). It remains unknown whether this G-protein-dependent PLA_2 activation is operative in TC cells. Moreover, TC cells express in variable amounts prostaglandin-endoperoxide H synthase-2 (38), the enzyme responsible for the generation of prostaglandin H2 (PGH2) by arachidonic acid. Of note, PGH2 and its metabolite thromboxane A2 (TXA2) has been implicated in cancer progression and emergence of metastatic potential in assorted malignancies (39). With regard to the role of other G-proteins in thyroid oncogenesis, although it was initially suggested that neither G_q nor G_{11} played a critical role in TC development (40), subsequent studies showed that a novel $G_{q/11}$-coupled receptor, the metastin receptor, is overexpressed in PTC, and activates the mitogen-activated protein kinase (MAPK) in the ATC-derived cell line ARO. Of note, metastin signaling does not involve Akt/protein kinase B (PKB) (41). No data exist on the role in TC development of other G-proteins to which the TSHR couples, such as G_{12}, or G_{13} (42).

Finally, proteins known as arrestins have been shown to exert potent regulatory control upon GPCR-dependent signaling, usually inducing termination of G-protein activation. Thus, changes in their expression level or activity can have profound effects upon TSHR signaling (43). The amount of β-arrestin-2 was found to be increased in hyperfunctioning ("hot") thyroid nodules, but decreased in hypofunctioning ("cold") thyroid nodules, as compared to the neighboring perinodular, normal-appearing tissue (44). For more details on other regulators of the intrathyrocyte cAMP levels within the context of the complex TSHR-dependent signaling system, we refer the reader to two recently published excellent reviews on this subject (45, 46).

Adenylyl cyclase, protein kinase A, and CREB

As alluded to above, TSHR signaling eventually leads to AC activation and production of cAMP. A subset of TC's has been shown to manifest increased AC activity. Earlier studies had shown that this phenomenon was not due to an increase in the number or affinity of the TSHR's (47), but to quantitatively greater amount of G-proteins in TC cells (48). Of interest, the exact opposite phenomenon has been observed in a subgroup of TC's, i.e. decrease in the cAMP production capacity of the malignant *vs.* normal thyrocytes, probably due to defective "coupling" of the TSHR to the G-protein in these tumors (49). Along the TSHR-dependent cascade, cAMP activates protein kinase A (PKA).

PKA belongs to a large family of proteins, whose members are heterotetramers, consisting of two regulatory (R-) subunits and two catalytic (C-) subunits. When the protein is in the fully complexed configuration (i.e., exists as the tetramer), it is inactive. Binding of cAMP to the R-subunits causes dissociation of the C-subunits. Once liberated from the inhibition of the R-subunits, the catalytic sites on the two dissociated C-subunits phosphorylate serine and threonine residues of various acceptor proteins, both in the cytoplasm and the nucleus. In the nucleus, the acceptor proteins are transcription factors, able to modulate the rate of DNA transcription of cAMP-responsive genes (50) (see below). Moreover, several PKA variants are themselves able to translocate to the nucleus, in order to exert their actions. Because there are four R-subunit isoforms (RI, RI, RII, RII), and three C-subunit isoforms (α, gβ, and γ), assorted combinations of holoenzyme complexes with different functional properties exist, a feature that confers considerable complexity to the cAMP/PKA signaling system. Although there is paucity of activating mutations of PKA C-subunits in TC (51), inactivating mutations of the PKA RIα subunit gene, which – when they occur in the germline – are associated to a rare multiple neoplasia syndrome named Carney complex (52), has been identified in a subgroup of TC's (53). It is believed that in these malignancies, the PKA RIαgene (*PRKAR1A*) seems to be functioning as a tumor suppressor.

In turn, TSH is also able to control the magnitude of its own signal along this pathway, by increasing the activity of the cyclic nucleotide phosphodiesterases (54, 55), as well as the expression level of certain PKA-anchoring proteins on subcellular organelles (56), events which prevent nuclear entry of PKA (56).

In thyrocytes, PKA phosphorylates a number of substrates, including the p85 phosphoprotein, leading to enhancement of the interaction between phosphatidylinositol-3-phospokinase (or PI3 kinase, PI3K) and p21/Ras (see below). Simultaneously, cAMP can also inhibit Raf1 kinase signaling by decreasing Raf1 availability to Ras. Hence, under conditions of strong cAMP activation, it is believed that PI3K-dependent signaling is favored (57). In addition to the above moleculart interactions, activated PKA also phosphorylates other proteins with fundamentally important functions, such as CREB (*c*AMP-*R*esponsive *E*lement *B*inding protein). CREB is a nuclear transcription factor that belongs to the large family of leucine zipper (b-ZIP) DNA binding proteins. CREB binds to cAMP response elements (CRE's) on the promoter of cAMP-responsive genes. CREB expression is reduced in human "toxic" thyroid adenomas (58), but unchanged in non-functioning (scintigraphically "cold") thyroid adenomas, when compared to normal thyroid tissue (59). On the other hand, CREB expression is markedly downregulated in TC, but this decrease in the amount of CREB seems unrelated to the functional state of differentiation of the malignancy, as assessed by NIS expression levels (60). Additionally, PKA phosphorylates the following nuclear target substrates, which – of note – are all CREB analogues: inducible cAMP early repressor (ICER; a.k.a. *c*AMP-*R*esponsive *E*lement *M*odulator or CREM), and activating transcription factors (ATF)-1 and -3. (60). Phosphorylated CREB binds to a protein called CREB-binding protein (CBP), which in turn interacts with the transcription factor TFIIB to recruit RNA polymerase II onto the preinitiation complex, thus promoting transcription of defined genes (reviewed in [61]). Although PKA can also also directly phosphorylate nuclear transcription factors AP-2 and junD (62), the role of these PKA-dependent effectors in TC initiation and progression remains unknown to-date.

Finally, TSH-dependent cAMP accumulation can lead to phosphorylation of high mobility protein (HMG)-14, which is a nuclear factor associated with transcriptionally active chromatin, thus altering its interactions with nucleosomes (63). The role of HMG-14 on transcriptional regulation has been recently reviewed in (64).

Phospholipase C and protein kinase C

TSHR activation can also result in stimulation of pathways dependent on the γ-isoforms of phospholipase C (PLC-γ), via coupling of the receptor to members of the $G_{q/11}$ family (34). The level of plasma membrane PLC activity is increased in neoplastic thyroid tissue, with the level of increase correlating to the degree of tumoral de-differentiation (65). PLC stimulation results in hydrolysis of phosphatidylinositol 4,5-biphosphate (PIP$_2$), which generates IP$_3$ and diacylglycerol (DAG). IP$_3$ increases the concentration of intracellular ionized calcium (iCa^{++}) by favoring its release from the endoplasmic reticulum, while DAG activates protein kinase C (PKC). In turn, PKC, which under certain conditions can also activated directly by iCa^{++}, phosphorylates several target proteins (66). With regard to PKC itself, a naturally occurring inhibitor of the PCK isoenzyme PKCε has been found in one TC cell line (WRO), whereas transfection of normal thyroid cells with this inhibitor, generated a neoplastic phenotype (67). Moreover, a selective impairment in PKCε was noted in several human PTC's and FTC's (68). Both these observations seem to be consistent with a protective role of PKC against the development of TC. In general, activation of the PKA pathway in thyroid tissue antagonizes the PI3-iCa^{++}-PKC pathway. A pertinent example of this antagonism in TC cells is the differential effects of the activation of PKA vs. PKC on the expression of two transcription factor proto-oncogenes, namely c-fos and c-jun (69).

Miscellanea

There are at least another four TSH-independent G-protein-mediated signaling pathways that could be putatively active in TC. These signaling systems are progressively better characterized, and are dependent on the following receptors: the adrenergic receptor (AR), the P1-purinergic (adenosine) receptor, the endothelin (ET) receptor, and (possibly) the ghrelin receptor (GHS-R1a).

In more detail, the expression level β2-AR is increased in TC, in proportion to the extent of de-differentiation (70). The functional significance of the β-AR system in controlling TC growth remains unknown, although it has been suggested cAMP overproduction due to preferential activation of the β-AR vs. the TSHR system may lead in growth inhibition in selected TC cell lines (71). Normal thyroid tissue also expresses α1-AR and α2-AR (72, 73). Constitutive activation of α1B-AR in transgenic mice leads to TC development with invasive features, probably via simultaneous activation of AC and PLC (74).

Regarding the effects of adenosine on cAMP accumulation in thyroid cells, such effects have been shown in earlier studies (75) and have been subsequently verified (76). Further, transgenic mouse models of thyroid hypertrophy have been developed with targeted overexpression of the adenosine-A2a receptor (reviewed in [77]). The above notwithstanding, the exact role of the adenosine receptor signaling system in native human TC's remains unknown.

ET-1, a potent vasoconstrictor, mitogen, and infammation mediator, also has effects upon thyroid cells. These were initially thought to be independent of cAMP or cGMP generation, and were mainly expressed as an ET-1-dependent decrease in Tg production *in vitro* (78). More recent studies showed that ET-1, secreted by porcine thyrocytes, was acting in an autocrine manner to inhibit TSH-induced iodine metabolism (79). It is assumed that in TC the two major subtypes of ET receptors, i.e., ET_AR and ET_BR, are coupled to their cognate effector systems by several distinct types of G-proteins, as is the case in other malignancies (reviewed in [80]), although this issue has not been specifically addressed in TC systems. Very recently, ET-1 and ET_AR overexpression has been observed in TC, commensurate with a mitogenic role of ET-1 (81).

Ghrelin, the endogenous ligand for the growth hormone secretagogue-receptor (GHS-R1a) (82) is also present in minute amounts in normal fetal (yet not adult) thyroid tissue (83). Ghrelin protein and mRNA are present, in variable amounts, in both benign and malignant thyroid tumors. TC tissues expressed ghrelin binding sites, and ghrelin induced dose-dependent inhibition of growth in TC cell lines. Nevertheless, specific GHS-R1a expression has not been convincingly demonstrated in either benign or malignant thyroid tissues (84).

Finally, receptors for both glucagon (85), and vasoactive intestinal peptide (VIP) (receptor subtype VPAC-1) (86) have been identified in normal thyroid tissue, but (to-date) not in TC. At this point, there is a paucity of data regarding the expression of other neuropeptide receptors in either normal or neoplastic thyroid tissue.

Enzyme-coupled membrane receptor systems

Receptor-tyrosine kinases (RTK's) and downstream effectors

RTK's are membrane receptors that have intrinsic tyrosine kinase (TK) activity and, hence, can independently phosphorylate tyrosine residues. These receptors can phosphorylate downstream intracellular substrate proteins or can undergo autophosphorylation. These modifications can result in the provision of docking sides for a variety of SH2-domain – containing proteins, which then bind either onto to the phosphorylated RTK itself or phosphorylated downstream effectors (87). Downstream molecules along RTK-dependent pathways include the elements of the Ras – Mitogen-Activated Protein (MAP) kinase (MAPK) pathway, the PI3 kinase (PI3K)-protein kinase B (PKB)/Akt system, phospholipase C-γ (PLC-γ), and GTPase-activating proteins (GAP's) (Reviewed in [88]).

SIGNALING DEPENDENT ON RECEPTORS FOR INSULIN AND GROWTH FACTORS. Insulin and insulin-like growth factor-1 (IGF-1) acting via the IGF-1 receptor (IGF-1R) synergize with TSH to promote follicular cell growth (89). Several patterns of expression have been also reported for IGF-1-binding proteins (IGFBP)-1 and -4 in thyroid tumors, thus adding further layers of complexity in the IGF-1 signaling pathway in thyrocytes (90). Of note, recent studies in transgenic mouse models of TC have suggested an important role of IGFBP-3 and –5 in the development of benign thyroid nodules, possibly through paracrine mechanisms (91). IGF-1R's are overexpressed in well-differentiated PTC's, but not in poorly differentiated TC's or ATC's, whereas insulin receptors (IR's) are greatly overexpressed in all TC histologic types, with a trend for higher values in de-differentiated tumors. As a consequence of IR overexpression, high amounts of IR/IGF-1R hybrid receptors, which bind IGF-1 with high affinity, have been detected in TC (92). Further, a novel autocrine loop involving IGF-2 and the IR-A isoform has been reported recently (93). Recently, IGF-1 has been shown to increase the expression of vascular endothelial growth factor (VEGF) in TC cells, via both AP-1/ hypoxia inducible factor-1α (HIF-1α)- and PI3K-dependent mechanisms, with obvious implications on the role of IGF-1 in peritumoral angiogenesis (94).

Several other signal molecules (growth factors), such as basic fibroblast growth factor (bFGF) (95, 96), VEGF (97), epidermal growth factor (EGF) (98, 99), and transforming growth factor-α (TGF-α) (100) have also been shown to stimulate thyroid epithelial growth, while nerve growth factor (NGF) (101) seems to inhibit such growth. EGF, well as phorbol esters, activate the PKC pathway, and may either stimulate thyrocyte growth or antagonize the effects of TSH, depending upon the system studied (99, 100). Although TC cells may rarely produce colony-stimulating factors (CSF) (102), to-date no cognate receptors for these factors (CSF-1R or FMS, the protein product of the *c-fms* proto-oncogene) have been identified in either normal or neoplastic thyroid tissue (103). Various reports have proposed the role of activating mutations, amplification or abnormal glycosylation patterns of assorted RTK's, including EGFR, various subtypes of NGFR, and platelet-derived growth factor receptor (PDGFR) in TC, which have been summarized in a recent review (104).

TC cells also express a variety of other RTK's, including c-erbB-2/HER-2/neu (104), FGFR-1 (or Flg) and FGFR-3 (105, 106), hepatocyte growth factor receptor (HGFR)/c-met (107), a spliced variant of c-ret (108), NTRK-1 (a.k.a. trkA, or p75/LNGFR) (109, 110), and VEGFR (existing in various subtypes and isoforms thereof, e.g. KDR, Flt-1, Flt-4, Tek, etc.) (111, 112). Specifically for the type-1 VEGFR (Flt-1), the level of its expression has been found to correlate with size in pediatric patients with PTC (113). With regard to HGFR expression, occult PTC's ("microcarcinomas") have been shown to overexpress this receptor, thus indicating that HGFR signaling may be involved in early stages of PTC formation (114), as well as also be associated with multicentricity, a common feature of PTC's (115). Interestingly, the level of HGFR expression was inversely correlated with the tendency of the tumors for angioinvasion (116), as well as risk for metastasis and clinical recurrence (117). Recently, the HGFR system has been shown to be universally and specifically active in PTC's, with STAT3 (rather than PI3K-dependent molecules) utilized preferentially as the intermediate effector molecule (118). Further, the levels of another RTK, KIT, the stem-cell factor receptor (SCFR, i.e., the protein product of the oncogene *c-kit*) (119) have been shown to be decreased in TC's, predating the decrease in thyroid-specific markers observed during de-differentiation (120, 121).

The progressive elucidation of the initial and intermediate steps along the RTK-dependent signal transduction pathways have led to the identification of the Grb2 adaptor molecule and Sos protein, a nucleotide exchange factor, as well as other downstream molecules, such as Shc, FRS-2, and insulin receptor substrate-1 (IRS-1) (122). These discoveries have led to new hypotheses on the tumorigenic potential of activating mutations of such molecules in TC, as well as their "cross-talk" with other oncoproteins, such as the RET/PTC molecules (123).

RAS AND THE MAPK KINASE/MAPK PATHWAY. Ligand-induced stimulation of RTK's results in the activation of the Ras—*M*itogen-*A*ctivated *P*rotein (MAP) kinase pathway, via modulation of Shc and Grb2/Sos (see above). Ras is the protein product of the *p21/ras* oncogene and has intrinsic GTPase activity. In its activated form, Ras is able to recruit other kinases to the cell membrane, where they are in turn activated themselves. This leads to transmission of the growth signal to the genome via nuclear transcription factors (reviewed in [124]). Indeed, Ras leads to activation of the Raf kinase family (including Raf-1 and B-raf), and subsequently the successive activation of MAPK kinase (MAPKK or *M*AP/*E*RK *K*inase [MEK]), MAPK (or *E*xtracellular signal-*R*egulated *K*inase [ERK]), and p90 *R*eceptor-activated *S*ignal *C*ascade *K*inase (p90/RSK) (reviewed in [125]). The latter intermediate enzymes ultimately transmit the growth signal to final nuclear effectors, which remain largely unknown, although MAPK activation has been shown to modulate the activity of the AP-1 complex (*c-fos/c-jun*), the *c-myc* gene (126), and members of the Ets family of transcription factors (127) in assorted (non-thyroid) cell systems.

The nuclear transcription factors/oncoproteins c-fos and c-myc do not seem to play a significant role in the initial stages of thyroid oncogenesis, as no mutations, deletions, rearrangement, or amplification involving these genes have been described to-date in TC (128, 129). The level of expression of c-fos seems to be increased in PTC's and FTC's (130). The oncogene *c-myc* is a reliable proliferative marker in a variety of neoplasms, hence, the level of its expression in TC has been positively correlated with the degree of tumor de-differentiation, as well as poor prognosis (130). The oncogene *ets-1* is also expressed in various types of TC in the context of both human tissue and cell lines (131). More recently, it has been shown that induction of ETS-1 and ETS-2 oncoproteins is required for thyroid cell transformation, and leads to modulation of *c-myc* activity (132).

Ras and selected RTK's can also lead to activation of p38/MAPK, a serine/threonine kinase responsible for the mediation of stress-activated cell responses, such as "generic" responses to ionizing radiation, ultraviolet light, heat, and osmotic shock (reviewed in [133]). Of note, the p38 MAPK kinase pathway can be activated by cytokines and other inflammatory mediators, although the isoenzymes involved are different than those pertinent to the Ras/RTK-induced activation. The final effectors of p38 MAPK signaling include ribosome protein S6 kinase-B (RSK-B), as well as nuclear proteins, such as CREB and ATF (134). The p38-α isoenzyme is expressed in normal thyroid tissue (135). Although activation of this isoenzyme though Ras, RTK's and cytokines is suspected in TC, it has not been demonstrated firmly. Interestingly, p38/MAPK is activated by TSHR in immortalized thyroid cells via a cAMP/PKA/Rac1 pathway (136).

The significance of the ras signaling pathway in TC is reviewed extensively herein in Chapter 7. We would just like to mention that downstream from ras are the Raf kinases, with main representatives being Raf-1 and b-Raf (the product of the *BRAF* gene). Very recently, mutations in the *BRAF* gene have been demonstrated as the most common genetic change in the tumors of adult patients with PTC. A single type of mutation was found, leading to mutation of the Val599 residue (137), and formation of the BRAF^{V599} oncoprotein. Additionally, BRAF mutations have been found in ATC's and poorly-differentiated variants of PTC's (thought to emanate from de-differentiation of pre-existing PTC's), but not in FTC's (of any histologic grade) or follicular adenomas (138). These recent findings indicate that *BRAF* activation may be one of the key determinants of the expression of the PTC phenotype.

SIGNALING DEPENDENT ON PHOSPHOLIPIDS AND OTHER LIPID MOIETIES. In addition to activation of the Ras-MAPK pathway, RTK's can also activate PI3K signaling, leading to the generation of D-3-phosphoinositides, such as phosphatidylinositol-3,4,5-trisphosphate (PIP3) (reviewed in [139]). A fact that renders the picture more complex is that PI3K can also be stimulated by both integrin-dependent cell adhesion and GPCR's (139); this type of PI3K activation has not been studied to-date in TC. D-3-phosphoinositides are able to recruit a subset of signaling proteins with pleckstrin homology domains (PHD's) to the submembranic space, where they are activated. Examples of such proteins include: Akt/Protein Kinase B (PKB), PDK1, intracellular protein tyrosine kinases (such as the members of the Tec family), GTP-binding "exchange factors" (such as Grp1 and Rac), and numerous Ras-associated adaptor proteins (such as GAB-1) (reviewed in [140]). Ultimately, these proteins initiate complex sets of events that control protein synthesis, actin polymerization, cell survival, and cell cycle entry.

In regards to the modulation of PI3K-dependent signaling, the following comments are pertinent: The *PTEN* (or *MMAC1/TEP1*) gene encodes a dual specificity phosphatase with high homology to tensin, which appears to function as a tumor suppressor in patients with Cowden disease (141). The latter is an inherited syndrome characterized by the development of a wide variety of malignancies and hamartomas of ectodermal, mesodermal, and endodermal origin. Patients with Cowden disease characteristically develop FTC's (142). *PTEN* appears to negatively control the PI3K signaling by dephosphorylating the D-3-position of phosphoinositides (143). The *PTEN* gene is inactivated in up to 10% of sporadic follicular neoplasms, including a similar proportion of sporadic FTC's (144). Based on the background presented above, inactivation of *PTEN* should lead to enhancement of PI3K signaling. Indeed, this is the case in Cowden disease. In the context of sporadic TC's, increased levels of phosphorylated total Akt were identified in FTC's, but not PTC's, when compared with normal tissue. Levels of Akt-1 and -2 proteins and Akt-2 mRNA were elevated only in FTC's. Additionally, in assorted TC cell lines, Akt-1,-2, and -3 proteins were expressed, total Akt was activated by insulin (via PI3K), and inhibition of PI3K activity reduced cell viability, suggesting that Akt activation may play a significant role in the etiopathogenesis and/or progression of TC (145). Interestingly, although overactivity of Akt (through constitutive myristoylation) leads to a definite growth advantage, it does not seem to be sufficient for the induction of thyrocyte de-differentiation (146).

Activation of the PI3K pathway results in putative second lipid messengers other than glycolipipids, i.e., sphingolipids. In assorted non-thyroidal malignancies, various growth factors can effectively induce sphingomyelinase activation, and subsequent sphingomyelin cleavage to yield ceramide and phosphocholine. In turn, these molecules can exert complex cellular actions (reviewed in [140] and [147]). In human TC cell lines, exogenous C2-ceramide was capable of activating *c-JUN* N-terminal Kinase (JNK), leading to apoptosis (148). More recently, lysophosphatidic acid, via binding to its cognate high-affinity receptor edg 4 (a GPCR), has been reported to promote growth in thyroid cell systems, in synergism with TSH. Significant overexpression of edg4 has been observed in both PTC's and FTC's *vs.* normal or goitrous thyroid tissue (149).

SIGNALING VIA FUSION ONCOPROTEINS WITH TK ACTIVITY. Although formally not a part of membrane-associated RTK systems, TC cells express specific intracellular fusion proteins that are produced in an aberrant fashion and possess TK activity. These are the protein products of the *RET/PTC* and *trk* oncogenes. The pathways dependent on these oncoproteins and their significance in TC are reviewed extensively in the Chapters 11 & 12, as well as in (150) and (151). Of note, activated RET/PTC and Trk proteins can interact with both Shc and Grb2 adaptor proteins, thus establishing "cross-talk" with RTK-dependent signaling cascades (152).

Tyrosine kinase (TK)-associated receptors (TKAR's) and downstream effectors

TKAR's represent a large family of receptors, which lack an intrinsic TK domain, but are able to activate various intracellular TK's following ligand binding, thus leading *indirectly* to the phosphorylation of downstream target substrates.

CYTOKINE SIGNALING AND THE JAK-STAT PATHWAY. The major TKAR-dependent systems pertinent to thyroid growth and differentiation are those related to cytokine signaling. This is a rapidly expanding field, but suffice it to say that an ever-increasing list of interleukins (IL's) is expressed or secreted by TC cells in *in vitro* systems (153–158), with their secretion being modulated by retinoids (159) or TSH (160) in selected cases. These immune peptides have important actions upon the regulation of cell cycle entry, induction of mitotic arrest in TC (161, 162), and modulation of TC cell responses to cytotoxic agents (163).

Activation of cytokine receptors leads to phosphorylation and activation of Janus kinases (Jak), usually via prior phosphorylation of the gp130 glycoprotein. Jak's subsequently phosphorylate and activate differentially members of the signal transducer and activator of transcription (STAT) proteins, eventually resulting in the regulation of transcription of specific genes, along a cascade known as the Jak-STAT pathway (reviewed in [164]).

Specifically for TC, IL-6 and its receptor (IL-6R) have been shown in less than 50% of PTC's studied (118). Interestingly, the downstream effector of the IL-6R system, STAT-3, seemed to be much better correlated with HGFR (MET) expression in these PTC's (118). At any rate, STAT-3 activation may be a great part of the mechanism relevant to the establishment of the specific morphologic phenotype in PTC's, as it is present in virtually 100% of these malignancies (118). Following activation by phosphorylation, STAT's translocate to the nucleus (165), where they can bind to three different classes of DNA sequences, IL-6-like cytokine response elements, interferon-activated sequences (GAS) and *sis*-inducible elements (SIE's) (166) on specifically targeted gene promoters.

TNF AND APOPTOSIS-RELATED MOLECULES. Closely related to TKAR's are the members of the tumor necrosis factor (TNF) receptor (TNFR) family. These heterotrimeric receptor systems are responsible for induction of apoptosis (or programmed cell death), and, hence, are also collectively known as "death receptors". Downstream effectors of the death receptor-dependent signaling cascades include the following (reviewed in [167] and [168]): (i). the adaptor molecules, which are interacting directly with the death receptors via pairs of molecular domains, known as the death domain (DD), death effector domain (DED), and caspase recruitment domain (CARD). Examples of adaptor molecules include: the Fas-associating death domain protein/mediator of receptor-induced toxicity-1 (FADD or MORT1), the TNFR1-associated death domain protein (TRADD), and the receptor-interacting protein (RIP). Activation of the adaptor molecules leads to subsequent conversion of the pro-enzyme of caspase-8 (a.k.a. FLICE) to its active form (see below). This pathway can be blocked by FLICE-inhibitory proteins (FLIP's); (ii). the caspases, a family of at least 14 *c*ysteinyl *a*spartate-specific prote*ases*, the prototypal members of which is the interleukin-1β-converting enzyme (ICE). Caspases constitute the common final pathway of all apoptotic signals, as they virtually dismantle the cell (leading to cell lysis); and (iii). the proteins of the Bcl-2 (for B-cell lymphoma leukemia-2) family. This family has diverse members that can have either pro-apoptotic or anti-apoptotic properties. Signaling through bcl-2 and other anti-apoptotic members of this protein family eventually involves inhibition of caspases, thus leading to promotion of cell survival (169).

The role of these receptor systems in apoptosis regulation in thyroid tissues has been recently reviewed exhaustively (94, 170). Without delving in depth, the following points are pertinent: TNF-α is detectable in PTC's, although its presence in normal thyrocytes remains debatable (171, 172). In addition, functional receptors for TNF-α have been shown in several TC cell lines (173). Activation of TNFR induces the activation of stress-activated protein kinase (SAPK) (a variant of p38-MAPK) (174), and c-*J*un *N*-terminal *k*inase (JNK) (175). Upon activation, JNK translocates to the nucleus and enhances the transcriptional activity of transcription factors, among which are c-jun and ATF-2 (176).

The significance of thyroidal TNFR-dependent signaling has been dwarfed recently by the crucial ability of death receptors other than the TNFR in controlling thyrocyte apoptosis. Indeed, one of these "death receptors", namely Fas (or CD95/Apo-1), seems to be of seminal importance in promoting apoptosis in assorted cell systems. The interaction of Fas with its ligand (FasL) initiates a number of processes along the pathway of cell death, via activation of caspases (177, 178). Whether normal thyrocytes constitutively express significant amounts of FasL remains controversial (179), while they have been shown not to express Fas (at least in the presence of ambient TSH) (180, 181). The identification of a possible Fas-FasL interaction in thyroid follicles during the development of Hashimoto thyroiditis, leading to thyrocyte apoptosis (179, 182), renders this system of immediate relevance for TC formation. In fact, apoptosis in TC could ensue either via infiltrating cytotoxic lymphocytes or as part of the natural course of rapidly growing tumors outstripping their growth resources. Induction of Fas expression in malignant thyrocytes can lead to their destruction via the coupling of Fas to either its constitutively expressed ligand *in situ* or FasL derived from cytotoxic lymphocytes in the vicinity of the malignant cells (183). FasL has been demonstrated in abundance in both PTC's and FTC's, and may help these cancers evade the immune system by eliminating Fas-sensitive tumor-infiltrating immunocytes. Additionally, FasL may have prognostic implications in PTC, as, when expressed in high levels, it is associated with a more aggressive phenotype in this subtype of TC (94, 184). Of note, recently it has been demonstrated that loss of FADD expression, along the Fas-dependent cascade, is strongly associated with TC development (185). Regarding other death receptors in TC, TNF-related apoptosis-inducing ligand (TRAIL/Apo2L), through cognate TRAIL receptors, has been proven to induce strong cytotoxicity in various TC cell lines (186).

With regard to the final effectors of death receptor signaling in TC, the following comments are of pertinence: Both Bcl-x (anti-apoptotic moiety) and Bax (pro-apoptotic moiety) have been detected with high frequence in FTC's. In these tumors, the levels of expression of Bax and Bcl-2 are inversely correlated with the degree of cellular dedifferentiation; the converse is true for Bcl-x (187, 188). In contrast, another study showed (paradoxically?) increased expression of Bcl-2 in ATC's, which are by definition undifferentiated malignancies, in which the level of pro-apoptotic moieties would have been expected to be low (189). Thus, the relationship of the expression the final effector molecules of the apoptotic pathways with the degree of TC differentiation has not been firmly established. The expression pattern and significance of other elements of the death receptor pathways in TC, including various caspases and mitochondrial effectors, remain largely unknown.

Serine-threonine kinase (STK) receptors and downstream effectors

The ligands for this group of receptors are members of the transforming growth factor-β (TGF-β) superfamily. The STK receptor-dependent signaling systems play a seminal role during embryonic development, but also participate in adult tissue homeostasis (reviewed in [190]). The expression of several members of this family of ligands, and their cognate receptors, has been identified in both normal and neoplastic thyroid tissues, including TGF-β (191–194), activin (191, 195), and bone morphogenetic proteins (BMP)'s (196).

STK receptors consist of a single TM domain, with STK activity within their intracellular part, which is activated upon receptor dimerization. Two types (I and II) of STK receptors have been described, the only known function of type II receptors being the activation of type I receptors via phosphorylation (reviewed in [197]). The "downstream" signal transduction cascade includes activation (via phosphorylation) of cytoplasmic SMAD proteins (SMAD-1 to -8), which then translocate to the cell nucleus and regulate the transcription of a variety of specific target genes (198). The STK receptor-dependent signaling system is under tight control by multiple other intracellular regulators, as this pathway is not only relevant to transduction of selected hormonal signals, but is also closely implicated in the initiation and promotion of tumorigenesis, as demonstrated *in vitro* for assorted malignancies (reviewed in [199]).

Specifically in TC, loss of the cell growth inhibition induced by TGF-β leads to loss of differentiated phenotype of thyrocytes *in vitro* (200, 201), while SMAD-2 expression is downregulated in FTC's, even in the presence of intact TGF-β receptors (192). In ATC-derived cell lines, despite the great degree of cell de-differentiation, all elements of the TGF-β-dependent signaling cascades have been demonstrated as intact. Nevertheless, in one of the cell lines studied, there was indication of a novel mechanism for TGF-β insensitivity, with escape from its growth inhibiting effects, despite maintainance of expression of TGFR and SMAD proteins (202). A very recent study showed maintenance of normal levels of SMAD-4 in cell lines derived from PTC, FTC and ATC, and upregulation of SMAD-7 in the ATC-derived cell line ARO (203). Regarding the mechanism of TGF-β-induced growth inhibition (eventually leading to apoptosis) in normal thyrocytes, it is believed that it involves reduction in the levels of p27/kip1 (a cyclin-dependent kinase [cdk] inhibitor). This reduction in p27/kip1 is overridden in malignant thyrocytes by NF-κB activation (204). Of note, p53 also modulates cellular responses to TGF-β in TC *in vitro* systems (205). Finally, TGF-β1 affected IGF-1-stimulated IRS-1 phosphorylation and its association with Grb2 protein, as well as decreased the activation of the adaptor protein CrkII and its association with the IGF-1R, actions that provide the basis for "cross-talk" between RTK- and STK-dependent signaling cascades in TC (206).

COMMENTARY

TC is one of the most well studied endocrine neoplasms at the molecular level. It also expresses a remarkable repertoire of ligands, cognate receptors, and downstream effectors, thus representing a "model malignancy" for the investigation of the molecular pathobiology of cancer cell signaling. In this chapter, we focused specifically on the description of the signal transducing receptors at the level of the cell membrane, their cognate ligands, the post-receptor downstream elements propagating the signal, as well as known or suspected "final effectors" of each pathway. We also presented in global terms the functional connections among various key molecules, as well as the current theories on the relevance of these signaling systems to TC formation, progression, and biological behavior. It is our belief that intimate knowledge of the elements of these systems and their interaction with other constituents of the cell proliferation machinery (cell cycle, protein synthesis and degradation, gene transcription) increases their potential as future targets for therapy, especially in the context of TC patients harbor disease currently refractory to standard treatment modalities.

ACKNOWLEDGMENTS

We wish to thank Dr. Steven I. Sherman, of the University of Texas – M. D. Anderson Cancer Center, Houston, Texas, and Dr. Derek LeRoith, of NIDDK, National Institutes of Health, Bethesda, Maryland, for their thorough review of the manuscript, as well as constructive comments and suggestions.

LIST OF ABBREVIATIONS

AA	arachidonic acid
AC	adenylyl cyclase
AR	adrenergic receptor
ATC	anaplastic thyroid carcinoma
ATF	activating transcription factor
ATP	adenosine triphosphate
bcl	B-cell lymphoma leukemia
BMP	bone morphogenetic proteins
b-ZIP	leucine zipper
cAMP	cyclic adenosine 3′,5′-monophosphate
CARD	caspase recruitment domain

CBP	CREB binding protein
cdk	cyclin-dependent kinase
CRE	cAMP response element
CREB	cAMP-responsive element binding protein
CREM	cAMP-responsive element modulator (a.k.a. ICER)
CSF	colony-stimulating factor
CSF-1R	CSF-1 receptor (the protein product of the *c-fms* proto-oncogene)
DAG	diacylglycerol
DED	death effector domain
DD	death domain
EGF	epidermal growth factor
EGFR	epithelial growth factor receptor
ET	endothelin
ETR	endothelin receptor
FADD	Fas-associating death domain protein (a.k.a. MORT-1)
FAP	familial adenomatous polyposis
FasL	Fas ligand
(b)FGF	basic fibroblast growth factor
FLIP	FLICE-inhibitory protein
FTC	follicular thyroid carcinoma
GAP	GTPase-activating protein
GAS	interferon-activated sequence
GDP	guanosine diphospate
GF	growth factor
GH	growth hormone
GHS-R1a	ghrelin receptor-1a
GPCR	G-protein coupled receptor
GRK	G-protein-coupled kinase
gsp	G-stimulatory protein
GTP	guanosine triphosphate
HIF-1α	hypoxia inducible factor-1α
HGFR	hepatocyte growth factor receptor (c-met product: MET)
HMG	high mobility protein
iCa^{++}	intracellular ionized calcium
ICE	interleukin-1 – converting enzyme
ICER	inducible cAMP early repressor (a.k.a. CREM)
IFN	interferon
IGF-1	insulin-like growth factor-1
IGF-1R	IGF-1 receptor
IGFBP	IGF-1 binding protein
IL	interleukin
IP3	inositol triphosphate
IR	insulin receptor
IRS	insulin receptor substrate

JAK	Janus kinase
MAPK	mitogen-activated protein kinase
MORT-1	mediator of receptor-induced toxicity-1 (a.k.a. FADD)
NGF	nerve growth factor
NGFR	NGF receptor
NIS	sodium-iodide symporter
PDGFR	platelet-derived growth factor receptor
PGH2	prostaglandin H2
PHD	pleckstrin homology domain
PI3K	phosphatidylinositol-3-phospokinase
PIP_2	phosphatidylinositol 4,5-biphosphate
PKA	protein kinase A
PKB	protein kinase B (AKT)
PKC	protein kinase C
PLA_2	phospholipase A_2
PLC	phospholipase C
PPAR	peroxisome proliferator-activated receptor
PTC	papillary thyroid carcinoma
RGS	regulators of G-protein signaling
RIP	receptor-interacting protein
RSK-B	ribosome protein S6 kinase-B
RTK	receptor tyrosine kinase
SAPK	stress-activated protein kinase
SCFR	stem cell factor receptor (c-kit product: KIT)
SIE	*sis*-inducible element
STAT	signal transducer and activator of transcription
STK	serine-threonine kinase
Tg	thyroglobulin
TGF	transforming growth factor
TC	thyroid cancer
TK	tyrosine kinase
TKAR	tyrosine kinase (TK)-associated receptor
TM	transmembrane
TNF	tumor necrosis factor
TNFR	tumor necrosis factor receptor
TRADD	TNFR1- associated death domain protein
TRAIL	TNF-related apoptosis-inducing ligand (a.k.a. Apo2L)
TSH	thyroid stimulating hormone (thyrotropin)
TSHR	TSH receptor
TK	tyrosine kinase
TXA2	thromboxane A2
VEGF	vascular endothelial growth factor
VIP	vasoactive intestinal peptide

REFERENCES

1. Usmani B.A. Genomic instability and metastatic progression. Pathobiology 1993; 61:109–16.
2. Jimenez E., Pavia J., Morell V., Martin E., Montiel M. Muscarinic receptor subtypes and calcium signaling in Fischer rat thyroid cells. Biochem Pharmacol 2001; 61:337–42.
3. Danowski J., Kmiec B.L. Histochemical and biochemical studies on the secretory mechanisms of some glands of guinea-pigs treated with histamine. Folia Histochem Cytobiol 2002; 40:213–4.
4. Kiang J.G., Wang X.D., Ding X.Z., Gist I.D., Smallridge R.C. Heat shock inhibits the hypoxia-induced effects on iodide uptake and signal transduction and enhances cell survival in rat thyroid FRTL-5 cells. Thyroid 1996; 6:475–83.
5. Karbownik M., Lewinski A. The role of oxidative stress in physiological and pathological processes in the thyroid gland; possible involvement in pineal-thyroid interactions. Neuroendocrinol Lett 2003; 24:293–303.
6. Suzuki K., Mori A., Lavaroni S., Ulianich L., Miyagi E., Saito J., Nakazato M., Pietrarelli M., Shafran N., Grassadonia A., Kim W.B., Consiglio E., Formisano S., Kohn L.D. Thyroglobulin regulates follicular function and heterogeneity by suppressing thyroid-specific gene expression. Biochimie 1999; 81:329–40.
7. Ulianich L., Suzuki K., Mori A., Nakazato M., Pietrarelli M., Goldsmith P., Pacifico F., Consiglio E., Formisano S., Kohn L.D. Follicular thyroglobulin (TG) suppression of thyroid-restricted genes involves the apical membrane asialoglycoprotein recepto and TG phosphorylation. J Biol Chem 1999; 274:25099–107.
8. Lewinski A., Pawlikowski M., Cardinali D.P. Thyroid growth-stimulating and growth-inhibiting factors. Biol Signals 1993; 2:313–51.
9. Kohn L.D., Shimura H., Shimura Y., Hidaka A., Giuliani C., Napolitano G., Ohmori M., Laglia G., Saji M. The thyrotropin receptor. Vitam Horm 1995; 50:287–384.
10. McGriff N.J., Csako G., Gourgiotis L., Lori C.G., Pucino F., Sarlis N.J. Effects of thyroid hormone suppression therapy on adverse clinical outcomes in thyroid cancer. Ann Med 2002; 34:554–64.
11. Lalli E., Sassone-Corsi P. Thyroid-stimulating hormone (TSH)-directed induction of the CREM gene in the thyroid gland participates in the long-term desensitization of the TSH receptor. Proc Natl Acad Sci U S A 1995; 92:9633–7.
12. Metaye T., Menet E., Guilhot J., Kraimps J.L. Expression and activity of G protein-coupled receptor kinases in differentiated thyroid carcinoma. J Clin Endocrinol Metab 2002; 87:3279–86.
13. Nagayama Y., Tanaka K., Hara T., Namba H., Yamashita S., Taniyama K., Niwa M. Involvement of G protein-coupled receptor kinase-5 in homologous desensitization of the thyrotropin receptor. J Biol Chem 1996; 271:10143–8.
14. Iacovelli L., Franchetti R., Masini M., De Blasi A. GRK2 and beta-arrestin 1 as negative regulators of thyrotropin receptor-stimulated response. Mol Endocrinol 1996; 10:1138–46.
15. Cai W.Y., Lukes Y.G., Burch H.B., Djuh Y.Y., Carr F., Wartofsky L., Rhooms P., D'Avis J., Baker J.R., Jr., Burman K.D. Analysis of human TSH receptor gene and RNA transcripts in patients with thyroid disorders. Autoimmunity 1992; 13:43–50.
16. Holzapfel H.P., Bergner B., Wonerow P., Paschke R. Expression of G(alpha)(s) proteins and TSH receptor signalling in hyperfunctioning thyroid nodules with TSH receptor mutations. Eur J Endocrinol 2002; 147:109–16.
17. Paschke R., Ludgate M. The thyrotropin receptor in thyroid diseases. N Engl J Med 1997; 337:1675–81.
18. Baloch Z., Livolsi V.A. Detection of an activating mutation of the thyrotropin receptor in a case of an autonomously hyperfunctioning thyroid insular carcinoma. J Clin Endocrinol Metab 1997; 82:3906–8.
19. Cetani F., Tonacchera M., Pinchera A., Barsacchi R., Basolo F., Miccoli P., Pacini F. Genetic analysis of the TSH receptor gene in differentiated human thyroid carcinomas. J Endocrinol Invest 1999; 22:273–8.
20. Russo D., Wong M.G., Costante G., Chiefari E., Treseler P.A., Arturi F., Filetti S., Clark O.H. A Val 677 activating mutation of the thyrotropin receptor in a Hurthle cell thyroid carcinoma associated with thyrotoxicosis. Thyroid 1999; 9:13–7.
21. Matsuo K., Friedman E., Gejman P.V., Fagin J.A. The thyrotropin receptor (TSH-R) is not an oncogene for thyroid tumors: structural studies of the TSH-R and the alpha-subunit of G_s in human thyroid neoplasms. J Clin Endocrinol Metab 1993; 76:1446–51.
22. Derwahl M., Broecker M., Kraiem Z. Clinical review 101: Thyrotropin may not be the dominant growth factor in benign and malignant thyroid tumors. J Clin Endocrinol Metab 1999; 84:829–34.

23. Gustavsson B., Hermansson A., Andersson A.C., Grimelius L., Bergh J., Westermark B., Heldin N.E. Decreased growth rate and tumour formation of human anaplastic thyroid carcinoma cells transfected with a human thyrotropin receptor cDNA in NMRI nude mice treated with propylthiouracil. Mol Cell Endocrinol 1996; 121:143–51.
24. Farfel Z., Bourne H.R., Iiri T. The expanding spectrum of G protein diseases. N Engl J Med 1999; 340:1012–20.
25. Hepler J.R. Emerging roles for RGS proteins in cell signalling. Trends Pharmacol Sci 1999; 20: 376–82.
26. Suarez H.G., du Villard J.A., Caillou B., Schlumberger M., Parmentier C., Monier R. gsp mutations in human thyroid tumours. Oncogene 1991; 6:677–9.
27. Hamacher C., Studer H., Zbaeren J., Schatz H., Derwahl M. Expression of functional stimulatory guanine nucleotide binding protein in nonfunctioning thyroid adenomas is not correlated to adenylate cyclase activity and growth of these tumors. J Clin Endocrinol Metab 1995; 80:1724–32.
28. Feuillan P.P. McCune-Albright syndrome. Curr Ther Endocrinol Metab 1997; 6:235–9.
29. Mastorakos G., Mitsiades N.S., Doufas A.G., Koutras D.A. Hyperthyroidism in McCune-Albright syndrome with a review of thyroid abnormalities sixty years after the first report. Thyroid 1997; 7:433–9.
30. Yang G.C., Yao J.L., Feiner H.D., Roses D.F., Kumar A., Mulder J.E. Lipid-rich follicular carcinoma of the thyroid in a patient with McCune-Albright syndrome. Mod Pathol 1999; 12:969–73.
31. Collins M.T., Sarlis N.J., Merino M.J., Monroe J., Crawford S.E., Krakoff J.A., Guthrie L.C., Bonat S., Robey P.G., Shenker A. Thyroid carcinoma in the McCune-Albright syndrome: contributory role of activating Gs alpha mutations. J Clin Endocrinol Metab 2003; 88:4413–7.
32. Michiels F.M., Caillou B., Talbot M., Dessarps-Freichey F., Maunoury M.T. Schlumberger M., Mercken L., Monier R., Feunteun J. Oncogenic potential of guanine nucleotide stimulatory factor alpha subunit in thyroid glands of transgenic mice. Proc Natl Acad Sci U S A 1994; 91:10488–92.
33. Zeiger M.A., Saji M., Gusev Y., Westra W.H., Takiyama Y., Dooley W.C., Kohn L.D., Levine M.A. Thyroid-specific expression of cholera toxin A1 subunit causes thyroid hyperplasia and hyperthyroidism in transgenic mice. Endocrinology 1997; 138:3133–40.
34. Coppee F., Gerard A.C., Denef J.F., Ledent C., Vassart G., Dumont J.E., Parmentier M. Early occurrence of metastatic differentiated thyroid carcinomas in transgenic mice expressing the A2a adenosine receptor gene and the human papillomavirus type 16 E7 oncogene. Oncogene 1996; 13:1471–82.
35. Allgeier A., Laugwitz K.L., Van Sande J., Schultz G., Dumont J.E. Multiple G-protein coupling of the dog thyrotropin receptor. Mol Cell Endocrinol 1997; 127:81–90.
36. Ekokoski E., Dugue B., Vainio M., Vainio P.J., Tornquist K. Extracellular ATP-mediated phospholipase A(2) activation in rat thyroid FRTL-5 cells: regulation by a G(i)/G(o) protein, Ca(2+), and mitogen-activated protein kinase. J Cell Physiol 2000; 183:155–62.
37. Balsinde J., Winstead M.V., Dennis E.A. Phospholipase A(2) regulation of arachidonic acid mobilization. FEBS Lett 2002; 531:2–6.
38. Smith T.J., Jennings T.A., Sciaky D., Cao H.J. Prostaglandin-endoperoxide H synthase-2 expression in human thyroid epithelium. Evidence for constitutive expression in vivo and in cultured KAT-50 cells. J Biol Chem 1999; 274:15622–32.
39. Rodrigues S., Nguyen Q.D., Faivre S., Bruyneel E., Thim L., Westley B., May F., Flatau G., Mareel M., Gespach C., Emami S. Activation of cellular invasion by trefoil peptides and src is mediated by cyclooxygenase- and thromboxane A2 receptor-dependent signaling pathways. FASEB J 2001; 15:1517–28.
40. Ringel M.D., Saji M., Schwindinger W.F., Segev D., Zeiger M.A., Levine M.A. Absence of activating mutations of the genes encoding the alpha-subunits of G11 and Gq in thyroid neoplasia. J Clin Endocrinol Metab 1998; 83:554–9.
41. Ringel M.D., Hardy E., Bernet V.J., Burch H.B., Schuppert F., Burman K.D., Saji M. Metastin receptor is overexpressed in papillary thyroid cancer and activates MAP kinase in thyroid cancer cells. J Clin Endocrinol Metab 2002; 87:2399..
42. Laugwitz K.L., Allgeier A., Offermanns S., Spicher K., Van Sande J., Dumont J.E., Schultz G. The human thyrotropin receptor: a heptahelical receptor capable of stimulating members of all four G protein families. Proc Natl Acad Sci U S A 1996; 93:116–20.
43. Luttrell L.M., Lefkowitz R.J. The role of beta-arrestins in the termination and transduction of G-protein-coupled receptor signals. J Cell Sci 2002; 115:455–65.
44. Voigt C., Holzapfel H., Paschke R. Expression of beta-arrestins in toxic and cold thyroid nodules. FEBS Lett 2000; 486:208–12.

45. Kimura T., Van Keymeulen A., Golstein J., Fusco A., Dumont J.E., Roger P.P. Regulation of thyroid cell proliferation by TSH and other factors: a critical evaluation of in vitro models. Endocr Rev 2001; 22:631–56.
46. Dremier S., Coulonval K., Perpete S., Vandeput F., Fortemaison N., Van Keymeulen A., Deleu S., Ledent C., Clement S., Schurmans S., Dumont J.E., Lamy F., Roger P.P., Maenhaut C. The role of cyclic AMP and its effect on protein kinase A in the mitogenic action of thyrotropin on the thyroid cell. Ann N Y Acad Sci 2002; 968:106–21.
47. Clark O.H. Gerend P.L. Thyrotropin regulation of adenylate cyclase activity in human thyroid neoplasms. Surgery 1985; 97:539–46.
48. Siperstein A.E., Miller R.A., Landis C., Bourne H., Clark O.H. Increased stimulatory G protein in neoplastic human thyroid tissues. Surgery 1991; 110:949–55.
49. Kimura H., Yamashita S., Namba H., Usa T., Fujiyama K., Tsuruta M., Yokoyama N., Izumi M., Nagataki S. Impairment of the TSH signal transduction system in human thyroid carcinoma cells. Exp Cell Res 1992; 203:402–6.
50. Sveshnikov P.G., Grozdova I.D., Nesterova M.V, Severin E.S. Protein kinase A: regulation and receptor-mediated delivery of antisense oligonucleotides and cytotoxic drugs. Ann NY Acad Sci 2002; 968:158–72.
51. Esapa C.T., Harris P.E. Mutation analysis of protein kinase A catalytic subunit in thyroid adenomas and pituitary tumours. Eur J Endocrinol 1999; 141:409–12.
52. Kirschner L.S., Carney J.A., Pack S.D., Taymans S.E., Giatzakis C., Cho Y.S., Cho-Chung Y.S., Stratakis C.A. Mutations of the gene encoding the protein kinase A type I-alpha regulatory subunit in patients with the Carney complex. Nat Genet 2000; 26:89–92.
53. Sandrini F., Matyakhina L., Sarlis N.J., Kirschner L.S., Farmakidis C., Gimm O., Stratakis C.A. Regulatory subunit type I-alpha of protein kinase A (PRKAR1A): a tumor-suppressor gene for sporadic thyroid cancer. Genes Chromosomes Cancer 2002; 35:182–92.
54. Grange M., Sette C., Cuomo M., Conti M., Lagarde M., Prigent A.F., Nemoz G. The cAMP-specific phosphodiesterase PDE4D3 is regulated by phosphatidic acid binding. Consequences for cAMP signaling pathway and characterization of a phosphatidic acid binding site. J Biol Chem 2000; 275:33379–87.
55. Sette C., Conti M. Phosphorylation and activation of a cAMP-specific phosphodiesterase by the cAMP-dependent protein kinase. Involvement of serine 54 in the enzyme activation. J Biol Chem 1996; 271:16526–34.
56. Scott J.D. A-kinase-anchoring proteins and cytoskeletal signalling events. Biochem Soc Trans 2003; 31:87–9.
57. Ciullo I., Diez-Roux G., Di Domenico M., Migliaccio A., Avvedimento E.V. cAMP signaling selectively influences Ras effectors pathways. Oncogene 2001; 20:1186–92.
58. Brunetti A., Chiefari E., Filetti S., Russo D. The 3′,5′-cyclic adenosine monophosphate response element binding protein (CREB) is functionally reduced in human toxic thyroid adenomas. Endocrinology 2000; 141:722–30.
59. Luciani P., Buci L., Conforti B., Tonacchera M., Agretti P., Elisei R., Vivaldi A., Cioppi F., Biliotti G., Manca G., Vitti P., Serio M., Peri A. Expression of cAMP response element-binding protein and sodium iodide symporter in benign non-functioning and malignant thyroid tumours. Eur J Endocrinol 2003; 148:579–86.
60. Rosenberg D., Groussin L., Jullian E., Perlemoine K., Bertagna X., Bertherat J. Role of the PKA-regulated transcription factor CREB in development and tumorigenesis of endocrine tissues. Ann N Y Acad Sci 2002; 968:65–74.
61. Goldman P.S., Tran V.K., Goodman R.H. The multifunctional role of the co-activator CBP in transcriptional regulation. Recent Prog Horm Res 1997; 52:103–20.
62. Montminy M. Transcriptional regulation by cyclic AMP. Annu Rev Biochem 1997; 66:807–22.
63. Spaulding S.W., Fucile N.W., Bofinger D.P., Sheflin L.G. Cyclic adenosine 3′,5′-monophosphate-dependent phosphorylation of HMG 14 inhibits its interactions with nucleosomes. Mol Endocrinol 1991; 5:42–50.
64. Bustin M., Trieschmann L., Postnikov Y.V. The HMG-14/-17 chromosomal protein family: architectural elements that enhance transcription from chromatin templates. Semin Cell Biol 1995; 6:247–55.
65. Kobayashi K., Shaver J.K., Liang W., Siperstein A.E., Duh Q.Y., Clark O.H. Increased phospholipase C activity in neoplastic thyroid membrane. Thyroid 1993; 3:25–9.
66. Osborne N.N., Tobin A.B., Ghazi H. Role of inositol trisphosphate as a second messenger in signal transduction processes: an essay. Neurochem Res 1988; 13:177–91.

67. Mochly-Rosen D., Fagin J.A., Knauf J.A., Nikiforov Y., Liron T., Schechtman D. Spontaneous occurrence of an inhibitor of protein kinase C localization in a thyroid cancer cell line: role in thyroid tumorigenesis. Adv Enzyme Regul 2001; 41:87–97.
68. Knauf J.A., Ward L.S., Nikiforov Y.E., Nikiforova M., Puxeddu E., Medvedovic M., Liron T., Mochly-Rosen D., Fagin J.A. Isozyme-specific abnormalities of PKC in thyroid cancer: evidence for post-transcriptional changes in PKC-epsilon. J Clin Endocrinol Metab 2002; 87: 2150–9.
69. Heinrich R., Kraiem Z. The protein kinase A pathway inhibits c-jun and c-fos proto-oncogene expression induced by the protein kinase C and tyrosine kinase pathways in cultured human thyroid follicles. J Clin Endocrinol Metab 1997; 82:1839–44.
70. Francis-Lang H., Zannini M., De Felice M., Berlingieri M.T., Fusco A., Di Lauro R. Multiple mechanisms of interference between transformation and differentiation in thyroid cells. Mol Cell Biol 1992; 12:5793–800.
71. Ohta K., Pang X.P., Berg L., Hershman J.M. Growth inhibition of new human thyroid carcinoma cell lines by activation of adenylate cyclase through the beta-adrenergic receptor. J Clin Endocrinol Metab 1997; 82:2633–8.
72. Kosugi S., Mori T., Iwamori M., Nagai Y., Imura H. Alpha 2- and beta-adrenergic receptors and adenosine A1 receptor of FRTL-5 rat thyroid cells in relation to fucosyl GM1-ganglioside. Endocrinology 1989; 124:2707–10.
73. Shimura H., Endo T., Tsujimoto G., Watanabe K., Hashimoto K., Onaya T. Characterization of alpha 1-adrenergic receptor subtypes linked to iodide efflux in rat FRTL cells. J Endocrinol 1990; 124:433–41.
74. Ledent C., Denef J.F., Cottecchia S., Lefkowitz R., Dumont J., Vassart G., Parmentier M. Co-stimulation of adenylyl cyclase and phospholipase C by a mutant alpha 1B-adrenergic receptor transgene promotes malignant transformation of thyroid follicular cells. Endocrinology 1997; 138: 369–78.
75. Fradkin J.E., Hardy W., Wolff J. Adenosine receptor-mediated accumulation of adenosine 3′,5′-monophosphate in guinea pig thyroid tissue. Endocrinology 1982; 110:2018–23.
76. Sho K., Narita T., Okajima F., Kondo Y. An adenosine receptor agonist-induced modulation of TSH-dependent cell growth in FRTL-5 thyroid cells mediated by inhibitory G protein, Gi. Biochimie 1999; 81:341–6.
77. Ledent C., Parmentier M., Vassart G., Dumont J.E. Models of thyroid goiter and tumors in transgenic mice. Mol Cell Endocrinol 1994; 100:167–9.
78. Jackson S., Tseng Y.C., Lahiri S., Burman K.D., Wartofsky L. Receptors for endothelin in cultured human thyroid cells and inhibition by endothelin of thyroglobulin secretion. J Clin Endocrinol Metab 1992; 75:388–92.
79. Tsushima T., Arai M., Isozaki O., Nozoe Y., Shizume K., Murakami H., Emoto N., Miyakawa M., Demura H. Interaction of endothelin-1 with porcine thyroid cells in culture: a possible autocrine factor regulating iodine metabolism. J Endocrinol 1994; 142:463–70.
80. Nelson J., Bagnato A., Battistini B., Nisen P. The endothelin axis: emerging role in cancer. Nat Rev Cancer 2003; 3:110–6.
81. Donckier J.E., Michel L., Van Beneden R., Delos M., Havaux X. Increased expression of endothelin-1 and its mitogenic receptor ETA in human papillary thyroid carcinoma. Clin Endocrinol (Oxf) 2003; 59:354–60.
82. Gualillo O., Lago F., Gomez-Reino J., Casanueva F.F., Dieguez C. Ghrelin, a widespread hormone: insights into molecular and cellular regulation of its expression and mechanism of action. FEBS Lett 2003; 552:105–9.
83. Gnanapavan S., Kola B., Bustin S.A., Morris D.G., McGee P., Fairclough P., Bhattacharya S., Carpenter R., Grossman A.B., Korbonits M. The tissue distribution of the mRNA of ghrelin and subtypes of its receptor, GHS-R, in humans. J Clin Endocrinol Metab 2002; 87:2988.
84. Volante M., Allia E., Fulcheri E., Cassoni P., Ghigo E., Muccioli G., Papotti M. Ghrelin in fetal thyroid and follicular tumors and cell lines: expression and effects on tumor growth. Am J Pathol 2003; 162:645–54.
85. Hansen L.H., Abrahamsen N., Nishimura E. Glucagon receptor mRNA distribution in rat tissues. Peptides 1995; 16:1163–6.
86. Reubi J.C. In vitro evaluation of VIP/PACAP receptors in healthy and diseased human tissues. Clinical implications. Ann N Y Acad Sci 2000; 921:1–25.
87. Schlessinger J. Cell signaling by receptor tyrosine kinases. Cell 2000; 103:211–25.

88. Sarlis, Nicholas J., Gourgiotis Loukas. "Molecular Endocrinology." In *Endocrine Surgery*, Arthur E. Schwartz, Demetrius Pertsemlides, and Michel Gagner, eds. pp. 1–10, New York, NY, Marcel Dekker, Inc., 2004..
89. Farid N.R., Shi Y., Zou M. Molecular basis of thyroid cancer. Endocr Rev 1994; 15:202–32.
90. Bachrach L.K., Nanto-Salonen K., Tapanainen P., Rosenfeld R.G., Gargosky S.E. Insulin-like growth factor binding protein production in human follicular thyroid carcinoma cells. Growth Regul 1995; 5:109–18.
91. Goffard J.C., Jin L., Mircescu H., Van Hummelen P., Ledent C., Emile Dumont J., Corvilain B. Gene expression profile in thyroid of transgenic mice over-expressing the adenosine receptor 2a. Mol Endocrinol 2003;
92. Vella V., Sciacca L., Pandini G., Mineo R., Squatrito S., Vigneri R., Belfiore A. The IGF system in thyroid cancer: new concepts. Mol Pathol 2001; 54:121–4.
93. Vella V., Pandini G., Sciacca L., Mineo R., Vigneri R., Pezzino V., Belfiore A. A novel autocrine loop involving IGF-II and the insulin receptor isoform-A stimulates growth of thyroid cancer. J Clin Endocrinol Metab 2002; 87:245–54.
94. Mitsiades C.S., Poulaki V,. Mitsiades N. The role of apoptosis-inducing receptors of the tumor necrosis factor family in thyroid cancer. J Endocrinol 2003; 178:205–16.
95. Eggo M.C., Hopkins J.M., Franklyn J.A., Johnson G.D., Sanders D.S., Sheppard M.C. Expression of fibroblast growth factors in thyroid cancer. J Clin Endocrinol Metab 1995; 80:1006–11.
96. Shingu K., Fujimori M., Ito K., Hama Y., Kasuga Y., Kobayashi S., Itoh N., Amano J. Expression of fibroblast growth factor-2 and fibroblast growth factor receptor-1 in thyroid diseases: difference between neoplasms and hyperplastic lesions. Endocr J 1998; 45:35–43.
97. Viglietto G., Chiappetta G., Martinez-Tello F.J., Fukunaga F.H., Tallini G., Rigopoulou D., Visconti R., Mastro A., Santoro M., Fusco A. RET/PTC oncogene activation is an early event in thyroid carcinogenesis. Oncogene 1995; 11:1207–10.
98. Duh Q.-Y., Gum E.T., Gerend P.L., Raper S.E., Clark O.H. Epidermal growth factor receptors in normal and neoplastic thyroid tissue. Surgery 1985; 98:1000–7.
99. Gabler B., Aicher T., Heiss P., Senekowitsch-Schmidtke R. Growth inhibition of human papillary thyroid carcinoma cells and multicellular spheroids by anti-EGF-receptor antibody. Anticancer Res 1997; 17:3157–9.
100. Haugen D.R., Akslen L.A., Varhaug J.E., Lillehaug J.R. Demonstration of a TGF-alpha-EGF-receptor autocrine loop and c-myc protein over-expression in papillary thyroid carcinomas. Int J Cancer 1993; 55: 37–43. .
101. Paez Pereda M., Missale C., Grubler Y., Arzt E., Schaaf L., Stalla G.K. Nerve growth factor and retinoic acid inhibit proliferation and invasion in thyroid tumor cells. Mol Cell Endocrinol 2000; 167:99–106.
102. Nakada T., Sato H., Inoue F., Mizorogi F., Nagayama K., Tanaka T. The production of colony-stimulating factors by thyroid carcinoma is associated with marked neutrophilia and eosinophilia. Intern Med 1996; 35:815–20.
103. Aust G., Hofmann A., Laue S., Ode-Hakim S., Scherbaum W.A. Differential regulation of granulocyte-macrophage colony-stimulating factor mRNA and protein expression in human thyrocytes and thyroid-derived fibroblasts by interleukin-1 alpha and tumor necrosis factor-alpha. J Endocrinol 1996; 151:277–85.
104. Tanaka K., Nagayama Y., Nakano T., Takamura N., Namba H., Fukada S., Kuma K., Yamashita S., Niwa M. Expression profile of receptor-type protein tyrosine kinase genes in the human thyroid. Endocrinology 1998; 139:852–8.
105. Thompson S.D., Franklyn J.A., Watkinson J.C., Verhaeg J.M., Sheppard M.C., Eggo M.C. Fibroblast growth factors 1 and 2 and fibroblast growth factor receptor 1 are elevated in thyroid hyperplasia. J Clin Endocrinol Metab 1998; 83:1336–41.
106. Onose H., Emoto N., Sugihara H., Shimizu K., Wakabayashi I. Overexpression of fibroblast growth factor receptor 3 in a human thyroid carcinoma cell line results in overgrowth of the confluent cultures. Eur J Endocrinol 1999; 140:169–73.
107. Ruco L.P., Stoppacciaro A., Ballarini F., Prat M., Scarpino S. Met protein and hepatocyte growth factor (HGF) in papillary carcinoma of the thyroid: evidence for a pathogenetic role in tumourigenesis. J Pathol 2001; 194:4–8.
108. Fluge O., Haugen D.R., Akslen L.A., Marstad A., Santoro M., Fusco A., Varhaug J.E., Lillehaug J.R. Expression and alternative splicing of c-ret RNA in papillary thyroid carcinomas. Oncogene 2001; 20:885–92.

109. Koizumi H., Morita M., Mikami S., Shibayama E., Uchikoshi T. Immunohistochemical analysis of TrkA neurotrophin receptor expression in human non-neuronal carcinomas. Pathol Int 1998; 48:93–101.
110. Meakin S.O., Shooter E.M. The nerve growth factor family of receptors. Trends Neurosci 1992; 15:323–31.
111. Bunone G., Vigneri P., Mariani L., Buto S., Collini P., Pilotti S., Pierotti M.A., Bongarzone I. Expression of angiogenesis stimulators and inhibitors in human thyroid tumors and correlation with clinical pathological features. Am J Pathol 1999; 155:1967–76.
112. Shushanov S., Bronstein M., Adelaide J., Jussila L., Tchipysheva T., Jacquemier J., Stavrovskaya A., Birnbaum D., Karamysheva A. VEGFc and VEGFR3 expression in human thyroid pathologies. Int J Cancer 2000; 86:47–52.
113. Fenton C., Patel A., Dinauer C., Robie D.K., Tuttle R.M., Francis G.L. The expression of vascular endothelial growth factor and the type 1 vascular endothelial growth factor receptor correlate with the size of papillary thyroid carcinoma in children and young adults. Thyroid 2000; 10:349–57.
114. Trovato M., Villari D., Bartolone L., Spinella S., Simone A., Violi M.A., Trimarchi F., Batolo D., Benvenga S. Expression of the hepatocyte growth factor and c-met in normal thyroid, non-neoplastic, and neoplastic nodules. Thyroid 1998; 8:125–31.
115. Di Renzo M.F., Olivero M., Ferro S., Prat M., Bongarzone I., Pilotti S., Belfiore A., Costantino A., Vigneri R., Pierotti M.A, et al. Overexpression of the c-MET/HGF receptor gene in human thyroid carcinomas. Oncogene 1992; 7:2549–53.
116. Belfiore A., Gangemi P., Costantino A., Russo G., Santonocito G.M., Ippolito O., Di Renzo M.F., Comoglio P., F iumara A., Vigneri R. Negative/low expression of the Met/hepatocyte growth factor receptor identifies papillary thyroid carcinomas with high risk of distant metastases. J Clin Endocrinol Metab 1997; 82:2322–8.
117. Ramirez R., Hsu D., Patel A., Fenton C., Dinauer C., Tuttle R.M., Francis G.L. Over-expression of hepatocyte growth factor/scatter factor (HGF/SF) and the HGF/SF receptor (cMET) are associated with a high risk of metastasis and recurrence for children and young adults with papillary thyroid carcinoma. Clin Endocrinol (Oxf) 2000; 53:635–44.
118. Trovato M., Grosso M., Vitarelli E., Ruggeri R.M., Alesci S., Trimarchi F., Barresi G., Benvenga S. Distinctive expression of STAT3 in papillary thyroid carcinomas and a subset of follicular adenomas. Histol Histopathol 2003; 18:393–9.
119. Zsebo K.M., Williams D.A., Geissler E.N., Broudy V.C., Martin F.H., Atkins H.L., Hsu R.Y., Birkett N.C., Okino K.H., Murdock D.C., et al. Stem cell factor is encoded at the Sl locus of the mouse and is the ligand for the c-kit tyrosine kinase receptor. Cell 1990; 63:213–24.
120. Tanaka T., Umeki K., Yamamoto I., Kotani T., Sakamoto F., Noguchi S., Ohtaki S. c-Kit proto-oncogene is more likely to lose expression in differentiated thyroid carcinoma than three thyroid-specific genes: thyroid peroxidase, thyroglobulin, and thyroid stimulating hormone receptor. Endocr J 1995; 42:723–8.
121. Natali P.G., Berlingieri M.T., Nicotra M.R., Fusco A., Santoro E., Bigotti A., Vecchio G. Transformation of thyroid epithelium is associated with loss of c-kit receptor. Cancer Res 1995; 55:1787–91.
122. LeRoith D. Insulin-like growth factor I receptor signaling – overlapping or redundant pathways? Endocrinology 2000; 141:1287–8.
123. Mercalli E., Ghizzoni S., Arighi E., A lberti L., Sangregorio R., Radice M.T., Gishizky M.L., Pierotti M.A., Borrello M.G, Key role of Shc signaling in the transforming pathway triggered by Ret/ptc2 oncoprotein. Oncogene 2001; 20:3475–85.
124. Barbacid M. ras oncogenes: their role in neoplasia. Eur J Clin Invest 1990; 20:225–35.
125. Blalock W.L., Weinstein-Oppenheimer C., Chang F., Hoyle P.E., Wang X.Y., Algate P.A., Franklin R.A., Oberhaus S.M., Steelman L.S., McCubrey J.A. Signal transduction, cell cycle regulatory, and anti-apoptotic pathways regulated by IL-3 in hematopoietic cells: possible sites for intervention with anti-neoplastic drugs. Leukemia 1999; 13:1109–66.
126. Monje P., Marinissen M.J., Gutkind J.S. Phosphorylation of the carboxyl-terminal transactivation domain of c-Fos by extracellular signal-regulated kinase mediates the transcriptional activation of AP-1 and cellular transformation induced by platelet-derived growth factor. Mol Cell Biol 2003; 23:7030–43.
127. Yordy J.S., Muise-Helmericks R.C. Signal transduction and the Ets family of transcription factors. Oncogene 2000; 19:6503–13.
128. Terrier P., Sheng Z.M., Schlumberger M., Tubiana M., Caillou B., Travagli J.P., Fragu P., Parmentier C., Riou G. Structure and expression of c-myc and c-fos proto-oncogenes in thyroid carcinomas. Br J Cancer 1988; 57:43–7.

129. del Senno L., Gambari R., degli Uberti E., Barbieri R., Bernardi F., Buzzoni D., Marchetti G., Pansini G., Perrotta C., Conconi F. c-myc oncogene alterations in human thyroid carcinomas. Cancer Detect Prev 1987; 10:159–66.
130. Farid N.R. Molecular pathogenesis of thyroid cancer: the significance of oncogenes, tumor suppressor genes, and genomic instability. Exp Clin Endocrinol Diabetes 1996; 104 Suppl 4:1–12.
131. Nakayama T., Ito M., Ohtsuru A., Naito S., Nakashima M., Sekine I. Expression of the ets-1 proto-oncogene in human thyroid tumor. Mod Pathol 1999; 12:61–8.
132. de Nigris F., Mega T., Berger N., Barone M.V., Santoro M., Viglietto G., Verde P., Fusco A. Induction of ETS-1 and ETS-2 transcription factors is required for thyroid cell transformation. Cancer Res 2001; 61:2267–75.
133. Dent P., Yacoub A., Contessa J., Caron R., Amorino G., Valerie K., Hagan M.P., Grant S., Schmidt-Ullrich R. Stress and radiation-induced activation of multiple intracellular signaling pathways. Radiat Res 2003; 159:283–300.
134. Kumar S., Boehm J., Lee J.C. p38 MAP kinases: key signalling molecules as therapeutic targets for inflammatory diseases. Nat Rev Drug Discov 2003; 2:717–26.
135. Wang X.S., Diener K., Manthey C.L., Wang S., Rosenzweig B., Bray J., Delaney J., Cole C.N., Chan-Hui P.Y., Mantlo N., Lichenstein H.S., Zukowski M., Yao Z. Molecular cloning and characterization of a novel p38 mitogen-activated protein kinase. J Biol Chem 1997; 272:23668–74.
136. Pomerance M., Abdullah H.B., Kamerji S., Correze C., Blondeau J.P. Thyroid-stimulating hormone and cyclic AMP activate p38 mitogen-activated protein kinase cascade. Involvement of protein kinase A, rac1, and reactive oxygen species. J Biol Chem 2000; 275:40539–46.
137. Kimura E.T., Nikiforova M.N., Zhu Z., Knauf J.A., Nikiforov Y.E., Fagin J.A. High prevalence of BRAF mutations in thyroid cancer: genetic evidence for constitutive activation of the RET/PTC-RAS-BRAF signaling pathway in papillary thyroid carcinoma. Cancer Res 2003; 63:1454–7.
138. Nikiforova M.N., Kimura E.T., Gandhi M., Biddinger P.W., Knauf J.A., Basolo F., Zhu Z., Giannini R., Salvatore G., Fusco A., Santoro M., Fagin J.A., Nikiforov Y.E. BRAF mutations in thyroid tumors are restricted to papillary carcinomas and anaplastic or poorly differentiated carcinomas arising from papillary carcinomas. J Clin Endocrinol Metab 2003; 88:5399–404.
139. Cantley L.C. Growth factors bind receptor tyrosine kinases to stimulate cell survival, cell division, cell growth, and cytoskeletal rearrangement. Sci STKE 2003; 2003:tr8.
140. Cantley L.C. The phosphoinositide 3-kinase pathway. Science 2002; 296:1655–7.
141. Li J., Yen C., Liaw D., Podsypanina K., Bose S., Wang S.I.,,Puc J., Miliaresis C., Rodgers L., McCombie R., Bigner S.H., Giovanella B.C., Ittmann M., Tycko B., Hibshoosh H., Wigler M.H., Parsons R. PTEN, a putative protein tyrosine phosphatase gene mutated in human brain, breast, and prostate cancer. Science 1997; 275:1943–7.
142. Longy M., Lacombe D. Cowden disease. Report of a family and review. Ann Genet 1996; 39:35–42.
143. Cantley L.C., Neel B.G. New insights into tumor suppression: PTEN suppresses tumor formation by restraining the phosphoinositide 3-kinase/AKT pathway. Proc Natl Acad Sci U S A 1999; 96:4240–5.
144. Halachmi N., Halachmi S., Evron E., Cairns P., Okami K., Saji M., Westra W.H., Zeiger M.A., Jen J., Sidransky D. Somatic mutations of the PTEN tumor suppressor gene in sporadic follicular thyroid tumors. Genes Chromosomes Cancer 1998; 23:239–43.
145. Ringel M.D., Hayre N., Saito J., Saunier B., Schuppert F., Burch H., Bernet V., Burman K.D., Kohn L.D., Saji M. Overexpression and overactivation of Akt in thyroid carcinoma. Cancer Res 2001; 61:6105–11.
146. De Vita G., Berlingieri M.T., Visconti R., Castellone M.D., Viglietto G., Baldassarre G., Zannini M., Bellacosa A., Tsichlis P.N., Fusco A., Santoro M. Akt/protein kinase B promotes survival and hormone-independent proliferation of thyroid cells in the absence of dedifferentiating and transforming effects. Cancer Res 2000; 60:3916–20.
147. Lemonnier L.A., Dillehay D.L., Vespremi M.J., Abrams J., Brody E., Schmelz E.M. Sphingomyelin in the suppression of colon tumors: prevention versus intervention. Arch Biochem Biophys 2003; 419:129–38.
148. Sautin Y., Takamura N., Shklyaev S., Nagayama Y., Ohtsuru A., Namba H., Yamashita S. Ceramide-induced apoptosis of human thyroid cancer cells resistant to apoptosis by irradiation. Thyroid 2000; 10:733–40.
149. Schulte K.M.,, Beyer A., Kohrer K., Oberhauser S., Roher H.D. Lysophosphatidic acid, a novel lipid growth factor for human thyroid cells: over-expression of the high-affinity receptor edg4 in differentiated thyroid cancer. Int J Cancer 2001; 92:249–56.

150. Alberti L., Carniti C., Miranda C., Roccato E., Pierotti M.A. RET and NTRK1 proto-oncogenes in human diseases. J Cell Physiol 2003; 195:168–86.
151. Sarlis N.J. Expression patterns of cellular growth-controlling genes in non-medullary thyroid cancer: basic aspects. Rev Endocr Metab Disord 2000; 1:183–96.
152. Borrello M.G., Pelicci G., Arighi E., De Filippis L., Greco A., Bongarzone I., Rizzetti M., Pelicci P.G., Pierotti M.A. The oncogenic versions of the Ret and Trk tyrosine kinases bind Shc and Grb2 adaptor proteins. Oncogene 1994; 9:1661–8.
153. Asakawa H., Kobayashi T. The secretion of cytokines and granulocyte colony stimulating factor by anaplastic and poorly differentiated thyroid carcinoma cell lines. Anticancer Res 1999; 19:761–4.
154. Scarpino S., Stoppacciaro A., Ballerini F., Marchesi M., Prat M., Stella M.C., Sozzani S., Allavena P., Mantovani A., Ruco L.P. Papillary carcinoma of the thyroid: hepatocyte growth factor (HGF) stimulates tumor cells to release chemokines active in recruiting dendritic cells. Am J Pathol 2000; 156: 831–7.
155. Basolo F., Fiore L., Pollina L., Fontanini G., Conaldi P.G., Toniolo A. Reduced expression of interleukin 6 in undifferentiated thyroid carcinoma: in vitro and in vivo studies. Clin Cancer Res 1998; 4:381–7.
156. Fiore L., Pollina L.E., Fontanini G., Casalone R., Berlingieri M.T., Giannini R., Pacini F., Miccoli P., Toniolo A., Fusco A., Basolo F. Cytokine production by a new undifferentiated human thyroid carcinoma cell line, FB-1. J Clin Endocrinol Metab 1997; 82:4094–100.
157. Ruggeri R.M., Villari D., Simone A., Scarfi R., Attard M., Orlandi F., Barresi G., Trimarchi F., Trovato M., Benvenga S. Co-expression of interleukin-6 (IL-6) and interleukin-6 receptor (IL-6R) in thyroid nodules is associated with co-expression of CD30 ligand/CD30 receptor. J Endocrinol Invest 2002; 25:959–66.
158. Chang J.W., Yeh K.Y., Shen Y.C., Hsieh J.J.,Chuang C.K., Liao S.K., Tsai L.H., Wang C.H. Production of multiple cytokines and induction of cachexia in athymic nude mice by a new anaplastic thyroid carcinoma cell line. J Endocrinol 2003; 179:387–94.
159. Kurebayashi J., Tanaka K., Otsuki T., Moriya T., Kunisue H.,U no M., Sonoo H. All-trans-retinoic acid modulates expression levels of thyroglobulin and cytokines in a new human poorly differentiated papillary thyroid carcinoma cell line, KTC-1. J Clin Endocrinol Metab 2000; 85:2889–96.
160. Weetman A.P., Bright-Thomas R., Freeman M. Regulation of interleukin-6 release by human thyrocytes. J Endocrinol 1990; 127:357–61.
161. Zeki K., Morimoto I., Arao T., Eto S., Yamashita U. Interleukin-1alpha regulates G1 cell cycle progression and arrest in thyroid carcinoma cell lines NIM1 and NPA. J Endocrinol 1999; 160:67–73.
162. Matsumura M., Banba N., Motohashi S., Hattori Y. Interleukin-6 and transforming growth factor-beta regulate the expression of monocyte chemoattractant protein-1 and colony-stimulating factors in human thyroid follicular cells. Life Sci 1999; 65:PL129–35.
163. Stassi G., Todaro M., Zerilli M., Ricci-Vitiani L., Di Liberto D., Patti M., Florena A., Di Gaudio F., Di Gesu G., De Maria R. Thyroid cancer resistance to chemotherapeutic drugs via autocrine production of interleukin-4 and interleukin-10. Cancer Res 2003; 63:6784–90.
164. Yeh T.C., Pellegrini S. The Janus kinase family of protein tyrosine kinases and their role in signaling. Cell Mol Life Sci 1999; 55:1523–34.
165. Hirano T. Interleukin 6 and its receptor: ten years later. Int Rev Immunol 1998; 16:249–84.
166. Ogata A., Chauhan D., Teoh G., Treon S.P., Urashima M., Schlossman R.L., Anderson K.C. IL-6 triggers cell growth via the Ras-dependent mitogen-activated protein kinase cascade. J Immunol 1997; 159:2212–21.
167. Wang S., El-Deiry W.S. TRAIL and apoptosis induction by TNF-family death receptors. Oncogene 2003; 22; 8628–33..
168. Yu J., Zhang L. Apoptosis in human cancer cells. Curr Opin Oncol 2004; 16: 19–24..
169. Griffith T.S., Chin W.A., Jackson G.C., Lynch D.H., Kubin M.Z. Intracellular regulation of TRAIL-induced apoptosis in human melanoma cells. J Immunol 1998; 161:2833–40.
170. Sarlis N.J., Gourgiotis L. Molecular elements of apoptosis-regulating pathways in follicular thyroid cells: mining for novel therapeutic targets in the treatment of thyroid carcinoma. Curr Drug Targets Immune Endocr Metabol Disord 2004 (in press)..
171. Yamakawa M., Yamada K., Orui H., Tsuge T., Ogata T., Dobashi M., Imai Y. Immunohistochemical analysis of dendritic/Langerhans cells in thyroid carcinomas. Anal Cell Pathol 1995; 8:331–43.
172. Aust G., Heuer M., Laue S., Lehmann I., Hofmann A., Heldin N.E., Scherbaum W.A. Expression of tumour necrosis factor-alpha (TNF-alpha) mRNA and protein in pathological thyroid tissue and carcinoma cell lines. Clin Exp Immunol 1996; 105:148–54.

173. Pang X.P., Hershman J.M., Chung M., Pekary A.E. Characterization of tumor necrosis factor-alpha receptors in human and rat thyroid cells and regulation of the receptors by thyrotropin. Endocrinology 1989; 125:1783–8.
174. Wajant H., Pfizenmaier K., Scheurich P. Tumor necrosis factor signaling. Cell Death Differ 2003; 10:45–65.
175. Shaulian E., Karin M. AP-1 as a regulator of cell life and death. Nat Cell Biol 2002; 4:E131–6.
176. Chang L., Karin M. Mammalian MAP kinase signalling cascades. Nature 2001; 410:37–40.
177. Thatte U., Dahanukar S. Apoptosis: clinical relevance and pharmacological manipulation. Drugs 1997; 54:511–32.
178. Fisher D.E. Pathways of apoptosis and the modulation of cell death in cancer. Hematol Oncol Clin North Am 2001; 15:931–56.
179. Giordano C., Stassi G., De Maria R., Todaro M., Richiusa P., Papoff G., Ruberti G., Bagnasco M., Testi R., Galluzzo A. Potential involvement of Fas and its ligand in the pathogenesis of Hashimoto's thyroiditis. Science 1997; 275:960–3.
180. Baker J.R., Jr. Dying (apoptosing?) for a consensus on the Fas death pathway in the thyroid. J Clin Endocrinol Metab 1999; 84:2593–5.
181. Mitsiades N., Poulaki V., Tseleni-Balafouta S., Koutras D.A., Stamenkovic I. Thyroid carcinoma cells are resistant to FAS-mediated apoptosis but sensitive tumor necrosis factor-related apoptosis-inducing ligand. Cancer Res 2000; 60:4122–9.
182. Borgerson K.L., Bretz J.D., Baker J.R., Jr. The role of Fas-mediated apoptosis in thyroid autoimmune disease. Autoimmunity 1999; 30:251–64.
183. Lin J.D. The role of apoptosis in autoimmune thyroid disorders and thyroid cancer. Br Med J 2001; 322:1525–7.
184. Ogasawara J., Watanabe-Fukunaga R., Adachi M., Matsuzawa A., Kasugai T., Kitamura Y., Itoh N., Suda T., Nagata S. Lethal effect of the anti-Fas antibody in mice. Nature 1993; 364:806–9.
185. Tourneur L., Mistou S., Michiels F.M., Devauchelle V., Renia L., Feunteun J., Chiocchia G. Loss of FADD protein expression results in a biased Fas-signaling pathway and correlates with the development of tumoral status in thyroid follicular cells. Oncogene 2003; 22:2795–804.
186. Mitsiades N., Poulaki V., Mitsiades C.S., Koutras D.A., Chrousos G.P. Apoptosis induced by FasL and TRAIL/Apo2L in the pathogenesis of thyroid diseases. Trends Endocrinol Metab 2001; 12:384–90.
187. Manetto V., Lorenzini R., Cordon-Cardo C., Krajewski S., Rosai J., Reed J.C., Eusebi V. Bcl-2 and Bax expression in thyroid tumours. An immunohistochemical and western blot analysis. Virchows Arch 1997; 430:125–30.
188. Pestereli H.E., Ogus M., Oren N., Karpuzoglu G., Karpuzoglu T. Bcl-2 and p53 expression in insular and in well-differentiated thyroid carcinomas with an insular pattern. Endocr Pathol 2001; 12:301–5.
189. Ito Y., Yoshida H., Nakano K., Takamura Y., Miya A., Kobayashi K., Yokozawa T., Matsuzuka F., Matsuura N., Kakudo K., Kuma K., Miyauchi A. Bag-1 expression in thyroid neoplasm: its correlation with Bcl-2 expression and carcinoma dedifferentiation. Anticancer Res 2003; 23: 569–76.
190. Shi Y., Massague J. Mechanisms of TGF-beta signaling from cell membrane to the nucleus. Cell 2003; 113:685–700.
191. Franzen A., Piek E., Westermark B., ten Dijke P., Heldin N.E. Expression of transforming growth factor-beta1, activin A, and their receptors in thyroid follicle cells: negative regulation of thyrocyte growth and function. Endocrinology 1999; 140: 4300–10.
192. West J., Munoz-Antonia T., Johnson J.G., Klotch D., Muro-Cacho C.A. Transforming growth factor-beta type II receptors and smad proteins in follicular thyroid tumors. Laryngoscope 2000; 110: 1323–7.
193. Jasani B., Wyllie F.S., Wright P.A., Lemoine N.R., Williams E.D., Wynford-Thomas D. Immunocytochemically detectable TGF-beta associated with malignancy in thyroid epithelial neoplasia. Growth Factors 1990;2: 149–55.
194. Kimura E.T., Kopp P., Zbaeren J., Asmis L.M., Ruchti C., Maciel R.M., Studer H. Expression of transforming growth factor beta1, beta2, and beta3 in multinodular goiters and differentiated thyroid carcinomas: a comparative study. Thyroid 1999; 9: 119–25.
195. Schulte K.M., Jonas C., Krebs R., Roher H.D. Activin A and activin receptors in thyroid cancer. Thyroid 2001; 11: 3–14.
196. Hatakeyama S., Gao Y.H., Ohara-Nemoto Y., Kataoka H., Satoh M. Expression of bone morphogenetic proteins of human neoplastic epithelial cells. Biochem Mol Biol Int. 1997; 42: 497–505.
197. Attisano L., Wrana J.L. Signal transduction by the TGF-beta superfamily. Science 2002; 296: 1646–7.
198. Miyazawa K., Shinozaki M., Hara T., Furuya T., Miyazono K. Two major Smad pathways in TGF-beta superfamily signalling. Genes Cells 2002; 7: 1191–204.

199. Ellenrieder V., Buck A., Gress T.M. TGFbeta-regulated transcriptional mechanisms in cancer. Int J Gastrointest Cancer 2002; 31: 61–9.
200. Lazzereschi D., Ranieri A., Mincione G., Taccogna S., Nardi F., Colletta G. Human malignant thyroid tumors displayed reduced levels of transforming growth factor beta receptor type II messenger RNA and protein. Cancer Res 1997; 57: 2071–6.
201. Blaydes J.P., Wynford-Thomas D. Loss of responsiveness to transforming growth factor beta (TGFbeta) is tightly linked to tumorigenicity in a model of thyroid tumour progression. Int J Cancer 1996; 65: 525–30.
202. Heldin N.E., Bergstrom D., Hermansson A., Bergenstrahle A., Nakao A., Westermark B., ten Dijke P. Lack of responsiveness to TGF-beta1 in a thyroid carcinoma cell line with functional type I and type II TGF-beta receptors and Smad proteins, suggests a novel mechanism for TGF-beta insensitivity in carcinoma cells. Mol Cell Endocrinol 1999; 153: 79–90.
203. Cerutti J.M., Ebina K.N., Matsuo S.E., Martins L., Maciel R.M., Kimura E.T. Expression of Smad4 and Smad7 in human thyroid follicular carcinoma cell lines. J Endocrinol Invest 2003; 26: 516–21.
204. Bravo S.B., Pampin S., Cameselle-Teijeiro J., Carneiro C., Dominguez F., Barreiro F., Alvarez C.V. TGF-beta-induced apoptosis in human thyrocytes is mediated by p27kip1 reduction and is overridden in neoplastic thyrocytes by NF-kappaB activation. Oncogene 2003; 22: 7819–30.
205. Blaydes J.P., Schlumberger M., Wynford-Thomas D., Wyllie F.S. Interaction between p53 and TGF beta 1 in control of epithelial cell proliferation. Oncogene 1995; 10: 307–17.
206. Mincione G., Esposito D.L., Di Marcantonio M.C., Piccirelli A., Cama A., Colletta G. TGF-beta 1 modulation of IGF-I signaling pathway in rat thyroid epithelial cells. Exp Cell Res 2003; 287: 411–23.

15. GENE EXPRESSION IN THYROID TUMORS

LASZLO PUSKAS[1] AND NADIR R. FARID[2]

Laboratory of Functional Genomics, Biological Research Center of the Hungarian Academy of Sciences, Szeged, Hungary[1] *& Osanor Biotech Inc, 31 Woodland Drive, Watford, Herts WD17 3BY,UK*[2]

INTRODUCTION

Endocrinologists and pathologists would welcome a simple reliable test of the nature and potential of thyroid nodules at the first encounter. Even with satisfactory fine needle aspirations a definitive cytological diagnosis may not be always be possible and prognostication is thus limited. As discussed in other chapters in this book (2 & 16), several molecular markers examined in surgical specimens have been proposed to be specific for histologic types of thyroid tumors and/or malignancy. None, however, is diagnostic.

In the event the approaches to examine a limited number of molecular markers at a time are by means not robust enough to apply to the cytological harvest of thyroid FNA. Because of the very nature of malignant transformation (see Chapter 1), it is expected that gene products in many cellular pathways would be involved, only some of which turn out to be tissue-specific or tumor-subtype specific.

The exploration of the transcriptome of tumors or normal tissue during development, or following treatment with drugs or hormones holds much promise to the better understanding of physiologic and pathologic processes (1–4).

This chapter discusses the application of this technique to thyroid tumors.

DNA MICROARRAYS

In essence, cDNA or oligonucleotides are spotted onto glass slides, silicon wafers or nylon membranes and are then exposed to florescently-labelled mix of RNA (or cDNA made thereof) from biological specimens. Each DNA latches onto the RNA or cDNA that matches its sequence. Based on the location and intensity of the signal the source gene and its activity can be detected. Many protocol refinements and software programs have been introduced to ensure internal consistency, reproducibility, statistical analysis, gene annotation and ontological linkages of the huge amounts of raw data (3,4).

THE APPLICATIONS OF DNA MICROARRAYS

DNA microarray is a tool most commonly used to monitor levels of gene expression levels. DNA chip technology can be helpful in documenting DNA copy number, DNA/protein interactions and genetic polymorphisms (4). It holds promise in the search for gene promotor regions and screening DNA/chromosomes for gene expression (4).

One of the first and still most used tools applied to microarray data visualization is hierarchical clustering. In one dimension, sample output is grouped to similarity and in the other according to the overall similarity of expression across samples. An important objective of this approach is to identify similarly regulated genes across specimens examined (3). Sophisticated computational treatment of the data has, however, failed to establish this "guilt by association" as a valid spin-off from microarray analysis (5). An evolutionary approach identifying orthologs that have retained their function goes a long way to answering the criticism of the identification of co-expressed genes by microarrays (6).

Cluster analysis of differentially expressed genes has, nevertheless, been helpful in a number of areas of clinical medicine, particular in oncology (3,7,8). Hierarchical clustering has been helpful in:

1. Tumor classification or subclassification
2. Identification of potentially important genes characterizing a tumor, susceptibility to drugs and metastatic potential
3. Identification of new drug targets to provide new therapeutic tools.
4. Identifying biomarkers for establishing or confirming diagnosis and outcome of therapy.

Microarray technology as currently used has provided novel insight into B-cell lymphoma, breast cancer, melanoma and other human malignancies (2,8–11)

GENE EXPRESSION PROFILING IN THYROID CANCER

A limited number of studies have reported on DNA microarray studies in thyroid cancer: two on follicular tumors, one on papillary carcinoma (PTC) and only one that examined a range of benign and malignant thyroid disease. The numbers of samples analyzed in each study was small to moderate in size. Most of the studies quoted are, however, robust and pass muster for the stringent rules stipulated for reporting of gene expression studies (4).

Papillary thyroid carcinoma

Huang et al. (12) used oligonucleotide DNA chips containing more than 12,000 genes to profile 8 papillary carcinomas and matching normal thyroid tissue. They found the expression of 8 genes to be suppressed in 7/8 samples and that of 19 genes in 6/8 samples. The genes whose expression was suppressed fell in a number of categories: tumor suppressor genes (e.g. *bcl-2, gas-1* and *fos-B*), thyroid metabolism (e.g. *dio-1, dio-2, tpo*), cell adhesion (*dpt* and *fgl-2*), fatty acid binding (*apo-B* and *fabp-4*) and signal transduction (*stc-1* and *itpr-1*).

24 genes were overexpressed in all 8 papillary thyroid cancer samples and an additional 22 genes in 7/8 specimens. Among the genes found to be overexpressed were several previously reported and include fibronectin-1, the *met* oncogene, *dipeptidylpeptidase IV, α-1-antitrypsin, keratin-19* and *galectin 3*. Other overexpressed genes fell in the categories of cellular adhesion/extracellular matrix, cytoskeleton, growth factors and their receptors as well as those involved in signal transduction.

Several genes found to be over-expressed in papillary carcinoma were not previously reported in any neoplasia or the thyroid and include: *ADORA1* (adenosine A1 receptor), *SCEL* (sciellin), *ODZ1* (Odz 1, Drosophila), *PROS1* (vitamin K-dependent plasma protein S), *KIAA0937*, *CST6* (cystatin E/M), *SDC4* (ryudocan core protein), *P4HA2* (propyl-4-hydroxylase alpha (II) subunit), *DUSP6* (dual specificity phosphatase 6), *TSSC3* (tumor suppressing subtransferable candidate 3). Changes in gene expression of selected genes were confirmed by multiplex semiquantitative RT PCR and consistent and highly correlated patterns of gene expression pattern in tumor samples relative to normal was also verified by hierarchial cluster analysis. The latter aspect of the results was unexpected given the previously noted heterogeneity of individual gene expression in PTC.

Specificity for PTC of two gene products (Cbp/p300-interacting transactivator [*CITED1*] and surfactant, pulmonary–associated protein B [*SFTPB*]) previously associated with other neoplasia was explored by immunoflorescence in a large number archival of PTC tissue and other thyroid malignant tumors (12).

Follicular tumors

Using the same array system as did Huang et al. (12), Barden et al. (13) compared RNA from 10 follicular adenomas with those from 9 follicular carcinomas (FTC), two minimally invasive, one poorly differentiated and one Hürthle cell carcinomas. The authors identified 105 genes whose expression significantly differed between adenomas and carcinomas (overexpressed in one or the other). They found that many previously unidentified genes contributed to the distinction between adenomas and carcinomas. Interestingly, very few of the genes suppressed or overexpressed in follicular tumors were identified as important in the Huang et al. study (12).

The authors (13) chose 5 genes with >3 fold overexpression for further verification of expression by semiquantitative RT-PCR and in the case of one gene, product extracellular matrix metalloproteinase inducer (EMMPRIN), by Western blotting of the extracted protein. The gene products overexpressed in follicular carcinomas compared to adenomas were adrenomedullin, autotoxin, EMMPRIN, transforming growth factor β II receptor and the *met* oncogene. *Met* was previously reported to be relevant to thyroid carcinogenesis (12,14, also see below). Adrenomedullin is important in growth and survival of several human cancers whereas autoxin promotes tumor cell growth and angiogenesis. EMMPRIN is a surface glycoprotein that is associated with metastatic behavior.

Aldred et al. (15,16) selected genes found to be differentially regulated in 19 FTCs. They chose genes mapping to regions of loss of heterozygozity (LOH), previously reported in FTC (15). They also monitored the downregulation of peroxisome proliferator-activated receptor gamma [PPAR γ] (16). Because of the questions asked, the authors focussed on down-regulated genes. In contrast to the initial study from this group (12), there was not enough material to test the samples in duplicate nor was there enough paired normal thyroid tissues for samples. The authors had, therefore, to respectively normalize their results to mean intensity and to carry out pairwise comparisons between all normal and tumorous thyroid tissue (15).

Three genes coordinately downregulated, caveolin-1, caveolin-2 and GDF10/BMP3b were further studied on the basis of their localization to two chromosomal regions, 7q31.1 and 10q11.1, that commonly show LOH in FTC. The authors also selected for further analysis two additional genes (glypican-3: Xq26.1 and a novel chordin-like:Xq22) involved in bone morphogenesis signalling and possible interaction with *GDF10*. Each of the 5 genes was downregulated in at least 15/19 of samples by RT-PCR. The authors followed in greater detail the relevance of *caveolin-1*, thought to be involved in the regulation of the dual-specificity phosphatase PTEN, suppressed in FTC. They found that it is the β isoform of *calveolin-1* that is specifically downregulated and that the reduced expression is specific to FTC, including insular and Hürthle-cell varieties (15). On the other hand, the expression of the 3 genes involved in bone morphogenesis signalling were downregulated also in benign adenomas and multinodular goitre and glypican-3 in PTC suggesting that they are early events in pathologic thyroid cell growth.

In apparently the same set of tumors, Aldred et al (16) found that whereas only 2/19 FTC exhibited the *PAX8/PPARγ* re-arrangement (see Chapter 4), the majority (13/17) of the remainder showed greatly reduced expression of PPARγ by microarray and semiquantitative RT-PCR. Reduction of PPARγ immunoreactivity was found not only in FTCs but also in Hürthe cell carcinomas and PTCs. Down regulation of PPARγ is probably related to repression by one or more upstream regulatory protein, as the results could not be explained on the basis of gene deletion, mutation or hypermethylation of the PPARγ regulatory sequences

A spectrum of thyroid tumors

We have used human cDNA microarray constructed in-house by spotting previously PCR-amplified and purified gene-specific samples to study RNA from a range of thyroid tissues. We examined samples from multinodular goitre (MNG), Graves' disease, Hashimoto's thyroiditis, papillary carcinoma, follicular carcinoma and follicular adenoma and compared these to normal perinodular thyroid tissue. Hierarchical cluster analysis (Figure 1) showed clear separation of various clinical pathological entities according to variation in the expression of 1322 genes, many of which were unidentified at the time.

We selected 26 genes whose expression showed variation in thyroid tumors for further examination using semiquantitative RT-PCR. Given that we used a completely

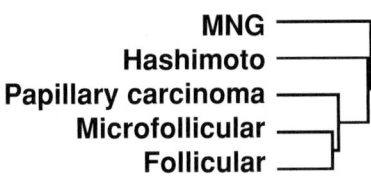

Figure 1. Hierarchical clustering of 1322 genes separates the thyroid diseases studied. Specific clusters were arrived at according to thyroid disease. The closest relatives were mircofollicular adenomas and follicular carcinoma, while papillary carcinoma exhibited some relationship to this subfamily. Multinodular goiter and Hashimoto's thyroiditis were distinct from each other and from other thyroid disease types.

Hierarchical cluster analysis was done using the Omniviz Gene Expression software package (Omniviz Inc.)

different panel of genes than did Huang et al. (12), we found remarkable agreement in genes differentially regulated in PTC. The expression of some of these genes was, however, also regulated in other thyroid tissues studied, thus (and as expected) *met* expression was increased in FTC, as was that of *galacetin3* whereas that of *cartilage glycoprotein3* was overexpressed in adenomas, MNG and FTC. That of Cpb/p300-interacting protein was overexpressed in FTC but 5 fold less in PTC.

Type I iodothyronine deiodinase which is down-regulated in PTC was enhanced in FTC and benign nodular tissue, *CRAB1 cellular retinoic acid binding protein* expression was also reduced in adenoma, FTC and MNG but less than in PTC whereas *fatty acid binding protein* 4, suppressed in PTC, appears to up-regulated in MNG.

We found the C8FW phosphoprotein, regulated in the thyroid gland by TSH and EGF (17), to be specifically overexpressed in FTC and so was *proprotein convertase subtilisin/kexin 2*. The latter is a furin involved in the processing of prohormones (18) but which is also involved in the digestion of pre-metalloproteases and cadherins and might be involved in tumor invasion and metastatic behavior. S100 calcium binding protein (*mts1* or metastasin), the subject of intense recent interest in carcinogensis (19), was specifically increased in PTC. By contrast the *small GTPase Rap1* (20), which is involved in the regulation of cell-adhesion and Glycerol kinase 2 (testis specific), a key enzyme in adipose tissue metabolism are increased in FTC.

The 15 Kda selenoprotein (21) whose abundance is modified in transformed cells was increased in PTC but not in FTC and less so in MNG.

We found *secreted frizzled related protein* (22,23), that is involved in the regulation of wnt signalling, to be specifically reduced in PTC. In contrast, the expression of *tight junction protein* 1, important in maintaining cellular polarity (24) was curiously suppressed specifically in FTC. *Eosinophil-derived neurotoxin*, which plays a role in allergic reactions and has an anti retroviral activity is reduced in all tumorous tissues studied (25,26). We speculate that it may be involved in evasion by tumors of immune cells. *Keratin, Type II cytoskeletal 7* important in maintaining cellular structure is reduced in all except follicular adenomas (27). In an independent study (28), we found that the cannabinoid receptor 2 (*CNR2*) as well as *met* to relevant to the metastatic behavior of anaplastic thyroid carcinoma.

CONCLUSIONS AND PERSPECTIVE

The study of gene expression by microarray technology (just as the earlier use of serial analysis of gene expression [SAGE, 29]) has yet to yield the answer to the proposition posited at the beginning of this chapter. While the protocols for performing gene expression are relatively easy, the analysis and interpretation of the results are time consuming and may be difficult to interpret in our current state of knowledge of functional genomics. Independent corroboration of differential expression is necessary by different techniques and, in our opinion, by replication in different sample sets in the same or independent laboratories. Some of the studies reviewed have limited themselves to circumscribed issues e.g overexpression of genes in two sets of tumors one benign and one malignant (13) and generalization from any of the studies is hampered by the small number of samples examined in each. Given the diverse pathways to malignancy it would be naïve to adopt a "candidate gene panel" approach in trying to develop robust tests to diagnose malignancy in a thyroid nodule, predict histology and subsequent tumor behavior and response to therapy.

A concerted multicenter effort in which large numbers (30–50) of thyroid tumors whose histology has been verified by expert thyroid pathologists is necessary to provide us with the data-base that can satisfy our diagnostic needs. The application of statistical methods such as that described by Wright et al. (30), will allow comparison of the results from the bank of tumors proposed above to previously studied tumors whose array results are in the public domain, and from tumors that may be independently studied in the future to hone in on a limited number of genes important in tumor classification, prognostication and adjuvant therapy targeting. The validity of these genes (probably 15–20) can then be prospectively validated in a large series of FNA specimens.

It is also important to reflect in a broader sense that genes overexpressed in a tumor, with poor prognosis for example, may not represent an appropriate target for therapeutic intervention or for targeted drug design. On the other hand, we may have to look to pathways upstream from those genes for the most vulnerable targets, usually enzymes or receptors.

ACKNOWLEDGMENTS

We thank Dr Yufei Shi for critical review of the manuscript and for helpful suggestions.

REFERENCES

1. Zvara A, Heckler L Jr, Nagy ZB, Micsik T, Puskas LG (2002) New Molecular methods for classification, diagnosis and therapy prediction of hemtological malignancies *Pathol. Oncol. Res.* 8, 231–140.
2. Macgregor PF (2003) Gene expression in cancer: The application of microarrays *Expert Rev. Mol. Diagn.* 3, 185–200.
3. Staudt LM, Brown PO 2000 Genomic view of the immune system *Annu. Rev. Immunol.* 18. 829–859.
4. Baldi P, Hatfield GW 2002 DNA microarrays and Gene exptression from experiments to data analysis Cambridge University Press.
5. Quackenbush J 2003 Microarrays—guilt by association *Science* 302, 240–241.
6. Stuart JM, Segal E, Koller D, Kim SK 2003 A gene-coexpression network for global discovery of conserved genetic module *Science* 302, 249–255.
7. Guo QM 2003 DNA microarray and cancer *Curr. Opin. Oncol.* 15, 36–43.

8. Macgregor PF, Squire JA 2002 Application of microarrays to analysis of gene expression in cancer *Clin. Chem.* 48, 1170–1177.
9. Schwaenen C, Wessendorf S , Kestler HA, Dohner H, Lichter P, Bentz, M 2003 DNA microarray analysis in malignant lymphomas *Ann. Hematol.* 82, 323–332.
10. Cooper CS 2001 Application of microarray technology in breast cancer research *Breast Cancer Res.* 3,158–175.
11. Carr KM, Bittner M, Trent JM 2003 Gene-expression profiling in human cutaneous melanoma *Oncogene* 22, 3076–3080.
12. Huang Y, Prasad M, Lemon WJ, Hempel H, Wright FA, Kornacker K, LiVolsi V, Frankel W, Kloos RT, Eng C, Pellegata, NS, de la Chapelle A 2001 Gene expression in papillary thyroid carcinoma reveals highly consistent profiles *Proc. Natl. Acad. Sci.U.S.A.* 98, 15044–15049.
13. Barden CB, Shister KW, Zhu B, Guiter G, Greenblatt DY, Zeiger MA, Fahey III TJ 2003 Classification of follicular thyroid tumors by molecular signature: results of gene profiling Clin. Cancer Res 9, 1792–1800.
14. Farid NR, Shi Y, Zou M 1994 Molecular basis of thyroid cancer Endocr. Rev. 15:202–232.
15. Aldred MA, Ginn-Pease ME, Morrison CD, Popkie AP, Gimm O, Hoang-Vu C, Krause U, Dralle H, Jhiang SM, Plass, C, Eng C 2003 *Caveolin-1* and *Caveolin-2*, together with three bone morphogenetic protein-related genes, amy encode novel tumor suppressors down-regulated in sporadic follicular thyroid carcinogenesis *Cancer Res.* 63, 2864–2871.
16. Aldred MA, Morrison C, Grimm O, Hoang-Vu C, Krause U, Dralle H, Jhiang S, Eng C 2003 Perxisome proliferators-activated receptor gamma is frequently downregulated in a diversity of sporadic nonmedullary thyroid carcinoma *Oncogene* 22, 3412–3416.
17. Wilkin F, Suarez-Huerta N, Robaye B, Peetermans J, Libert F, Dumont JE, Maenhaut C 1997 Characterization of a phosphoprotein whose mRNA is regulated by the mitogenic pathways in dog thyroid cells *Eur. J. Biochem* 248, 660–668.
18. Bassi DE, Mahloogi H, Klein-Szanto AJ 2000 The proprotein furin and PACE-4 play a significant part in tumor progression *Mol. Carcino.* 28, 63–69.
19. Mazzucchelli L 2001 Protein S100A4: Too long overlooked by pathologists *Am. J Pathol.* 160, 7–13.
20. De Buryn KM, Rangarajan S, Reedquist KA, Figdor CG, Bos JL 2003 The small GTPase Rap1 is required for Mn (2+)- and antibody-induced LFA-1 and VLA-4-mediated cell adhesion *J. Biol. Chem.* 277, 29468–29476.
21. Kumaraswamy E, Malykh A, Korotkov KV, Kozyavkin S, HuY , Kwon SY, Moustafa, ME, Carlson BA, Berry MJ, Lee BJ, Hatfied DL, Diamond AM, Gladyshev VN 2000 Structure-relationship of the 15-kDa seleoprotein gene. Possible role of the protein in cancer *J. Biol. Chem* 275, 45540–35547.
22. Uren A, Reichsman F, Anest V, Taylor WG, Muraiso K, Bottaro DP, Cumberledge S, Rubin JS 2000 Secreted frizzled-related protein-1 binds directly to Wingless and is a biphasic modulator of wnt signalling *J. Biol. Chem* 275, 4374–4382.
23. Ko J, Ryu KS, Lee YH, Na DS, Kim YS, Oh YM, Kim IS, Kim JW 2002 Human frizzled-related protein is down-regulated and induces apoptosis in human cervical cancer *Exp. Cell Res.* 280, 280–287.
24. Rao RK, Baurov S, Rao VU, Karnaky Jr KJ, Gupta A 2002 Tyrosine phosphorylation and dissociation of occludin-ZO-1 and E-cadherin-beta-catenin complexes from the cytoskeleton by oxidative stress *Biochem. J* 368, 471–481.
25. McDevitt AL, Deming MS, Rosenberg HF, Dyer KD 2001 Gene structure and enzymatic activity of mouse eosinophil-associated ribonuclease 2 *Gene* 267:23–30.
26. Brenner SA 2002 The past as the key to the present: Resurrection of ancient proteins from eosinophils *Proc. Natl. Acad Sci USA* 99, 4760–4761.
27. Kirfel J, Magin TM, Reichelt J. 2003 Keratins: a structural scaffold with emerging functions *Cell. Mol. Life Sci.* 60, 56–71.
28. Shi, Y, Parhar RS, Zou M , Baieti E, Kessie G, Farid NR, Alzahrani A, Al-Mohanna FA Gene therapy of anaplastic carcinoma with a single chain interleukin 12 fusion protein *Hum. Gene Therapy* (in press).
29. Takano T, Hasegawa y, Matsuzuka F, Miyauchi A, Yoshida H, Higaashiyama T, Kuma K, Amino N 2000 Gene expression profiles in thyroid carcinomas *Br J Cancer* 83, 1495–14502.
30. Wright G, Tan B, Rosenwald A, Hurt EH, Wiester A, Staudt LM A gene expression-based method to diagnose clinically distinct subgroups of diffuse large B cell lymphoma *Proc. Natl Acad. Sci. USA*, 100, 9991–9996.

16. ANIMAL MODELS OF THYROID CARCINOGENESIS

CARSTEN BOLTZE

Department of Pathology, Otto Van Guericke University, Leipziger Strasse 44,
D-39120 Magdeburg, Germany

INTRODUCTION

Thyroid nodules affect approximately 20% to 45% of the population during their lifetime, but only a minority of nodular goiters bear a clinically relevant malignant potential. A simple diagnostic approach solving this problem does not exist. Cytological evaluation after fine needle aspiration obtained from thyroid nodules allows only for the detection of thyroid carcinoma in 80% to 90% of the cases. Thus, better methods predicting the malignant potential of thyroid nodules and/or diagnosing existing malignancies are urgently needed. To solve this problem the first step was designating animal models of thyroid carcinogenesis that help to understand this process in more detail. Last century's investigations in this field showed that the thyroid gland serves as a useful experimental model for understanding tumor formation not only in endocrine systems but, in epithelial tissues in general. Since the mid-1930s, the study of experimental carcinogenesis in rats, mice, hamsters, guinea pigs, sheep and swine has been focus of attention. In vivo, the growth of the follicular epithelium is controlled by a single tropic stimulus, the thyroid-stimulating hormone (TSH), which is secreted by the anterior pituitary gland at a rate dependent on the serum concentration of thyroid hormones (T3 and T4). Inhibition of this feedback loop by reduction or abolition of T3/T4 production leads to an increase in serum TSH. This initially induces an uniform hyperplasia of thyroid follicular epithelium, the first step of tumorigenesis. The discovery of the thyrostatic effect of some naturally occurring substances and the subsequent development of numerous synthetic preparations with the same action gave an impetus to and provided an opportunity for the systematic investigation of morphological and functional changes in thyroids of experimental animals.

HISTORICAL OVERVIEW

In 1909, McCoy was the first to systematically investigate thyroids of animals. He searched for tumors in 23,000 wild rats, but failed to detect them. Eight years later, Bullock and Rhodenburg identified nine tumors in 4,300 rats. In 1926, Slye at al found 12 so-called carcinomas in 51,700 mice. All these tumors were spontaneous tumors. After the description of goiter in man (Marine 1924), the era of experiments in the field of thyroid carcinogenesis started sporadically with the investigations of Wegelin (1928), Hellwig (1935), and Hercus & Purves (1936). In the following time, each decade was influenced by leading research groups. In the 1940s, Purves, Bielschowsky, Kennedy and Griesbach (New Zealand, Germany) described the role of low iodine intake and continued the investigation of other positive goitrogenic agents. Kennedy, therefore, synthesized a quantity of allylthiocyanate (mustard oil), from a glucoside in mustard seeds, which were also goitrogenic. This compound was too toxic to be fed to rats, but when treated with ammonia, it was converted to allylthiourea and could be incorporated in the rat diet. It was shown that such drugs are goitrogenic, as is a deficiency of iodine, because they block the production of thyroid hormone. In the 1950s-1970s, Lindsay, Chaikoff (USA) and Doniach (U.K.) described the effects of external and internal irradiation on thyroid tumor production and gave evidence of a dose-dependent relationship. In the 1980s, Hesch, von zur Mühlen (Germany) and Dumont (Belgium) searched for tumor-initiating mechanisms through hormone dysbalances (TSH vs. TRH) and detected morphological changes by electron microscopy. Williams and Wynford-Thomas (U.K.) clarified the functional role of TSH and described differential gene expression (*ras*) in experimental thyroid tumors for the first time (Lemoine et al 1988). In the 1990s, Brabant, Dralle and Hoang-Vu (Germany) conducting short-term and long-term studies, investigated the regulatory mechanisms of thyroid tumorigenesis and described the changes of histology, ultrastructure, function, and proliferation in detail. In the present time, experiments performed by Japanese and Russian groups (Hirose, Hoshi, Hiasa, Nadolnik) focus on testing the carcinogenic potential of several parts of nutrition and diverse environmental factors.

THE PROBLEM OF TUMOR CLASSIFICATION

All the difficulties encountered in the classification of human thyroid tumors have to be faced in an attempt to classify thyroid tumors in animals, particularly in the rat. In early experiments, the well-known absence of clear-cut histological criteria for distinguishing reactive hyperplasia from neoplasia or benign from malignant tumorous growth has been reflected in publications describing corresponding lesions in the rat. In most cases, the authors have tried to apply the nomenclature of human pathology to the lesions observed in the rat thyroid. This approach has not only some easily recognizable advantages, but also some disadvantages. On the one hand, the use of similar terms would provide an opportunity for conducting a comparative analysis of

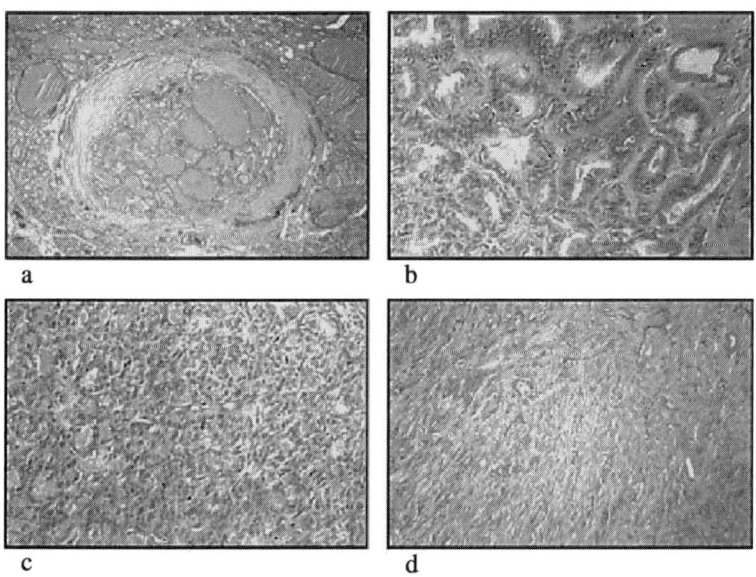

Figure 1. Experimental thyroid tumors in rats induced by x-ray irradiation: Low power view of a follicular adenoma with surrounding capsule (a), high power view of papillary carcinoma (b), follicular carcinoma (c) and squamous cell (epidermoid) carcinoma.

experimental and clinical observations. On the other hand, the same terms might be, and have already been, applied to morphological lesions that are superficially similar, but whose biological behavior is different. The broadest definition applicable to both benign and malignant neoplasms was formulated by Axelrad and Leblond (1955). It fits in with the criteria applied to rat tumors by most experimentalists and can be paraphrased as follows: a pathological change in the rat thyroid can be regarded as a neoplasm when it is focal; it is distinct from the rest of the gland cytologically and architecturally and shows evidence of progressive growth. As to the definition of such terms as "adenoma" and "carcinoma", the wording suggested here is based on the above definition of a neoplasm and on personal experience gained in studying the peculiarities of behavior of rat thyroid tumors.

An encapsulated epithelial neoplasm without evidence of invasive growth or distant metastasis can be considered an adenoma (Figure 1a). A carcinoma in the rat thyroid is an epithelial neoplasm of any histological structure that shows destructive invasive growth, which leads to metastasis to the body (Figure 1b–d). Apart from clear proof of local invasive growth, there is no convincing evidence of malignant growth except the demonstration of metastases. The tendency to overestimate the malignancy of rat thyroid neoplasms and to diagnose them as carcinomas simply on the grounds of their "malignant" appearance is discernable in many publications. The classification given below, was drawn up under consideration of certain data on embryogenesis of this gland, heterogeneity of its epithelial cell population, and the already mentioned peculiarities of normal growth of the thyroid epithelium. However, to make this classification more practicable and comparable with that of WHO for human tumors microscopic morphology rather than histogenesis has been selected as a basis:

Benign tumors:

Follicular adenoma (including microfollicular, polymorphofollicular and trabecular adenoma), papillary adenoma, simple solid adenoma, light-cell solid adenoma, and squamous cell (epidermoid) cystadenoma.

Malignant tumors:

Follicular carcinoma (including microfollicular and polymorphofollicular carcinoma), papillary carcinoma, solid carcinoma (including small cell, polymorphous solid and light-cell solid carcinoma), squamous cell carcinoma, sarcomas and mixed tumors (carcinosarcoma).

This classification does not include such entities as leiomyoma, hemangioma, lymphoma, teratoma, neurogenous tumors, and some other neoplasms that have been observed in humans and several animal species other than the rat. An attempt has also been made to avoid the use of proper names that have already led to some diagnostic confusion (for instance Hürtle cell tumor or Lindsay tumor). Of the characteristic and predominant histological patterns observed in neoplastic epithelial nodules, the three most common ones (follicular, solid and epidermoid) were selected to designate the main categories of tumors. As mentioned earlier, the proliferation of rat thyroid epithelial cells in solid aggregations must be considered a normal feature. The listed tumors are rarely found in their pure morphological form. Most experimental tumors in animals represent virtually different transitional variations in between these artificially separated entities. The vast majority of follicular neoplasms contain solitary or numerous foci of solid cell nests, and it is the rare solid tumor that does not show areas of follicular structure. An introduction of all the subdivisions covering even the most frequent transitional forms of tumors would make this classification useless. An attempt to classify the endless variety of histological pictures produced by physiological shifts in this correlation is hardly justifiable.

SPONTANEOUS THYROID TUMORS IN ANIMALS

Roe (1965) defined a spontaneous thyroid tumor as a neoplasm that had developed without any influence exerted by internal or external carcinogens. Data on the incidence of spontaneous thyroid tumors in animals are contradictory. McCoy (1909) and Woolley & Wherry (1912) were the first to systematically investigate thyroids of animals. They searched for tumors in 23,000 and 100,000 wild rats, but failed to detect them. In 1917, Bullock and Rhodenburg firstly described nine tumors found in 4,300 rats; in 1926, Slye at al detected 12 so-called carcinomas in 51,700 mice. They are seen more often in laboratory rats, but have a predilection for older animals. Many of these tumors are derived from the C-cell component of the thyroid gland. Lindsay et al (1968) coined the term "naturally occurring carcinoma of the rats thyroid" for these medullary tumors. In the following years, many studies described spontaneous tumors in various rat strains: For example, van Dyke (1944) reported on nine cystadenomas in 16 Wistar rats that died at the age of more than 800 days. According to other reports, the incidence of spontaneous thyroid neoplasms in Wistar rats is much lower (about 5%; Bielschowsky 1953, van Dyke 1953). In a large group of female Sherman rats kept for more than two years, Axelrad and Leblond (1955) came across only one solid nodule that was composed of light cells. In 1960, Isler et al showed that approximately 40% of female Sherman rats had developed small nodules of light cells at the age of 14 months. In a careful study of serial sections of thyroid glands from Sprague-Dawley rats (mean age 637 days), Thompson & Hunt (1963) observed C-cell tumors in 39% of animals. In contrast, Schardein et al (1968) recorded only 20 follicular adenomas in 5,086 Sprague-Dawley rats. Boorman et al (1972) reported on 123 cases of naturally occurring medullary carcinomas among 334 WAG/Rij rats, 84% of which were older than two years. Lindsay et al (1968) investigated various rat strains and found medullary carcinomas in 19% of Wistar, 22% of Fischer, 22% of Sprague-Dawley, and 40% of Long-Evans rats. Hamsters were also occasionally used for experimental tumorigenesis; Pour et al (1976) found spontaneous thyroid adenomas in 5–10% and carcinomas in 1% of untreated Syrian hamsters. Summarizing the data of the above-mentioned studies, one can draw the following conclusions: the vast majority of spontaneous thyroid tumors so far observed in rats maintained under conventional conditions, i.e., not subjected to factors that either continuously increase the output of TSH or have direct carcinogenic effects, is represented by solid neoplasms. These tumors appear as nodules of different sizes, composed of several varieties of large, oval or polygonal pale cells that neither form follicular structures nor produce colloid. Such nodules usually grow slowly, despite the fact that growth is infiltrative in many cases. The incidence of the neoplasms increases with age. Most of them are revealed in two-year-old or even older rats. The origin of spontaneous solid thyroid tumors in rats has been attributed to the intrafollicular light cells (Askanazy/Hürthle-cells) and to the parafollicular C-cells. In normal rats, spontaneous tumors of follicular, adenomatous and papillary pattern have been observed much less frequently than the above mentioned neoplasms, and in these rare cases, they were consisted of colloid cysts or small hyperplastic nodules.

EXPERIMENTAL INDUCTION OF THYROID TUMORS

Methods for inducing thyroid tumors in animals can be subdivided into two groups according to the mechanism of action. The first group comprises methods based on the application of substances with a direct oncogenic effect on thyroid cells, i.e., proper carcinogenic agents. The methods in the second group aim primarily at establishing a hormonal imbalance that, in turn, will lead to tumor development. Such a division, however, is rather artificial. Some known carcinogenic agents with a direct mechanism of action may also produce profound and irreversible hormonal disturbances that lead to thyroid carcinogenesis. Vice versa, many of the agents used to disturb the hormonal balance may exert a direct carcinogenic effect.

Tumor induction by elevation of TSH

As a result of numerous investigations, a consistent concept of experimental thyroid tumor pathogenesis was established to explain the tumorigenic effect of antithyroid drugs (Bielschowsky 1955). According to this concept, the first stage in the development of thyroid tumors is inhibition of hormone production by the thyroid tissue under the influence of goitrogens. The second stage is the sustained intensification of synthesis and release of TSH. Continuous excessive secretion of TSH is assumed to be one of the basic pathogenic factors responsible for thyroid tumor development.

Goitrogen-induced tumors

Experimental goitrogen-induced tumorigenesis began with the observation that prolonged feeding of a diet containing plants of the Brassica species produced goiter in rats (Hercus & Purves 1936) leading to a high yield of adenomas (Griesbach et al. 1945). Kennedy (1942) suggested that the active agent in the rape seed was a urea derivative. Numerous investigations have previously revealed that in the thyroid the family of thiourea derivatives is both goitrogenic and carcinogenic. For example, Paschkis et al (1948), Kuzell et al. (1949), Clausen (1953), Wollman (1961), and Grundman & Seidel (1965) used thiouracil; Doniach (1950), Christov (1968), and Jemec (1977) used methylthiouracil (MTU); Van Dyke (1953) and Sellers & Schonbaum (1957) used propylthiouracil (PTU); Ulland et al. (1972), Graham et al. (1975), and Arnold et al. (1983) used ethylenethiourea (ETU); tetramethylthioura (TMTU) was used by Stula et al. (1979). Although there is some variation in the goitrogenic activity of the different thioureas, subsequent development of tumors appears to be a uniform finding for all members of this family of thiourea derivatives. They all inhibit steps in hormone synthesis (coupling of iodotyrosines, iodination of thyrosines and monoiodotyrosines) and some, such as PTU, also inhibit deiodination. Daily intake of 5–10mg PTU or 10–20mg MTU is considered an optimum dose for tumor development. Another compound with goitrogenic and carcinogenic activity is the herbicide aminotriazole (ATA). Jukes & Shaffer (1960) and Napalkov (1967) found a similarly high tumor frequency (25% adenomas) in rats of both sexes following lifelong 0.01% ATA administration. Tsuda et al. (1976) and Steinhoff et al. (1983) were able to produce carcinomas in Wistar rats. ATA has turned out to be an experimental goitrogen because the level of general toxicity was lower, than that observed in the thiourea group (Gibson & Doniach 1967). In contrast to mice and rats, hamsters appear to be relatively resistant to tumorigenesis caused by goitrogenic agents. Steinhoff et al. (1983) showed that irrespective of the amount of dosage given to hamsters ATA produced no increase in thyroid neoplasia, while PTU produced thyroid hyperplasia but no neoplasia (Kirkman 1972). However, MTU is reported to produce adenomas and carcinomas in hamsters with frequency and latent intervals similar to those in rats and mice (Akimova et al. 1969, Christov & Raichev 1972). In addition, Hellwig & Welch (1963) described the development of thyroid tumors in 15% of guinea pigs after 14 months PTU intake.

Tumor induction by low-iodine intake

Thyroid tumors have been induced in rats by prolonged over-stimulation of the gland with endogenous TSH only. This method involves maintaining the animals in a state of chronic iodine deficiency. The first observations of rats kept in such a state can be traced back to Bircher (1910, 1911). Since then, the method has been perfected by several groups (Hellwig 1935, Bielschowsky 1953, Isler 1959, Al-Saadi 1968 a.o.), but the most detailed examination was performed by Axelrad & Leblond (1955). These authors found that the changes seen in the thyroid gland and pituitary gland with a low-iodine diet are identical to those seen under long-term goitrogen administration. Thyroid adenomas could be induced in almost all experimental rats when maintaining an iodine-restricted diet with daily intake of about 0.7μg for two years. However, the malignancy of the follicular neoplasms that arise in the rat thyroid as a result of chronic iodine deficiency is questionable. In all cases reported so far, the frequency of carcinomas originating from follicular epithelium is clearly lower in rats kept on a low-iodine diet than in animals treated with goitrogens. In rats, iodine deficiency is a much more effective tumor promoter than is a carcinogen, suggesting that a similar relationship may exist in human populations (Ward & Oshima 1986). In C3H/Hey strain-mice, Schaller & Stevenson (1966) used low-iodine diet to induce benign and malignant thyroid tumors; after one year of treatment, carcinomas developed in 14%. In hamsters, Fortner et al. (1959) found well-differentiated, metastatic follicular tumors in 18% of females, but no lesions in males after a 70-week iodine-deficient diet.

Tumor growth after partial thyroidectomy

Although it has been claimed that subtotal thyroidectomy is a potent method that raises the level of trophic stimulus to the thyroid, the yield of tumors in animals treated in this way is lower than in animals given a low-iodine diet or long-term goitrogen (Doniach 1970). Doniach & Williams (1962) and Goldberg et al. (1964) induced 14% adenomas and 4% carcinomas in Lister rats 15 months after 85%-excision of thyroid mass. In contrast, Ird (1968) found that subtotal thyroidectomy alone did not increase the incidence of tumors above that seen in control rats, and that surgery reduced the incidence of tumors in rats treated with MTU (25% vs. 74%). The relatively low yield of tumors obtained by this method may be explained by the fact that owing to surgery most part of the target gland responsible for the trophic stimulus is removed. This, of course, reduces the population of cells that might undergo neoplastic change.

Tumor induction by ionizing radiation

Radiation affecting the thyroid gland is possible via two routes: external or internal. External administration of radiation is achieved by using either X- or gamma-emitting radiation sources. Theoretically, this route has the advantage of permitting delivery of a precisely calculable amount of rads (Gray), but suffers from several practical problems. Firstly, given the size of the thyroid of the rat or mice, it is difficult both to localize the target and to avoid damaging the surrounding tissue. Secondly, it is also essential, but difficult, to avoid unirradiated parts of the thyroid, leading to an overestimation of the dose delivered. These problems may be solved by lightly anaesthetizing animals and by carefully placing a lead collar with a small window over the neck region, both to protect the surrounding tissue and to hold the animal in position. Internal irradiation is usually given in form of sodium salts of I^{131} or I^{125} by intraperitoneal or intrathyroidal injection. This method is much more convenient than external irradiation, although different problems arise. Accurate calculation of the dose received is difficult, since it is dependent both on percentage uptake and retention of the isotope. The amount of

Table 1. Review of the literature: incidence of thyroid tumors in rats following a single irradiation with radio-iodine (I^{131})

Dosage ($\mu Ci\ I^{131}$)	Age (days)	Latent period (month)	Adenoma (%)	Carcinoma (%)	Authors
1	—	6	0		Lindsay et al. (1968b)
1	—	12	1		Lindsay et al. (1968b)
1	—	24	2		Lindsay et al. (1968b)
1.1	4	12	26		Doniach (1969)
2.9	4	12	39		Doniach (1969)
5	70	15	50		Doniach (1953)
5	—	6	0		Lindsay et al. (1968b)
5	—	12	9		Lindsay et al. (1968b)
5	—	24	12		Lindsay et al. (1968b)
5.5	4	12	48		Doniach (1969)
10	42–84	32	33	16	Lindsay et al. (1957)
25	42	12	11	3	Lindsay et al. (1966)
25	56	24	96	26	Potter et al. (1960)
25	42–84	32	35	15	Lindsay et al. (1957)
30	70	15	50		Doniach (1953)
30	84	15	18		Doniach (1956)
100	70	15	0		Doniach (1953)
100	42–84	31	0	10	Lindsay et al. (1957)
200	42–84	32	13		Lindsay et al. (1957)
400	42–84	28	0.7		Lindsay et al. (1957)

isotope retained by the gland is dependent on the biological, as well as on the physical, half-life. The biological half-life is difficult to predict and may vary with the strain of animal species, diet and sex. Even the surrounding temperature has been shown to influence iodine uptake (Doniach 1950).

Tumor growth following internal radio-iodine application

The destructive effect of variable amounts of radioactive iodine on the normal thyroid was shown for the first time in 1942 by Hamilton & Lawrence in the dog and rabbit and in 1948 by Findlay & Leblond in the adult rat. Experimentally induced neoplasms of the rat thyroid following I^{131}-irradiation were first produced by Doniach (1950). He reported that the administration of $32\mu Ci\ I^{131}$ significantly increased the formation of adenomas, as compared with untreated groups. In 1951, Goldberg & Chaikoff showed that a single dose of I^{131} would cause benign and malignant tumors after a period of 1.5–2 years. Since these initial experiments, several pieces of evidence have shown that as little as $5\mu Ci\ I^{131}$ is tumorigenic to the rat thyroid, and that the administration of doses ranging from 5–$400\mu Ci\ I^{131}$ can produce benign and malignant neoplasms. However, with increasing dose, a larger percentage of cells is sterilized, thus reducing the number of tumors produced (Table 1). The optimal carcinogenic radiation dose to young adult rats is approximately 5–$50\mu Ci\ I^{131}$. One important factor affecting the dose-response curve for tumor production is the age at which radiation is given. Doniach (1969) showed that after administration of $2.9\mu Ci\ I^{131}$ at birth tumor yield was similar to that following $30\mu Ci\ I^{131}$ given to adult rats. Taking into account the weight

Table 2. Review of the literature: incidence of thyroid tumors in rats following a single bilateral irradiation with X-rays

Dosage (Gy)	Age (days)	Latent period (month)	Adenoma (%)	Carcinoma (%)	Authors
1	70	18–20	14		Doniach (1974)
2.5	70	18–20	10		Doniach (1974)
3	10	15	38		Christov (1978)
3	60	15	15		Christov (1978)
4	40	13	70		Boltze et al. (2002)
4	40	25	80		Boltze et al. (2002)
5	70	18–20	0	6	Doniach (1958)
5	56–84	24	18	4	Lindsay et al. (1961)
10	56–84	24	54	22	Lindsay et al. (1961)
11	92	15	23	8	Doniach (1956)
20	56–84	24	75	25	Lindsay et al. (1961)

of the animals, his results do not reveal any increased susceptibility of the newborn rat to the carcinogenic action of radioactive iodine compared with adults. There is also no marked difference in weanling rats (28 days) as compared with young adults (70 days) (Doniach 1957).

Tumor induction after external X-ray irradiation

Experimentally, the effects of external irradiation on thyroid tumor production have mostly been assessed in rats. In several studies, doses ranged from 1Gy to 20Gy, including various intermediate doses. Table 2 shows that the optimum dose for the development of tumors is dependent on the age at which the radiation is initially administered and, obviously, the age at which the animal is examined. For 3-month-old rats, the optimal dose for thyroid tumor induction using only X-rays lies between 5 and 10Gy. A lower dose of X-rays given to the neck region of 10-day old rats has induced more tumors with a shorter latent period than the same dose given to 60-day-old animals (Christov 1978). This increase in tumorigenicity in younger animals is possibly due to the higher mitotic index of the thyroid in younger rats.

Comparisons of X-ray and I^{131} doses, which are able to produce thyroid tumors have shown a ratio of 1:8 to 1:10 (Doniach 1956, 1963). Abbatt et al. (1957) investigated the inhibition of goitrogenesis in rats, produced by varying doses of X-rays and radioactive iodine. After giving either 30µCi I^{131} or 10Gy of X-rays their results showed a similar effect. They suggested that compared with I^{131} the apparent ten-fold increased sensitivity of the thyroid to X-rays as may be due to the overall uneven distribution of radiation with I^{131} so that some follicles possibly receive a smaller amount than those absorbed by others.

Thyroid tumorigenesis induced by chemical carcinogens

In 1942, Esmarch was the first to use chemical carcinogens for the production of thyroid tumors in experiments. He applied methylcholanthrene directly to thyroid glands of rats. The direct application of other carcinogenic polycyclic hydrocarbons was studied later and, as expected, such an approach produced more sarcomas and squamous cell carcinomas than adenocarcinomas. Money & Rawson (1950, 1965) found that administration of dimethylbenzanthracene either directly to the thyroid gland or by subcutaneous injection did not significantly alter the incidence or type of produced tumors.

Tumor induction by aromatic amines and azo dyes

Thyroid adenomas can be produced by systemic administration of acetylaminofluorene (AAF, formerly used as an insecticide), which can also produce a high yield of tumors in other organs of rats, including mammary gland, liver, kidney, intestine and uterus (Bielschowsky 1944). Murthy (1980) found that continuous administration of the dye intermediate, 4,4'-methylene-bis-(N,N-dimethyl)-benzenamine (MDBA), to F344 rats of both sexes produced follicular tumors after 80 weeks. The incidence was higher in animals receiving larger doses, and it was in these animals only that hyperplastic changes were seen in the thyroid. Murthy et al. (1985), taking up earlier studies of 4,4'-oxydianiline (ODA) that had shown evidence of a goitrogenic and carcinogenic effect on the thyroid in rodents (Hayden et al. 1978), in whom it also caused a high incidence of liver tumors. They reported that the incidence of thyroid hyperplasia and neoplasia was high in animals given 0.04%–0.05% ODA in the diet. The earliest follicular tumor was seen at 28 weeks, and after two years, neoplasms were present in 86% of the survivors of these groups. Thyroid hyperplasia and changes in thyrotroph population in the pituitary glands of rats with follicular tumors suggested that the carcinogenic effect of ODA was at least partly mediated through an elevation of TSH.

Tumor growth induced by nitrosamines

Diisopropanolnitrosamine (DIPN) is one member of a family that belongs to the carcinogenic nitrosamines, i.e., postulated intermediates of the parent compound di-n-propylnitrosamine, with broad-spectrum activity in most species tested. When given weekly subcutaneous injection to Sprague-Dawley rats for life, there was up to 50% incidence of thyroid tumors, with short latent intervals of 23 weeks for adenomas and 26 weeks for carcinomas (Mohr et al. 1977). N-bis-(2-hydroxypropyl)nitrosamine (DHPN) can also initiate thyroid tumors, although the frequency is lower in the absence of a promoting agent. Obviously, there is a difference in the sensitivity of rat strains to this agent: equitoxic doses resulted in thyroid tumors in 50% of Sprague-Dawley rats and in 20% of MRC rats (Mohr et al. 1977, Pour et al. 1979). N-nitrosobis (2-oxopropyl)amine (BOP) is a nitrosamine closely related to DHPN, with a high yield of thyroid tumors in rats: Pour & Salmasizadeh (1978) found 50% incidence in MRC rats following a single dose, and 60% after weekly treatment for life. When given in equitoxic doses, BOP produced thyroid neoplasms in 60% and DHPN in 20% of MRC rats (Pour et al. 1979). In 1986, Pour also showed that intrauterine exposure of hamsters to BOP results in 50% incidence of thyroid adenomas in female animals, but 0% in male animals; this is of particular interest as in adult hamsters, the carcinogenic effect is almost entirely confined to the pancreas.

Tumor induction by nitrosoureas

Thyroid carcinogenesis with N-nitroso-N-methylurea (NMU) was first described by Jobst (1967). He treated rats during their intrauterine development and after birth with weekly injections and found thyroid carcinomas in some of the survivors. NMU (3 injections of 30mg/kg) was given to Wistar rats by Thomas & Bollman (1974), who reported a 100% incidence of follicular cell carcinomas after 7–8 months. Takizawa & Nishihara (1971) reported the induction of a thyroid carcinoma in a female rat given the powerful neurocarcinogen N-nitrosobutylurea (NBU). N-ethyl-N-nitrosourea (ENU) has been extensively applied as a transplacental neurocarcinogen in several species, but the use of high doses in young rats can produce thyroid tumors, mostly of encapsulated papillary type, in a small portion (Stoica & Koestner 1984). Warzok et al. (1977) and Napalkov et al. (1981) reported that transplacental administration of ENU to dogs causes not only early development of thyroid tumors in a minority of cases, but also to late tumors.

Studies with combination of tumor-inducing factors

The methods of thyroid tumor induction outlined above, i.e., treatment with antithyroid or carcinogenic substances, restriction of iodine consumption and irradiation, are often used in various combinations. For instance, pre-irradiation of the thyroid significantly increased the tumor development in rats kept on a low iodine diet (Nadler et al. 1969). Similar effects have been observed in experiments with the combining irradiation with antithyroid drugs or certain chemical carcinogens (Lindsay 1969). The combination of antithyroid drugs or a low-iodine diet with chemical carcinogens (AAF was usually used) also resulted in accelerated tumor developmemt (Bielschowsky 1944, Hall & Bielschowsky 1949, Axelrad & Leblond 1955). Hall (1948) made the interesting observation that even relatively small doses of AAF given for a period as short as 1 week were sufficient to produce an enhancing effect on tumorigenesis, and this effect was still observed when goitrogen treatment with allylthiourea was delayed for up to 18 weeks. There is evidence that AAF causes neoplastic progression of thyroid epithelium only under conditions of excess TSH stimulation. Otherwise no detectable effect was observed by Bielschowsky & Griesbach (1950) a finding not confirmed by other studies (Grundmann & Seidel 1965). It is possible that owing to a toxic alteration of hepatic cells normally responsible for hormone degradation AAF itself might indirectly raise TSH levels. Hiasa et al. (1982) found that treatment of rats with either repeated small doses of DHPN or treatment with aminotriazole (ATA) did not produce tumors, but combination therapy with both agents could yield neoplasms in up to 100% of animals after 12 weeks. PTU has also been used successfully in combination with DHPN by this group (Kitahori et al. 1984). Several studies have given evidence of the promoting effect of barbiturates on thyroid carcinogenesis by DHPN. Whereas single or multiple administrations of DHPN alone resulted in 0% tumors at week 20 in rats, additional treatment with barbital for 12 weeks produced thyroid neoplasms in 45% of animals; phenobarbital treatment was even more effective, leading to an incidence of up to 100% of animals at week 20 (Hiasa et al. 1983). Schaffer & Müller (1980) found invasive thyroid tumors by 16 weeks and pulmonary metastases by 30 weeks after 3-times NMU injection in combination with long-term MTU treatment. Similar results were obtained by combining NMU with PTU in F344 rats (Milmore et al. 1982), and NMU with phenobarbital (Tsuda et al. 1983). Ohshima & Ward (1984) found that iodine-deficient diet was also an efficient promoter for NMU-initiated tumors, with 100% incidence of thyroid tumors in F344 rats after 20-week treatment. Even without the additional influence if iodine-deficient diet, NMU treatment resulted in 10% incidence of adenomas after 20 weeks, 70% incidence after 33 weeks, and 10% incidence of carcinomas after 33 weeks. Diwan et al. (1985) used NMU in combination with barbiturates and demonstrated that the incidence and multiplicity of thyroid tumors are greater in male rats, because in this sex phenobarbital seems to be a more effective promoter, as shown by the higher incidence of liver tumors in male animals in the same experiment.

Long term study for investigating changes in morphology, function and proliferation of thyrocytes after varying nutrition iodine and external radiation in rats

Several studies mentioned above have addressed the question of a predominant iodide-dependent regulation in the development of hyperplasia and proliferation of thyroid follicle cells *in vivo*, or have reported a major contribution of TSH in this respect. However, most of these studies, based on severe iodide depletion, used a short observation period for defining iodide-dependent effects. Only few reports have dealt with the ontogenesis of morphological and hormonal changes during moderate long-term iodine deficiency, which more closely parallels the situation of humans in an iodine-deficient area. The long-term effects of iodine excess in humans have not been studied in detail, but recent reports suggest that iodine excess also induces goitrogenesis and benign thyroid tumors.

One study (Boltze et al. 2002) aimed at systematically monitoring the influence of a long-term increase or decrease in daily iodine supply on the morphology of the thyroid of rats. To develop a reproducible model of thyroid tumorigenesis, this treatment was combined with short-term external radiation of the thyroid using known environmental hazards. It is expected that such a model helps to define the relevant genetic alterations causing thyroid tumor formation in a subsequent step, and may thus contribute to the diagnosis of thyroid adenomas.

Experimental design

Three groups of 80 male Sprague-Dawley rats (28d old), each differing in daily iodine supply, were investigated: 1. normal iodine intake (7000ng Iodine/100g body weight/day)(In), 2. low iodine diet (420ng Iodine/100g bw/d (I-) and 3. high iodine diet (72000ng Iodine/100g bw/d. On day 40, the thyroid region of half of each group was externally irradiated with a single dose of 4Gy X-rays (InR, I-R, I+R). Weekly, the animals were monitored as for their body weight, and blood samples for determining TSH, T3 and T4 were obtained. Of each of the six groups, 10 animals were killed at weeks 15, 35, 55 and 110; the thyroids were removed and investigated by histology

Table 3. Number of benign and malignant thyroid tumors after and without nutrition pretreatment and radiation ($n = 10$)

Group and tumors	55th week	110th week
Normal iodine		
In		
B	2 dermoid cyts	3 dermoid cysts
C	0	0
P	0	0
InR		
B	7 adenomas	8 adenomas
C	0	0
P	0	1 squamous carcinoma
Iodine deficiency		
I-		
B	5 adenomas	9 adenomas
C	0	0
P	0	0
I-R		
B	7 adenomas	9 adenomas
C	0	2 FTC / 3 PTC
P	1 adenocarcinoma	1 adenocarcinoma
Iodine supplementation		
I+		
B	5 adenomas	9 adenomas
C	0	0
P	0	0
I+R		
B	9 adenomas	10 adenomas
C	0	3 FTC / 5 PTC
P	0	1 squamous carcinoma

B, benign thyroid tumors; C, thyroid carcinomas; PTC, papillary thyroid carcinoma; FTC, follicular thyroid carcinoma. Parathyroid carcinomas (P) were also induced: squamous cell carcinomas of the cervical soft tissue and adenocarcinomas of salivary glands.

and immunohistochemistry. The following parameters were detected: follicles/mm^2, colloid diameter, index of fibrosis, proliferation rate and number of tumors.

Results

Iodine-dependent changes without radiation:

Iodine deficiency led to lower daily growth rates and a significantly lower final mean body weight of 430g (I-) vs. 501g (In) vs. 475g (I+). The growth process was finished after 18 weeks in I+ and after 21 weeks in In and I-. Long-term iodine deficiency significantly decreased plasma T3 and T4 concentrations after week 9. In contrast, the high iodine diet did not change thyroid function. All changes manifested themselves in alterations in thyroid morphology. Iodine deficiency was associated with significantly large, but fewer, follicles, whereas the high iodine diet led to a significant decrease in the diameter, but to an increase in the number of follicles. The mitotic activity of thyrocytes was very low under normal iodine intake conditions (<1±0.2%). Not only iodine deficiency, but also higher iodine intake significantly increased proliferation

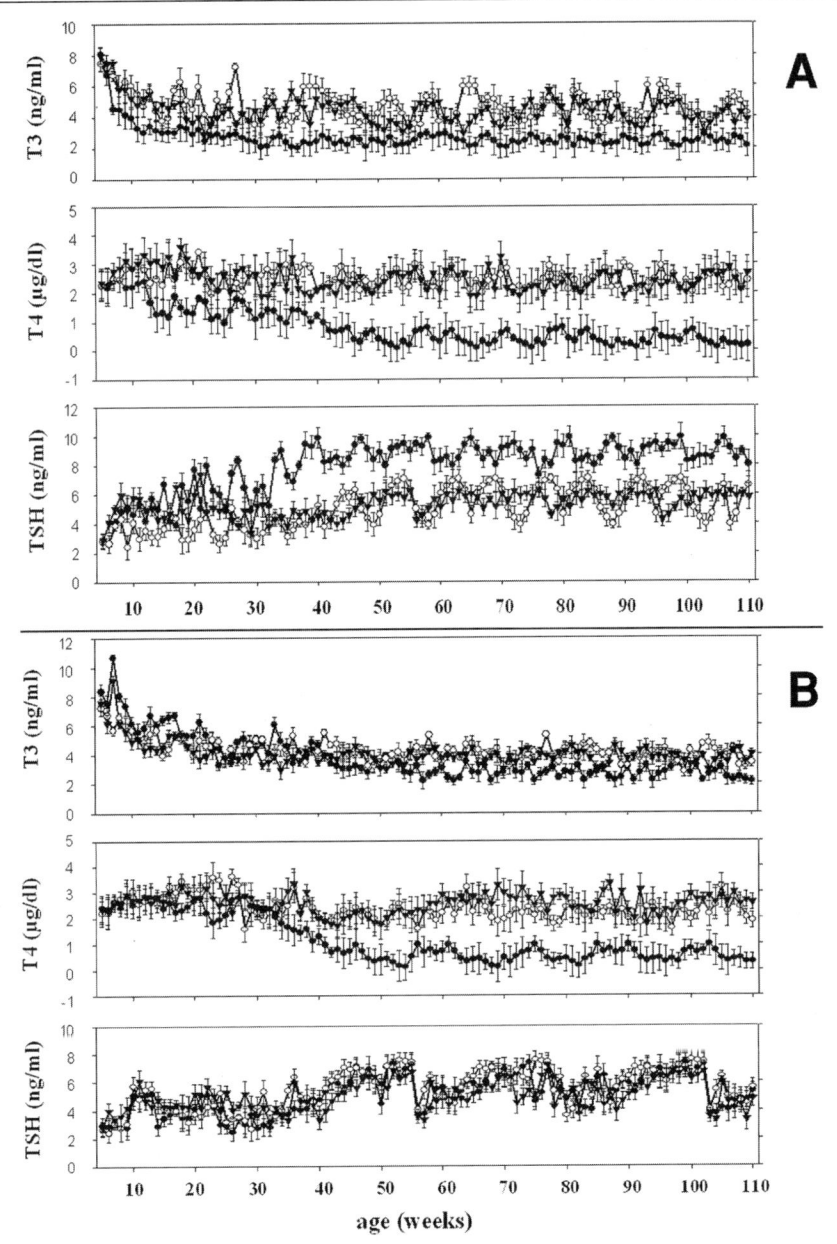

Figure 2. Changes of T3, T4 and TSH plasma concentrations in rats without (A) and after radiation with 4Gy (B) under normal nutrition iodine conditions (white circle (o)), iodine deficiency (black circles (•)) and iodine supplementation (black triangles (▲)).

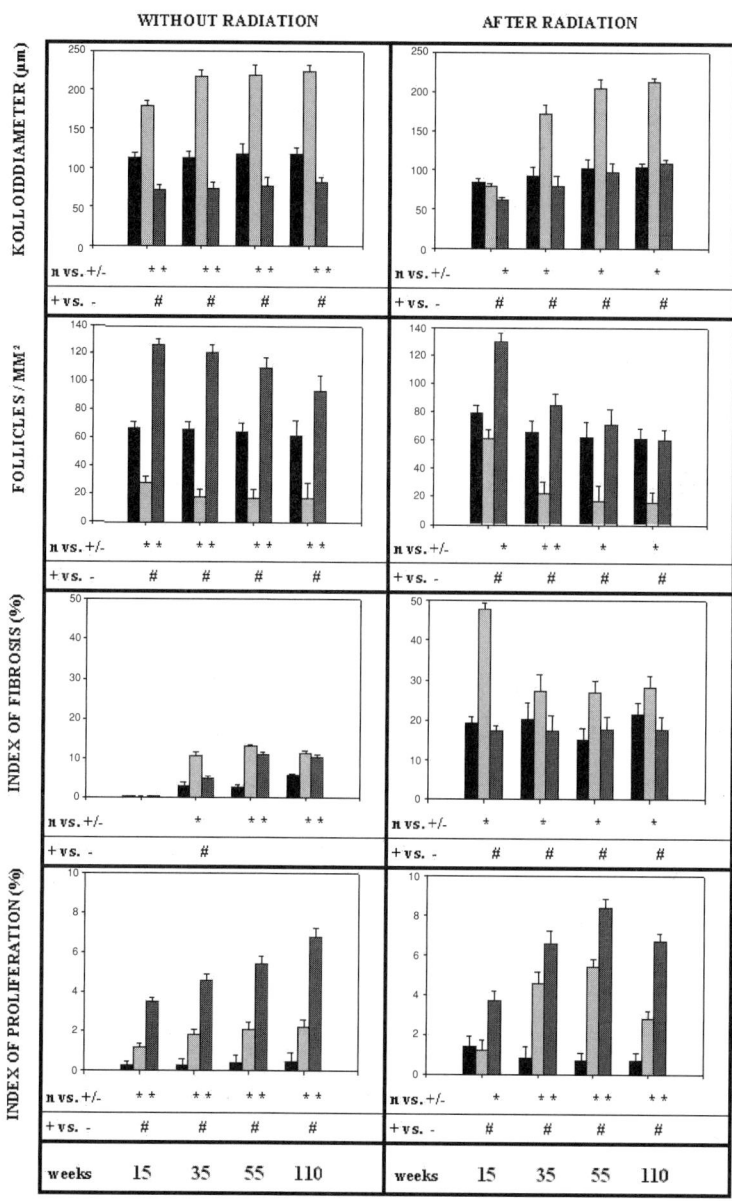

Figure 3. Histological data of the thyroids after 15, 35, 55 and 110 weeks under normal iodine conditions (In; black bars ■), iodine deficiency (I−; gray bars ☐) and iodine supplement (I+; dark-grey bars ▨) with or without irradiation (n = 10; mean±SEM).
(* = statistical significance In vs. I− or I+, $p < 0.05$; # = statistical significance I+ vs. I−, $p < 0.05$)

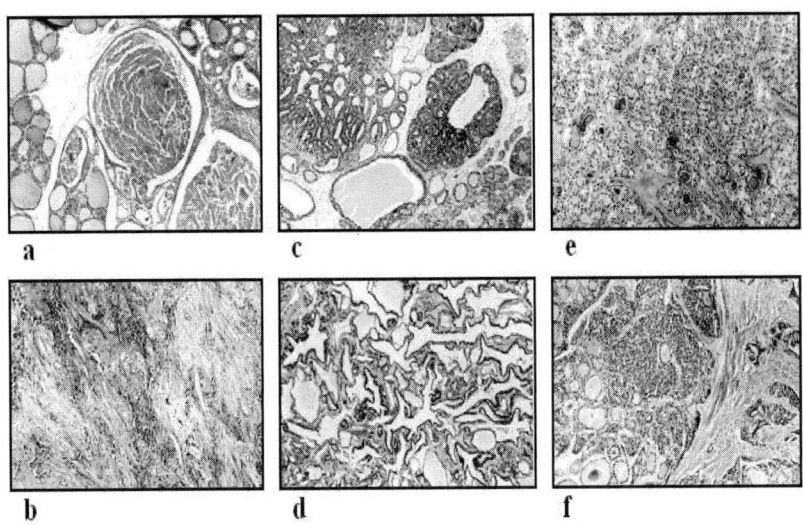

Figure 4. Histological examples of tumors induced after 4Gy radiation of the thyroid region under normal nutrition iodine conditions (A and B), iodine deficiency (C and D) and iodine supplementation (E and F; magnification x100). A, Metaplasia of squamous epithelium with dermoid cysts (55 weeks). B, Squamous cell carcinoma of the cervical soft tissue beside the thyroid gland (55 weeks). C, Adenocarcinoma of a salivary gland (glandula submandibularis; 55 weeks). D, Follicular thyroid carcinoma with a bizarre pattern (110 weeks). E, Follicular thyroid carcinoma, small follicular/insular type (110 weeks). F, Papillary thyroid carcinoma, predominant follicular pattern, sporadic papillae (110 weeks).

rates. At week 55 and 110, all non-irradiated animal groups were free of malignant tumors, and benign tumors were not detected until week 55.

Iodine-dependent changes after radiation:

After radiation, there were increases in T3 and T4, and a significant decrease in TSH in the group with iodine deficiency. The hormone concentrations of the normal iodine and high iodine groups were not significantly altered. In all groups, thyroid weight was not significantly influenced by radiation. Histologically, the most important finding in irradiated low iodine diet thyroids was the total destruction of follicles observed at week 15. After this destruction, a short-term increase in T3 (7th week) was measured. After the 55th week, a complete restitution of the follicle structure was seen. In contrast to the sole manipulation of iodine intake, radiation treatment led to a higher number of benign tumors, starting 55 weeks after having changed nutritional iodine supply, and to malignant tumors after 110 weeks. Parathyroid carcinomas were also induced: squamous cell carcinomas of the cervical soft tissue and adenocarcinomas of the salivary glands. The thyroid carcinomas were solitary tumors, their size ranged between 0.1 and 1.5mm. Neither local lymph node metastasis nor distant metastasis was found.

Conclusions

This animal model clearly supports the concept that in thyroid carcinogenesis, there is a very long latency period between the mutational event and the developement of malignant changes. This contradicts previous studies using a higher stimulation of thyrocyte proliferation by iodine deficiency, where malignancies were detected after much shorter time intervals (Axelrad & Leblond 1955). Large doses of iodine may induce thyroid carcinomas (Correa & Welsh 1960). We showed that mild iodine excess is not necessarily associated with the formation of thyroid malignant neoplasms, but when combined with a mutagen, carcinomas arise with high frequency. These data on mild forms of high iodine intake thus put a note of caution to a long term-use of high iodine. It was shown that euthyreosis is best protection against thyroid cancer before environmental hazards are effective.

The well-defined setting in these experiments clearly demonstrates that mutational lesions acquired by radiation are clinically silent over a long period of time. It is tempting to use such a model to search for candidate genes altered by mutagens, but which are not changed in thyroid adenomas found under control conditions. The definition of such changes may then have important implications for the characterization of the malignant potential of a given adenoma well before cytological or histological changes occur.

FUTURE OF ANIMAL MODELS INVESTIGATING THYROID CARCINOGENESIS

In the last 75 years, very different models investigating thyroid carcinogensis have been developed. The concept of initiation and promotion of carcinogenesis is well demonstrated by the studies reviewed in this chapter. The initiation step may be produced by diverse agents, including ionizing radiation and many classes of carcinogens. The action of these agents is promoted by raising the level of trophic stimulation (TSH), which can also be achieved in a variety of ways (for instance goitrogen therapy or low-iodine diet). All these models successfully described the changes in morphology and function of thyrocytes during carcinogenesis. However, the time in which these kind of models were used is over. Therefore, in the last ten years, such studies were published only sporadically. The molecular basis of thyroid neoplastic processes involved in experimental tumors is now being elucidated by investigations of the changes associated with developing tumors, and also by the reconstruction of the tumor phenotype through the introduction of genes into thyroid cells. In the last few years, many new methods (including chip- and array technology, or proteomics) have been developed to clarify tumor-related mechanisms and to search for tumor-associated genes. The tumor induction models mentioned above can serve as the basis for yielding material of different stages of thyroid carcinogenesis. A factor limiting these forthcoming gene expression studies is the small amount of relevant material. The use of more sensitive methods will solve this problem in future.

REFERENCES

1. Abbatt JD, Doniach I, Howard-Flanders P, Logothetopoulos JH: Comparison of the inhibition of goitrogenesis in the rat produced by X-rays and radioactive iodine. Br J Radiol 1957; 30:86–88.
2. Akimova P, Gonina R, Zotikov LA, Kulik GI: Results of a biochemical, histochemical and ultrastructural study of the thyroid gland in the process of experimental carcinogenesis. In: Hedinger C (ed) Thyroid cancer. UICC Monograph series, volume 12, Springer-Verlag Berlin, 1969, pp. 149–154.

3. Al-Saadi: Precursor genetic changes of transplantable thyroid carcinoma in iodine deficient goitres. Cancer Res 1968; 28:739–745.
4. Arnold DL, Krewski DR, Junkins DB, McGuire PF, Moodie CA, Munro IC: Reversibility of ethylenethiourea-induced thyroid lesions. Toxicol Appl Pharmacol 1983; 67:264–273.
5. Axelrad AA, Leblond CP: Induction of thyroid tumors in rats by a low iodine diet. Cancer 1955; 8:339–367.
6. Bielschowsky F: Tumors of the thyroid produced by 2-acetyl-amino-fluoren and allyl-thiourea. Brit J Exp Path 1944; 25:90–94.
7. Bielschowsky F: Chronic iodine deficiency as cause of neoplasia in thyroid and pituitary of aged rats. Br J Cancer 1953; 7:203–213.
8. Bielschowsky F: Neoplasia and internal environment. Br J Cancer 1955; 9:80–116.
9. Bielschowsky F, Griesbach WE: Effect of acetoaminofluorene on the thyroids of rats treated with methylthiouracil and thyroxine. Br J Cancer 1950; 4:133–138.
10. Bircher E: On the experimental induction of goitre and a contribution on its histogenesis. Dtsch Z Chir 1910; 103:276–364.
11. Bircher E: Further histological findings on goitre induced by water in the rat. Dtsch Z Chir 1911; 112:368–424.
12. Boltze C, Brabant G, Dralle H, Gerlach R, Roessner A, Hoang-Vu C: Radiation-induced thyroid carcinogenesis as function of time and dietary iodine supply—An in-vivo model of tumorigenesis in the rat. Endocrinology 2002; 143:2584–2592.
13. Boorman GA, van Noord MJ, Hollander CF: Naturally occurring medullary carcinoma in the rat. Arch Pathol 1972; 94:35–41.
14. Bullock FD, Rhodenberg GL: Tumors of the rat. J Cancer Res 1917; 2:39–60.
15. Christov K: Experimental tumours of the thyroid gland in rats treated with 2-acetylaminofluorene and methylthiouracil. Oncologia 1968; 5:49–60.
16. Christov K: Radiation induced thyroid tumours in infant rats. Radiat Res 1978; 73:330–339.
17. Christov K, Raichev R: Experimental thyroid carcinogenesis. Curr Top Pathol 1972; 56:79–114.
18. Clausen HJ: Further studies on the thyroid gland of the rat following the administration of thiouracil. Anatomical Record 1953; 117:535–536.
19. Correa P, Welsh RA: The effect of excessive iodine intake on the thyroid gland of the rat. Arch Pathol 1960; 70:247–251.
20. Diwan BA, Palmer AE, Ohshima M, Rice JM: N-Nitroso-N-methylurea initiation in multiple tissues for organ-specific tumor promotion in rats by phenobarbital. J Natl Cancer Inst 1985; 75:1099–1105.
21. Doniach I: The effect of radioactive iodine alone and in combination with methylurea and acetylaminofluorene upon tumour production in the rats thyroid gland. Br J Cancer 1953; 7:181–202.
22. Doniach I: Comparison of the carcinogenetic effect of X-irradiation with radioactive iodine on the rats thyroid. Br J Cancer 1956; 11:67–76.
23. Doniach I: Sensitivity of the weanling rat thyroid to radiation. Br J Cancer 1957; 11:253–257.
24. Doniach I: Experimental induction of tumours of the thyroid by radiation Br Med Bull 1958; 14:181–183.
25. Doniach I: Effects including carcinogenesis of I^{131} and X-rays on the thyroid of experimental animals: a review. Health Phys 1963; 9: 1357–1362.
26. Doniach I: Tumor production in thyroids of rats given varying dosis of radioactive iodine at birth. In: Hedinger C (ed) Thyroid cancer. UICC Monograph series, volume 12, Springer Verlag, Berlin, 1969, pp. 174–182.
27. Doniach I: Experimental thyroid tumors. Monogr Neoplast Dis Var Sites 1970; 6:73–99.
28. Doniach I: Carcinogenic effect of 100, 250 and 500 rad X-rays on the rat thyroid gland. Br J Cancer 1974; 30:487–495.
29. Doniach I, Williams ED: Development of thyroid and pituitary tumours in the rat two years after partial thyroidectomie. Br J Cancer 1962; 16:222–231.
30. Esmarch O: Deposition of methylcholanthrene in some organs of the rat. Acta Path Microbiol Scand 1942; 19:79–99.
31. Findlay D, Leblond CP: Partial destruction of the rat thyroid by large doses of radio-iodine. Am J Roentgenol 1948; 59:387–395.
32. Fortner JG, George PA, Sternberg SS: The development of thyroid cancer and other abnormalities in Syrian hamsters maintained on an iodine-deficient diet. Surg Forum 1959; 9:646–650.
33. Gibson JM, Doniach I: Correlation of dose of X-radiation to the rat thyroid gland with degree of subsequent impairment of response to goitrogenic stimulus. Br J Cancer 1967; 21:525–530.

34. Goldberg RC, Chaikoff IL: Development of thyroid neoplasms in the rat following a single injection of radioactive iodine. Proc Soc Exp Biol 1951; 76:560–563
35. Goldberg RC, Lindsay S, Nichols CW, Chaikoff IL: Induction of neoplasms in thyroid glands of rats by subtotal thyroidectomy and by injection of one microcurie of I^{131}. Cancer Res 1964; 24:35–43.
36. Graham SL, Davis KJ, Hansel WH, Graham CH: Effects of prolonged ethylene thiourea ingestion on the thyroid of the rat. Food Cosmet Toxicol 1975; 13:493–499
37. Griesbach WE, Kennedy TH, Purves HD: Studies on experimental goitre. Thyroid adenomata in rats on Brassica seed diet. Br J Exp Pathol 1945; 26:18–24.
38. Grundmann E, Seidel HJ: Die Entstehung des Schilddrüsenkarzinoms bei der Ratte unter Thiouracil und 2-acetaminofluoren. Beitr Pathol Anat Allg Pathol 1965; 132:188–219.
39. Hall WH: The role of initiating and promoting factors in the pathogenesis of tumours of the thyroid. Br J Cancer 1948; 2:273–280.
40. Hall WH, Bielschowsky F: The development of malignancy in experimentally induced adenomata of the thyroid. Br J Cancer 1949; 3:534–541.
41. Hamilton JG, Lawrence JH: Recent clinical advances in the therapeutic application of radiophosphorus and radio-iodine. J Clin Invest 1942; 21:624.
42. Hayden DW, Wade G, Handler AH: The goitrogenic effect of 4,4′-oxydianiline in rats and mice. Vet Pathol 1978; 15:649–662.
43. Hellwig CA: Thyroid adenoma in experimental animals. Am J Cancer 1935; 23:550–555.
44. Hellwig CA, Welch JW: Drug induced tumors of the thyroid in guinea pigs with experimental thyroiditis. Growth 1963; 27:305–315.
45. Hercus CE, Purves HD: Studies on endemic and experimental goitre. J Hyg 1936; 36:182–203.
46. Hiasa Y, Kitahori Y, Konishi N, Enoki N, Fujita T: Effect of varying the duration of exposure to phenobarbital on its enhancement of N-bis(2-hydroxypropyl)nitrosamine-induced thyroid tumorigenesis in male Wistar rats. Carcinogenesis 1983; 4:935–937.
47. Hiasa Y, Ohshima M, Kitahori Y, Yuasa T, Fujita T, Iwata C: Promoting effects of 3-amino-1,2,4-triazole on the development of thyroid tumors in rats treated with N-bis(2-hydroxypropyl)nitrosamine. Carcinogenesis 1982; 3:381–384
48. Hoang-Vu C, Brabant G, Leitolf H, von zur Mühlen A, Dralle H, Schroder S, Sierralta WD: Functional an morphological changes of the thyroid gland following 5 days of pulsatile TRH infusion in male rats. J Endocrinol 1995; 146:339–348.
49. Ird EA: Effect of subtotal thyroidectomy on the development of thyroid tumours in rats treated with methylthiouracil. Probl Endokrinol 1968; 14:87-94.
50. Isler H: Effect of iodine tumors induced in the rat by low-iodine diet. J Natl Cancer Inst 1959; 23:675–693.
51. Isler H, Thompson B, Tonkin R, Sarkar SK: Three-dimensional structure of the thyroid gland with reference to the basement membrane of the follicles and to the location of the light cell. Anat Rec 1960; 136:338.
52. Jemec B: Studies of the tumorigenic effect of two goitrogens. Cancer 1977; 40:2188–2202.
53. Jobst K: Teratogenous changes and tumors in rats following treatment with methylnitrosourea (MNU). Neoplasma 1967; 14:435–436.
54. Jukes TH, Schaffer CB: Antithyroid effects of aminotriazole. Science 1960; 132:296–297
55. Kennedy TH: Thioureas as goitrogenic substances. Nature 1942; 150:233–234.
56. Kirkman H: Hormone-related tumors in Syrian hamsters. Prog Exp Tumors Res 1972; 16:201–240.
57. Kitahori Y, Hiasa Y, Konishi N, Enoki N, Shimoyama T, Miyashiro A: Effect of propylthiouracil on the thyroid tumorigenesis induced by N-bis(2-hydroxypropyl) nitrosamine in rats. Carcinogenesis 1984; 5:657–660.
58. Kuzell WC, Tripi HB, Gardner GM, Laqueur GL: Diffuse and nodular hyperplasia of the thyroid gland in thiuracil-treated rats. Sience 1949; 107:374–375.
59. Larsen PR, Merker A, Parlow AF: Immunoassay of human TSH using dried blood samples. J Clin Endocrinol Metab 1976; 42:987–990
60. Lemoine NR, Mayall ES, Williams ED, Thurston V, Wynford-Thomas D: Agent-specific ras oncogene activation in rat thyroid tumours. Oncogene 1988; 3:541–544.
61. Lindsay S: Ionizing radiation and experimental thyroid neoplasms: A review. In: Hedinger C (ed) Thyroid cancer. UICC Monograph series, volume 12, Springer-Verlag, Berlin, 1969, pp. 161–171.
62. Lindsay S, Potter GD, Chaikoff IL: Thyroid neoplasms in the rat: a comparison of naturally occuring and I^{313}-induced tumours. Cancer Res 1957; 17:183–189.

63. Lindsay S, Sheline GE, Potter GD, Chaikoff IL: Induction of neoplasms in the thyroid gland of the rat by X-irradiation of the gland. Cancer Res 1961; 21:9–16
64. Lindsay S, Potter GD, Chaikoff IL: Induction of benign and malignant thyroid neoplasms in the rat. Arch Pathol 1966; 81:308–317.
65. Lindsay S, Nichols CW, Chaikoff IL: Naturally-occurring thyroid carcinoma in the rat: similarities to human medullary carcinoma Arch Pathol 1968; 86:353–364.
66. Lindsay S, Nichols CW, Chaikoff IL: Carcinogenic effect of irradiation. Arch Pathol 1968b; 86:487–492.
67. Marine D: Etiology and prevention of simple goiter. Medicine 1924; 3:453.
68. McCoy GW: A preliminary report on tumors found in wild rats. J Med Res 1909; 21:285–296.
69. Milmore JE, Chandrasekaran V, Weisburger JH: Effects of hypothyroidism on development of nitrosomethylurea-induced tumors of the mammary gland, thyroid gland, and other tissues. Proc Soc Exp Biol Med 1982; 169:487–493.
70. Mohr U, Reznik G, Pour P: Carcinogenic effects of diisopropanolnitrosamine in Sprague-Dawley rats. J Natl Cancer Inst 1977; 58:361–366.
71. Money WL, Rawson RW: The experimental production of thyroid tumors in the rat exposed to prolonged treatment with thiouracil. Cancer 1950; 3:321–335
72. Money WL, Rawson RW: Intrathyroidal implantation of chemical carcinogens in the rat. Arch Pathol 1965; 79:470–474
73. Murthy AS: Morphology of the neoplasms of the thyroid gland in Fischer 344 rats treated with 4,4'-methylene-bis-(N,N-dimethyl)-benzenamine. Toxicol Lett 1980; 6:391–397
74. Murthy AS, Russfield AB, Snow GJ: Effect of 4,4'-oxydianiline on the thyroid and pituitary glands of F344 rats: a morphologic study with the use of the immunoperoxidase method. J Natl Cancer Inst 1985; 74:203–208.
75. Nadler NJ, Mandavia MG, Leblond CP: Influence of preirradiation on thyroid tumorigenesis by low-iodine diet in the rat. In: Hedinger C (ed) Thyroid cancer. UICC Monograph series, volume 12, Springer-Verlag, Berlin, 1969, pp. 125–130.
76. Napalkov NP: On blastogemic effect of antithyroid drugs. In: Truhaut R (ed) Potential carcinogenesis hazards from drugs. UICC Monograph series, volume 7, Springer-Verlag Berlin, 1967, pp172–179
77. Napalkov NP, Alexandrov VA, Anisimov VN: Transplacental carcinogenic effect of N-nitrosoethylurea in dogs. Cancer Lett 1981; 12:161–167
78. Ohshima M, Ward JM: Promotion of N-methyl-N-nitrosourea-induced thyroid tumors by iodine deficiency in F344/NCr rats. J Natl Cancer Inst 1984; 73:289–296
79. Paschkis KE, Cantarow A, Stasney J: Influence of thiouracil on carcinoma induced by 2-acetylaminofluorene. Cancer Res 1948; 8:257–263.
80. Potter GD, Lindsay S, Chaikoff IL: Induction of neoplasms in rat thyroid glands by low doses of radio-iodine. Arch Pathol 1960; 69:257–269
81. Pour P, Mohr U, Althoff J, Cardesa A, Kmoch N: Spontaneous tumors and common diseases in two colonies of Syrian hamsters. J Natl Cancer Inst 1976; 56:949–961
82. Pour P, Salmasizadeh S: Induction of thyroid follicular adenomas and carcinomas by N-nitrosobis(2-oxopropyl)amine. Cancer Lett 1978; 5:13–18
83. Pour P, Salmasi S, Runge R, Gingell R, Wallcave L, Nagel D, Stepan K: Carcinogenicity of N-nitrosobis(2-hydroxypropyl)amine and N-nitrosobis(2-oxopropyl)amine in MRC rats. J Natl Cancer Inst 1979; 63:181–90
84. Roe FJ: Spontaneous tumors in rats and mice. Food Cosmet Toxicol 1965; 3:707–720.
85. Schaffer R, Muller HA: On the development of metastasizing tumors of the rat thyroid gland after combined administration of nitrosomethylurea and methylthiouracil. J Cancer Res Clin Oncol 1980; 96:281–285
86. Schaller RT, Stevenson JK: Development of carcinoma of the thyroid in iodine-deficient rats. Cancer 1966; 19:1063–1080
87. Schardein JL, Fitgerald JE, Kaump DH: Spontaneous tumours in Holtzman-source rats of various ages. Pathologia Veterinaria 1968; 5:238–252
88. Sellers EA, Schonbaum E: Enhancement of goitrogenic action of propylthiouracil by thyroxine. Science 1957; 126:1342–1345.
89. Slye M, Holmes HF, Wells HG: Studies in the incidence and inheritability of spontaneous thyroid tumors in mice. J Cancer Res 1926; 10:175–194.
90. Steinhoff D, Weber H, Mohr U, Boehme K: Evaluation of amitriole (aminotriazole) for potential carcinogenicity in orally dosed rats, mice and golden hamsters. Toxicol Appl Pharmacol 1983; 60:161–169.

91. Stoica G, Koestner A: Diverse spectrum of tumors in male Sprague-Dawley rats following single high doses of N-ethyl-N-nitrosourea (ENU). Am J Pathol 1984; 116:319–326.
92. Stula EF, Sherman H, Barnes JR: Thyroid tumors in rats from tetramethylthiourea. J Environ Pathol Toxicol 1979; 2:889–906.
93. Takizawa S, Nishihara H: Induction of tumors in the brain, kidney and other extra-mammary gland organs by continuous oral administration of N-nitrosobutylurea in Wistar-Furth rats. Jap J Cancer Res 1971; 62:495–503.
94. Thomas C, Bollmann R: Zur kausalen Pathogenese und Morphologie der Schilddrüsen-tumoren bei der Ratte. Z Krebsforschung 1974; 81:243–249.
95. Thompson SW, Hunt RD: Spontaneous tumors in the Sprague-Dawley rat: incidence in rats of some types of neoplasms as determined by serial sections versus single section techniques. Ann N Y Acad Sci 1963; 108:832–845.
96. Tsuda H, Hananouchi M, Tatematsu M, Hirose M, Hirao K: Tumorigenic effect of 3-amino-1H-1,2-4-triazole on rat thyroid. J Natl Cancer Inst 1976; 57:861–864.
97. Tsuda H, Fukushima S, Imaida K, Kurata Y, Ito N: Organ-specific promoting effect of phenobarbital and saccharin in induction of thyroid, liver, and urinary bladder tumors in rats after initiation with N-nitrosomethylurea. Cancer Res 1983; 43:3292–3296.
98. Ulland BM, Weisburger JH, Weisburger EK, Rice JM, Cypher R: Thyroid cancer in rats from ethylene thiourea intake J Natl Cancer Inst 1972; 49:583–584.
99. Van Dyke JH: Behavior of ultimobranchial tissue in the postnatal thyroid gland: The origin of thyroid cystadenomata in rat. Anat Rec 1944; 88:369–391.
100. Van Dyke JH: Experimental tumorigenesis in rats. Predominance of neoplasm type and influence of age. Arch Path 1953; 56:613–628.
101. Ward JM, Ohshima M: The role of iodine in carcinogenesis. Adv Exp Med Biol 1986; 206:529–542.
102. Warzok R, Schneider J, Thust R, Scholtze P, Potzsch HD: On the transplacental induction of tumours by N-ethyl-N-nitrosourea in different species. Zentralbl Allg Pathol 1977; 121:54–60.
103. Wegelin C: Malignant disease of the thyroid gland and ist relation to goitre in man and animals. Cancer Res 1928; 3:297–313.
104. Wollman SH: Effects of feeding thiouracil on thyroid glands of rats. J Natl Cancer Inst 1961; 26:473–487.
105. Wooley PG, Wherry WB: On twenty-two spontaneous tumors in wild rats (M. norvegiens). J Med Res 1912; 25:205–216.

17. DIAGNOSTIC MOLECULAR MARKERS IN THYROID CANCER

MATTHEW D. RINGEL, M.D.

Associate Professor of Medicine Department of Medicine, Divisions of Endocrinology and Oncology The Ohio State University, Columbus, Ohio

INTRODUCTION

Thyroid cancer is the commonest classical endocrine tumor, accounting for approximately 1% of all cancers. The diagnosis of thyroid cancer is typically made on cytopathologic features on fine needle aspiration or histological features on surgical samples. Following treatment of patients with thyroidectomy, and in some cases radioiodine, patients are monitored for disease recurrence using a variety of scanning modalities and serum thyroglobulin. The accuracy of both the preoperative testing and postoperative monitoring is excellent in many cases; however, there are some important deficiencies that have led to the development new tools for clinical use. Specifically, the application of molecular methods to the analysis of pathology and blood samples has led to the development of highly sensitive markers for the diagnosis of new cases of thyroid cancer, and in the evaluation of patients for recurrent disease. In this review, the molecular analysis of thyroid nodules, lymph nodes and peripheral blood as adjunctive tests for thyroid cancer will be discussed.

PREOPERATIVE EVALUATION OF THYROID NODULES

Thyroid nodules are extremely common with prevalence rates approaching 50–60% of adults under 60 years old. Because only approximately 5% of thyroid nodules are malignant, accurate pre-operative characterization of thyroid nodules is critical in selecting patients appropriate for surgical thyroidectomy. Fine needle aspiration (FNA) is the single most important diagnostic procedure in the evaluation of thyroid nodules.

Table 1. Molecular markers for thyroid nodules and lymph nodes

Potential diagnostic markers for thyroid nodules and lymph nodes	
Telomerase	GLUT-1
Galectin-3	CA 19-9
Thyroid peroxidase	CD 15
Thyroglobulin	HBME-1
Oncofetal fibronectin	CD 30
ret/PTC oncogenes	CD 57
Pax8/PPARγ oncogene	CD 97
B-Raf mutations	Leu-7
Nm23	Epithelial Membrane Antigen
High mobility Group I (Y) Protein	Cyclooxygenase 2
Ceruloplasmin	Cytokeratin 19
Survivin	Cytokeratin 20
	TSH Receptor Hypermethylation

For small, solid nodules, experienced cytopathologists can accurately distinguish most benign nodules and papillary cancers. However, cytological features do not distinguish benign from malignant follicular neoplasms, and cystic papillary thyroid cancers are a common cause of false negative results. Importantly, only 15% of cytological follicular neoplasm will ultimately be follicular carcinomas; therefore, 85% of individuals that undergo surgery for these nodules will have done so unnecessarily. Finally, by its nature, cytopathologic interpretation of FNA samples is subjective. For these reasons, the application of molecular analysis to better characterize thyroid nodule cytologic samples has been an area of intense interest.

With the advent of methods, such as reverse transcriptase-polymerase chain reaction (RT-PCR), in which tiny amounts of samples are suitable for analysis, and increases in the number of antibodies suitable for immunocytochemistry, the possibility of improving FNA-based characterization of thyroid nodules is now possible. In the initial section of this review, several of the most carefully studied molecular markers (Table 1) for thyroid FNA will be discussed.

Telomerase

Telomeres are chromosomal end structures, consisting of tandem repeats of TTAGGG that play a critical role in the protection of chromosomes during cell division and are important in chromosome positioning during replication (1). Chromosomes typically lose about 50 to 200 nucleotides of telomeric sequence from chromosomal ends per cell division because DNA polymerase is unable to replicate the ends of linear DNA. The resultant progressive shortening of chromosomes as cells divide has been described a cellular "biological clock"; once the chromosomes are shortened to a critical length through telomeric loss, cell growth stops and apoptosis is induced. Therefore, preservation of chromosomal end length during division would be expected to retard this natural "aging" of cells and result in continuous cell growth.

Telomerase is an enzyme that extends telomeres, thereby preserving chromosomal length. Structurally, telomerase is a ribonucleic acid-protein complex containing a catalytic component, the human telomerase reverse transcriptase (hTERT) (2). Telomerase expression and activity have been identified in immortalized human cell lines and cells and in bone marrow cells that normally divide, but not in normal human adult epithelial cells. However, expression of telomerase and demonstration of telomerase activity using a PCR-based assay (TRAP; Telomeric Repeat Amplification Protocol) has been described in a variety of malignancies and other dividing cells, such as germinal cells of the ovary and testis (1). Based on these results, detection of telomerase activity and expression of hTERT have been explored as potential distinguishing markers for the presence of malignant thyroid cells.

Saji et al. (3) evaluated surgical pathology samples from thirty papillary thyroid cancers, three benign nodules and ten normal thyroid specimens for telomerase activity by TRAP and found that 67% of the malignant tissues had telomerase activity compared to 0% of the benign nodules. In this study, 64% of the papillary thyroid cancers that had a non-diagnostic preoperative FNA were positive for telomerase activity. Haugen et al. (4) and Onoda, et al. (5) obtained similar results when they investigated surgical thyroid specimens.

The ability of telomerase help differentiate follicular adenoma from carcinoma was reported by Umbricht et al. (6) who studied frozen tissue samples from patients undergoing thyroidectomy for follicular neoplasm on FNA. TRAP assays were performed on 44 follicular thyroid tissue specimens and 22 normal thyroid tissue samples. The authors reported a sensitivity of 100% and a specificity of 76% for detecting follicular carcinoma. The false positive samples occurred mostly in tumors that also had lymphocytic infiltration, as lymphocytes are known to have detectable telomerase activity. However, it is possible that the presence of telomerase activity in histologically benign specimens may represent an early step in the development of an invasive tumor. This issue of potentially creating an assay that is more sensitive than the clinical gold standard is a problem for many RT-PCR-based assays.

De Deken et al. (7) demonstrated a decrease of telomere length as well as increased variability in the telomere size in benign nodules without measurable telomerase activity, as compared to normal thyroid tissues. These data suggest that the benign nodular cells may have progressed through more mitotic divisions than the adjacent normal tissue and therefore may be closer to their limit for further growth, consistent with benign tumor growth.

The cloning of the human telomerase reverse transcriptase cDNA allowed for RT-PCR analysis of expression of its mRNA in clinical samples. This created an opportunity to design a more user-friendly telomerase assay that could be applied to FNA samples. Saji et al. (8) studied 19 malignant and 18 benign thyroid surgical samples for evidence of hTERT gene expression by RT-PCR. HTERT mRNA was detected in 15 (79%) of the malignant and 5 (28%) of the benign tumors; all 5 benign lesions with demonstrable hTERT gene expression had lymphocytic infiltration on final pathology. HTERT mRNA was not detected in any of the normal thyroid specimens. The results correlated with TRAP assay results from the same samples. Similar results were reported by the same authors using thyroid FNA samples (9).

Fine needle aspiration specimens have also been investigated for telomerase activity using TRAP assay. Sebesta et al. (10) failed to show any additional usefulness of measuring telomerase activity in a small study of FNA samples. It is likely that RT-PCR of hTERT is more sensitive than TRAP assay due to the logarithmic amplification inherent in RT-PCR, thus accounting for a greater sensitivity when used to analyze FNA samples.

The frequency of telomerase-positive results, either by RT-PCR or TRAP assay for papillary thyroid cancer varies between studies. For example, some report that as many as 67% of papillary thyroid cancers are positive (3), while others indicate a much lower percentage of about 20% (11). The small number of cases in many of these studies makes interpretation quite difficult. Similarly, results regarding the association between telomerase activity and tumor aggressiveness also vary; some studies demonstrate a correlation between telomerase activity and tumor progression (5, 12) while others do not (3). It is clear that larger, more extensive studies are needed before telomerase can be considered an effective diagnostic tool.

Galectin-3

Galectin-3 is a member of the lectin family that regulates the functions of its protein targets by interacting with attached galactose-containing glycoprotein side chains. As a group, galectins regulate cell growth and differentiation, intercellular recognition and adhesion, as well as malignant transformation. Galectin-3 levels have been directly correlated with metastatic potential in fibrosarcoma and melanoma cell lines. In vitro studies have indicated that expression of galectin proteins is elevated in thyroid cancer cell lines and microarray analysis has demonstrated increased levels of galectin-3 in papillary thyroid cancers (13) This led to their investigation as molecular markers used to distinguish between benign and malignant thyroid tissues.

Xu, et al. (14) evaluated protein derived from 41 surgical thyroid specimens for galectin-1 and galectin-3 expression by Western blot. Elevated levels of both proteins were demonstrated in thyroid cancer compared to normal thyroid tissue. Similarly, normal thyroid tissue did not express galectin 1 or 3 by immunohistochemical analysis, but high levels of both proteins were detected in both papillary and follicular thyroid cancers, and in regional nodal metastases. A second group evaluated 41 malignant and 35 benign thyroid tissue specimens (15) for both galectin-3 protein and RNA levels. Galectin-3 expression was identified in 18 of 18 of papillary cancer samples, 4 of 8 follicular cancers, 2 of 3 poorly differentiated cancers, 5 of 5 anaplastic cancers, 3 of 6 medullary, and 1 of 1 Hurthle cell cancers. By contrast, none of the normal or benign nodular tissues expressed galectin-3, other than those with lymphocytic infiltration. Levels of galectin-3 mRNA appeared to correlate with protein levels in papillary cancers and normal tissue (15).

To determine if galectin-3 immunocytochemistry could be applied to FNA samples, Orlandi, et al. (16) evaluated FNA and surgical pathology specimens from 64 patients who had undergone thyroidectomy whose preoperative diagnosis was malignant (n = 15), indeterminate (n = 37), and benign (n = 12). The final histologic diagnosis included 18 papillary and 17 follicular cancers, as well as 29 follicular adenomas. All papillary thyroid cancers expressed galectin-3 in both FNA and surgical specimens. For the follicular cancers, immunoactive galectin-3 was detected in all surgical specimens in a heterogeneous pattern, and in all but 3 FNA samples. By contrast, only 3 of 29 benign follicular adenomas expressed galectin-3.

In a more recent study (17), different antibodies against human galectin-3 were used in an immunohistochemical study of thyroid surgical specimens (13 benign and 62 malignant). Immunoactive galectin-3 was most prevalent in the papillary thyroid cancers (33 of 45), but some benign lesions were 3 of 8 benign adenomas demonstrated immunoactive galectin-3.

Finally, Bernet, et al. (18) applied quantitative RT-PCR to galectin-3 analysis to determine if a particular "cut-point" of galectin-3 gene expression correlated best with malignancy. In this study, markedly elevated levels of galectin-3 mRNA were identified in papillary cancers compared with normal tissue. There was no difference between the galectin-3 mRNA levels in follicular adenomas and carcinomas.

Based on the above results, galectin-3 immunocytochemistry seems to be a promising new marker of thyroid cancer that could be applied to FNA analysis. It appears that classic molecular approaches, such as quantitative RT-PCR may not be helpful for the conundrum of follicular neoplasm FNA results. However, additional studies are still required.

Thyroid peroxidase

Thyroid peroxidase (TPO) is a thyroid-specific enzyme that catalyzes iodide oxidation, thyroglobulin iodination, and iodothyronine coupling. Reduced expression of TPO impairs thyroid follicular cell function correlates with a loss of differentiated thyroid function and has been well described in thyroid cancer cell lines and tumor samples. Thus, immunohistochemical staining for TPO expression and molecular analysis of the TPO gene have been studied for use as diagnostic tools for thyroid cancer.

DeMicco, et al. reported a retrospective study of 150 FNA samples including 125 benign tissues (19), and demonstrated that 113 of 125 benign lesions were characterized by immunoactive TPO in more than 80% of cells while <80% of the cells expressed TPO in all 25 malignant lesions. Thus, using this level of TPO-expressing cells as a positive, they reported a sensitivity of 100% and a specificity of 90%.

Christensen, et al. reported their prospective experience using this method in 124 consecutive FNAs using the same anti-TPO primary antibody (20). In their hands, TPO immunohistochemistry (>80% cut-off) correctly identified all cases of cancer. Only one benign follicular adenoma was identified as malignant by this immunohistochemical criterion. These investigators concluded that TPO immunohistochemistry of FNA samples using the 80% cut-off values has a sensitivity of 100% and a specificity of 99%. These results are obviously subjective and may be antibody dependent.

Because germline mutations of the TPO gene that cause functional loss of TPO activity cause of congenital hypothyroidism, loss of heterozygocity (LOH) at the TPO gene locus has been implicated as a cause of the organification defect typical of benign and malignant thyroid tumors. However, in a study of 40 hypoactive thyroid nodules (21), LOH of the TPO gene was noted in only 6, making this an unlikely method for evaluating thyroid nodules preoperatively.

Thus, it appears that immunostaining for thyroid peroxidase may be a valuable addition to the analysis of FNA samples. Studies with additional available antibodies may be useful from a practical standpoint.

Oncofetal fibronectin

Fibronectins are high-molecular-weight glycoproteins found in the extracellular matrix. Oncofetal fibronectin is characterized by the presence of the oncofetal domain (IIICS domain), which is absent in normal fibronectin. Overexpression of this variant of fibronectin has been demonstrated in many epithelial cancers and it has been studied as a molecular marker of malignancy. Several investigators have evaluated the utility of the oncofetal fibronectin mRNA as a marker of thyroid malignancy.

Higashiyama, et al. (22) evaluated 19 malignant and 33 benign surgical thyroid specimens by competitive RT-PCR and demonstrated elevated levels in papillary and anaplastic cancers versus benign tissues. Levels were variable in follicular carcinomas and were not clearly different from follicular adenomas. The same group also reported detection of oncofetal fibronectin mRNA on surgical samples using in situ hybridization and reported similar results (23).

Takano et al. (24) examined 72 FNA samples (23 normal, 14 adenomatous goiters, 13 follicular adenomas, 3 follicular carcinomas, 18 papillary carcinomas and 1 anaplastic cancer) for expression of oncofetal fibronectin mRNA using RT-PCR. 95% of the papillary or anaplastic carcinomas by cytology also expressed oncofetal fibronectin mRNA compared to only 4% (n = 109) of benign specimens. In contrast, none of the 6 follicular tumors expressed oncofetal fibronectin. Fifty of these patients underwent surgery, based on the results of the surgical histology, oncofetal fibronectin RT-PCR was 97% sensitive and 100% specific. These results are similar to Higashiyama, et al. as all but one cancer sample included in this study was papillary. These results suggested that oncofetal fibronectin mRNA amplification was an accurate marker of papillary, but not follicular carcinoma. A potential cause of false positive results is the expression of oncofetal fibronectin in thyroid fibroblasts (25). Despite the fibroblast data, the results of the immunhistochemical and molecular studies suggest that measurement of oncofetal fibronectin expression may be useful as an adjunctive test for identifying papillary thyroid carcinoma.

Ret/PTC

Ret/PTC oncogenes are genomic rearrangments that couple the tyrosine kinase domain of the Ret receptor to different 5′ regions leading to aberrant expression and activation of Ret. To date, there are 8 Ret/PTC proteins, however, the prevalence is greatest for Ret/PTC 1, 2, and 3. Translocations involving Ret are particularly prevalent in papillary carcinomas that develop following exposure to radiation. Because these rearrangements are largely limited to thyroid carcinomas, the expression of PTC oncogenes has been studied as molecular markers for thyroid malignancy.

In a study of 73 thyroid specimens from which both FNA and surgically obtained tissue was available, Cheung, et al. (26) evaluated the presence of PTC1-5 by RT-PCR. Only Ret/PTC 1, 2 or 3 were detected in the samples; Ret/PTC translocations were not detected on FNA and surgical samples from 39 benign tissue samples, including 11 follicular adenomas, 25 nodular hyperplasia's and 3 Hashimoto's thyroiditis cases. In contrast, Ret/PTC1, 2, or 3 expression was detected in 17 FNA samples and 21 surgical specimens derived from 33 malignant thyroid tumors. Of importance, this molecular method was more accurate than routine cytopathology in these samples.

Conflicting results were reported by Elisei, et al. (27) who studied 154 patients referred to surgery for FNA-characterized benign nodules (n = 65) or papillary thyroid cancer (n = 89). Expression of Ret/PTC-1 and Ret/PTC-3, the most common Ret/PTC oncogenes, was identified in both benign and malignant nodules. RET protein expression has been evaluated by immunohistochemistry in papillary thyroid cancers (28). Overall, expression of Ret was heterogenous and was demonstrated in regions of cellular atypia in both malignant and benign lesions. Thus, based on these data, it appears that Ret/PTC may not be helpful in pre-operative diagnosis due to a relatively low prevalence in many populations with papillary thyroid cancer and potential issues with specificity. However, more studies are needed to clarify a role for Ret/PTC rearrangement or Ret overexpression in the diagnosis of thyroid nodules.

Pax8-PPARγ

Kroll, et al. (29) identified a chromosomal translocation t(2;3)(q13;p25) causing a fusion gene between Pax8 and the peroxisome proliferator activated receptor gamma (PPARγ) in follicular thyroid carcinomas. Specifically, 5 of 8 follicular cancers expressed the fusion gene, while all of the 20 follicular adenomas, 10 papillary thyroid carcinomas and 10 other benign nodules did not express the rearranged gene, suggesting that detection of Pax 8-PPARγ fusion gene expression might accurately identify follicular carcinomas preoperatively.

The specificity of the Pax 8-PPARγ may not be complete, as other groups (30, 31) have reported expression of PAX8-PPARγ in benign follicular adenomas, albeit at a lower frequency than follicular carcinomas. The importance of expression of Pax8-PPARγ in follicular adenomas on malignant transformation is uncertain. It has been speculated that overexpression of PPARγ alone, even in the absence of a defined chromosomal rearrangement, may be a marker of malignant transformation. Detection of PPARγ overexpression by immunohistochemistry appears to be more sensitive, but also, less specific for detection of follicular carcinoma (31).

B-Raf

Mutations in the serine-threonine kinase, B-Raf have been described in 35–70% of papillary thyroid carcinomas, with almost no overlap with other known oncogenes or other benign or malignant thyroid lesions (32–34). Because this mutation appears quite specific for papillary thyroid cancer, and it is limited to two specific mutations, detection of the mutations has been proposed as an adjunctive test for FNA analysis (32). This method would likely be useful only for papillary thyroid cancer detection, however.

Nm23

Re-expression of the Nm23 tumor suppressor gene has been demonstrate to reduce the metastatic potential of malignant cells in-vitro and reduced expression of Nm23 occurs in aggressive forms of breast cancer (35) . In thyroid tissues, the interesting finding of increased expression has been demonstrated, primarily in stage IV papillary cancers and anaplastic carcinomas (36). Farley et al. (37) also evaluated 34 thyroid tumors, including 4 follicular adenomas, 19 papillary carcinomas, 6 follicular carcinomas and 5 medullary carcinomas for Nm23 mRNA levels. In this study, overexpression of Nm23 was noted in follicular and medullary cancers, although there was overlap between benign and malignant samples. Similarly, Berthau, et al. (38) reported that immunocytochemical analysis of Nm23 protein expression did not accurately distinguish between benign and malignant lesions. Mechanistically, the finding that overexpression of nm23, rather than reduction of loss of nm23 expression were demonstrated suggests an alternative function for this protein in thyroid cancer (39).

High mobility group I(Y) protein—HMGI(Y)

The high mobility group I (HMGI) proteins are nuclear proteins that regulate chromatin structure and function. HMGI(Y) is particularly highly expressed during embryogenesis, and its reexpression has been described in cancers, but not in normal adult tissues. Chiappetta et al. (40) reported evaluated expression of HMGI(Y) protein by immunohistochemistry on 358 thyroid tissue samples. HMGI(Y) was detected in 18 of 19 follicular carcinomas, 92 of 96 papillary tumors and 11 of 11 anaplastic cancers, but in only 1 of 20 hyperplastic nodules, 44 of 200 benign follicular adenomas and 0 of 12 normal thyroid tissue samples. HMGI(Y) mRNA was detected in 4 of 4 malignant tumors while eight benign FNA samples (6 follicular adenomas and 2 normal thyroid tissue) were negative. Thus, HMGI(Y) may be a potentially useful diagnostic tool for thyroid cancer that warrants further identification.

Ceruloplasmin

Because ceruloplasmin, a copper transport protein that shares homology with lactoferrin (a molecular marker for several tumor types), it has been investigated as a tumor marker in thyroid cancer. Tuccari et al. (41) evaluated 56 surgical thyroid specimens for ceruloplasmin expression by immunohistochemistry. None of the 15 follicular adenomas expressed ceruloplasmin, while two of two Hurthle cell tumors, all 21 follicular, and all 6 papillary carcinomas were positive. All of the medullary thyroid cancers were negative for ceruloplasmin, as was the normal thyroid tissue surrounding the thyroid cancers. The functional role of ceruloplasmin in thyroid tumors as its potential role as a marker for malignancy require further clarification.

Cytokeratins

Cytokeratins are structural proteins found in all epithelial cells; several types of keratins have been identified with altered expression patterns in malignancies. In thyroid cancer, immunocytochemical expression for prekeratin was detected in papillary thyroid cancer but not normal thyroid tissues, follicular adenomas and follicular thyroid carcinomas (42). With the development of more specific antibodies that identify cytokeratin subtypes, a more comprehensive evaluation was able to be performed. Schelfhout et al. (43) used monoclonal antibodies against cytokeratin 8, 18 and 19 to characterize cytokeratin expression in different thyroid histologies. Of these, cytokeratin-19 was overexpressed 12 of 12 papillary cancers, while follicular cancers, follicular adenomas, colloid nodules and normal thyroid tissue were negative or had only weak staining. The authors concluded that staining with antibodies against cytokeratin 19 is a useful diagnostic tool for papillary thyroid cancer. However, these promising results were not able to be confirmed. Sahoo, et al. (44) evaluated 35 surgical thyroid specimens for cytokeratin 19 expression. Although papillary cancers tended to display more intense staining than other tumors, the presence or absence of immunoactive cytokeratin 19 did not distinguish the tumor histologic subtypes. Technical issues could account for the discrepant results and further studies are needed. Cytokeratin 20 has also been evaluated in lymph nodes and peripheral blood of patients with medullary and follicular cell-derived thyroid cancer (see below).

GLUT 1

Because malignant cells typically are characterized by an increased rate of glucose utilization, overexpression of glucose transporters has been identified in malignancies, particularly overexpression of Glut-1. In thyroid cancer, Haber, et al. (45) reported the absence of immunoactive Glut-1 in 38 benign thyroid tissues, but its presence in 9 of 17 papillary, 2 of 6 follicular and 2 of 2 anaplastic cancers. These results suggest that Glut-1 could be potentially useful marker of malignancy. These results concur with clinical studies that demonstrate enhanced glucose uptake using [18F]-2-fluorodeoxyglucose (FDG) PET in aggressive thyroid tumors with a worse prognosis (46). Thus, determination of Glut-1 expression levels may be important both diagnostically and prognostically in thyroid cancer.

CA 19-9 and CD15

CA 19-9 and CD15 (Leu-M1) are have markers for a variety of epithelial tumors and Hodgkin's disease, respectively, that have been evaluated in thyroid cancer. Immunohistochemical expression of both CA19-9 and CD15 were identified in benign thyroid tumors and in papillary carcinomas, suggesting these would not be useful markers in the clinical setting (47).

HBME-1

In contrast to CA 19-9 and CD 15, HBME-1, a tumor suppressor gene whose product is involved in signal transduction, has been reported to have a pattern of expression suggesting it would be a potential marker of papillary thyroid cancer (48). Of importance is a recent report that demonstrated that papillary and follicular cancers with apocrine or Hurthle cell features, respectively, have distinctly lower levels of HBME-1 expression than more typical papillary and follicular tumors (49). The biological impact of this finding is uncertain. Mase, et al. recently published data demonstrating that HBME-1 expression was detected in 23% of follicular adenomas, 27% of benign goiters, but in 85% of follicular and 97% of papillary cancers (50). Based on these results, HMBE-1 is a potentially useful marker FNA samples, although follicular carcinomas require initial evaluation and the papillary cancer data require confirmation.

CD30

The CD30 antigen (Ki-1) is a cytokine receptor that is expressed in activated B and T lymphocytes, but not normal adult epithelial cells. Its expression has been demonstrated in Hodgkin's disease and Burkitt's lymphoma. The presence and distribution of both CD30 and the CD30 ligand in the thyroid were investigated using immunohistochemistry in 131 thyroid specimens and 6 normal thyroid glands (51). Normal thyroid tissue did not express CD30 or the CD30 ligand including tissue adjacent to benign nodules or follicular cancer did not express either molecule, while tissue adjacent to papillary and medullary cancer expressed CD30 ligand. Of thyroid tumors examined, 20% of follicular adenomas showed coexpression of CD30 and CD30L, while 7% of the follicular, 33% of the anaplastic, 76% of the papillary and 67% of the medullary cancers expressed both proteins. The overlap in expression between benign and malignant thyroid tissues may ultimately limit the use of this marker in identifying thyroid cancer, however, the regulation of these proteins may be very interesting for thyroid cancer biology.

Epithelial membrane antigen and Leu-7 (CD57)

Epithelial membrane antigen (EMA) is a glycoprotein that is expressed by malignant epithelial cells, while Leu-7 is an antigen expressed by immune cells whose expression has been demonstrated in a variety of tumors. Cheifetz et al. (52) evaluated the expression of these proteins in 40 benign and malignant nodules by immunohistochemistry of surgical specimens. For EMA, 16 of 22 malignant (73%) and 5 of 18 benign (28%) tumors were positive, and Leu-7 expression was detected in 20 of 22 malignant tumors and 6 of 18 benign tumors, both of which were significantly different statistically. Leu-7 expression as a marker of thyroid malignancy was also evaluated by Khan, et al. (53) who found that 95% of 83 malignant and 21% of 77 benign surgical specimens were positive. This results in an overall sensitivity of 98% and a specificity of 82%, but, as with other immunhistochemical markers, differences in the intensity and distribution of the staining were noted.

Cyclooxygenase-2

Cyclooxygenase type 2 (Cox-2) is a highly inducible enzyme in the phospholipase A2 pathway that appears to be involved in carcinogenesis. Cox-2 mRNA and protein levels are upregulated in many epithelial cell-derived malignancies. Similarly, in thyroid cancer, Cox-2 gene and protein expression are also elevated both in surgical and FNA samples (54). These data suggest that in addition to being a treatment target, Cox-2 mRNA and/or protein levels could distinguish benign from malignant thyroid tumors.

Hypermethylation of the TSH receptor

Gene silencing can occur through a variety of mechanisms. One of the most common is hypermethylation of CPG islands in promoter regions that cause reduced expression of genes. This phenomenon has been shown to occur in thyroid cancer. Xing, et al. (55) demonstrated that detection of TSH receptor gene methylation by PCR was an accurate adjuct in the evaluation of thyroid tumors. Further work in this area is required to determine if this method is useful in a clinical setting.

MOLECULAR MARKERS OF TUMOR RECURRENCE OR PROGRESSION

The use of highly sensitive molecular tests to identify recurrent or progressive disease using tissue and/or tumor-specific markers have been used to detect metastases in bone marrow, lymph nodes, peripheral blood, and other sites. Methods employed include RTT-PCR amplification of tissue or tumor-specific transcripts or isolation of cancer cells directly using cell sorting. These approaches are particularly attractive for thyroid cancer because, in comparison to other solid tumors, initial therapy of thyroid cancer frequently results in the removal and ablation of all thyroid tissue, making both tumor and tissue-specific markers useful for early diagnosis. Several markers have been applied to nodes (Table 1) and peripheral blood (Table 2).

Lymph node recurrence

The most common sites of tumor metastases in thyroid cancer are local-regional lymph nodes, particularly for papillary cancer. These metastases are frequently present at diagnosis and can be difficult to isolate and eradicate. Standard approaches to diagnosis of local nodes include the level of elevation of serum thyroglobulin concentrations, the presence of abnormally sized or appearing nodes on anatomic imaging often with abnormal cytology on FNA, or iodine uptake in an extrathyroidal location. The diagnosis of metastatic thyroid cancer within a node frequently is confirmed by FNA, but

Table 2. Published diagnostic peripheral blood markers for thyroid cancer

Marker	References
Thyroglobulin	(66–77, 82–85, 87,88)
Thyroid Peroxidase	(67, 74, 84)
Ret/PTC Oncogenes	(67)
Cytokeratin 20	(58)
TSH Receptor	(76)
Human Kallikrein 2	(86)

this method is difficult for small nodes in the neck bed where the amount of aspirated tissue may be small. To enhance diagnostic sensitivity, there has been an interest in developing RT-PCR based approaches to amplify thyroid-specific transcripts from node FNA for both thyroid cancer derived from for papillary and follicular thyroid cancer and for medullary thyroid cancer.

Arturi, et al. (56) reported their experience using RT-PCR amplification of thyroglobulin and TSH-receptor mRNAs from nodal tissue obtained by FNA of 46 lymph nodes and compared them to cytopathology, thyroglobulin immunoassay of the aspirate fluid, and final histopathology. RT-PCR detected thyroid transcripts in 41 of 41 histopathologically confirmed metastatic tumor samples, including 45% that were inadequate or false negative by standard cytopathology. Similar results were obtained by Gubala, et al. (57) who reported their experience in 70 nodes aspirated from 60 patients with suspected thyroid cancer recurrence. Taken together, these data confirm that thyroid-specific mRNAs can be amplified from nodes in patients with metastatic thyroid cancer, that false positives from ectopic transcription in lymphocytes appears to be uncommon using these particular primers, and the overall accuracy may be adequate for clinical use. Weber, et al. (58, 59) used a slightly different approach, amplifying cytokeratin 20, an epithelial cell tumor marker, mRNA using RT-PCR from nodes suspected of harboring metastatic differentiated thyroid cancer. In comparison to cytokeratin 20 immunohistochemistry and cytology, the molecular diagnostic approach was more sensitive.

This group has also reported similar data for patients suspected to have recurrent medullary thyroid cancer in cervical nodes. The report that amplification of cytokeratin 20 and preprogastrin mRNA, a marker of neuroendocrine tumors, by RT-PCR demonstrated enhanced sensitivity and specificity over routine cytology (60, 61). These results, in combination with detection of medullary cancer-related mRNAs in peripheral blood of patients suggest this approach may be useful for patients with medullary cancer (62).

The importance of detecting metastases earlier has not been clarified in thyroid cancer, a disease that typically follows an indolent course. However, for patients with malignant melanoma, amplification of tyrosinase mRNA from sentinel lymph node tissue removed at surgery correlates with development of metastatic melanoma and subsequent prognosis (63, 64). With time, it is likely that early detection will result in better prognosis. The development of markers of aggressiveness, such as p53 mutation analysis, may provide additional predictive data that will help clinicians stratify patients for appropriate treatment paradigms. Other markers derived from cDNA array analysis may also be particularly useful in the future.

Detection of distant metastases

The most frequently employed tests for monitoring patients with thyroid cancer for tumor recurrence are measurements of circulating serum thyroglobulin concentrations and radioiodine scanning, both of which rely on thyroid-specific gene transcription or function. Non-thyroid specific monitoring methods include ultrasound, magnetic resonance imaging, computed tomography, positron emissions tomography, and physical examination. Thyroid-specific monitoring, rather than tumor-specific monitoring is particularly useful for patients treated with thyroidectomy and radioiodine ablative therapy who are, theoretically, devoid of all thyroid tissue, benign or malignant.

The development of more sensitive and specific thyroglobulin assays has led to increased dependence on this test in monitoring paradigms. The ease of a simple blood test and the lack of exposure to radiation are two advantages of this method. However, there are several important limitations of serum thyroglobulin monitoring; 1) circulating autoantibodies directed against thyroglobulin (anti-thyroglobulin antibodies) interfere with clinical assays in approximately 20% of patients, and 2) stimulation of thyroglobulin transcription and release with either endogenous or exogenous thyrotropin (TSH) is required for adequate clinical sensitivity (65). There has therefore been an interest in developing new assays for thyroid cell detection that are not altered by antibodies and are sensitive enough to not require TSH stimulation.

Qualitative thyroid mRNA assays

Ditkoff, et al. (66) reported results from 100 individuals including 87 with thyroid cancer, 6 with benign thyroid disease (nontoxic goiters), and 5 normal subjects following total thyroidectomy (except normal subjects). Total RNA was isolated from the macrophage layer of peripheral blood, and, using RT-PCR amplification of thyroglobulin mRNA, they detected thyroid transcripts in blood from 9 of 9 patients with metastatic thyroid cancer, but from only 7 of 78 patients thought to be free of disease, and no patients having surgery for benign disease or normal control subjects. Detailed clinical information was not included regarding the clinical status of the patients and TSH levels were not reported. However, these investigators clearly demonstrated that thyroglobulin mRNA could be amplified from peripheral blood and that its presence appeared to correlate with stage of disease.

Tallini, et al. (67) subsequently reported data using different RT-PCR assays for detection of thyroid transcripts from peripheral blood. In this study, the investigators evaluated 44 patients including 24 with thyroid cancer (16 with metastases and 8 free of disease), either pre-operatively, postoperatively, or at both time points for peripheral blood expression of thyroglobulin, thyroid peroxidase, and the RET/PTC1 thyroid oncogene. 56% of the patients with either local or distant metastases had positive assays, compared to 63% of those thought to be free of disease. Of those thought to be free of disease that had positive assays, 80% had cervical adenopathy at diagnosis and were felt to be at high risk of tumor recurrence. Of the patients with benign disease, 2 of 20 patients had a positive mRNA assay, both of which reverted to negative after surgery. The in vitro sensitivities of this assay were approximately 50 cells/ml of blood. Technically, these authors isolated total RNA from whole blood drawn into EDTA-containing tubes and did not isolate a buffy coat layer.

Ringel, et al. (68) also developed a thyroglobulin mRNA assay designed for detection of circulating thyroid cells. The method employed in this study used whole blood placed directly into an RNA-stabilization solution and resulted in a more sensitive assay. In this study, 87 individuals with thyroid cancer were evaluated. Thyroglobulin mRNA was detected in all 14 cervical or distant metastases during L-T4 therapy, while 65% of patients with thyroid bed uptake and 20% of patients with no uptake had detectable thyroglobulin mRNA. These data suggested both a high sensitivity and lower specificity of the assay than the prior studies. Of concern was that similar to the patients with multinodular goiter analyzed by Tallini et al. circulating thyroglobulin mRNA was detectable in all of the normal subjects evaluated and in 20% of athyreotic patients. These results raised the possibility that thyroglobulin may not represent a truly thyroid-specific transcript and that this more sensitive assay detected ectopically transcribed of thyroglobulin in non-thyroid cells. Alternatively, the assay could have been detecting very early minimal residual or recurrent disease.

Additional data have been published from many groups using similar qualitative approaches to amplify thyroglobulin and other mRNA transcripts from peripheral blood. The results have been remarkably variable, with some groups demonstrating excellent correlation between tumor stage and results (69–72), while others demonstrate no correlation with tumor stage (73–75). Several have concluded that the assay is more useful for papillary rather than follicular cancer (69), while others have demonstrated optimal screening by combining thyroglobulin mRNA with new highly sensitive thyroglobulin immunoassays (71). Taken together, nearly all groups have confirmed the presence of circulating thyroglobulin mRNA in peripheral blood of normal subjects, and in a subset of athyreotic patients, suggesting that ectopic transcription of thyroglobulin or splice variants of thyroglobulin can be detected.

The importance of assay methodology has been highlighted in several recent studies. Bojunga, et al. (73) reported data using low and high sensitivity qualitative thyroglobulin mRNA assays in patients with thyroid cancer. Using a lower sensitivity assay, they detected circulating thyroglobulin mRNA in 69% of patients with metastatic disease, 46% of patients with thyroid cancer thought to be free of disease, 25% of patients with benign thyroid disease and 18% of control patients. The more sensitive assay increase sensitivity modestly, but resulted in the complete loss of specificity. Gupta, et al. (76) created PCR primers designed to carefully avoid amplification of all known splice variants of thyroglobulin and the TSH receptor. Using these PCR primers, these authors reported detection of thyroid transcripts in 83% of thyroid cancer patients with positive compared to 5% of patients with negative radioiodine scans. All normal volunteers were negative. The specificity was slightly greater for TSH mRNA detection rather than thyroglobulin mRNA detection. Similarly, Savagner, et al. (77) designed thyroglobulin primers that amplified known splice variants and others that did not. They determined that the splice variants account for approximately 1/3 of the total amplified thyroglobulin mRNA, and that when the primers that do not amplify the region are used, the results correlated with the volume of thyroid tissue and TSH concentration. Taken together, these data clearly demonstrate the importance of methodology in performing these assays, and in proper evaluation of the published data. Differences in sensitivity could be due to the method of sample collection, storage of samples between the phlebotomy and RNA isolation, the specific method for reverse transcription and the PCR primers employed.

Quantitative thyroid mRNA assays

Due to the subjective nature of PCR and the apparent discrepancy in the results of studies using qualitative RT-PCR systems, there has been interest in attempting to quantify peripheral blood RT-PCR assays in order to define a clinically relevant level of detection. The advent of real-time quantitative PCR has enabled testing of this approach in clinical trials. Similar to quantitative RT-PCR, the methodological issues are considerable, particularly when attempting to detect very rare transcripts within a particular sample. Other major issues when considering quantitation of RNA is normalization to a control transcript. Traditionally, normalization to glyceraldehyde-3-phosphate-dehydrogenase (GAPDH) or beta actin has been employed; however, tremendous variability in these control transcripts has been reported (72–74). An alternative is normalization to total RNA (18S), while others have chosen not to normalize transcripts at all and normalize to the original blood volume (78–80). This also may not be an accurate method and the use of a "geometric" panel of markers has recently been suggested (81). Thus, it is apparent that normalizing to different control transcripts clearly will alter the reported results and, to date, no standard method has been applied by all laboratories; however, it appears clear that normalizing to a single "housekeeping" gene such as GAPDH or beta actin is likely not appropriate for these samples (81).

Wingo, et al. (82) reported the first quantitative thyroglobulin mRNA assay. In this study, total RNA was derived from peripheral blood samples and the assay was extensively tested. Calibration assays revealed interassay variability of 17–22% due primarily to RNA stability, RNA handing and the reverse transcriptase reaction. The assay displayed reproducible results over a three log concentration range. Ringel, et al. (83) subsequently used this assay to analyze peripheral blood RNA from 107 patients with thyroid cancer; including 84 during L-T4 therapy, 14 following L-T4 withdrawal, and 9 before and after thyroxine withdrawal. Twenty-three patients had circulating anti-thyroglobulin antibodies. Using an arbitrary cut-point to identify patients as either positive or negative for detection (36 PCR cycles), thyroglobulin mRNA measurement assay was more sensitive than thyroglobulin immunoassay, but was less specific at detecting the presence of local and distant metastases. In addition, while there was a statistical correlation between the level of thyroglobulin mRNA and the presence of thyroid tissue on scan, the level of thyroglobulin mRNA did not correlate well with stage of disease. Importantly, the assay appeared to be unaffected by circulating anti-thyroglobulin antibodies, suggesting that perhaps Thyroglobulin mRNA could be used as an adjunctive test to identify patients with recurrent or residual thyroid tissue in the presence of anti-thyroglobulin antibodies. However, the authors cautioned that there was significant overlap between the patients with positive results without definable disease and those with disease, a factor which may limit the usefulness of this particular assay method in clinical practice. Thus, for individual patients, the absolute value of thyroglobulin mRNA did not appear to be diagnostically useful, but the presence or absence of thyroglobulin mRNA might be useful. In addition, similar to other studies, even using a cut-point, a significant minority (38%) of patients with no evidence of disease had positive results and many had detectable values below the cut-point. The relevance of an isolated thyroglobulin mRNA level is uncertain as it might reflect a false positive result from ectopic expression, or the presence of bona fide residual thyroid tissue.

Savagner, et al. (77) developed a quantitative assay for measurement of thyroglobulin mRNA in peripheral blood. In this study, the cut point of a positive or negative assay was determined to be the amount of circulating prostate specific antigen mRNA as a control transcript, no internal normalization was performed and results were reported per total RNA amount. The results in this study were similar to those of Ringel, et al. in that using a mean value, there was a statistical correlation with the absence or presence of residual or recurrent thyroid tissue, but there was significant overlap between all groups for individual data.

Similar to the experience with qualitative thyroglobulin mRNA assays, variable results have also been reported with the quantitative approach. Some of these differences are methodological (different primers, use of DNase I, normalization), inherent in the assay method (instability of RNA), while others may be interpretive. Takano, et al. (84) performed a study evaluating thyroglobulin mRNA from peripheral blood and similar to Ringel, et al. identified this transcript in all patients. Unlike the prior study, they were not able to correlate levels with stage of disease. However, in this study, the normalization was performed in a different manner (GAPDH), different PCR primers were utilized, and DNase I treatment was not performed, all different from Ringel, et al. Takano, et al. (84) also report similar data amplifying thyroid peroxidase (TPO) as a tumor marker, results that did not agree with those of Roddiger, et al. (74) who reported a better correlation using TPO mRNA amplification than thyroglobulin mRNA in patients with thyroid cancer. Eszlinger, et al. (85) also did not demonstrate correlation between thyroglobulin mRNA levels and the presence or absence of thyroid tissue. They evaluated several different methods of blood collection and also describe important differences in results depending on the types of tubes used for phlebotomy and the time between the sample collection and RNA isolation. These authors used a new set of primers and normalized to beta actin, factors that distinguish their method from others. To further clarify the importance of recognition of assay differences between groups, Span, et al. (75) used the same thyroglobulin PCR primers as earlier reports and were not able to confirm a relationship between stage of disease and level of thyroglobulin mRNA. However, distinct from those reports, the authors used a different method of RNA isolation and normalize their results to beta actin, both important differences in assay methods that can alter results.

Tumor-specific mRNA assays

Additional markers, such as cytokeratin 20 and human kallikrein 2 mRNA amplification have recently been reported to have potential diagnostic benefit for thyroid cancer patients (58, 86). These are not thyroid-specific, but may be cancer-specific. These preliminary data require confirmation, but may be an interesting alternative approach to molecular diagnosis of metastatic disease.

Thus, based on these data, it seems that there is clear evidence of ectopic expression of thyroglobulin, or at least splice variants of thyroglobulin in non-thyroid tissues. Assay quantitation to "subtract out" this amplification is of uncertain value due to differences in the reported methods and the challenges of normalization of results. Further study and clarification of these issues, in particular, the use of primers that do not amplify splice variants, determination of the best processing protocol for blood RNA isolation, and whether an appropriate form of normalization exists are required before a clear assessment regarding the clinical usefulness of this approach to molecular diagnosis can be made.

SUMMARY

The use of molecular assays to analyze clinical tissues in the diagnosis and management of thyroid cancer, similar to other tumors, will likely allow for more accurate characterization of the aggressiveness of individual tumors and may allow for the early diagnosis of recurrence. The application of these methods to thyroid nodules and nodal metastases is less encumbered by difficulties arising from amplification of transcripts in non-thyroid cells. For these tissues, these assays are likely to be used clinically in the near-future. New data arising from cDNA arrays identifying novel markers of malignancy or tumor aggressiveness make this a growing area of interest. The use of molecular assays in diagnosing distant metastases is more problematic due to issues with ectopic expression of either full length or splice variants of genes thought to be thyroid-specific. Assay quantitation is a complex problem owing to variability in the level of expression of "housekeeping" genes and the variety of phlebotomy and RT-PCR methods reported. Additional research in this area is clearly required before a recommendation can be given regarding clinically applicability of these tests.

REFERENCES

1. Kim, N. W., Piatyszek, M. A., Prowse, K. R., Harley, C. B., West, M. D., Ho, P. L., Coviello, G. M., Wright, W. E., Weinrich, S. L., and Shay, J. W. Specific association of human telomerase activity with immortal cells and cancer. Science, 266: 2011–2015, 1994.
2. Feng, J., Funk, W. D., Wang, S. S., Weinrich, S. L., Avilion, A. A., Chiu, C. P., Adams, R. R., Chang, E., Allsopp, R. C., Yu, J., and et al. The RNA component of human telomerase. Science, 269: 1236–1241, 1995.
3. Saji, M., Westra, W. H., Chen, H., Umbricht, C. B., Tuttle, R. M., Box, M. F., Udelsman, R., Sukumar, S., and Zeiger, M. A. Telomerase activity in the differential diagnosis of papillary carcinoma of the thyroid. Surgery, 122: 1137–1140, 1997.
4. Haugen, B. R., Nawaz, S., Markham, N., Hashizumi, T., Shroyer, A. L., Werness, B., and Shroyer, K. R. Telomerase activity in benign and malignant thyroid tumors. Thyroid, 7: 337–342, 1997.
5. Onoda, N., Ishikawa, T., Yoshikawa, K., Sugano, S., Kato, Y., Sowa, M., and Hirakawa-Yong Suk Chung, K. Telomerase activity in thyroid tumors. Oncol Rep, 5: 1447–1450, 1998.
6. Umbricht, C. B., Saji, M., Westra, W. H., Udelsman, R., Zeiger, M. A., and Sukumar, S. Telomerase activity: a marker to distinguish follicular thyroid adenoma from carcinoma. Cancer Res, 57: 2144–2147, 1997.
7. De Deken, X., Vilain, C., Van Sande, J., Dumont, J. E., and Miot, F. Decrease of telomere length in thyroid adenomas without telomerase activity. J Clin Endocrinol Metab, 83: 4368–4372, 1998.
8. Saji, M., Xydas, S., Westra, W. H., Liang, C. K., Clark, D. P., Udelsman, R., Umbricht, C. B., Sukumar, S., and Zeiger, M. A. Human telomerase reverse transcriptase (hTERT) gene expression in thyroid neoplasms. Clin Cancer Res, 5: 1483–1489, 1999.

9. Siddiqui, M. T., Greene, K. L., Clark, D. P., Xydas, S., Udelsman, R., Smallridge, R. C., Zeiger, M. A., and Saji, M. Human telomerase reverse transcriptase expression in Diff-Quik-stained FNA samples from thyroid nodules. Diagn Mol Pathol, *10*: 123–129, 2001.
10. Sebesta, J., Brown, T., Williard, W., Dehart, M. J., Aldous, W., Kavolius, J., and Azarow, K. Does telomerase activity add to the value of fine needle aspirations in evaluating thyroid nodules? Am J Surg, *181*: 420–422, 2001.
11. Brousset, P., Chaouche, N., Leprat, F., Branet-Brousset, F., Trouette, H., Zenou, R. C., Merlio, J. P., and Delsol, G. Telomerase activity in human thyroid carcinomas originating from the follicular cells. J Clin Endocrinol Metab, *82*: 4214–4216, 1997.
12. Cheng, A. J., Lin, J. D., Chang, T., and Wang, T. C. Telomerase activity in benign and malignant human thyroid tissues. Br J Cancer, *77*: 2177–2180, 1998.
13. Huang, Y., Prasad, M., Lemon, W. J., Hampel, H., Wright, F. A., Kornacker, K., LiVolsi, V., Frankel, W., Kloos, R. T., Eng, C., Pellegata, N. S., and de la Chapelle, A. Gene expression in papillary thyroid carcinoma reveals highly consistent profiles. Proc Natl Acad Sci U S A, *98*: 15044–15049, 2001.
14. Xu, X. C., el-Naggar, A. K., and Lotan, R. Differential expression of galectin-1 and galectin-3 in thyroid tumors. Potential diagnostic implications. Am J Pathol, *147*: 815–822, 1995.
15. Fernandez, P. L., Merino, M. J., Gomez, M., Campo, E., Medina, T., Castronovo, V., Sanjuan, X., Cardesa, A., Liu, F. T., and Sobel, M. E. Galectin-3 and laminin expression in neoplastic and non-neoplastic thyroid tissue. J Pathol, *181*: 80–86, 1997.
16. Orlandi, F., Saggiorato, E., Pivano, G., Puligheddu, B., Termine, A., Cappia, S., De Giuli, P., and Angeli, A. Galectin-3 is a presurgical marker of human thyroid carcinoma. Cancer Res, *58*: 3015–3020, 1998.
17. Herrmann, M. E., LiVolsi, V. A., Pasha, T. L., Roberts, S. A., Wojcik, E. M., and Baloch, Z. W. Immunohistochemical expression of galectin-3 in benign and malignant thyroid lesions. Arch Pathol Lab Med, *126*: 710–713, 2002.
18. Bernet, V. J., Anderson, J., Vaishnav, Y., Solomon, B., Adair, C. F., Saji, M., Burman, K. D., Burch, H. B., and Ringel, M. D. Determination of galectin-3 messenger ribonucleic Acid overexpression in papillary thyroid cancer by quantitative reverse transcription-polymerase chain reaction. J Clin Endocrinol Metab, *87*: 4792–4796, 2002.
19. De Micco, C., Zoro, P., Garcia, S., Skoog, L., Tani, E. M., Carayon, P., and Henry, J. F. Thyroid peroxidase immunodetection as a tool to assist diagnosis of thyroid nodules on fine-needle aspiration biopsy. Eur J Endocrinol, *131*: 474–479, 1994.
20. Christensen, L., Blichert-Toft, M., Brandt, M., Lange, M., Bjerregaard Sneppen, S., Ravnsbaek, J., Mollerup, C. L., Strange, L., Jensen, F., Kirkegaard, J., Sand Hansen, H., Sorensen, S. S., and Feldt-Rasmussen, U. Thyroperoxidase (TPO) immunostaining of the solitary cold thyroid nodule. Clin Endocrinol (Oxf), *53*: 161–169, 2000.
21. Krohn, K. and Paschke, R. Loss of heterozygocity at the thyroid peroxidase gene locus in solitary cold thyroid nodules. Thyroid, *11*: 741–747, 2001.
22. Higashiyama, T., Takano, T., Matsuzuka, F., Liu, G., Miyauchi, A., Yokozawa, T., Morita, S., Kuma, K., Shiba, E., Noguchi, S., and Amino, N. Measurement of the expression of oncofetal fibronectin mRNA in thyroid carcinomas by competitive reverse transcription-polymerase chain reaction. Thyroid, *9*: 235–240, 1999.
23. Takano, T., Matsuzuka, F., Miyauchi, A., Yokozawa, T., Liu, G., Morita, S., Kuma, K., and Amino, N. Restricted expression of oncofetal fibronectin mRNA in thyroid papillary and anaplastic carcinoma: an in situ hybridization study. Br J Cancer, *78*: 221–224, 1998.
24. Takano, T., Miyauchi, A., Yokozawa, T., Matsuzuka, F., Liu, G., Higashiyama, T., Morita, S., Kuma, K., and Amino, N. Accurate and objective preoperative diagnosis of thyroid papillary carcinomas by reverse transcription-PCR detection of oncofetal fibronectin messenger RNA in fine-needle aspiration biopsies. Cancer Res, *58*: 4913–4917, 1998.
25. Takano, T., Miyauchi, A., Matsuzuka, F., Kuma, K., and Amino, N. Expression of oncofetal fibronectin messenger ribonucleic acid in fibroblasts in the thyroid: a possible cause of false positive results in molecular-based diagnosis of thyroid carcinomas. J Clin Endocrinol Metab, *85*: 765–768, 2000.
26. Cheung, C. C., Carydis, B., Ezzat, S., Bedard, Y. C., and Asa, S. L. Analysis of ret/PTC gene rearrangements refines the fine needle aspiration diagnosis of thyroid cancer. J Clin Endocrinol Metab, *86*: 2187–2190, 2001.
27. Elisei, R., Romei, C., Vorontsova, T., Cosci, B., Veremeychik, V., Kuchinskaya, E., Basolo, F., Demidchik, E. P., Miccoli, P., Pinchera, A., and Pacini, F. RET/PTC rearrangements in thyroid nodules: studies in irradiated and not irradiated, malignant and benign thyroid lesions in children and adults. J Clin Endocrinol Metab, *86*: 3211–3216, 2001.

28. Fusco, A., Chiappetta, G., Hui, P., Garcia-Rostan, G., Golden, L., Kinder, B. K., Dillon, D. A., Giuliano, A., Cirafici, A. M., Santoro, M., Rosai, J., and Tallini, G. Assessment of RET/PTC oncogene activation and clonality in thyroid nodules with incomplete morphological evidence of papillary carcinoma: a search for the early precursors of papillary cancer. Am J Pathol, *160*: 2157–2167, 2002.
29. Kroll, T. G., Sarraf, P., Pecciarini, L., Chen, C. J., Mueller, E., Spiegelman, B. M., and Fletcher, J. A. PAX8-PPARgamma1 fusion oncogene in human thyroid carcinoma [corrected]. Science, *289*: 1357–1360, 2000.
30. Marques, A. R., Espadinha, C., Catarino, A. L., Moniz, S., Pereira, T., Sobrinho, L. G., and Leite, V. Expression of PAX8–PPARgamma1 Rearrangements in Both Follicular Thyroid Carcinomas and Adenomas. J Clin Endocrinol Metab, *87*: 3947-3952, 2002.
31. Cheung, L., Messina, M., Gill, A., Clarkson, A., Learoyd, D., Delbridge, L., Wentworth, J., Philips, J., Clifton-Bligh, R., and Robinson, B. G. Detection of the PAX8-PPAR gamma fusion oncogene in both follicular thyroid carcinomas and adenomas. J Clin Endocrinol Metab, *88*: 354–357, 2003.
32. Cohen, Y., Xing, M., Mambo, E., Guo, Z., Wu, G., Trink, B., Beller, U., Westra, W. H., Ladenson, P. W., and Sidransky, D. BRAF mutation in papillary thyroid carcinoma. J Natl Cancer Inst, *95*: 625–627, 2003.
33. Kimura, E. T., Nikiforova, M. N., Zhu, Z., Knauf, J. A., Nikiforov, Y. E., and Fagin, J. A. High prevalence of BRAF mutations in thyroid cancer: genetic evidence for constitutive activation of the RET/PTC-RAS-BRAF signaling pathway in papillary thyroid carcinoma. Cancer Res, *63*: 1454–1457, 2003.
34. Xu, X., Quiros, R. M., Gattuso, P., Ain, K. B., and Prinz, R. A. High prevalence of BRAF gene mutation in papillary thyroid carcinomas and thyroid tumor cell lines. Cancer Res, *63*: 4561–4567, 2003.
35. Bevilacqua, G., Sobel, M. E., Liotta, L. A., and Steeg, P. S. Association of low nm23 RNA levels in human primary infiltrating ductal breast carcinomas with lymph node involvement and other histopathological indicators of high metastatic potential. Cancer Res, *49*: 5185–5190, 1989.
36. Zou, M., Shi, Y., al-Sedairy, S., and Farid, N. R. High levels of Nm23 gene expression in advanced stage of thyroid carcinomas. Br J Cancer, *68*: 385–388, 1993.
37. Farley, D. R., Eberhardt, N. L., Grant, C. S., Schaid, D. J., van Heerden, J. A., Hay, I. D., and Khosla, S. Expression of a potential metastasis suppressor gene (nm23) in thyroid neoplasms. World J Surg, *17*: 615–620; discussion 620–611, 1993.
38. Bertheau, P., De La Rosa, A., Steeg, P. S., and Merino, M. J. NM23 protein in neoplastic and non-neoplastic thyroid tissues. Am J Pathol, *145*: 26–32, 1994.
39. Shi, Y., Zou, M., and Farid, N. R. The mystery of nm23H1 in thyroid cancer. J Endocrinol Invest, *25*: 663–664, 2002.
40. Chiappetta, G., Tallini, G., De Biasio, M. C., Manfioletti, G., Martinez-Tello, F. J., Pentimalli, F., de Nigris, F., Mastro, A., Botti, G., Fedele, M., Berger, N., Santoro, M., Giancotti, V., and Fusco, A. Detection of high mobility group I HMGI (Y) protein in the diagnosis of thyroid tumors: HMGI (Y) expression represents a potential diagnostic indicator of carcinoma. Cancer Res, *58*: 4193–4198, 1998.
41. Tuccari, G. and Barresi, G. Immunohistochemical demonstration of ceruloplasmin in follicular adenomas and thyroid carcinomas. Histopathology, *11*: 723–731, 1987.
42. Permanetter, W., Nathrath, W. B., and Lohrs, U. Immunohistochemical analysis of thyroglobulin and keratin in benign and malignant thyroid tumours. Virchows Arch A Pathol Anat Histopathol, *398*: 221–228, 1982.
43. Schelfhout, L. J., Van Muijen, G. N., and Fleuren, G. J. Expression of keratin 19 distinguishes papillary thyroid carcinoma from follicular carcinomas and follicular thyroid adenoma. Am J Clin Pathol, *92*: 654–658, 1989.
44. Sahoo, S., Hoda, S. A., Rosai, J., and DeLellis, R. A. Cytokeratin 19 immunoreactivity in the diagnosis of papillary thyroid carcinoma: a note of caution. Am J Clin Pathol, *116*: 696–702, 2001.
45. Haber, R. S., Weiser, K. R., Pritsker, A., Reder, I., and Burstein, D. E. GLUT1 glucose transporter expression in benign and malignant thyroid nodules. Thyroid, *7*: 363–367, 1997.
46. Wang, W., Larson, S. M., Tuttle, R. M., Kalaigian, H., Kolbert, K., Sonenberg, M., and Robbins, R. J. Resistance of [18f]-fluorodeoxyglucose-avid metastatic thyroid cancer lesions to treatment with high-dose radioactive iodine. Thyroid, *11*: 1169–1175, 2001.
47. van Hoeven, K. H., Kovatich, A. J., and Miettinen, M. Immunocytochemical evaluation of HBME-1, CA 19-9, and CD-15 (Leu-M1) in fine-needle aspirates of thyroid nodules. Diagn Cytopathol, *18*: 93–97, 1998.

48. Casey, M. B., Lohse, C. M., and Lloyd, R. V. Distinction between papillary thyroid hyperplasia and papillary thyroid carcinoma by immunohistochemical staining for cytokeratin 19, galectin-3, and HBME-1. Endocr Pathol, *14*: 55–60, 2003.
49. Mai, K. T., Bokhary, R., Yazdi, H. M., Thomas, J., and Commons, A. S. Reduced HBME-1 immunoreactivity of papillary thyroid carcinoma and papillary thyroid carcinoma-related neoplastic lesions with Hurthle cell and/or apocrine-like changes. Histopathology, *40*: 133–142, 2002.
50. Mase, T., Funahashi, H., Koshikawa, T., Imai, T., Nara, Y., Tanaka, Y., and Nakao, A. HBME-1 immunostaining in thyroid tumors especially in follicular neoplasm. Endocr J, *50*: 173–177, 2003.
51. Trovato, M., Villari, D., Ruggeri, R. M., Quattrocchi, E., Fragetta, F., Simone, A., Scarfi, R., Magro, G., Batolo, D., Trimarchi, F., and Benvenga, S. Expression of CD30 ligand and CD30 receptor in normal thyroid and benign and malignant thyroid nodules. Thyroid, *11*: 621–628, 2001.
52. Cheifetz, R. E., Davis, N. L., Robinson, B. W., Berean, K. W., and LeRiche, J. C. Differentiation of thyroid neoplasms by evaluating epithelial membrane antigen, Leu-7 antigen, epidermal growth factor receptor, and DNA content. Am J Surg, *167*: 531–534, 1994.
53. Khan, A., Baker, S. P., Patwardhan, N. A., and Pullman, J. M. CD57 (Leu-7) expression is helpful in diagnosis of the follicular variant of papillary thyroid carcinoma. Virchows Arch, *432*: 427–432, 1998.
54. Specht, M. C., Tucker, O. N., Hocever, M., Gonzalez, D., Teng, L., and Fahey, T. J., 3rd Cyclooxygenase-2 expression in thyroid nodules. J Clin Endocrinol Metab, *87*: 358–363, 2002.
55. Xing, M., Usadel, H., Cohen, Y., Tokumaru, Y., Guo, Z., Westra, W. B., Tong, B. C., Tallini, G., Udelsman, R., Califano, J. A., Ladenson, P. W., and Sidransky, D. Methylation of the thyroid-stimulating hormone receptor gene in epithelial thyroid tumors: a marker of malignancy and a cause of gene silencing. Cancer Res, *63*: 2316–2321, 2003.
56. Arturi, F., Russo, D., Giuffrida, D., Ippolito, A., Perrotti, N., Vigneri, R., and Filetti, S. Early diagnosis by genetic analysis of differentiated thyroid cancer metastases in small lymph nodes. J Clin Endocrinol Metab, *82*: 1638–1641, 1997.
57. Gubala, E., Handkiewicz-Junak, D., Zeman, M., Chmielik, E., Wiench, M., and Jarzab, B. [Thyroglobulin RT-PCR method for detection of lymph node metastases during the course of differentiated thyroid cancers]. Wiad Lek, *54 Suppl 1*: 349–356, 2001.
58. Weber, T., Lacroix, J., Weitz, J., Amnan, K., Magener, A., Holting, T., Klar, E., Herfarth, C., and von Knebel Doeberitz, M. Expression of cytokeratin 20 in thyroid carcinomas and peripheral blood detected by reverse transcription polymerase chain reaction. Br J Cancer, *82*: 157–160, 2000.
59. Weber, T. and Klar, E. Minimal residual disease in thyroid carcinoma. Semin Surg Oncol, *20*: 272–277, 2001.
60. Weber, T., Amann, K., Weckauf, H., Lacroix, J., Weitz, J., Schonfuss, T., Holting, T., Klar, E., Herfarth, C., and von Knebel Doeberitz, M. Detection of disseminated medullary thyroid carcinoma cells in cervical lymph nodes by cytokeratin 20 reverse transcription-polymerase chain reaction. World J Surg, *26*: 148–152, 2002.
61. Weber, T., Lacroix, J., Worner, S., Weckauf, H., Winkler, S., Hinz, U., Schilling, T., Frank-Raue, K., Klar, E., and Knebel Doeberitz Mv, M. Detection of hematogenic and lymphogenic tumor cell dissemination in patients with medullary thyroid carcinoma by cytokeratin 20 and preprogastrin-releasing peptide RT-PCR. Int J Cancer, *103*: 126–131, 2003.
62. Saller, B., Feldmann, G., Haupt, K., Broecker, M., Janssen, O. E., Roggendorf, M., Mann, K., and Lu, M. RT-PCR-based detection of circulating calcitonin-producing cells in patients with advanced medullary thyroid cancer. J Clin Endocrinol Metab, *87*: 292–296, 2002.
63. Bostick, P. J., Morton, D. L., Turner, R. R., Huynh, K. T., Wang, H. J., Elashoff, R., Essner, R., and Hoon, D. S. Prognostic significance of occult metastases detected by sentinel lymphadenectomy and reverse transcriptase-polymerase chain reaction in early-stage melanoma patients. J Clin Oncol, *17*: 3238–3244, 1999.
64. Hochberg, M., Lotem, M., Gimon, Z., Shiloni, E., and Enk, C. D. Expression of tyrosinase, MIA and MART-1 in sentinel lymph nodes of patients with malignant melanoma. Br J Dermatol, *146*: 244–249, 2002.
65. Torrens, J. I. and Burch, H. B. Serum thyroglobulin measurement. Utility in clinical practice. Endocrinol Metab Clin North Am, *30*: 429–467, 2001.
66. Ditkoff, B. A., Marvin, M. R., Yemul, S., Shi, Y. J., Chabot, J., Feind, C., and Lo Gerfo, P. L. Detection of circulating thyroid cells in peripheral blood. Surgery, *120*: 959–964; discussion 964–955, 1996.
67. Tallini, G., Ghossein, R. A., Emanuel, J., Gill, J., Kinder, B., Dimich, A. B., Costa, J., Robbins, R., Burrow, G. N., and Rosai, J. Detection of thyroglobulin, thyroid peroxidase, and RET/PTC1 mRNA

transcripts in the peripheral blood of patients with thyroid disease. J Clin Oncol, *16*: 1158–1166, 1998.
68. Ringel, M. D., Ladenson, P. W., and Levine, M. A. Molecular diagnosis of residual and recurrent thyroid cancer by amplification of thyroglobulin messenger ribonucleic acid in peripheral blood. J Clin Endocrinol Metab, *83*: 4435–4442, 1998.
69. Bellantone, R., Lombardi, C. P., Bossola, M., Ferrante, A., Princi, P., Boscherini, M., Maussier, L., Salvatori, M., Rufini, V., Reale, F., Romano, L., Tallini, G., Zelano, G., and Pontecorvi, A. Validity of thyroglobulin mRNA assay in peripheral blood of postoperative thyroid carcinoma patients in predicting tumor recurrences varies according to the histologic type: results of a prospective study. Cancer, *92*: 2273–2279, 2001.
70. Biscolla, R. P., Cerutti, J. M., and Maciel, R. M. Detection of recurrent thyroid cancer by sensitive nested reverse transcription-polymerase chain reaction of thyroglobulin and sodium/iodide symporter messenger ribonucleic acid transcripts in peripheral blood. J Clin Endocrinol Metab, *85*: 3623–3627, 2000.
71. Fugazzola, L., Mihalich, A., Persani, L., Cerutti, N., Reina, M., Bonomi, M., Ponti, E., Mannavola, D., Giammona, E., Vannucchi, G., di Blasio, A. M., and Beck-Peccoz, P. Highly sensitive serum thyroglobulin and circulating thyroglobulin mRNA evaluations in the management of patients with differentiated thyroid cancer in apparent remission. J Clin Endocrinol Metab, *87*: 3201–3208, 2002.
72. Grammatopoulos, D., Elliott, Y., Smith, S. C., Brown, I., Grieve, R. J., Hillhouse, E. W., Levine, M. A., and Ringel, M. D. Measurement of thyroglobulin mRNA in peripheral blood as an adjunctive test for monitoring thyroid cancer. Mol Pathol, *56*: 162–166, 2003.
73. Bojunga, J., Roddiger, S., Stanisch, M., Kusterer, K., Kurek, R., Renneberg, H., Adams, S., Lindhorst, E., Usadel, K. H., and Schumm-Draeger, P. M. Molecular detection of thyroglobulin mRNA transcripts in peripheral blood of patients with thyroid disease by RT-PCR. Br J Cancer, *82*: 1650–1655, 2000.
74. Roddiger, S. J., Bojunga, J., Klee, V., Stanisch, M., Renneberg, H., Lindhorst, E., Usadel, K. H., Kusterer, K., Schumm-Draeger, P. M., and Kurek, R. Detection of thyroid peroxidase mRNA in peripheral blood of patients with malignant and benign thyroid diseases. J Mol Endocrinol, *29*: 287–295, 2002.
75. Span, P. N., Sleegers, M. J., van den Broek, W. J., Ross, H. A., Nieuwlaat, W. A., Hermus, A. R., and Sweep, C. G. Quantitative detection of peripheral thyroglobulin mRNA has limited clinical value in the follow-up of thyroid cancer patients. Ann Clin Biochem, *40*: 94–99, 2003.
76. Gupta, M., Taguba, L., Arciaga, R., Siperstein, A., Faiman, C., Mehta, A., and Sethu, S. Detection of Circulating Thyroid Cancer Cells by Reverse Transcription-PCR for Thyroid-stimulating Hormone Receptor and Thyroglobulin: The Importance of Primer Selection. Clin Chem, *48*: 1862–1865, 2002.
77. Savagner, F., Rodien, P., Reynier, P., Rohmer, V., Bigorgne, J. C., and Malthiery, Y. Analysis of Tg transcripts by real-time RT-PCR in the blood of thyroid cancer patients. J Clin Endocrinol Metab, *87*: 635–639, 2002.
78. Bustin, S. A. Quantification of mRNA using real-time reverse transcription PCR (RT-PCR): trends and problems. J Mol Endocrinol, *29*: 23–39, 2002.
79. Lossos, I. S., Czerwinski, D. K., Wechser, M. A., and Levy, R. Optimization of quantitative real-time RT-PCR parameters for the study of lymphoid malignancies. Leukemia, *17*: 789–795, 2003.
80. Tricarico, C., Pinzani, P., Bianchi, S., Paglierani, M., Distante, V., Pazzagli, M., Bustin, S. A., and Orlando, C. Quantitative real-time reverse transcription polymerase chain reaction: normalization to rRNA or single housekeeping genes is inappropriate for human tissue biopsies. Anal Biochem, *309*: 293–300, 2002.
81. Vandesompele, J., De Preter, K., Pattyn, F., Poppe, B., Van Roy, N., De Paepe, A., and Speleman, F. Accurate normalization of real-time quantitative RT-PCR data by geometric averaging of multiple internal control genes. Genome Biol, *3*: RESEARCH0034, 2002.
82. Wingo, S. T., Ringel, M. D., Anderson, J. S., Patel, A. D., Lukes, Y. D., Djuh, Y. Y., Solomon, B., Nicholson, D., Balducci-Silano, P. L., Levine, M. A., Francis, G. L., and Tuttle, R. M. Quantitative reverse transcription-PCR measurement of thyroglobulin mRNA in peripheral blood of healthy subjects. Clin Chem, *45*: 785–789, 1999.
83. Ringel, M. D., Balducci-Silano, P. L., Anderson, J. S., Spencer, C. A., Silverman, J., Sparling, Y. H., Francis, G. L., Burman, K. D., Wartofsky, L., Ladenson, P. W., Levine, M. A., and Tuttle, R. M. Quantitative reverse transcription-polymerase chain reaction of circulating thyroglobulin messenger ribonucleic acid for monitoring patients with thyroid carcinoma. J Clin Endocrinol Metab, *84*: 4037–4042, 1999.

84. Takano, T., Miyauchi, A., Yoshida, H., Hasegawa, Y., Kuma, K., and Amino, N. Quantitative measurement of thyroglobulin mRNA in peripheral blood of patients after total thyroidectomy. Br J Cancer, 85: 102–106, 2001.
85. Eszlinger, M., Neumann, S., Otto, L., and Paschke, R. Thyroglobulin mRNA quantification in the peripheral blood is not a reliable marker for the follow-up of patients with differentiated thyroid cancer. Eur J Endocrinol, 147: 575–582, 2002.
86. Roddiger, S. J., Renneberg, H., Martin, T., Tunn, U. W., Zamboglou, N., and Kurek, R. Human kallikrein 2 (hK2) mRNA in peripheral blood of patients with thyroid cancer: a novel molecular marker? J Cancer Res Clin Oncol, 129: 29–34, 2003.
87. Fenton, C., Anderson, J. S., Patel, A. D., Lukes, Y., Solomon, B., Tuttle, R. M., Ringel, M. D., and Francis, G. L. Thyroglobulin messenger ribonucleic acid levels in the peripheral blood of children with benign and malignant thyroid disease. Pediatr Res, 49: 429–434, 2001.
88. Haber, R. S. The diagnosis of recurrent thyroid cancer–a new approach. J Clin Endocrinol Metab, 83: 4189–4190, 1998.

18. THYROID CANCER IMAGING

T.T.H PHAN*, P.L. JAGER*, K.M. van TOL, T.P. LINKS
*Department of Nuclear Medicine * and Endocrinology #, University Hospital Groningen, Groningen, The Netherlands*

INTRODUCTION

Molecular imaging in thyroid cancer using nuclear medicine methods is based on specific cellular characteristics. These characteristics can be derived from common cell features, but can also be based on specific properties of thyroid cancer cells. While in the diagnosis of thyroid cancer these methods have not found great potential, many applications can be found in treatment and follow up of the papillary, follicular and medullary thyroid carcinoma patients. In anaplastic thyroid carcinoma the experience with nuclear imaging is scarce, but the clinical relevance in this aggressive tumor is low.

The broad spectrum of radioactive tracer methods is associated with a great variety in sensitivity and specificity. This variation is partly based on cellular or tumor cell characteristics but also can be explained by the different technical factors and techniques. For example, where radioiodine imaging is among the cornerstones of thyroid cancer treatment, this tracer is of limited value in medullary thyroid cancer. This difference illustrates the importance of the specific cell characteristics that governs uptake of radiotracers. C-cells do not take up radioiodine, while follicular thyroid cells do. Another example can be found in the uptake of the tracer 18 FluoroDeoxyGlucose (FDG), which can be used in conjunction with the Positron Emission Tomography (PET) technique. Uptake of this tracer is based on the glucose metabolism that is present in benign and malignant cells. However, the demand for glucose is considerably higher in malignant cells, which results in higher tracer uptake and adequate imaging of thyroid cancer lesions. Also other nuclear imaging techniques have their additional value in the diagnosis and sometimes treatment of thyroid cancer. For some tracers the discovery of its value in the diagnosis of thyroid cancer is a matter of serendipity and the mechanisms of action are not always fully understood.

In this chapter nuclear medicine tracers methods, commonly used in thyroid cancer patients, will be reviewed, with a special emphasis on the general uptake mechanism, followed by the method of scanning and the clinical applications.

IODINE

General mechanism

The synthesis of thyroid hormone depends on the supply and metabolism of iodine in the thyroid gland and on the synthesis of thyroglobulin (a receptor protein for iodine). Iodine is taken up by the thyroid follicular cells as inorganic iodide and is transformed through a sequence of metabolic process into thyroid hormones (thyroxine (T4) and triiodothyronine (T3)).

The recommendations of the World Health Organization (WHO) for the iodine intake is 90–200 μg/day (90 μg/day for the newborn, 200 μg/day for the pregnant and lactating women) to maintain growth, development and normal thyroid function (1). The average daily dietary intake of iodide varies greatly per area or country. An average of 190–300 μg iodide per person is ingested daily in the United States. In Europe the average daily intake varies greatly from 50 μg (Belgium) to 430 μg (Great Britain) (2,3). About 60 to 80 μg of iodide is taken up daily by the thyroid from the circulating pool that ranges from 250 to 750 μg. If this extrathyroidal iodide pool is labeled with radioactive iodine (^{131}I or ^{123}I), the percentage of uptake of this tracer in 24 hours (8 to 35%) gives a dynamic index of the thyroid gland activity. The total iodide content of the thyroid gland averages 7500 μg, virtually all of which is in the form of iodothyronines (secretory products of the thyroid gland). In a steady state condition 60 to 80 μg (approximately 1% of the total) iodide is released from the thyroid gland daily. Of this amount 75% is secreted as thyroid hormones, and the remainder is free iodide. The large ratio of iodide stored in the form of hormone to the amount of tuned over daily, can protect the individual from the effects of iodide deficiency for about 2 months (4).

Iodide is actively transported into the thyroid follicular cells against chemical and electrical gradients, the iodide trapping. The site of active iodide transport in thyroid follicular cells is the basolateral membrane. The transport of iodide across this membrane is linked to the transport of sodium (Na+/I symporter (NIS)), generated by Na+/K+-ATPase as the driving force. Iodide trapping is stimulated by the thyroid-stimulating hormone (TSH).

Once in the thyroid follicular cell, iodide moves to the apical surface of the cell and seems to be translocated across the apical membrane by the chloride/iodide transporter molecule pendrin (encoded by PDS-gene) into the lumen (colloid) of the follicle cell (5,6,7). The function of pendrin in the thyroid is currently not precisely determined (5,6,8). Once in the follicular lumen, iodide is immediately incorporated into tyrosine residues of thyroglobulin (a glycoprotein synthesized on the rough endoplasmatic reticulum). Within the follicle thyroglobulin is iodinated and via monoiodotyrosine (MIT) and diiodotyrosine (DIT) T_4 and T_3 are formed.

Radioactive iodide (^{131}I and ^{123}I) can be used to visualize the thyroid gland and to measure the iodide trapping function. Only the follicular and the papillary variants of thyroid carcinomas, together called differentiated thyroid carcinoma (DTC), have the ability to concentrate radioiodine. Nevertheless, the iodine metabolism is profoundly altered in DTC. Iodine uptake is quantitatively decreased compared with the uptake in normal thyroid tissue. Furthermore, the iodine organification process is defective in thyroid cancer tissue, resulting in shorter biological half-life within the thyroid. Thyroid hormone synthesis is also usually absent. These abnormalities in organification and hormone synthesis are related to decreased NIS-expression and peroxidase genes and the impairment of the pendrin- PDS gene pathway (7). PDS-gene and pendrin expression seems to be dramatically decreased only in DTC (6,7).

Stimulation of TSH will induce uptake of in tumors that are able to concentrate radioiodine and increase Tg production by all tumor tissues, even in lesions unable to concentrate radioiodine (9). In order to be detectable by gammacamera imaging, lesions must have a critical combination of size and tracer uptake. Thus, the ability to visualize thyroid cancer remnants or metastatic tissue with radioiodine depends on several factors: a critical cell mass; the activity of the iodine trapping and organification mechanisms and incompletely defined mechanism (e.g. pendrin) that export or clear iodine from the cells.

Delivery of radioiodine to the thyroid tissue therefore requires stimulation by high level of endogenous TSH, induced after an adequate period of withdrawal from thyroid hormones causing hypothyroidism.

Iodine isotopes

Several iodine isotopes play an important role in nuclear medicine, as well for in vivo imaging as for in vitro investigations. Radioiodine can be used as a tracer itself, but is also very suitable to label other molecules. Three kinds of iodine isotopes, including iodine-123 (^{123}I), iodine-125 (^{125}I) and iodine-131 (^{131}I), are widely applied in nuclear medicine. ^{123}I and ^{131}I are used for imaging, ^{125}I is unsuitable for imaging, but often used for in in vitro applications and radiolabeling of other substances. Iodine-124 (^{124}I) is a positron emitting isotope, which is suitable for positron emission tomography (PET) imaging. A summary of the properties of these iodine isotopes is presented in Table 1.

Table 1. Characteristics of iodine isotopes

Iodine isotopes	$T^{1/2}$	Decay	Energy (keV)	Application
^{123}I	13 hours	EC, γ	159	diagnostic
^{124}I	4.1 days	ß+	511	PET
^{125}I	60 days	EC, γ	28 + 35	radioimmunoassay
^{131}I	8.04 days	ß$^-$	330 (max)	therapeutic
		γ	364	diagnostic

For diagnostic purposes the gamma emissions are important. The distribution of the radiopharmaceutical inside the body can be externally measured through imaging with gamma cameras. For therapeutic purposes the beta energy emission is important because of the destructive character in tissue. The path length of the beta particle depends on the energy and ranges from several mm to 1 cm.

Iodine-131

An important property of ^{131}I is that it can both be used for imaging purposes (high energy gamma ray) as well as for therapeutic purposes (medium-energy beta emission) while most of other radionuclides only have diagnostic utility. ^{131}I has however suboptimal imaging characteristics, including high energy gamma ray (364 keV), which is not optimal for most gamma cameras. The long half-life (8.04 days) and high beta emission limit the administered dose for diagnostic purpose only. The path length of the beta particle is about 0.5 mm, the toxic effects are limited to the thyroid tissue, with therefore sparing of adjacent normal tissue. The normal biodistribution of iodine includes salivary glands, stomach and renal tract including the bladder.

The long half-life is advantageous in the detection of functioning metastatic thyroid cancer lesions, because imaging can be done for many days after administration. This enables long take up periods in metastatic tissue and adequate clearance of background activity.

The radiation dose delivered by ^{131}I concentrated in a tissue depends on two factors: the radioactive concentration (the ratio between total uptake and the volume of functioning tissue) and the effective half-life (time after which the radioactivity in the tissue has decreased by a factor of 2). The effective half-life is related to the physical half-life and the biological half-life, which is related to the elimination of ^{131}I from the concentrating tissue.

In normal thyroid tissue the concentration is about 1 to 2% of the administered ^{131}I activity per gram and effective half-life is about 8 days. Functional thyroid cancer tissues concentrate under favourable condition about 0.1 to 0.5% of the administered ^{131}I activity per gram and the effective half-life is shorter than 3 days (9).

Iodine-123

Like ^{131}I the chemical behavior of ^{123}I is identical to that of stable iodide. The half-life of ^{123}I is 13.2 hours. ^{123}I decays by electron capture and is a lower energy gamma emitter (159 keV) compared with ^{131}I. Therefore the resulting imaging quality is better than ^{131}I. In addition, ^{123}I delivers a lower radiation dose to the thyroid tissue due to the absence of beta particle emission which may prevent a possible 'stunning' effect (discussed below). The major disadvantages of ^{123}I are the high cost due to the facts that it is produced by cyclotron, the limited availability and furthermore, the short half-life.

Iodine-124

While the radioisotopes ^{123}I and especially ^{131}I are used on a wide scale in diagnosis and treatment of all thyroid disorders, the positron emitting isotope ^{124}I, which is suitable for PET, has received little attention. Chemically identical to non-radioactive iodine, this isotope would allow thyroid cancer imaging using the high resolution PET technique (10). ^{124}I, however, is difficult to obtain and only available at specific research centers, as it is produced in a cyclotron. The isotope has a relatively low yield of radiation (positron yield 23%) suitable for imaging, but also emits other high-energy gamma radiation that increases the radiation to the thyroid (when present) almost to the (therapeutic) level of ^{131}I. In addition, the high-energy byproducts may deteriorate image quality. For these reasons clinical use has been minimal. ^{124}I has been used for dosimetric purposes or thyroid volume measurements (11,12,13,14,15). Recent development of combined PET-CT scanners with a single gantry, may increase clinical application in thyroid cancer patients, as detailed anatomical information is combined with the location of iodine positive tissue (16). The clinical value, for example, as compared to ^{131}I scintigraphy, is currently unknown.

Iodine-125

^{125}I decays by electron capture and gamma emission. The very low energy gamma emission (28–35 keV) and the long half-life (60 days) of ^{125}I make this radionuclide less suitable for in-vivo application. The very low energy gamma ray is to weak to be detected by gamma cameras. However, ^{125}I is extremely suitable for in-vitro application. It is a common agent for use in radioimmunoassay.

Scan method

Patient preparation

Thyroid stimulating hormone (TSH), produced by the pituitary is essential for stimulation of thyroid cells for optimal imaging with radioiodine. There are two ways to prepare a patient for radioiodine imaging: thyroid hormone withdrawal or administration of recombinant human TSH (rhTSH) during thyroid hormone therapy. Standard thyroid hormone medication (l-thyroxine, T4) withdrawal is usually 4–6 weeks until the serum TSH is greater than 30 mU/l to permit maximum stimulation of thyroid tissue. L-triiodothyronine (T3, Cytomel) replacement therapy (25 µg BID or TID) can be given the first 4 weeks of a 6 weeks withdrawal due to the short half-life and the immediate effects of L-triiodothyronine. The transient thyroid hormone suppletion withdrawal is associated with morbidity of hypothyroidism and therefore decreases the quality of life and diminishing productivity (17).

Recombinant human TSH (rhTSH) prevents the profound symptoms of hypothyroidism as a consequence of thyroid hormone withdrawal. rhTSH increases serum TSH concentration sufficiently to stimulate thyroidal ^{131}I uptake and release of thyroglobulin (Tg) while patients are still taking thyroid hormone medication. The recommended protocol of rhTSH is two intramuscular injections of 0.9 mg given on 2 consecutive days followed by 148 MBq (4 mCi) ^{131}I on the third day and a WBS and Tg measurement on the fifth day. Whole body images were acquired after 30 minutes of scanning or after 140,000 counts. This is necessary because 4 mCi ^{131}I after rhTSH has about the same effect as 2 mCi given in the hypothyroid state with reduced renal clearance and raised ^{131}I body retention (18,19).

However, it must be emphasized that there is so far few experience concerning this issue especially on the long term effects on outcome, so the application of rhTSH in the diagnostics still a matter of discussion (20).

Diagnostic ^{131}I WBS

TECHNIQUES OF SCANNING. Imaging is performed using high-energy collimator. The bladder must be emptied before imaging. Supine anterior and posterior images of the neck, chest, abdomen and pelvis are acquired. Anatomic landmark or transmission scans using cobalt marker can be helpful in the interpretation of the images. Additional or delayed images can be obtained in patients with atypical findings on the scans.

INTERPRETATION. The correct interpretation of the radioiodine images is crucial in the therapy management of thyroid cancer. It requires knowledge and understanding of the normal biodistribution of radioiodine. Radioiodine uptake in the choroid plexus, nasal mucosa, salivary glands, mammary glands, gastric mucosa, gastrointestinal tract and urinary tract including bladder should be considered as physiological. These tissues contain like thyroid tissue NIS-transporter. Diffuse iodine uptake in the liver can also be seen on the post-treatment scans when there is functioning thyroid due to the incorporation of radioiodine into thyroid hormones which are degraded in the liver by de-iodination and conjugation. Uptake of radioiodine outside the above mentioned organs should be considered as residual and/or metastatic thyroid tissue (true positive) or as contamination (false positive) (21,22).

Clinical application

Pretherapeutic diagnostic scintigraphy

The goal of the diagnostic scan after total or near-total thyroidectomy is to quantify the residual thyroid and detect metastatic disease. It is also included as part of the follow-up procedures. The ablative or therapeutic dose of ^{131}I used for treatment can be based on the results of the diagnostic scan. The diagnostic WBS is usually acquired 48–72 hours after administration of a diagnostic dose of ^{131}I during hypothyroid state.

Performing diagnostic ^{131}I scans before ablation therapy (23) or during follow-up, up is controversial (24).

The reason to perform no pre-ablative diagnostic ^{131}I scintigraphy is, that it is known that nearly all patients show residual neck uptake after (near) total thyroidectomy. And some believe that low diagnostic dose of ^{131}I may impair the thyroid remnants uptake of the subsequent ablative dose of ^{131}I, the so-called stunning effect. This issue will be discussed further on. Carlisle et al. (22) support performing diagnostic scans prior to therapy for several reasons. First, patients with undectectable Tg and a normal diagnostic scan after total thyroidectomy need not to be treated with ^{131}I. Second, a correct treatment ^{131}I dose can be determined when the extent of the disease is known.

Discussions are continuing concerning performing diagnostic scans before ^{131}I treatment in patients with elevated serum Tg. Cailleux et al. (24) suggest that diagnostic scanning need not to be done when serum Tg is higher than 5 ng/ml and one rather should considered therapy and posttherapeutic scan after thyroid hormone withdrawal.

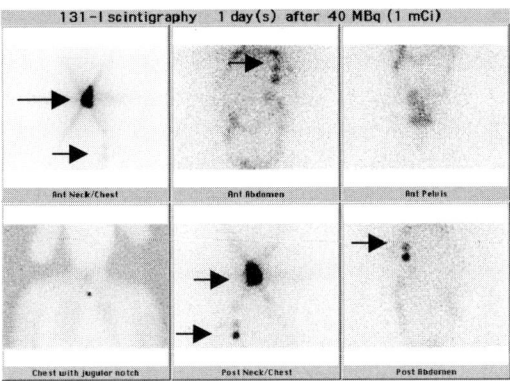

Figure 1.1. Pre-therapeutic diagnostic ^{131}I-WBS 1 day after 40 MBq in a 37-year-old patient with papillary thyroid carcinoma with elevated serum Tg after total thyroidectomy. It shows intense uptake in the neck (arrow) and uptake in the lung (arrow). Normal biodistribution in the gastrointestinal tract and bladder. This patient was subsequently treated with ablative dose of 1850 MBq ^{131}I.

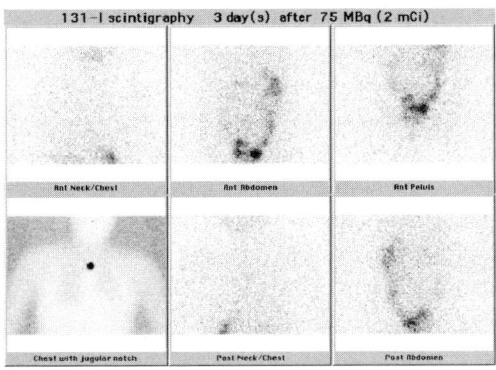

Figure 1.2. Posttherapeutic ^{131}I-WBS 10 days after a treatment dose of 5550 MBq in the same patient with papillary thyroid carcinoma with persistent elevated serum Tg and a negative diagnostic ^{131}I-WBS 3 months after ablative dose of 1850 MBq. This posttherapeutic ^{131}I-WBS was also negative, with only normal biodistribution in the gastrointestinal tract and bladder.

Pacini (25) suggest that diagnostic scanning is of low usefulness when the serum Tg-off T4 is undetectable after initial therapy.

Posttherapeutic (diagnostic) scintigraphy

A consensus for optimal dose of ^{131}I for ablation has not been reached. Some preferred a dosimetric approach by blood and whole-body and quantitative dosimetry to define the ablative dose. The majority use a standard fixed dose, which can range from 1110 MBq to 7400 MBq (30 mCi–200 mCi), depending on tumor characteristics (18,26), because of its simplicity and safety.

The timing of the acquisition of a post-therapy scan can vary widely. The interval varies from 1 day to 10 days after a therapeutic dose. However, shorter time interval allows less time for soft tissue clearance of radioiodine resulting in a relatively higher soft-tissue background which could make ^{131}I foci less visible and difficult to detect (27,28). More lesions are identified on the post-therapy scans than on the diagnostic scans. Carlisle (22) have found a discrepancy of 10% which alter the treatment management in 5% of the cases. These findings were similar with that of Fatourechi (29). The reasons of detecting more disease on the post-treatment scans compared with the diagnostic scans are probably due to the higher therapeutic doses and the longer time delay (22).

Post-therapy scans are most likely to yield important information when the serum Tg is elevated in a patient who is clinically disease-free with negative diagnostic scans or other conventional radiologic imaging (19,30).

Stunning

The timing and the amount of the diagnostic and therapeutic ^{131}I dose are controversial. There has been controversy concerning whether radiation of the diagnostic dose really has a suppressive effect on the uptake of subsequent therapeutic ^{131}I, the so-called stunning-effect (31). For extensive review of stunning see chapter 11.

The issue whether stunning is a real phenomenon and its clinical relevance/consequence is questionable (32). Our retrospective evaluation of 158 patients, who received a high-dose diagnostic scan with 370 MBq (10 mCi) because of a negative low-dose diagnostic scan with 74 MBq (2 mCi) ^{131}I, demonstrates that diagnostic ^{131}I scan with 74 MBq (2 mCi) is sufficient for correct clinical decision making with regards to further radioiodine treatment, when combined with Tg-off measurements. In 98% of the patients a 370 MBq (10 mCi) dose of ^{131}I for diagnostic WBS had no additional value (33).

rhTSH

The yield of ^{131}I scans seems to be slightly lower with rhTSH than following thyroid hormone withdrawal (17), although another study mentioned a similar diagnostic yield (34). ^{131}I scanning it self provides complementary information besides the measurement of Tg after withdrawal (24) or after rhTSH (35). For now it is unclear which specific patient group will have benefit of this follow-up policy with rhTSH (20).

The retrospective review of Robbins (35) showed no significant difference in the rate of complete ablation between a group of patients who were prepared with rhTSH or by thyroid hormone withdrawal. Other reports mention the effectiveness of rhTSH in ablative therapy (26,36). However, in the study of Menzel (37) there is a significant reduction in the effective half-life of ^{131}I in patients after rhTSH-stimulated TSH before radioiodine therapy compared with patients after endogenous stimulated TSH. Although the use of rhTSH in the follow up patients with thyroid cancer is proposed (38,39) proper prospective data concerning rhTSH applications are still very poor or even lacking (40).

Lithium

Lithium has an inhibitory effect on the release of iodine from the thyroid but does not change the uptake. The mechanism by which lithium inhibits the secretion of thyroid hormone is not well understood. In vitro, lithium decreases the droplet formation of the colloid of thyroid follicular cells, which is a reflection of a decreased pinocytosis of colloid from the follicular lumen (41). The efficiency of proteolytic digestion of thyroglobulin may also be impaired. For this feature lithium may be useful as an adjuvant for ^{131}I therapy of thyroid cancer.

However, there are very few experiences concerning the application of lithium in thyroid cancer. Only in one study was shown, that lithium prolonged the biological and effective half-lives and increased the accumulation of ^{131}I by 50% in tumors and 90% in thyroid remnants.

Thus, it is in tumors that are less likely to respond to ^{131}I therapy that lithium may be most useful but further experience is required (42).

Retinoic acid

Retinoic acids are biologically active metabolites of vitamin A. They play an important role in the morphogenesis, differentiation and proliferation of many cells (43,44). Retinoic acid has been used for cancer treatment due to their growth and differentiation effects.

Dedifferentiation changes can occurred in differentiated thyroid cancer. This is accompanied by loss of thyroid-specific function and loss of iodide uptake, which makes the therapy with radioiodine inaccessible. It seems that retinoic acids have the potential for redifferentiating therapy in these advanced stage of thyroid cancer (43,44). Nevertheless, the therapeutic effects of isotretinoin in thyroid cancer is so far very disappointing and further controlled clinical trials are required (45).

Sodium iodide symporter (NIS)

The human NIS gene is localized on chromosome 9p12–13.2. NIS is an integral protein of the basolateral membrane of thyroid gland follicular cells. Uptake of iodide from the interstitium into the cell through the NIS-transporter is an active process.

NIS-expression is inversely related to the degree of differentiation of thyroid cancer cells. NIS is more expressed in differentiated thyroid cancer and often negative in less well-differentiated thyroid cancer. Elucidating of the molecular mechanism of NIS expression in thyroid cancer might have the potential in enhancing the diagnostic and therapeutic management since thyroid cancer tissues with NIS expression take up more ^{131}I and subsequent show a high rate of response to radioiodine therapy than those without NIS expression (46,47) (see also chapter 11).

Blind therapy of ^{131}I

After total thyroidectomy and radioiodine ablation, an elevated serum Tg level as well as positive diagnostic radioiodine scanning, are good indicators of the presence of persistent, recurrent or metastatic thyroid cancer (48,49). However, there is a management dilemma in case of negative diagnostic radioiodine scanning and an elevated serum Tg. Negative diagnostic radioiodine scanning may be caused by factors such as an insufficient rise in serum TSH or iodine contamination (50). Another explanation for negative diagnostic scanning is dedifferentiation of the tumor leading to a loss of its iodine trapping ability while Tg production is still preserved. Finally, the presence of microscopic metastases that are too small to be visualized with a diagnostic ^{131}I dose, which can cause false negative scans. Nowadays in patients with negative diagnostic radioiodine scanning, an empirical therapeutic dose between 100–300 mCi ^{131}I, followed by a posttherapy whole-body scan (WBS) is advocated (24,28,38,51,52). The purpose of this approach is twofold. First, posttherapy radioiodine scanning after high-dose ^{131}I treatment is believed to be the most sensitive tool for localizing residual disease not shown by diagnostic scanning with 2–5 mCi ^{131}I (28,53,54). Thus detected residual disease can be treated with other forms of therapy, such as surgery or radiotherapy. Second, small metastases not seen on diagnostic scanning may accumulate sufficient ^{131}I after high-dose ^{131}I treatment, leading to a relevant reduction in tumor load. Several studies have shown a drop in serum Tg after high-dose ^{131}I treatment in patients with negative diagnostic radio-iodide scanning (54,55). Serum Tg remained the same or Tg increased (28,56). Since patient numbers in these studies are small and follow-up data are scarce, it is still unclear whether such high-dose ^{131}I treatment after negative diagnostic radio-iodide scanning is of benefit for the patient. Recently, several reports were published that show no additional effect of high-dose ^{131}I therapy (52,57,58), except for limited cases as lung metastases (52). High-dose ^{131}I treatment in patients with negative diagnostic ^{131}I WBS and detectable serum Tg during hypothyroidism can be used as a diagnostic and prognostic tool (59).

18 FLUORODEOXYGLUCOSE (FDG)

General mechanism

The glucose analogue FDG is a tracer of glucose metabolism, and enters cells by the same mechanisms both in benign and malignant tissue. However, the energy metabolism of malignant cells is considerably less efficient than the metabolism in their benign counterparts (60). For example anaerobic glycolysis is strongly increased in malignant cells, which is associated with less energy (ATP) production per molecule of glucose as compared to the energy production resulting from the citric acid cycle. Therefore, the need for glucose molecules and FDG is strongly increased in malignancy, which is the basis for the preferential uptake of FDG in malignancy. FDG is intracellularly phosphorylated by a hexokinase into FDG-6-phosphate, which is not further metabolized, in contrast with glucose-6-phosphate. In addition, the FDG-6-phosphate cannot leave the cell again, and the compound is therefore trapped intracellulary. The final accumulation of FDG-6-phosphate is proportional to the glycolytic rate of the involved cell. In some tissues however, the level of phosphatase activity may be variable, and FDG accumulation in liver, kidney, intestine, muscle and some tumor cells may be lower. Apart from the increased glycolysis, it has been demonstrated that levels of transmembrane glucose transporters (e.g. the GLUT-1 transporter) and possibly also of some hexokinase isoenzymes are also increased in malignancy and relate to FDG uptake (61,62,63,64). On the one hand, the uptake mechanism of FDG with selective irreversible trapping of the tracer in malignant tissue is ideal for Positron Emission Tomography (PET) imaging, which has generated the increasing clinical application in oncology. On the other hand, it can be understood that FDG uptake does not exclusively occur in malignant tissues, as also benign tissue requires glucose. Especially activated macrophages, as present in infection and inflammation, are known to accumulate much FDG, sometimes to a degree that interferes with oncological image interpretation (65,66).

Scan method

In PET imaging radioactive tracers are used that emit positrons. After positron emission, the positron annihilates with a ubiquitous electron, which causes emission of two 511 KeV photons, precisely under an 180 degree angle. These photons are simultaneously detected by a ring of detectors, which are the main component of the PET camera.

FDG uptake occurs rapidly after administration, and due to the uptake mechanism, the amount of FDG that is taken up in tumor tissue, increases over time. Due to excretion of FDG, which causes clearance of 'background' uptake, and the decay of the radioactivity ($T^1/_2 = 110$ min) the optimal moment for imaging is generally considered to be 60–90 min after tracer administration.

For precise patient preparation and image protocols we refer to dedicated PET papers or books (67). Briefly, patients are generally injected with FDG in a fasting condition and after oral prehydration. The injected dose varies between 2-8MBq/kg. The scan duration for a whole body scan varies largely, but is in general 30–60 min.

Clinical application

Papillary and follicular thyroid carcinoma

FDG PET is not considered to be a useful method in the primary diagnosis of thyroid cancer. Although this issue has not received much study, the uptake of FDG in thyroid cancer in general appears to be low, and image interpretation may suffer from interfering uptake in benign tumors, such as follicular adenoma. In addition, the diagnosis can nearly always be obtained by other diagnostic methods.

Much more data are available to underscore the value of PET in the follow-up of thyroid cancer patients, such as to detect recurrences or metastases, especially in cases where metastases do not trap radioiodine. Interestingly, there appears to be a complementary uptake of FDG and radioiodine, which has been termed the 'flip-flop' phenomenon. This means that some metastases within the same patient that do not trap radioiodine may accumulate FDG, and metastases that do not trap FDG, accumulate radioiodine. Some lesions accumulate both tracers. This observation was first described by Joensuu (68). It might be explained by the different degree of tissue differentiation. Well-differentiated thyroid cancer tissue has retained its iodine trapping capabilities, but is metabolically inactive, causing uptake of radioiodine and no or minimal FDG accumulation. Less differentiated thyroid cancer tissue, as may develop during treatment, loses its iodine trapping capability and becomes metabolically more active. This results in FDG positivity and iodine negativity. For this reason, most PET research has focussed on detection of thyroid cancer metastases in radioiodine negative patients with increased thyroglobulin levels, which currently seems to be the best clinical application.

In a recent meta-analysis the value of FDG PET in papillary and follicular thyroid cancer both in patients with negative radioiodine scans and in patients with known neoplastic foci was determined (69). They selected 14 studies that met quality criteria as described by the Cochrane Methods Group on Screening and Diagnostic Tests. Although general evidence levels appeared to be low, precluding quantitative summary, all these studies claimed a positive role for PET, especially in the group of patients with negative radioiodine scans. Sensitivity for finding tumor locations of PET varied between 70 and 95%, and specificity was between 77 and 100%. Considerable heterogeneity existed, however, in the pre-PET data risk profile, such as patient selection criteria concerning variations in TNM stage, Tg levels, radioactive radioiodine dose and levels of TSH. Although troubled by severe methodological problems, the performance of FDG PET appeared to be superior to 99mTc-Sestamibi or Tc99m-furifosmin, and probably Tl-201 scintigraphy. Also the impact on overall clinical outcome of PET was difficult to assess, but, due to the general slow disease progression, that may be true for many diagnostic studies in thyroid cancer.

A frequently observed issue whether PET should be performed during the hypothyroid state (e.g. after thyroid hormone withdrawal) or in euthyroid state (during thyroxine treatment). In a study van Tol (70) better performance of PET in hypothyroid state was found, but the issue is not clearly settled.

Furthermore, it has been hypothesized that exogenous TSH stimulation with rhTSH increases FDG uptake by differentiated thyroid cancer and seems apparently more accurate than FDG-PET under suppression, in terms of number of detected lesions and tumor/background contrast (71). In a small study this hypothesis has been confirmed (18).

Medullary thyroid cancer

Nearly all imaging modalities (Ultrasonography, CT, MRI, scintigraphy using In-111-octreotide, Tc99m-DMSA-V, MIBG) have limited sensitivies (40–70%) compared to the apparently very high sensitivity of the calcitonin tumor marker (72). Although the clinical course of metastatic medullary thyroid cancer can be mild in some patients, others develop clinically relevant metastases (in liver, bone, lungs) that remain undetected until a relatively late stage. Earlier detection of metastases during follow up after primary treatment might therefore have relevant therapeutic implications. Results of FDG PET studies in MTC demonstrate slightly better performance (sensitivity around 75%—specificity 79%) as compared to other imaging modalities, but patient selection probably influences these results (73,74).

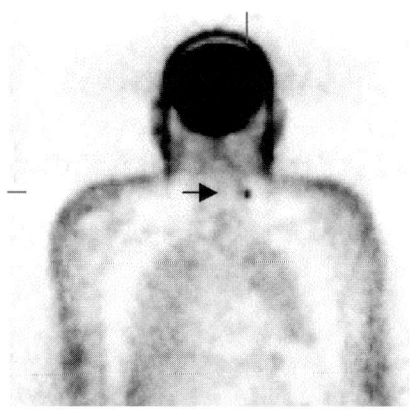

Figure 2. 50-year-old patient with papillar thyroid carcinoma, negative posttherapeutic ^{131}I-WBS 10 days after a treatment dose of 5550 MBq, thyroglobulin 25 ng/ml. FDG PET coronal slice showing a small lesion in the right neck (arrow) that proved to be a small metastasis of papillary thyroid cancer.

Other PET tracers

Similar to other neuroendocrine tumors as described above, uptake of FDG appears to be low, and theoretically radiolabeled amino acids might perform better in these calcitonin producing tumors (75). Preliminary experience using C11-methionine does not seem to confirm this expectation (76). Recent experience with the catecholamine precursor amino acid ^{18}F-DOPA and PET appears to be more promising. In a small group Hoegerle found more lymph node metastases of MTC using ^{18}F-DOPA PET than with any other modality (77). Also ^{18}F-DOPA PET was reported to be able to detect a medullary thyroid cancer lesion in a MEN2a patient (78).

THALLIUM-201 CHLORIDE

General mechanism

Thallium-201 (Tl-201) is a potassium analogue. This positively charged ion is actively transported over the cell membrane by an ATP-dependant sodium/potassium transport system and localizes non-specifically in thyroid cells, as well as in other tissues with high cellularity and high perfusion. Additional mechanisms of entry have not been excluded. Originally Tl-201 has been developed for myocardial perfusion imaging, for which it is still routinely used, but it also accumulates in kidney, stomach, liver, spleen, testes, salivary glands, large bowel and in thyroid tissue (79). Several reports have suggested that comparison between early and delayed Tl-201 images could distinguish between benign and malignant thyroid diseases, but usually results in benign and malignant tissues overlap and have not lead to sound clinical application (80,81).

Isotope characteristic

Tl-201 is an isotope that decays by electron capture to Mercury-201. Mercury 201 emits characteristic gamma rays of 68–90 keV and much smaller amount of gamma rays of 135 keV and 167 keV. The half-life of Tl-201 is 73.1 hours. Tl-201 is normally administered as thallium chloride and rapidly disappears from the blood with a half-life between 30 seconds and 3 minutes. Peak uptake in the thyroid occurs 5–10 minutes after injection.

The relative long half-life and the poor physical characteristic of the radiopharmaceutical limit the injected dose (3–5 mCi). The low photon energy causes a relatively large radiation burden and is also less suitable for imaging, because of scattered and absorbed radiation. This results in low image quality.

Scan method

Techniques of scanning

Tl-201 imaging for thyroid cancer does not require withdrawal of thyroid hormones or restriction of iodine intake. Imaging, using a low-energy collimator, is usually performed 10–20 minutes after intravenous injection of Tl-201, because at that time tumor/background ratio is highest. The accumulation in tumoral tissues remains constant between 20–60 minutes. Supine anterior and posterior whole-body scans are acquired. Additional or delayed images can be obtained 3–4 hours postinjection to differentiate malignant tissues (slower washout) from benign tissues (82).

Clinical application

Papillary and follicullar thyroid carcinoma

The primary value of Tl-201 is the analysis of patients with a negative ^{131}I scan and elevated thyroglobulin levels. Several studies discuss the usefulness of Tl-201 in the localization of metastatic disease (83,84,85,86). The combination of ^{131}I with Tl-201 scintigraphy resulted in a sensitivity for recurrent tumor of 90–100% at a specificity of 95%–100%. Adding also the information from thyroglobulin measurements even further increases diagnostic yield. Tl-201 alone generally depicts approximately half of all thyroid cancer lesions. Few reports have specifically addressed the value of Tl-201 scintigraphy in patients with negative ^{131}I scans.

Tl-201 scintigraphy seems to be most value in the localization of local metastases and in mediastinal lymph nodes. Sensitivity has been reported between 55–94%, specificity between 82–97% (85,86,87). The large variety in sensitivity can be attributed to the different methods of disease confirmation, the variability in location of metastases and the different selection of the patients.

Although most published studies were performed with planar images, SPECT imaging shows a 25% increase in sensitivity, especially for chest, neck and micronodular pulmonary metastases (88).

In the small study of Shiga et al. (89) Tl-201 scintigraphy seems to provide similar information in the detection of metastatic lesions after total thyroidectomy compared with FDG-PET.

Medullary thyroid carcinoma

There have been several studies of Tl-201 uptake in medullary thyroid carcinoma, most of them with a limited number of patients and in comparison with DMSA-V or

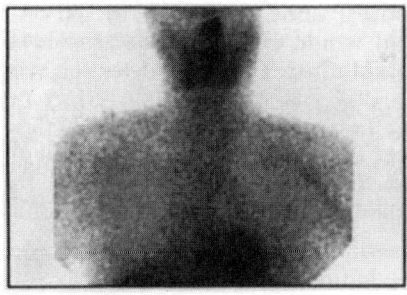
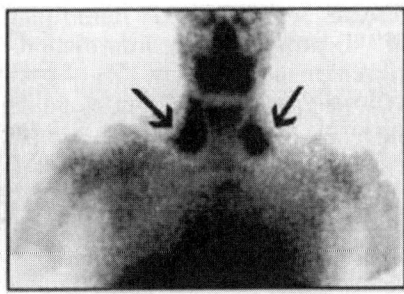

Figure 3. ^{201}Tl neck and chest scans. Normal scan taken when Tg was 4 ng/mL and ^{131}I scan was negative. Repeat ^{201}Tl scan when Tg was 75 ng/mL. Note uptake in the apices of the lungs (arrows). Iodine scan remained negative.

MIBG. The non-specific uptake of this tracer in background tissues and low tumoral uptake probably cause the relatively low sensitivity. DMSA-V scintigraphy has shown to be clearly superior to Tl-201 (90). Another study showed Tl-201 superior to MIBG. Although non-specific, Tl-201 may be be useful in individual clinical setting.

Although only limited comparison data of FDG PET and Tl-201 scintigraphy are available, but FDG PET is considered to be clearly superior.

TECHNETIUM-99M-SESTAMIBI (METHOXY-ISOBUTYL-ISONITRILE)

General mechanism

Technetium-99m-sestamibi (Tc-99m-sestamibi) is a lipophilic cationic agent that primary localizes in the mitochondria. Tc-99m-sestamibi accumulates in the mitochondria secondary to a negative potential of the mitochondria. Tc-99m-sestamibi uptake is driven by a negative transmembrane potential and up to 90% of the intracellular tracer is found in the mitochondria. The uptake is an energy dependant process. Tc-99m-sestamibi is also a substrate for the transmembrane P-glycoprotein drug efflux pump (91).

The affinity for mitochondria probably generates the specific uptake in Hürthle cell carcinoma, which is often poorly iodine concentrating, but rich in mitochondria. Similar to Tl-201, Tc-99m-sestamibi uptake in thyroid cancer cell is independent of TSH stimulation, although one report mentioned a TSH dependent uptake (92).

Isotope characteristic

Tc-99m-sestamibi is obtained by elution from a Tc generator, which contains the parent isotope molybdenum-99 (Mo-99). Mo-99 is a radionuclide with a half-life of 66 hours. The isolated 140 keV gamma emission of Tc-99m is ideally suited for gamma camera imaging. The 6 hr half life is very convenient for radiopharmaceutical production on a day to day basis. The commercial production of generators, which can be eluted up to 1 week, make Tc99m very easily available. These factors make Tc-99m the most used radioisotope in nuclear imaging in general. A kit preparation for radiolabeling of Tc-99m to sestamibi is commercially widely available.

Scan method

Tc-99m-sestamibi scintigraphy does not require any patient preparation and no thyroid hormone withdrawal. The favorable scan characteristics and the relative short half-life of Tc-99m (6 hours) in comparison to 131I (8 days) enable the use of relatively larger doses which increases image quality. This is a clear advantage over Tl-201.

Imaging is usually performed early, 10–30 minutes after tracer administration, and repeated 3 hours later. Others only image 60 minutes p.i., which might be less sensitive.

Clinical application

Tc-99m-sestamibi is only applied in papillary and follicular thyroid carcinoma.

The application of Tc-99m-sestamibi scanning is in patients with a negative 131-scan and an elevated thyroglobulin. In many instances Tc-99m-sestamibi has shown predilection to concentrate in the same abnormal sites as Tl-201.

Tc-99m-sestamibi scanning is particularly sensitive for the detection of nodal metastases. One study reported more sensitivity than high doses ^{131}I (93), another found the lowest sensitivity for lung metastases (94). Especially in high risk patient with a negative ^{131}I scan a combination of MIBI and ultrasound may be useful in detecting lymph node metastases (95).

Other Tc-99m based tracers

The data about the clinical application in thyroid cancer and value of Tc-99m Tetrofosmin, Tc-99m Pertechnate, Tc-99m Furifosmin is very limited and the results are conflicting. All three tracers are characterized by accumulation in the mitochondria by a different and not clearly understood mechanism.

Of the limited published data on Tc-99m tetrofosmin high sensitivities are mentioned (>85%) (96,97) in papillary and follicular thyroid carcinoma. No additional value is found in medullary thyroid carcinoma (90).

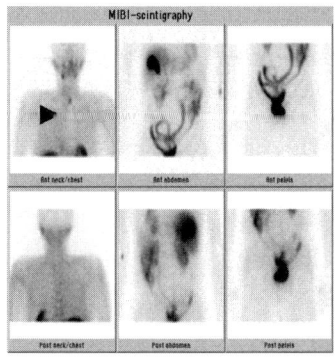

Figure 4. Technetium-99m-sestamibi scan 15 minutes after injection of 730 MBq in a 85-year-old patient with recurrent papillary thyroid carcinoma. It shows uptake in the neck (arrow). The ^{131}I-WBS was negative.

INDIUM-111 DTPA—PHE-1-OCTREOTIDE

General mechanism

Somatostatin receptors are present on many neuroendocrine tissues, both benign and malignant, also including normal thyroid cells and thyroid carcinoma cells. These receptors are the basis of scintigraphy using the radiolabelled somatostatin analogue, In-111-octreotide, which is an important diagnostic tool in neuroendocrine tumors in general. Five somatostatin receptors subtypes have been isolated. Somatostatin and its synthetic analogues act through specific binding to these receptors subtypes. Each subtype has its own tissue distribution pattern, and has specific pharmacological properties. After ligand—receptor interaction signals are transmitted (using G-proteins) to adenylate cyclase pathway, resulting in inhibitory effects on cell growth and proliferation. Normal thyroid tissue shows expression of all somatostatin receptor subtypes except somatostatin receptor subtype (SST) 2 in one study (98), while others found a high expression of SST3 and SST5, and only a weak expression of SST1 and SST2 (99). Thyroid cancer tissue shows a different SST expression. Papillar and follicular tumours have high expression of SST3, 4 and 5, while in Hürthle cell and medullary thyroid tumours SST2 expression is present.

Apart from different tissue distribution, ligand affinity also varies. The well-known somatostatin analogue, octreotide, has the highest affinity for SST2 and lower affinities for SST3 and SST5 and no affinity for SST1 and SST4. The lack or the low density of SST2 receptor is presumably the reason that only half of all thyroid cancers can be visualized by scintigraphy using radiolabelled octreotide (100).

Isotope characteristic

Indium-111 (In-111) has a half-life of 67.5 hours and is cyclotron-produced. It predominantly emits gamma photons with gamma-energy of 171 keV and 247 keV. Indium is coupled to the octreotid peptide using DTPA as a chelator (In-111-DTPA), and the ready-to-inject compound is commercially available. The tracer is also called In-111-pentreotide.

Scan method

Thyroid hormone suppression can be continued during scanning, although one study has shown a small increase in detection of positive lesions after thyroid hormone withdrawal (101). Whole-body imaging is performed 24 hours after intravenous injection of 200 MBq of In-111-octreotide, using a medium energy collimator. Laxation of patients is often performed to facilitate intestinal clearance. Normal distribution consists of intense uptake in kidneys and spleen, minor uptake in liver and intestine. Endocrine organs such as the thyroid and pituitary gland can also often be seen. Minor non-specific uptake can be observed in inflammatory lesions. Additional images, lateral views and/or SPECT, of the neck and upper abdomen improve the detection of smaller or equivocal lesions in those areas. Delayed images can be obtained 48 hours postinjection, mostly because of interfering accumulation of radioactivity in the bowel to differentiate pathological from physiological uptake.

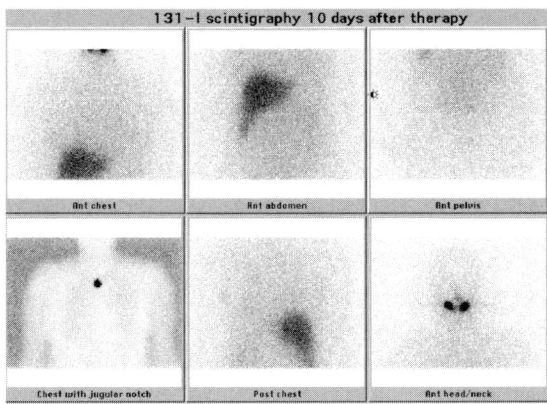

Figure 5.1. Negative posttherapeutic ^{131}I-WBS 10 days after a treatment dose of 5550 MBq in a 63-year-old patient with DTC with persistent elevated serum Tg and negative diagnostic ^{131}I-WBS 3 months after the ablative dose of 5550 MBq. Normal biodistribution in the liver and salivary glands. This patient showed on the first pre-ablative diagnostic ^{131}I-WBS, 6 weeks after total thyroidectomy, uptake in the neck and was subsequently treated with an ablative dose of 5550 MBq; the posttherapeutic ^{131}I-WBS 10 days after the ablative dose also showed uptake in the neck.

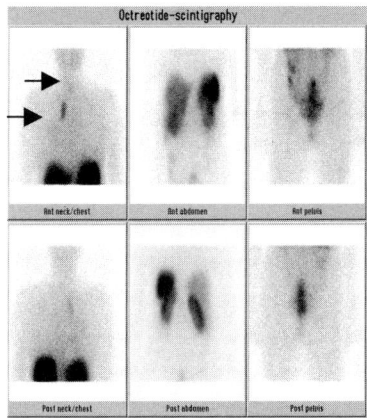

Figure 5.2. Indium-111-octreotide scan 24 hours after injection of 185 MBq in the same patient with DTC with persistent elevated serun Tg and negative ^{131}I-WBS. The indium-111-octreotide scan clearly shows uptake in the right lung (arrow) and faintly uptake in the neck (arrow).

Clinical application

Papillary and follicular thyroid carcinoma

In-111-Octreotide scintigraphy is especially useful in patients with 131-I negative scans and clinical suspicion on persistent tumor activity, as confirmed with recent studies (101,102,103). The uptake of In-111-Octreotide broadens the ability of the application of radiolabeled somatostatin analogues in general. High doses of Yttrium-90 (beta emitting) or the In-111 (gamma emitting) DOTA chelated somatostatin analogues have been applied in both patients with papillary and follicular thyroid cancer and with medullary thyroid cancer for therapeutic reasons. Currently response rates are around 35%. (104).

Medullary thyroid carcinoma

In medullary thyroid carcinoma In-111-octreotide scintigraphy can have a complementary value in individual cases. However, the somatostatin receptor density and the number of receptors appears to be lower in medullary thyroid carcinoma in comparison to other neuro-endocrine tumors. Also some medullary thyroid tumors can produce somatostatin which may be competitive in the receptor binding (105). However, In-111-octreotide can be a useful radiotracer for the detection of metastatic or recurrent medullary thyroid carcinoma. Especially in cases with minimal residual disease, as can be found by persistently elevated calcitonin levels, In-111-octreotide scintigraphy showed more tumor localisation than conventional techniques (106,107). Liver metastases are slightly less more difficult to visualise (108) because of the non specific background uptake in the liver. In-111 octreotide has the similar sensitivity ($\pm$80%) to CT and MRI for the detection of recurrent or metastatic medullary thyroid carcinoma (109).

META-IODOBENZYLGUANIDINE (MIBG)
General mechanism

Metaiodobenzylguanidine (MIBG) is a norepinephrine analogue that can be radiolabeled with ^{131}I or ^{123}I. MIBG is an aralkylguanidine, with combines the benzylgroup of bretylium and the guanidinegroup of guanethudine with an idione on the meta place. By competition with the energy dependent transport mechanism of norepinephrine MIBG is taken up in cells (110). Evidence has been found that probably a sodium-dependent and a sodium-independent uptake system is present. Differential expression of the uptake systems, may be responsible for the variations of the kinetic parameters for both norepinephrine and MIBG in different tumor cells. (111). It is especially sensitive in (nor)epinephrine producing tumors, such as pheochromocytoma, neuroblastoma or paraganglioma. In vitro experiments have shown that MIBG may act as a substrate for chromaffin granules. The vesicular mono-amine transporter (VMAT) type 2, that has extensively been expressed in pheochromocytomas seems to be responsible for MIBG transport and tumor visualization (112,113).

Scan method

MIBG can be radiolabeled with both ^{123}I or ^{131}I. Because of the unfavorable imaging characteristics and the higher radiotion dose, ^{123}I-MIBG is mostly used, although the ^{131}I labeled variant allows imaging up to several days after administration. In general thyroid uptake of (in small quantities liberated from the tracer) free iodine is blocked by administering non radioactive iodine or perchlorate at the time of injection. Imaging is generally performed 24 hrs after tracer administration. A large variety of medications

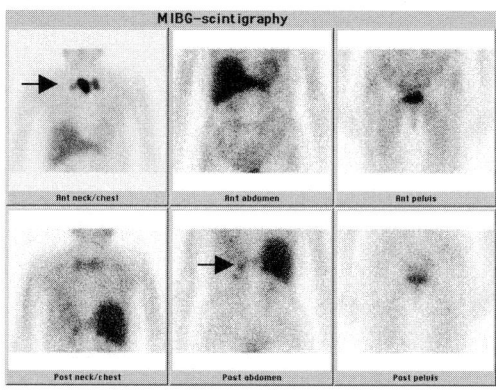

Figure 6. I-123 MIBG whole body scan 24 hours after injection of 185 MBq in a 78-year-old patient known with MTC, hyperparathyroidism and suspected of pheochromocytoma (MEN-2a). It shows intense uptake in the neck with bilateral paratracheal expansion (arrow); it also shows uptake in the left adrenal region (arrow).

may have some impact on tumoral uptake (e.g. alpha receptor blocking agents). Whole body and spot imaging may be supplemented by SPECT imaging.

Application

There is no place for MIBG scintigraphy in patients with differentiated thyroid cancer, but in medullary cancer the method may be helpful.

In medullary thyroid cancer, MIBG scans are positive in only a limited number of patients with medullary thyroid carcinoma with mentioned sensitivities of 12–30% (114,115).

A pitfall in imaging arises when liberated free iodine localizes in thyroid remnants (in the rare patients that were not ablated after thyroidectomy), but this can usually be differentiated from uptake in medullary thyroid cancer metastases. In cases of doubt Tc-pertechnetate imaging can be helpful.

A number of patients with medullary thyroid cancer have been treated with 131I-MIBG and a palliative response has been reported in 50% of the patients (116). Pentavalent 99m Technetium Dimercaptosuccinic Acid (99mTc (V)DMSA).

General mechanism

Pentevalent Tc-DMSA (called DMSA-V) is derived from DMSA, but includes the Tc99m label in a 5+ molecular charge, instead of 7+, as is the common chemical form of Tc99m. 99mTc(V) DMSA is not taken up by the normal thyroid gland, but can be applied in the diagnosis of medullary thyroid cancer due to an increased turnover of calcium and phosphate ions. The compound localizes in a number of tumours. The precise mechanism is not well known, uptake may be related to the intracellular phosphate concentration (117). 99mTc(V) DMSA exists in three isomeric forms and the biodistribution of the individual isomers differs from the whole radiopharmaceutical.

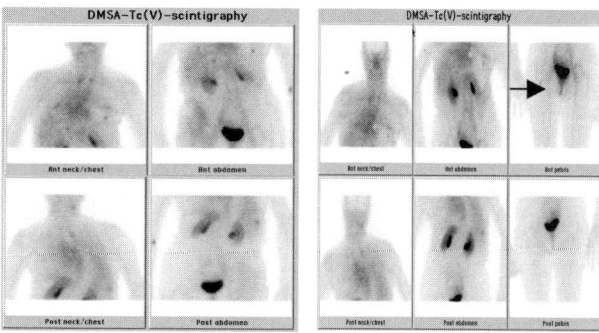

Figure 7. Tc-99m(V)-DMSA scan 2 hours after injection of 290 MBq in a patient known with MTC (MEN-2a) with persistent elevated serum calcitonin. The scan shows uptake in the neck, chest and in the right proximal femur (arrow). This patient also has severe scoliosis of the thoracal spine.

Scan method

Images are acquired 2–3 hours after injection. SPECT imaging of suspected areas may be helpful to improve the sensitivity of tumour detection.

The normal biodistribution is seen after 2 hours in the nasal mucosa and faintly in the skeleton, with breast uptake in women. Excretion is through the kidneys, liver uptake is not prominent. Some blood pool activity may also be present.

Clinical application

99mTc(v) DMSA is not commercially available in the United States but is well used in other countries. Tumor lesion sensitivity is reported to be between 50 and 95% (118,119).

RADIOLABELED ANTI CARCINOEMBRYONIC ANTIGEN ANTIBODY

General mechanism

Serum calcitonin and carcinoembryonic antigen (CEA) are used as tumormarkers in medullary thyroid carcinoma (MTC).

The specific positive immuno-histochemical property of a positive staining for calcitonin and carcinoembryonic antigen (CEA) and the expression of CEA levels at the surface of the cells were the basis for the development of specific anti-CEA monoclonal antibodies, the so-called radioimmunoscintigraphy, to image patients with MTC. Various anti-CEA antigen antibodies can be labeled with 99m-Tc, 111-In, ^{123}I or ^{131}I. The disadvantages of using monoclonal antibodies include the low tumor-background ratio and the forming of human anti-mouse antibodies (HAMA) making repeated studies difficult.

Scan method

The injected dose depends on the radionuclide the antibodies are labeled with, just like the timing of scanning and the choice of collimator (120,121,122). Injected activity are 555–1110 MBq (15–30 mCi) for 99m-Tc labeled antibodies, 74–370 MBq (2–10 mCi) for ^{131}I labeled antibodies and 111–185 MBq (3–5 mCi) for 111-In labeled antibodies. With the 99m-Tc labeled anti-CEA antibodies planar and SPECT imaging of the neck/chest, abdomen and pelvis can be acquired 4 and 24 hours postinjection with an LEHR-collimator. With the 111-In labeled anti-CEA antibodies imaging can be performed up to 72 hours postinjection with a medium energy collimator. Imaging of ^{131}I labeled anti-CEA antibodies can be performed 4 hours and up to 7 days postinjection. Blood pool activity may be prominent, kidney and bone marrow uptake can be seen.

Clinical application

Reported lesion based sensitivity of various anti-CEA antibodies in medullary thyroid carcinoma is around 70–100%, for both known and occult disease (121,122,123). However, only a limited number of groups have published about these results. Apart from the limited application in medullary thyroid cancer, the anti-CEA antibodies scan has been extensively used in the detection of metastatic colon cancer, where it appears to have a sensitivity of 50–70% and provides clinically relevant information, especially in combination with CT scanning.

REFERENCES

1. Delange F. Iodine deficiency in Europe and its consequences: an update. Eur J Nucl Med Mol Imaging 2002; 29, suppl 2:S404–S16.
2. Delange F., van Onderbergen A., Shabana W., Vandemeulebroucke E., Vertongen F., Gnat D., Dramaix M. Silent iodine profylaxis in Western Europe only partly corrects iodine deficiency; the case of Belgium. Eur J Endocrinol 2000; 143:189–96.
3. European Commission: Health & Consumer Protection Directorate-General. Opinion of the Scientific Committee on Food on the tolerable upper intake level of iodine.2002. B-1049 BruxellesBelgium. http://www.europa.eu.int/comm./food/fs/sc/scf/index e. html.
4. Berne R.M., Levy M.N. Physiology. Mosby Year Book, Missouri, USA. Third edition 1993: p932–937.
5. Yoshida A., Taniguchi S., Hisatome I., Royaux I.E., Green E.D., Kohn L.D., Suzuki K. Pendrin is an iodide-specific apical porter responsible for iodide efflux from thyroid cells. J Clin Endocrinol Metab 2002; 87:3356–61.
6. Kondo T., Nakamura N., Suzuki K., Murata S., Muramatsu A., Kawaoi A., Katoh R. Expression of human pendrin in diseased thyroids. J Histochem Cytochem 2003; 51:167–73.
7. Bidart J.M., Mian C., Lazar V., Russo D., Filetti S., Caillou B., Schlumberger M. Expression of pendrin and the Pendred Syndrome (PDS) gene in human thyroid tissues. J Clin Endocrinol Metab 2000; 85:2028–33.
8. Porra V., Bernier-Valentin F., Trouttet-Masson S., Berger-Dutrieux N., Peix J.L., Perrin A., Sehni-Ruby S., Rousset B. Characterization and semiquantitative analyses of pendrin expressed in normal and tumoral human thyroid tissues. J Clin Endocrinol Metab 2002; 87:1700–07.
9. Klain M., Ricard M., Leboulleux S., Baudin E., Schlumberger M. Radioiodine therapy for papillary and follicular thyroid carcinoma. Eur J Nucl Med Mol Imaging 2002; 29 suppl 2:S479–S85.
10. Pentlow K.S., Graham M.C., Lambrecht R.M., Daghighian F., Bacharach S.L., Bendriem B., Finn R.D., Jordan K., Kalaigian H., Karp J.S., Robeson W.R., Larson S.M. Quantitative imaging of iodine-124 with PET. J Nucl Med. 1996; 37:1557–62.
11. Eschmann S.M., Reischl G., Bilger K., Kupferschlager J., Thelen M.H., Dohmen B.M., Besenfelder H., Bares R. Evaluation of dosimetry of radioiodine therapy in benign and malignant thyroid disorders by means of iodine-124 and PET. Eur J Nucl Med Mol Imaging 2002; 29:760–7.
12. Crawford D.C., Flower M.A., Pratt B.E., Hill C., Zweit J., McCready V.R., Harmer C.L. Thyroid volume measurement in thyrotoxic patients: comparison between ultrasonography and iodine-124 positron emission tomography. Eur J Nucl Med 1997; 24:1470–8.

13. Flower M.A., al-Saadi A., Harmer C.L., McCready V.R., Ott R.J. Dose-response study on thyrotoxic patients undergoing positron emission tomography and radioiodine therapy. Eur J Nucl Med. 1994; 21:531–6.
14. Frey P., Townsend D., Jeavons A., Donath A. In vivo imaging of the human thyroid with a positron camera using 124I. Eur J Nucl Med. 1985; 10:472–6.
15. Frey P., Townsend D., Flattet A., De Gautard R., Widgren S., Jeavons A., Christin A., Smith A., Long A., Donath A. Tomographic imaging of the human thyroid using 124I. J Clin Endocrinol Metab 1986; 63:918–27.
16. Freudenberg L.S., Antoch G., Gorges R., Knust J., Pink R., Jentzen W., Debatin J.F., Brandau W., Bockisch A., Stattaus J. Combined PET/CT with iodine-124 in diagnosis of spread metastatic thyroid carcinoma: a case report. Eur Radiol 2003; May 8 [Epub ahead of print].
17. Ladenson P.W. Recombinant thyrotropin versus thyroid hormone withdrawal in evaluating patients with thyroid carcinoma. Semin Nucl Med 2000; 30:98–106.
18. Chin B.B., Patel P., Cohade C., Ewertz M., Wahl R., Ladenson P. Recombinant human thyrotropin stimulaton of fluoro-D-glucose positron emission tomography uptake in well-differentiated thyroid carcinoma. J Clin Endocrinol Metab 2004; 89:91–5.
19. Mazzaferri E.L., Kloos R.T. Clinical review 128: Current approaches to primary therapy for papillary and follicular thyroid cancer. J Clin Endocrinol 2001; 86:1447–63.
20. Mazzaferri E.L., Massoll N. Management of papillary and follicular (differentiated) thyroid cancer: new paradigms using recombinant human thyrotropin. Endoc-Relat Cancer 2002; 9:227–47.
21. Toft A., Beckett G. Use of recombinant thyrotropin. Lancet 2002; 359:1874–5.
22. Shapiro B., Rufini V., Jarwan A., Geatti O., Kearfott K.J., Fig L.M., Kirkwood I.D., Gross M.D. Artifacts, anatomical and physiological variants, and unrelated diseases that might cause false-positive whole-body 131-I scans in patients with thyroid cancer. Sem Nucl Med 2000; 30:115–32.
23. Carlisle M.R., Lu C., McDougall I.R. The interpretation of 131I scans in the evaluation of thyroid cancer, with an emphasis on false positive findings. Nucl Med Comm 2003; 24:715–5.
24. de Klerk J.M., de Keizer B., Zelissen P.M., Lips C.M., Koppeschaar H.P. Fixed dosage of 131I for remnant ablation in patients with differentiated thyroid carcinoma without pre-ablative diagnostic 131I scintigraphy. Nucl Med Comm 2000; 21:529–32.
25. Cailleux A.F., Baudin E., Travagli J.P., Ricard M., Schlumberger M. Is diagnostic iodine-131 scanning useful after thyroid ablation for differentiated thyroid cancer ? J Clin Endocrinol Metab 2000; 85: 175–8.
26. Pacini F., Capezzone M., Elisei R., Ceccarelli C., Taddei D., Pinchera A. Diagnostic 131-iodine whole body scan may be avoided in thyroid cancer patients who have undetectable stimulated serum Tg levels after initial treatment. J Clin Endocrinol Metab 2002; 87:1499–1501.
27. Pacini F., Molinaro E., Castagna M.G., Lippi F., Ceccarelli C., Agate L., Elisei R., Pinchera A. Ablation of the thyroid residues with 30 mCi (131)I: A comparison in thyroid cancer patients prepared with recombinant human TSH or thyroid hormone withdrawal. J Clin Endocrinol Metab 2002; 87: 4063–8.
28. Cholewinski S.P., Yoo K.S., Klieger P.S., O'Mara R.E. Absence of thyroid stunning after diagnostic whole-body scanning with 185 MBq 131I. J Nucl Med 2000; 41:1198–1202.
29. Pacini F., Lippi F., Formica N., Elisei R., Anelli S., Cecccarelli C., Pinchera A.Therapeutic doses of iodine-131 reveal undiagnosed metastases in thyroid cancer patients with detectable serum thyroglobulin levels. J Nucl Med. 1987; 8:1888–91.
30. Fatourechi V., Hay I.D., Mulan D.P., Wiseman G.A., Eghbali-Fatourechi G.Z., Thorson L.M., Gorman C.A. Are posttherapy radioiodine scans informative and do they influence subsequent therapy of patients with differentiated thyroid cancer? Thyroid 2000; 10:573–77.
31. Mazzaferri E.L. Long-term outcome of patients with differentiated thyroid carcinoma: effect of therapy. Endocr Pract 2000; 6:469–76.
32. Sabri O., Zimny M., Schreckenberger M., Meyer-Oelman A., Reinartz P., Buell U. Does thyroid stunning exist? A model with benign thyroid disease. Eur J Nucl Med 2000; 27:1591–7.
33. Coakley A.J. Thyroid stunning. Eur J Nucl Med 1998; 25:203–4.
34. Van Tol K.M. New insights in diagnosis and treatment of differentiated thyroid carcinoma. Thesis 2002. State University Groningen (a).
35. Robbins R.J., Tuttle R.M., Sharaf R.N., Larson S.M., Robbins H.K., Ghossein R.A., Smith A., Drucker W.D. Preparation by recombinant human thyrotropin or thyroid hormone withdrawal are comparable for the detection of residual differentiated thyroid carcinoma.J Clin Endocrinol Metab 2001; 86:619–25.

36. Robbins R.J., Larson S.M., Sinha N., Shaha A., Divgi C., Pentlow K.S., Ghossein R., Tuttle R.M. A retrospective review of the effectiveness of recombinant human TSH as a preparation for radioiodine thyroid remnant ablation. J Nucl Med 2002; 43:1482–88.
37. Barbaro D., Boni G., Meucci G., Simi U., Lapi P., Orsini P., Pasquini C., Piazza F., Caciagli M., Mariani G. Radioiodine treatment with 30 mCi after recombinant human thyrotropin stimulation in thyroid cancer: effectiveness for postsurgical remnants ablation and possible role of iodine content in L-thyroxine in the outcome of ablation. J Clin Endocrinol Metab 2003; 88:4110–5.
38. Menzel C., Kranert, Dorbert N., Diehl M., Fietz T., Hamscho N., Berner U., Grunwald F. RhTSH stimulation before radioiodine therapy in thyroid cancer reduces the effective half-life of ^{131}I. J Nucl Med 2003; 44:1065–68.
39. Wartofsky L. Editorial: Using baseline and recombinant human TSH-stimulated Tg measurements to manage thyroid cancer without diagnostic ^{131}I scanning. J Clin Endocrinol Metab 2002; 87:1486–89.
40. Mazzaferri E.L., Kloos R.T. Is diagnostic iodine-131 scanning with recombinant human TSH useful in the follow-up of differentiated thyroid cancer after thyroid ablation? J Clin Endocrinol Metab 2002; 87:1490–98.
41. Sherman S.I. Thyroid carcinoma. Lancet 2003; 361:501–11.
42. Williams J.A., Berens S.C., Wolff J. Thyroid secretion in vitro : inhibition of TSH and dibutyryl cyclic-AMP stimulated (131I) release by lithium. Endocrinology 1971; 88:1385–88.
43. Koong S.S., Reynolds J.C., Movius E.G., Keenan A.M., Ain K.B., Lakshmanan M.C., Robbins J. Lithium as a potential adjuvant to 131I therapy of metastatic, well differentiated thyroid carcinoma. J Clin Endocrinol Metab 1999; 84:912–16.
44. Simon D., Koehrle J., Reiners C., Boemer A.R., Schmutzler C., Mainz K., Goretzki P.E., Roeher H.D. Redifferentiation therapy with retinoids: therapeutic option for advanced follicular and papillary thyroid carcinoma. World J Surg 1998; 22:569–74.
45. Schmutzler C., Kohrle J. Retinoic acid redifferentiation therapy for thyroid cancer. Thyroid 2000; 10:393–406.
46. Gruning T., Tiepolt C., Zophel K., Bredow J., Kropp J., Franke W.G. Retinoic acid for redifferentiation of thyroid cancer: does it hold its promise? Eur J Endocrinol 2003 ; 148 :395–402.
47. Chung J.K. Sodium iodide symporter: its role in nuclear medicine. J Nucl Med 2002; 43:1188–1200.
48. Filetti S., Bidart J.M., Arturi F., Caillou B., Russo D., Schlumberger M. Sodium/iodide symporter: a key transport system in thyroid cancer cell metabolism. Eur J Endocrinol 1999; 141:443–57.
49. Ozata M., Suzuki S., Miyamoto T., Liu R.T., Fierro-Renoy F., DeGroot L.J. Serum thyroglobulin in the follow-up of patients with treated differentiated thyroid cancer. J Clin Endocrinol Metab 1994; 79:98–105.
50. Schlumberger M., Baudin E. Serum thyroglobulin determination in the follow-up of patients with differentiated thyroid cancer. Eur J Endocrinol 1998; 138:249–52.
51. Mazzaferri E.L. Treating high thyroglobulin with radioiodine: A magic bullet or a shot in the dark? J Clin Endocrinol Metab 1995; 80:1485–7.
52. Schlumberger M., Mancusi F., Baudin E., Pacini F. 131-I therapy for elevated thyroglobulin levels. Thyroid 1997; 7:273–6.
53. Pacini F., Agate L., Elisei R., Capezzone M., Ceccarelli C., Lippi F., Molinaro E. & Pinchera A. Outcome of differentiated thyroid cancer with detectable serum Tg and negative diagnostic ^{131}I whole body scan: Comparison of patients treated with high ^{131}I activities versus untreated patients. J Clin Endocrinol Metab 2001; 86:4092–7.
54. Schlumberger M., Arcangioli O., Pierkaski J.D., Tubiana M., Parmentier C. Detection and treatment of lung metastases of differentiated thyroid carcinoma in patients with normal chest X-rays. J Nucl Med 1988; 29:1790–4.
55. Pineda J.D., Lee T., Ain K., Reynolds J.C. & Robbins J. Iodine-131 therapy for thyroid cancer patients with elevated thyroglobulin and negative diagnostic scan. J Clin Endocrinol Metab 1995; 80:1488–92.
56. de Keizer B., Koppeschaar H.P.F., Zelissen P.M.J., Lips C.J.M., van Rijk R.P., van Dijk A., de Klerk J.M.H. Efficacy of high therapeutic doses of iodine-131 in patients with differentiated thyroid cancer and detectable serum thyroglobulin. European Journal of Nuclear Medicine 2001; 281:198–202.
57. McDougall I.R. 131-I treatment of 131-I negative whole body scans, and positive thyroglobulin in differentiated thyroid carcinoma: what is being treated? Thyroid 1997; 7:669–72.
58. Fatourechi V., Hay I.D., Javedan H., Wiseman G.A., Mullan B. & Gorman C.A. Lack of impact of radioiodine therapy in Tg-positive, diagnostic whole-body scan-negative patients with follicular cell-derived thyroid cancer. J Clin Endocrinol Metab 2002; 87:1521–26.

59. Schaap J., Eustatia-Rutten C.F.A., Stokkel M., Links T.P., Diamant M., van der Velde E., Romijn J.A., Smit J.W.A. Does radioiodine therapy have disadvantageous effects in non-radioiodine accumulating differentiated thyroid cancer? Clin Endocrinol 2002; 57:117–24.
60. Van Tol K.M., Jager P.L., De Vries E.G.E., Piers D.A., Boezen H.M., Sluiter W.J., Dullaart R.P.F., Links T.P. Outcome in patients with differentiated thyroid cancer with negative whole body scanning and detectable stimulated thyroglobulin. Eur J Endocrinol 2003; 148:589–96.
61. Warburg O. The metabolism of tumors. New York, NY: Richard R. Smith. 1931:129–6.
62. Brown R.S., Goodman T.M., Zasadny K.R., Greenson J.K., Wahl R.L. Expression of hexokinase II and Glut-1 in untreated human breast cancer. Nucl Med Biol. 2002; 29:443–53.
63. Higashi T., Saga T., Nakamoto Y., Ishimori T., Mamede M.H., Wada M., Doi R., Hosotani R., Imamura M., Konishi J. Relationship between retention index in dual-phase (18)F-FDG PET, and hexokinase-II and glucose transporter-1 expression in pancreatic cancer. J Nucl Med. 2002; 43: 173–80.
64. Muzi M., Freeman S.D., Burrows R.C., Wiseman R.W., Link J.M., Krohn K.A., Graham M.M., Spence A.M.. Kinetic characterization of hexokinase isoenzymes from glioma cells: implications for FDG imaging of human brain tumors. Nucl Med Biol 2001; 28:107–16.
65. Smith T.A. Mammalian hexokinases and their abnormal expression in cancer. Br J Biomed Sci. 2000; 57:170–8.
66. Kubota R., Yamada S., Kubota K., Ishiwata K., Tamahashi N., Ido T. Intratumoral distribution of fluorine-18-fluorodeoxyglucose in vivo: high accumulation in macrophages and granulation tissues studied by microautoradiography. J Nucl Med 1992; 33:1972–80.
67. Strauss L.G. Fluorine-18 deoxyglucose and false-positive results: a major problem in the diagnostics of oncological patients. Eur J Nucl Med 1996; 23:1409–15.
68. Wieler H.J., Coleman R.E. PET in Clinical Oncology. Springer, Steinkopff Verlag, Darmstadt, Germany. 2000 17–62. .
69. Joensuu H., Ahonen A. Imaging of metastases of thyroid carcinoma with fluorine-18 fluorodeoxyglucose. J Nucl Med. 1987;28:910–4.
70. Hooft L., Hoekstra O.S., Deville W., Lips P., Teule G.J., Boers M., van Tulder M.W. Diagnostic accuracy of 18F-fluorodeoxyglucose positron emission tomography in the follow-up of papillary or follicular thyroid cancer. J Clin Endocrinol Metab 2001; 86:3779–86.
71. Van Tol K.M., Jager P.L. Piers D.A., Pruim J., De Vries E.G.E., Dullaart R.P.F., Links T.P. Better yield of ^{18}Fluorodeoxyglucose-Positron Emission Tomography in patients with metastatic differentiated thyroid carcinoma during thyrotropin stimulation. Thyroid 2002; 12:381–7.
72. Petrich T., Borner A.R., Otto D., Hofmann M., Knapp W.H. Influence of rhTSH on [18F]fluorodeoxyglucose uptake by differentiated thyroid carcinoma. Eur J Nucl Med 2002; 29: 641–7.
73. James C., Starks M., MacGillivray D.C., White J. The use of imaging studies in the diagnosis and management of thyroid cancer and hyperparathyroidism. Surg Oncol Clin N Am 1999; 8:145–69.
74. Diehl M., Risse J.H., Brandt-Mainz K., Dietlein M., Bohuslavizki K.H., Matheja P., Lange H., Bredow J., Korber C., Grunwald F. Fluorine-18 fluorodeoxyglucose positron emission tomography in medullary thyroid cancer: results of a multicentre study. Eur J Nucl Med. 2001; 28:1671–6.
75. Szakall S. Jr., Esik O., Bajzik G., Repa I., Dabasi G., Sinkovics I., Agoston P., Tron L. 18F-FDG PET detection of lymph node metastases in medullary thyroid carcinoma. J Nucl Med 2002; 43:66–71.
76. Jager P.L., Vaalburg W., Pruim J., de Vries E.G., Langen K.J., Piers D.A. Radiolabeled amino acids: basic aspects and clinical applications in oncology. J Nucl Med 2001; 42:432–45.
77. Kienast O., Pirich C., Becherer A., Mitterhauser G., Dobrozemsky G., Dudczak R., Kletter K., Kurtaran A. Limited value of C11-methionine (MET)-PET for imaging of neuroendocrine tumors. Eur J Nucl Med 2003; 30:S203 [abstract].
78. Hoegerle S., Altehoefer C., Ghanem N., Brink I., Moser E., Nitzsche E. 18F-DOPA positron emission tomography for tumour detection in patients with medullary thyroid carcinoma and elevated calcitonin levels. Eur J Nucl Med. 2001; 28:64–71.
79. Gourgiotis L., Sarlis N.J., Reynolds J.C., VanWaes C., Merino M.J., Pacak K. Localization of medullary thyroid carcinoma metastasis in a multiple endocrine neoplasia type 2A patient by 6-[18F]-fluorodopamine positron emission tomography. J Clin Endocrinol Metab 2003; 88:637–41.
80. Tonami N., Hisada K. 201-Tl scintigraphy in postoperative detection of thyroid cancer: a comparative study with 131 I. Radiology 1980; 136:461–4.
81. Bleichrodt R.P., Vermey A., Piers D.A. de Langen Z.J. Early and delayed thallium 201 imaging: Diagnosis of patients with cold thyroid nodules. Cancer 1987; 60:2621–23.

82. Burman K.D., Anderson J.H., Wartofsky L., Mong D.P., Jellenik J.J. Management of patients with thyroid carcinoma: application of thallium-201 scintigraphy and magnetic resonace imaging. J Nucl Med 1990; 31:1958–64.
83. Murray I.P.C., Ell P.J. Nuclear medicine in clinical diagnosis and treatment. Churchill Livingstone. Second edition 1998: p832–p948.
84. Piers D.A., Sluiter W.J., Willemse P.H.B., Doorenbos H. Scintigraphy with 201 Tl for detection of thyroid cancer metastases. Eur J Nucl Med 1982; 7:515–7.
85. Brendel A.J., Guyot M., Jeandot R., Lefort G., Manciet G. Thallium-201 imaging in the follow-up of differentiated thyroid carcinoma. J Nucl Med 1988; 29:1515–20.
86. Hoefnagel C.A., Delprat C.C., Marcuse H.R., de Vijlder J.J. Role of thallium-201 total body scintigraphy in follow up of thyroid carcinoma. J Nucl Med 1986; 27:1854–57.
87. Van Sorge-Van Boxtel R.A., Van Eck-Smit B.L., Goslings B.M. Comparison of serum thyroglobulin, 131I and 201 Tl scintigraphy in the postoperative follow up of differentiated thyroid cancer. Nucl Med Commun 1993; 14:365–72.
88. Dadparvar S., Krishna L., Brady L.W., Slizofski W.J., Brown S.J., Chevres A., Micaily B. The role of iodine-131 and thallium -201 imaging and serum thyroglobulin in the management of differentiated thyroid carcinoma. Cancer 1993; 71:3767–73.
89. Charkes N.D., Vitti R.A., Brooks K. Thallium-201 SPECT increases detectability of thyroid cancer metastases. J Nucl Med 1990; 31:147–53.
90. Shiga T., Tsukamoto E., Nakada K., Morita K., Kato T., Mabuchi M., Yoshinaga K., Katoh C., Kuge Y., Tamaki N. Comparision of (18)F-FDG, 131I-Na, and 201Tl in diagnosis of recurrent or metastatic thyroid carcinoma. J Nucl Med 2001;42: 414–19.
91. Adalet I., Demirkale P., Unal S., Ouz H., Algol F., Cantez S. Disappointing results with Tc-99m tetrofosmin for detecting medullary thyroid carcinoma metastases comparison with Tc-99m VDMSA and Tl-201. Clin Nucl Med 1999; 24: 678–83.
92. Piwnica-Worms D., Chiu M.L., Budding M., Kronauge J.F., Kramer R.A., Croop J.M. Functional imaging of multidrug-resistant P-glycoprotein with an organotechnium complex. Cancer Res 1993; 53:977–84.
93. Seabold J., Gurll N., Schurrer M., Aktay R., Kirchner P.T. Comparison of 99mTc-methoxyisobutyl isonitrile and 201 Tl scintigraphy for detection of residual thyroid cancer after 131I ablative therapy. J Nucl Med 1999; 40:1434–40.
94. Ng D., Sundram F., Sin A. 99mTc-sestamibi and 131I whole-body scintigraphy and initial serum thyroglobulin in the management of differentiated thyroid carcinoma. J Nucl Med 2000; 41:631–5.
95. Miyamoto S., Kasagai K., Misaki T., Alam M.S., Konishi J. Evaluation of technetium-99m-MIBI in metastatic differentiated thyroid carcinoma J Nucl Med 1997; 38:352–6.
96. Rubello D., Mazzarotto R., Casara D. The role of technetium-99m methoxyisobutylisonitrile scintigraphy in the planning of therapy and follow-up of patients with differentiated thyroid carcinoma after surgery. Eur J Nucl Med 2000; 27:431–40.
97. Lind P., Gallowitsche H.J., Langsteger W., Kresnik E., Mikosh P., Gomez I. Technetium-99m-tetrafosmin whole body scintigrapy in the follow-up of differentiated thyroid carcinoma J Nucl Med 1997; 38:348–52.
98. Unal S. Menda Y., Adalet I., Boztepe H. et al. Thallium-201, technetium-99m-tetrofosmin and iodine-131 in detecting differentiated thyroid carcinoma metastases J Nucl Med 1998; 39:1897–1902.
99. Forsell-Aronsson E.B., Nilsson O., Bejegard S.A., Kolby L., Bernhardt P., Molne J., Hashemi S.H., Wangberg B., Tisell L.E., Ahlman H. 111 In-DTPA-D Phe1 octreotidebinding and somatostatin receptor subtype in thyroid tumors. J. Nucl Med 2000; 41:636–42.
100. Ain K.B., Taylor K.D., Tofiq S., Venkatamaran G. Somatostatin receptor subtypes expression in human thyroid and thyroid carcinoma cell lines. J Clin End Metab 1997; 82:1857–62.
101. Forsell-Aronsson E.B., Nilsson O., Benjegard S.A., Kölby L., Ahlman H. 111In-DTPA-D-Phel-octreotide binding and somatostatin receptor subtypes in thyroid tumors. J Nucl Med 1999; 41:636–42.
102. Haslinghuis L.M., Krenning E.P., De Herder W.W., Reijs A.E., Kwekkeboom D.J. Somatostatin receptor scintigraphy in the follow-up of patents with differentiated thyroid cancer J Endocrinol Invest 2001; 24:415–22.
103. Christian J.A., Cook G.J., Harmer C. Indium-111-labelled octreotide scintigraphy in the diagnosis and mangement of non-iodine avid metastatic carcinoma of the thyroid. Br J Cancer 2003; 89:258–61.
104. Stokkel M.P.M., Reigman H.I.E., Verkooyen R.B.P., Smit J.W.A. Indium −111-Octreotide scintigrapy in differentiated thyroid carcinoma metastases that do not respond to treatment with high-dose I-131 J Cancer Res Clin Oncol 2003; 129:287–94.

105. Waldherr C., Schumacher T., Pless M., Crazollara A., Maecke H.R., Nitzsche E.U., Haldemann A., Mueller Brand J. Radiopeptide transmitted internal irradiation of non-iodophil thyroid cancer and conventionally untreatable medullary thyroid cancer using. Nucl Med Commun 2001; 22:673–78.
106. Pacini F., Elisei R., Anelli S., Basolo F., Cola A., Pinchera A. Somatostatin in medullary thyroid cancer. In vitro and in vivo studies. Cancer 1989; 63:1189–95.
107. Dorr U., Wurstlin S., Frank-Raue K., Raue F., Hehrmann R., Iser G., Scholz M., Guhl L., Buhr H.J., Bihl H. Somatostatin receptor scintigraphy and magnetic resonance imaging in recurrent medullary thyroid carcinoma: a comparative study. Horm Metab Res (Suppl) 1993; 27:48–55.
108. Berna L., Chico A., Matias-Guiu X., Mato E. Catafau A., Alonso C., Mora J., Mauricio D., Rodriguez-Espinosa J., Mari C., Flotats A., Martin J.C., Estorch M., Carrio I. Use of somatostatin analogue scintigraphy in the localization of recurrent medullary thyroid carcinoma. Eur J Nucl Med 1998; 25:1482–88.
109. Frank-Raue K., Bihl H., Dorr U., Buhr H., Ziegler R., Raue F. Somatostatin receptor imaging in persistent medullary thyroid carcinoma Clin Endocrinol 1995; 42: 31–7.
110. Arslan N., Ilgan S., Yuksel E., Serdengecti M., Bulakbasi N., Ugur O., Ozguven M.A. Comparison of In-111 octreotide and Tc-99m (V) DMSA scintigraphy in the detection of medullary thyroid tumor foci in patients with elevated levels of tumor markers after surgery. Clin Nucl Med 2001; 26:683–8.
111. Sisson J.C., Frager M.S., Valk T.W., Gross M.D., Swanson D.P., Wieland D.M., Tobes M.C., Beierwaltes W.H., Thompson N.W. Scintigraphic localization of pheochromocytoma. N Eng J Med 1981; 305:12–7.
112. Jaquea Jr. S., Tobes M.C., Sisson J.C. Sodium dependency of uptake of norepinephrine and m-iodobenzylguanidine into cultured human pheochromocytoma cells: evidence for uptake –one. Cancer Res 1987; 47:3920–28.
113. Kimmig B.N. Radiotherapy for gastroenteropancreatic neuroendocrine tumors. Ann N Y Acad Sci 1994; 733:488–95.
114. Henry J.P., Gasnier B., Desnos C., Scherman D., Krejci E., Massoulie J. The catecholamine transporter of adrenal medulla chromaffin granules. Ann N Y Acad Sci 1994; 733:185–92.
115. Skowsky W.R., Wilf L.H. Iodine 131 metaiodobenzylguanidine scintigraphy of medullary carcinoma of the thyroid. South Med J 1991; 84:636–41.
116. Clarke S.E.M., Lazarus C.R., Wraight P., Sampson C., Maisey M.N. Pentavalent (99m-Tc) DMSA, (131-I) MIBG and (99m-Tc) MDP: an evaluation of three imaging techniques in patient with medullary carcinoma of the thyroid. J Nucl Med 1988; 29:33–8.
117. Clarke S.E.M. (131I)metaiodobenzylguanidine therapy in medullar thyroid cancer : Guy's Hospital experience. J Nucl Biol Med 1991; 35:323–6.
118. Chauhan P.S., Babbar A., Kashyap R., Prakash R. Evaluation of a DMSA kit for instant preparation of 99mTc-(V)-DMSA for tumour and metastases scintigraphy. Int J Rad Appl Instrum B 1992; 19: 825–30.
119. Guerra U.P., Pizzocara C., Terzi A. Giubbini R., Maira G., Pagliaini R., Bestagno M. New tracers for the imaging of the medullary thyroid carcinoma. Nucl Med Comm 1989; 10:285–89.
120. Verga V., Muratori F., Sacco G., Banfi F., Libroia A. The role of radiopharmaceuticals MIBG and (V) DMSA in the diagnosis of medullary thyroid carcinoma. H Ford Hosp Med J 1989; 37:175–77.
121. Behr T.M., Gratz S., Markus P.M., Dunn R.M., Hufner M., Schauer A., Fischer M., Munz D.L., Becker H., Becker W. Anti-carcinoembryonic antigen antibodies versus somatostatin analogs in the detection of metastatic medullary thyroid carcinoma: are carcinoembryonic antigen and somatostatin receptor expression prognostic factors? Cancer 1997; 80:2436–57.
122. Juweid M., Sharkey R.M., Behr T., Swayne L.C., Rubin A.D., Herskovic T., Hanley D., Markowitz A., Dunn R., Siegel. J., Kamal T., Goldenberg D.M. Improved detection of medullary thyroid cancer with radiolabeled antibodies to carcinoembryonic antigen. J Clin Oncol 1996; 14:1209–17.
123. Juweid M., Sharkey R.M., Swayne L.C., Goldenberg D.M. Improved selection of patients for reoperation for medullary thyroid cancer by imaging with radiolabeled anticarcinoembryonic antigen antibodies. Surgery 1997; 122:1156–65.
124. Barbet J., Peltier P., Bardet S., Vuillez J.P., Bachelot I. Denet S., Olivier P., Leccia F., Corcuff B., Huglo D., Proye C., Rouvier E., Meyer P., Chatal J.F. Radio immunodetection of medullary thyroid carcinoma using indium-111 bivalent hapten and anti CEA x anti-DTPA indium bispecific antibody. J Nucl Med 1998; 39:1172–78.

19. PAST, PRESENCE AND FUTURE OF THYROID-STIMULATING HORMONE (TSH) SUPERACTIVE ANALOGS

MARIUSZ W. SZKUDLINSKI

Trophogen, Inc., 6 Taft Court, Suite #150, Rockville, MD 20850, USA

INTRODUCTION

In recent years many new engineered protein therapeutics are being developed and tested in clinical trials (Marshall et al. 2003). Many early protein drugs showed limited applicability due to short half-life or low affinity to their receptors. Recombinant DNA technology permitted engineering protein molecules with specific chemical and biological characteristics. It is now anticipated that engineered hormone analogs will largely exceed clinical efficacy of existing products, including recombinant human TSH (rec-hTSH; Thyrogen^{TM}, Genzyme). Preclinical development of superactive TSH analogs can be divided into three phases: the TSH structure-function phase, the discovery phase and the optimization phase. It is apparent that detailed structure-function studies of TSH provided important foundation for rational modifications of human TSH molecule. This chapter describes the past, presence and future of superactive analogs of TSH with high receptor binding affinity. Such superactive analogs of TSH are expected to provide not only more efficacious diagnostic methods, but should also serve as indispensable tools in management of thyroid carcinomas with low TSH receptor number, impaired coupling and deficient ligand binding.

TSH STRUCTURE-FUNCTION

TSH is a key protein controlling thyroid function through its interaction with TSH receptor in thyroid. TSH is a member of glycoprotein hormone family produced by basophiles in the anterior pituitary (Pierce and Parsons 1981; Hearn and Gomme

2000). Human TSH is a heterodimer composed of two non-covalently linked subunits, α- and TSHβ-subunit. α-Subunit contains 92 amino acids and a sequence identical in all human glycoprotein hormones. TSHβ-subunit contains 118 amino acids and is unique for human TSH. The high-resolution structure of homologous to TSH human chorionic gonadotropin (hCG) has revealed that both subunits contain a central cystine-knot motif and three loops: two β-hairpin loops ($L1$ and $L3$) on one side of a cystine-knot and a long loop ($L2$) on the other (Lapthorn et al. 1994). The long loop in the α-subunit includes two-turn α-helix. The cystine-knot is made up of three central disulfide bonds, where one of the disulfide bonds threads through a ring formed by two other disulfide bonds. Similar to other glycoprotein hormones (LH, FSH and hCG), TSH hetero-dimers are stabilized by a unique segment of the β-subunit termed "seat-belt", because it wraps around the α-subunit. In light of the common α-subunit and 38% sequence identity between the hCGβ- and hTSHβ-subunit, homology modeling of hTSH was performed and showed expected similarities in the global conformation of these two hormones (Szkudlinski et al. 1996). Accordingly, assignment of disulfide bonds in bovine TSH β-subunit revealed bonding analogous to hCG (Fairlie et al. 1996). Thus, in hTSH β-subunit, three disulfide bonds (2–52, 27–83 and 31–85) form cystine-knot motif that determines the core structure, two disulfide bonds (19–105, 88–95) are involved in "seat-belt" formation and one (17–67) links two β-hairpin loops. Such structural features result in an increased interaction between two subunits and provide stability of heterodimer in physiological conditions.

Three carbohydrate chains constitute 15–25% of TSH molecular weight. The human α-subunit contains two carbohydrate chains linked to asparagine 52 and asparagine 78, and the human TSH β-subunit contains one carbohydrate chain attached at asparagine 23. Such asparagine-linked oligosaccharides are complex-type structures displaying notable hormone-, species-, source- and production-dependent differences in their core and terminal residues. Differences in oligosaccharide structure result in physiological heterogeneity of pituitary and recombinant TSH (Szkudlinski et al. 1993). It has been very well established that co-translational attachment of site-specific oligosaccharide chains is highly important in subunit folding, dimerization, TSH dimer secretion, stability, plasma half-life and bioactivity.

As reviewed previously, TSH contains several important domains that are tightly conserved among different species or homologous hormones (Grossmann et al. 1997, Szkudlinski et al. 2002). Even minor modifications of such domains result in decreased expression, impaired receptor binding and bioactivity. These domains located within a "composite binding domain" proposed by Lapthorn et al. (Lapthorn et al. 1994) include: α-helix (α40–46), αLys51, αAsn52, the α-carboxyl terminus (α 88–92), α33–38, "the Keutmann loop" (TSHβ31–52) and the "seat belt" in the β-subunit (TSHβ88–105) (Szkudlinski et al. 1996; Grossmann et al. 1997) (Figure 1). In addition to the stabilizing role of the "seat-belt", recent studies involving β-subunit chimeras have shown that this region is critical in conferring glycoprotein hormone specificity (Grossmann et al. 1997). Additional functionally critical residues have been identified

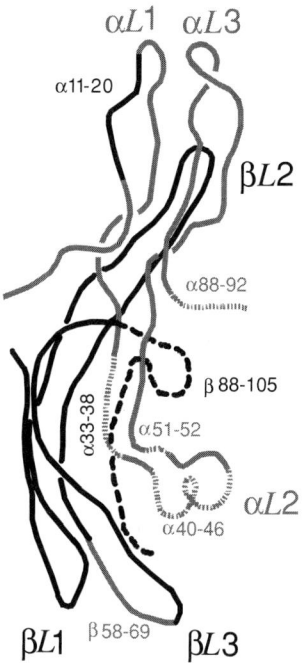

Figure 1. The schematic drawing of hTSH structure. For clarity the carbohydrate chains are not shown. The α-subunit backbone is shown as a gray line, the β-subunit chain as a black line. Important domains are marked directly within the line drawings. The peripheral β-hairpin loops are marked: αL1, αL3 in the α-subunit and βL1, βL3 in the β-subunit. Two long loops are αL2 with α-helical structure and βL2 or the "Keutmann loop."

by studies of patients with mutations in TSHβ subunit gene [see (Szkudlinski, et al. 2002)].

Several other domains involved in the modulation of TSH and gonadotropin function have been described in the last decade. Studies employing combination of alanine with proline scanning mutagenesis have revealed the importance of α-helical conformation (α40–46) in TSH bioactivity (Szkudlinski et al. 1996). Further, the 11–20 region in the α-subunit with a cluster of basic residues [(K-K/R–K—K/R); lysine(K), arginine (R)] present in all vertebrates except hominoids (apes and humans) has been recognized as an important motif in the evolution of TSH and gonadotropin bioactivity in primates (Szkudlinski et al. 1996; Szkudlinski et al. 2002). Selective elimination of basic residues in this domain of α-subunit resulted in a major decrease of receptor binding affinity and bioactivity of TSH in higher primates. Conversely, reconstitution of such basic motif resulted in a major increase in bioactivity of human TSH. It provided the first evidence that introduction of basic residues in selected sites in peripheral loops may permit design of a new class of TSH analogs (see below).

RECOMBINANT HUMAN TSH

Recombinant human TSH (rec-hTSH; Thyrogen®, Genzyme) has been produced in a large-scale bioreactor using Chinese hamster ovary (CHO) cells stably transfected with TSH genes (Cole et al. 1993). Since CHO cells, unlike the pituitary thyrotroph cells, have no capacity to add penultimate N-acetylgalactosamine or terminal sulfate, rec-hTSH is predominantly composed of oligosaccharide chains terminating in sialic acid. Rec-hTSH carbohydrate isoforms are similar to the sialylated forms of hTSH that are increased in primary hypothyroidism. Rec-hTSH has longer plasma half-life compared with normal pituitary hTSH. However, in several in vivo studies the bioactivity of rec-hTSH was found comparable to that of pituitary-derived hTSH (Cole et al. 1993; Szkudlinski et al. 1993; East-Palmer et al. 1995).

After cloning of human TSH beta gene (Wondisford et al. 1988) NIH researchers led by Bruce Weintraub initiated a collaborative research agreement with the Genzyme Corporation to produce and test rec-hTSH as a diagnostic agent to stimulate ^{131}I uptake in patients with differentiated thyroid carcinoma. An initial Phase I/II clinical trials showed that rec-hTSH is safe and efficacious in stimulating ^{131}I uptake and thyroglobulin secretion (Meier et al. 1994). Subsequent Phase III and confirmatory phase III trial with more than 100 patients indicated that rec-hTSH is almost as sensitive as conventional thyroid hormone withdrawal, but leads to considerable improvement of the quality of life because it avoids the symptoms of hypothyroidism (Ladenson et al. 1997). These major studies and case reports, including description of a patient with papillary thyroid carcinoma and hypopituitarism who had metastasis detected only after administration of rec-hTSH, exemplified the diagnostic potential of rec-hTSH (Ringel and Ladenson 1996). Thyrogen® has been approved by US FDA in 1998 for use in conducting thyroid scanning and thyroglobulin testing in the follow-up of patients with well differentiated thyroid carcinomas. Although many clinical studies demonstrated that the use of rec-hTSH is an effective strategy to increase ^{131}I uptake, rec-hTSH is considered not entirely equivalent to endogenous hTSH induction by thyroid hormone withdrawal (Utiger 1997; Robbins et al. 2002; Emerson and Torres 2003). Therefore, novel recombinant hTSH analogs with enhanced bioactivity may become long awaited component of improved follow-up, ablation of remnants and metastases in differentiated thyroid carcinoma.

DISCOVERY AND OPTIMIZATION OF SUPERACTIVE TSH ANALOGS

Protein engineering using recombinant DNA methods started in 1982, after the first results of oligonucleotide-directed mutagenesis had been published. Despite numerous site-directed mutagenesis studies, successful examples of engineering proteins with improved receptor binding affinity are quite rare. The first superactive analogs of hTSH with significant increases in receptor binding affinity, in vitro and in vivo bioactivity were constructed in 1994 (Table 1).

It was recognized previously that human TSH binding to TSH receptor is relatively a low-affinity interaction resulting in an extended 4–5 log unit competition curve for

Table 1. Chronology of superactive analog development and related projects

Year (Institution)	Achievements/Studies
1994 (NIH)	First TSH superactive analogs with single amino acid substitutions
1995 (NIH)	Superactive analogs with combined substitutions in TSH and hCG
1996 (NIH)	Initial superactive analogs of LH and FSH
1996 (NIH)	Biological activity of modified free-alpha subunit
1996–1998 (UMBI)	Rescuing "loss of function" mutations
1996–2001 (UMBI)	Studies on the mechanism of TSH receptor activation

TSH binding, with IC_{50} in high nanomolar range. However, Scatchard transformation of the equilibrium binding data produced a two-component curve which translates into a high and low affinity binding site, cellular bioassays always required low ionic strength buffer to achieve adequate sensitivity and reliability (Willey 1999). Although reasons for relatively low affinity of human TSH-TSH receptor interaction were not completely understood (Rommerts et al. 1992), in order to circumvent low affinity of human TSH all bindings studies were performed using ^{125}I-labeled bovine TSH. Interestingly, bovine and rat TSH were previously found 10–100 fold more potent than human TSH and such differences were observed at human and rodent TSH receptors, both in vitro and in vivo (Rapoport and Seto, 1985; East-Palmer et al. 1995). Thus, TSH from rodents was considered more bioactive than human TSH, but the exact mechanism of such differences were unknown. Some investigators attributed differences to variable purity, carbohydrate structures or other posttranslational modifications of pituitary TSH preparations.

Our studies on the role of carbohydrate residues in TSH bioactivity performed at NIH from 1990 to 1993 indicated that species- or production-dependent variability of TSH carbohydrate residues could not provide adequate explanation for observed differences in bioactivity between human TSH and TSH from various non-primate species (Szkudlinski et al. 1993). While exploring the role of carbohydrate residues by using subunit hybrids we observed that [(bovine alpha) – (human TSH beta)] heterodimer is at least 10-fold more bioactive in vitro that human TSH or [(human alpha—bovine TSH beta)] heterodimer (Szkudlinski, Thotakura - unpublished data). These and other studies led Szkudlinski et al. in 1994 to substitute various amino acids in human alpha subunit according to the amino acid sequence of the bovine alpha subunit. After the first three "gain of activity" mutations were identified (Q13K, P16K, Q20K) more detailed sequence alignments, homology modeling and sequencing of subunit genes in various species, including primates, were performed. This resulted in an identification of additional targets within the sequence of both subunits including residue 14 in the alpha and 69 in the TSH beta subunit. Further development included combination of single mutations, alternative substitutions with arginines or histidines as well as studies on cooperative effects of different substitutions. hTSH with quadruple mutations in the α-subunit (Q13K+E14K+P16K+Q20K) and an additional replacement in the hTSHβ-subunit (L69R) showed 95-fold higher potency and more than

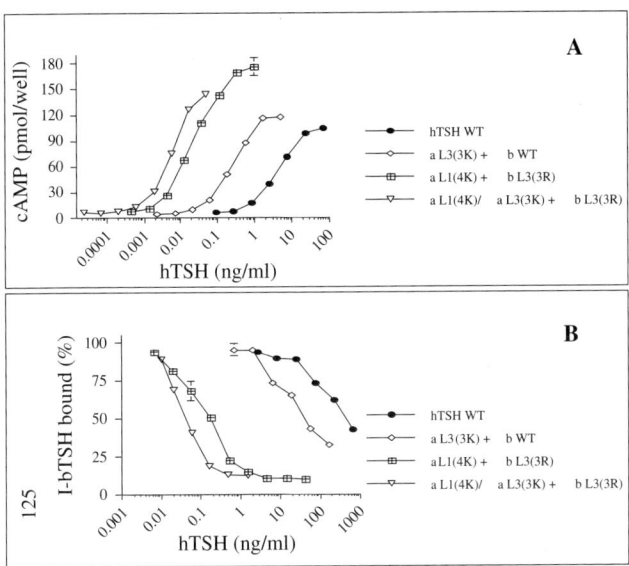

Figure 2. Superactive Analogs of TSH. Reprinted from Leitolf et al. (Leitolf et al. 2000). Gradual increase in the in vitro bioactivity (A) and receptor binding (B) for mutants with one, two and three engineered peripheral loops. Combination of the αL3 loop analog with our previously optimized αL1-βL3 loop combination (Grossmann, et al. 1998) results in a further gain of hormone potency.

1.5-fold increase in efficacy compared to the *in vitro* bioactivity of the wild-type hormone (Szkudlinski et al. 1996). Moreover, the combination of these 4 mutations in the α-subunit with 3 mutations in the β-subunit (I58R+E63R+L69R) resulted in an analog with greater than 1000-fold increase in receptor binding and in vitro bioactivity and 100-fold increase in the in vivo activity (Grossmann et al. 1998). Subsequently seven new site-specific "gain-of-activity" mutations were identified. Four in the αL3 loop (S64K, N64K, G73K, A81K) and three in the βL1 loop (Leitolf et al. 2000) (Figure 2). TSH analogs with optimized combinations of these substitutions are significantly more potent and efficacious than any known species of TSH and hold great promise as a second generation therapeutic forms of recombinant TSH. The relative increase in potency and efficacy (Vmax) of superactive analogs in comparison to the unmodified hormone are assay system dependent as illustrated in Figure 3. Because of the specious argument that increasing dose of the unmodified hormone should result in comparable to analog maximal effect, it is important to emphasize that such possibility is limited to extremely sensitive (rarely physiological) systems with high receptor number and/or highly efficient coupling.

MECHANISM OF ENHANCED BIOACTIVITY OF TSH ANALOGS

A long-standing postulate held that charge-charge interactions are of major importance in the interaction between TSH and TSH receptor (Rees Smith et al. 1988). Similar

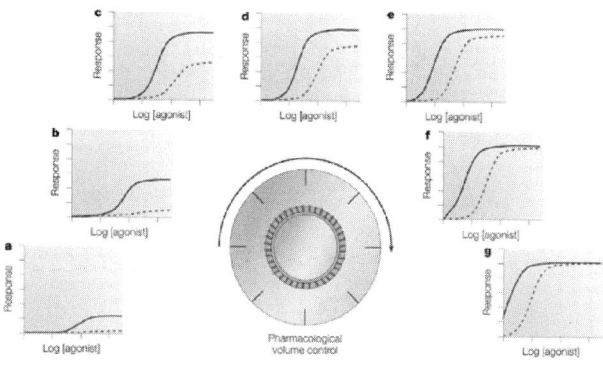

Figure 3. Schematic of a range of dose-response curves to two agonists (Kenakin 2003). Various degree of difference in potency and efficacy (Vmax) is dependent on assays sensitivity determined by coupling efficiency and receptor number. In poorly coupled systems (assay **a**), the lower-efficacy agonist (dotted line) shows almost no response. In intermediate-sensitivity assays (**b–d**), both are partial agonists, whereas in high-sensitivity assays (**f** and **g**) both are full agonists.

interactions between additional basic residues in TSH superactive analogs and specific acidic residues in the receptor, yet to be fully characterized, are likely involved in prolonged dissociation rates and enhanced receptor activation and signaling.

Largely unpublished studies indicated that new TSH superactive analogs are receptor specific and inactive at related LH and FSH receptors; analog concentrations up to 1000 fold higher than activating TSH receptors did not result in detectable stimulation. TSH analogs showed their enhanced activity at the TSH receptor from different species (i.e. human, rat, mouse), suggesting that various changes described during mammalian evolution of TSH receptor (Kaczur et al. 2003) are probably not involved in the phenomenon of analog "superactivity." In addition, an enhanced in vitro activity of TSH analogs was observed in normal media and in buffers with various salt concentrations. The effect of substitutions on the TSH in vitro bioactivity was in most cases highly correlated with their effect on receptor binding affinity. TSH superactive analogs are also more potent than standard rec-hTSH stimulators of inositol phosphate pathway. The difference in bioactivity between TSH analogs and wile-type hormone was demonstrated using cells with TSH receptor and largely depleted pool of the negatively charged cell surface proteoglycans. This further indicated that the mechanism of enhanced activity is not dependent on their interaction with heparan sulfate proteoglycans recognizing various motifs of basic residues (Cardin and Weintraub 1989; Bozon et al. 1998).

Although the exact mechanism of interaction of TSH analogs with TSH receptor has not yet been fully clarified specific interaction modes of TSH analogs with TSH receptor have been discovered. Our initial model of TSH-TSH receptor interaction was generally supported by "charge-reversal mutagenesis" and other approaches (Grossmann et al. 1997; Costagliola et al. 2002; Smits et al. 2003)) (Figure 4).

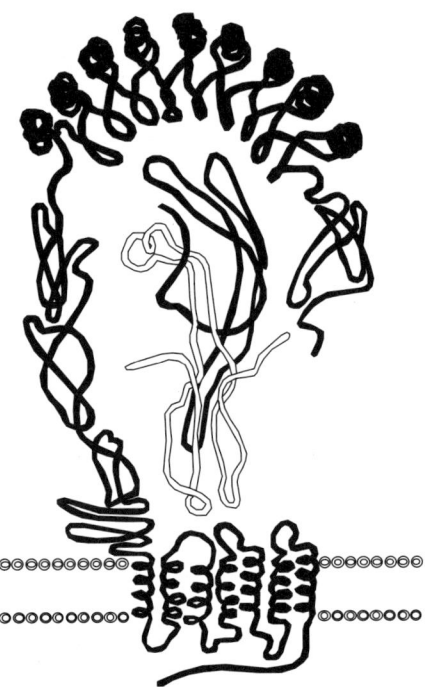

Figure 4. Schematic configuration of TSH-TSHR complex. Two parallel β-hairpin loops of the α-subunit (αL1, αL3) are located in the lower part of the model and may participate in the interaction with C-terminal portion of extracellular domain and the extracellular loops of the receptor transmembrane domain. Two loops of the β-subunit (βL1, βL3) are shown in the upper part with proposed binding site within the concave of leucine rich-repeats modeled by Kajava et al (Kajava et al. 1995).

Analogous amino acid substitutions in the α-subunit were also performed in hCG, LH and FSH. Although significant increases in respective gonadotropin affinities for their cognate receptors were observed, in contrast to TSH analogs, differences were smaller for both single and combined substitutions (Szkudlinski et al. 1996). Consequently the effects of single mutations were more difficult to detect and only selected combinations were later confirmed at various laboratories (Heikoop et al 1999).

FUTURE PERSPECTIVES OF TSH ANALOGS

The opportunities and challenges facing clinical development of rec-hTSH analogs are now being realized more clearly. Thyrogen® (wild-type recombinant human TSH) produced in Chinese hamster ovary cells exhibits relatively low affinity to the TSH receptor that translates into limited clinical efficacy. Despite quite apparent advantages of TSH superactive analogs, further development and clinical trails of such analogs are now dependent on commitment of biotech industry for a relatively small "thyroid market" (Table 2).

Table 2. Potential uses of superactive analogs of TSH

Clinical	Differentiated thyroid cancer follow-up (TSH analog stimulated thyroglobulin testing and radioiodine scanning)
	Differentiated thyroid cancer treatment (TSH analog induced radioiodine ablation)
	Large euthyroid goiter treatment (TSH analog induced radioiodine ablation)
	TSH analog stimulation tests (testing thyroid reserve, identifying "warm" thyroid nodules, detecting thyroid hemiagenesis, etc.)
	Management of patients with TSH receptor mutations associated with low ligand binding, impaired receptor expression or coupling
	TSH receptor-mediated delivery of therapeutic agents to the thyroid cancer cell (Figure 5)
Laboratory	^{125}I-hTSH analog in TSH binding inhibition (TBI) assay for autoantibodies to the TSH receptor (Kakinuma et al. 1997) and immunoassays (Ribela et al. 1996)
	TSH analog-stimulated thyroglobulin (Tg) mRNA testing in thyroid cancer patients with positive or negative anti-Tg antibodies
Basic Science	Structure-function studies of TSH-TSH receptor interaction, studies of TSH receptors in non-thyroidal tissue (Szkudlinski et al. 2002)

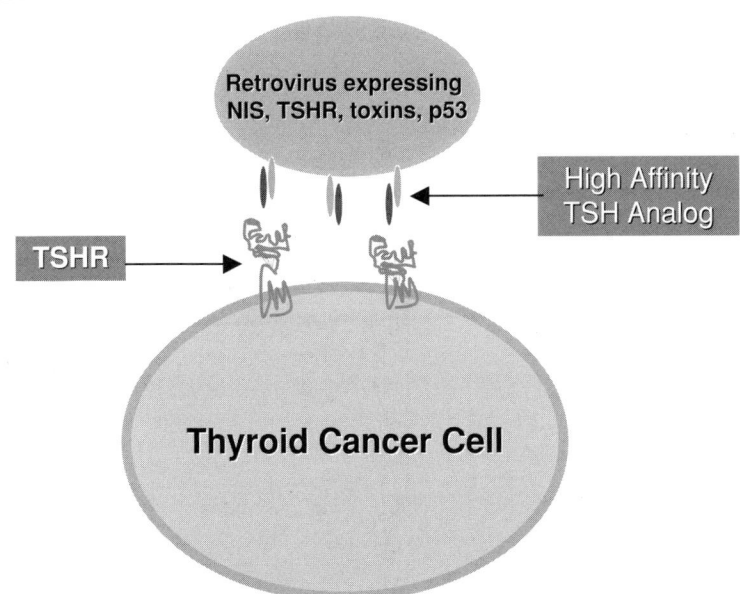

Figure 5. TSH receptor-mediated delivery of various therapeutic agents to the thyroid cancer cell. One of many possible scenarios includes restoration of cancer cell differentiation using high affinity interaction between TSH analog and largely depleted pool of TSH receptors. Another approach involves TSH analog-mediated targeted killing of thyrocyte originated carcinomas. TSHR, TSH receptor, NIS, sodium iodide symporter.

Since structural data on TSH receptor and other G protein-coupled receptors (GPCRs) are very limited, designing small molecules binding to TSH receptor that do not bind to non-targeted receptors poses a major problem. Although GPCR microarrays may narrow the number of useful agonistic compounds it is not clear if selected small molecule can be devoid of aberrant binding to other receptors that can lead to serious side effects (Fang et al. 2003). Therefore, TSH and TSH receptor structure based analogs appear far more promising. Recent studies on the mechanism of TSH receptor activation and their constitutive activity provide additional leads for the design of high affinity antagonist and inverse agonists (Gudermann et al. 1996; Zhang et al. 2000; Wonerow et al. 2001; Rodien et al. 2003).

Interestingly, another member of glycoprotein hormone family—thyrostimulin was recently identified by comparative genomic analysis (Hsu et al. 2002) and shown to be capable of activating TSH receptor (Nakabayashi et al. 2002). Structure-function studies of thyrostimulin and its analogs should provide new insights into mechanism of TSH receptor activation. Although, the intrinsic bioactivity of highly purified thyrostimulin should be studied in more details, it is possible that third or fourth generation TSH analogs will include TSH-thyrostimulin chimeras with their respective superactive components.

Current research, development pipelines and clinical trials in progress clearly suggest that the decade of recombinant proteins with a native amino acid sequence is coming to an end. The pharmaceutical industry and biotechnology companies are increasingly exploring new types of engineered proteins including superactive hormones. Diagnostic and therapeutic use of such engineered hormones with improved characteristics, tailored to specific patient needs (long and short acting variants) should represent an important milestone in medicine of 21st century.

ACKNOWLEDGEMENTS

I thank to Dr. Bruce Weintraub for continuous support, inspiration, enthusiasm and guidance. Drs. Rao Thotakura, Ines Bucci, Lata Joshi, Mathis Grossmann, Holger Leitolf, Meng Zhang and Valerie Fremont are acknowledged for their unique contributions, help and friendship.

REFERENCES

1. Bozon V., Pajot-Augy E., Vignon, X., Salesse, R. (1998). "Endocytosis of lutropin by Leydig cells through a pathway distinct from the high-affinity receptor." *Mol Cell Endocrinol 143: 33–42*.
2. Cardin, A. D., Weintraub H.J. (1989). "Molecular modeling of protein-glycosaminoglycan interactions." *Arteriosclerosis 9: 21–32*.
3. Cole, E.S., K. Lee, Lauziere, K., Kelton, C., Chappel, S., Weintraub, B., Ferrara, D., Peterson, P., Bernasconi, R., Edmunds, T. et al. (1993). "Recombinant human thyroid stimulating hormone: development of a biotechnology product for detection of metastatic lesions of thyroid carcinoma." *Biotechnology (N Y) 11: 1014–24*.
4. Costagliola, S., Panneels, V., Bonomi, M., Koch, J., Many, M. C., Smits, G., Vassart, G. (2002). "Tyrosine sulfation is required for agonist recognition by glycoprotein hormone receptors." *Embo J 21(4): 504–13*.
5. East-Palmer, J., Szkudlinski M.W., Lee, J., Thotakura, N. R., Weintraub, B. D. (1995). "A novel, nonradioactive in vivo bioassay of thyrotropin (TSH)." *Thyroid 5: 55–9*.
6. Emerson, C.H., Torres M.S. (2003). "Recombinant human thyroid-stimulating hormone: pharmacology, clinical applications and potential uses." *BioDrugs 17: 19–38*.
7. Fairlie, W. D., Stanton, P.G., Hearn M.T. (1996). "The disulphide bond structure of thyroid-stimulating hormone beta-subunit." *Biochem J 314: 449–55*.
8. Fang, Y., Lahiri, J., Picard L. (2003). "G protein-coupled receptor microarrays for drug discovery." *Drug Discov Today 8: 755–61*.

9. Grossmann, M., Szkudlinski, M. W., Wong, R., Dias, J. A., Ji, T. H., Weintraub, B. D. (1997). "Substitution of the seat-belt region of the thyrotropin (TSH)-ß subunit with the corresponding regions of choriogonadotropin or follitropin confers luteotropic, but not follitropic activity to chimeric TSH." J Biol Chem 272: 15532–15540.
10. Grossmann, M., Weintraub, B.D., Szkudlinski, M.W. (1997). "Novel insights into the molecular mechanisms of human thyrotropin action: structural, physiological and therapeutic implications for the glycoprotein hormone family." Endocr Rev 18: 476–501.
11. Grossmann, M., Leitolf, H., Weintraub, B.D., Szkudlinski, M.W. (1998). "A rational design strategy for protein hormone superagonists." Nature Biotechnol 16: 871–5.
12. Gudermann, T., Kalkbrenner F., Schultz, G. (1996). "Diversity and selectivity of receptor-G protein interaction." Annu Rev Pharmacol Toxicol 36: 429–59.
13. Hearn, M. T. and P. T. Gomme (2000). "Molecular architecture and biorecognition processes of the cystine knot protein superfamily: part I. The glycoprotein hormones." J Mol Recognit 13: 223–78.
14. Heikoop, J. C., Huisman-de Winkel, B., Grootenhuis, P.D. (1999). "Towards minimized gonadotropins with full bioactivity." Eur J Biochem 261: 81–4.
15. Hsu, S. Y., Nakabayashi,K., Bhalla, A. (2002). "Evolution of glycoprotein hormone subunit genes in bilateral metazoa: identification of two novel human glycoprotein hormone subunit family genes, GPA2 and GPB5." Mol Endocrinol 16: 1538–51.
16. Kaczur, V., Puskas, L. G. Takacs, M., Racz, I. A., Szendroi, A., Toth, S., Nagy, Z., Szalai, C., Balazs, C, Falus, A., Knudsen, B., Farid, N. R. (2003). "Evolution of the thyrotropin receptor: a G protein coupled receptor with an intrinsic capacity to dimerize." Mol Genet Metab 78: 275–90.
17. Kajava, A. V., Vassart, G., Wodak, S.J. (1995). "Modeling of the three-dimensional structure of proteins with the typical leucine-rich repeats." Structure 3: 867–77.
18. Kakinuma, A., Chazenbalk, G. D., Jaume, J. C., Rapoport, B., McLachlan, S. M. (1997). "The human thyrotropin (TSH) receptor in a TSH binding inhibition assay for TSH receptor autoantibodies." J Clin Endocrinol Metab 82: 2129–34.
19. Kenakin, T. (2003). "Predicting therapeutic value in the lead optimization phase of drug discovery." Nat Rev Drug Discov 2: 429–38.
20. Ladenson, P. W., Braverman, L.E., Mazzaferri, E., Brucker-Davis, F., Cooper, D.S., Garber, J.R., Wondisford, F.E., Davies, T.F., DeGroot, L.J., Daniels, G.H., Ross, D.S., Weintraub, B.D. (1997). "Comparison of administration of recombinant human thyrotropin with withdrawal of thyroid hormone for radioactive iodine scanning in patients with thyroid carcinoma." N Engl J Med 337: 888–930.
21. Lapthorn, A. J., Harris, D. C., Littlejohn, A., Lustbader, J. W., Canfield, R. E., Machin, K. J., Morgan, F. J., Isaacs, N. W. (1994). "Crystal structure of human chorionic gonadotropin" Nature 369: 455–61.
22. Leitolf, H., Tong, K. P., Grossmann, M., Weintraub, B. D., Szkudlinski, M. W. (2000). "Bioengineering of human thyrotropin superactive analogs by site-directed "lysine-scanning" mutagenesis. Cooperative effects between peripheral loops." J Biol Chem 275: 27457–65.
23. Marshall, S. A., Lazar, G. A., Chirino, A. J., Desjarlais, J. R. (2003). "Rational design and engineering of therapeutic proteins." Drug Discov Today 8: 212–21.
24. Meier, C. A., Braverman, L. E., Ebner, S. A., Veronikis, I., Daniels, G. H., Ross, D. S., Deraska, D. J., Davies, T. F., Valentine, M., DeGroot, L. J. et al., (1994). "Diagnostic use of recombinant human thyrotropin in patients with thyroid carcinoma (phase I/II study)." J Clin Endocrinol Metab 78: 188–96.
25. Nakabayashi, K., Matsumi, H., Bhalla, A., Bae, J., Mosselman, S., Hsu, S. Y., Hsueh, A. J. (2002). "Thyrostimulin, a heterodimer of two new human glycoprotein hormone subunits, activates the thyroid-stimulating hormone receptor." J Clin Invest 109: 1445–52.
26. Pierce, J. G. and Parsons T.F. (1981). "Glycoprotein hormones: structure and function." Annu Rev Biochem 50: 465–95.
27. Rapoport B, Seto, P. (1985). "Bovine thyrotropin has a specific bioactivity 5- to 10-fold that of previous estimates for highly purified hormone." Endocrinology 116: 1379–82.
28. Rees Smith B., McLachlan S.M., Furmaniak J. (1988) Autoantibodies to the TSH receptor. Endocr Rev 9: 106–121
29. Ribela, M. T., Bianco, A.C., Bartolini, P. (1996). "The use of recombinant human thyrotropin produced by Chinese hamster ovary cells for the preparation of immunoassay reagents." J Clin Endocrinol Metab 81: 249–56.
30. Ringel, M. D., Ladenson P.W. (1996). "Diagnostic accuracy of 131I Scanning with recombinant human thyrotropin versus thyroid hormone withdrawal in a patient with metastatic thyroid carcinoma and hypothyroidism." J Clin Endocrinol Metab 81: 1724–1725.

31. Robbins, R. J., Larson, S. M., Sinha, N., Shaha, A., Divgi, C., Pentlow, K. S., Ghossein, R., Tuttle, R. M. (2002). "A retrospective review of the effectiveness of recombinant human TSH as a preparation for radioiodine thyroid remnant ablation." *J Nucl Med 43: 1482–8*.
32. Rodien, P., Ho, S. C., Vlaeminck, V., Vassart, G., Costagliola, S. (2003). "Activating mutations of TSH receptor." *Ann Endocrinol (Paris) 64: 12–6*.
33. Rommerts, F. F., van Loenen, H.J., Schipper, I., Fauser, B.C. (1992). "FSH-receptor interactions and signal transduction: an alternative view." *in* "Follicle Stimulating Hormone: Regulation of Secretion and Molecular Mechanisms of Action." The Proceedings of the Symposium On Regulation and Actions of Follicle Stimulating Hormone, October 25–28, 1990, Evanston, Illinois. *Edited by M. Hunzicker-Dunn and N. B. Schwartz. Norwell, MA, Serono Symposia, USA: 61–81*.
34. Smits, G., Campillo, M., Govaerts, C., Janssens, V., Richter, C., Vassart, G., Pardo, L. Costagliola, S. (2003). "Glycoprotein hormone receptors: determinants in leucine-rich repeats responsible for ligand specificity." *Embo J 22: 2692–703*.
35. Szkudlinski, M. W., Thotakura, N. R., Bucci, I., Joshi, L. R., Tsai, A., East-Palmer, J., Shiloach, J., Weintraub, B. D. (1993). "Purification and characterization of recombinant human thyrotropin (TSH) isoforms produced by Chinese hamster ovary cells: the role of sialylation and sulfation in TSH bioactivity." *Endocrinology 133: 1490–503*.
36. Szkudlinski, M. W., Teh, N.G., Grossmann, M., Tropea, J.E., Weintraub, B.D. (1996). "Engineering human glycoprotein hormone superactive analogues." *Nature Biotechnol 14: 1257–63*.
37. Szkudlinski, M. W., Grossmann, M., Weintraub, B.D. (1996). "Structure-function studies of human TSH: new advances in the design of glycoprotein hormone analogs." *Trends Endocrinol Metab 7: 277–286*.
38. Szkudlinski, M., Teh, N.G., Grossmann, M., Tropea, J.E., Witta, J., Weintraub, B.D. (1996). "Role of the 40–51 region of the alpha-subunit in the bioactivity of human thyrotropin and gonadotropins: Implications for the design of new hormone analogs based on simultaneous mutagenesis of multiple domains." *10th International Congress of Endocrinology, San Francisco, CA, June 12–15th, 1996 (Abstract #OR1-4)*.
39. Szkudlinski, M. W., Fremont, V., Ronin, C., Weintraub, B.D. (2002). "Thyroid-stimulating hormone and thyroid-stimulating hormone receptor structure-function relationships." *Physiol Rev 82: 473–502*.
40. Utiger, R. D. (1997). "Follow-up of patients with thyroid carcinoma." *N Engl J Med 337: 928–30*.
41. Willey, K. P. (1999). "An elusive role for glycosylation in the structure and function of reproductive hormones." *Hum Reprod Update 5: 330–55*.
42. Wondisford, F. E., Usala, S. J., DeCherney, G. S., Castren, M., Radovick, S., Gyves, P. W., Trempe, J. P., Kerfoot, B. P., Nikodem, V. M., Carter, B. J. et al., (1988). "Cloning of the human thyrotropin beta-subunit gene and transient expression of biologically active human thyrotropin after gene transfection." *Mol Endocrinol 2: 32–9*.
43. Wonerow, P., Neumann, S., Gudermann, T., Paschke, R. (2001). "Thyrotropin receptor mutations as a tool to understand thyrotropin receptor action." *J Mol Med 79: 707–21*.
44. Zhang, M., Tong, K. P., Fremont, V., Chen, J., Narayan, P., Puett, D., Weintraub, B. D., Szkudlinski, M. W. (2000). "The extracellular domain suppresses constitutive activity of the transmembrane domain of the human TSH receptor: implications for hormone-receptor interaction and antagonist design." *Endocrinology 141: 3514–7*.

20. PATHOBIOLOGY OF ANTINEOPLASTIC THERAPY IN UNDIFFERENTIATED THYROID CANCER

KENNETH B. AIN, M.D.

Professor of Medicine; Director, Thyroid Oncology Program, Division of Hematology & Oncology, Department of Internal Medicine, University of Kentucky, Lexington, KY 40536

and

Director, Thyroid Cancer Research Laboratory, Veterans Affairs Medical Center, Lexington, KY 40511

INTRODUCTION

Undifferentiated thyroid carcinoma is a descriptive term often applied to the rare subset of thyroid cancers classified as anaplastic; however, there is a broad spectrum of tumors which show varying degrees of differentiated function and clinical aggressiveness. Among thyroid carcinomas derived from the thyroid follicular cell, differentiated functions include: expression and membrane localization of the sodium/iodide symporter (NIS; enabling intracellular concentration of iodide), expression of thyrotropin receptors (permitting both stimulation of the cell by rising thyrotropin levels and suppression of the cell by decreasing thyrotropin levels), organification of internalized iodide (enhancing iodide retention), and production of thyroglobulin (clinically useful as a specific tumor marker in thyroidectomized patients). Additional clinical features common to differentiated thyroid cancers include: a slow growth rate, limited metastatic potential (usually only local lymphatic spread in the majority of cases), and the ability of the host to tolerate a significant tumor burden for extraordinary lengths of time. As each of these functional features are lost and clinical aggressiveness is enhanced, therapeutic options decrease while, at the same time, the clinical situation becomes more desperate (1). This is epitomized by anaplastic carcinomas with median survival measured in months despite the most assertive therapeutic efforts (2, 3).

Although fewer than 400 cases of anaplastic thyroid carcinoma are expected in North America in a year, many-fold more patients will manifest poorly differentiated metastatic thyroid cancers with sufficient loss of differentiated function to make classical treatments (surgery, radioiodine, and thyroid hormone suppression of thyrotropin) ineffectual. Also, disseminated medullary thyroid carcinomas and rare histologies, such as mucoepidermoid carcinomas and angiosarcomas, have no known effective systemic therapies and are usually lethal. Patients with these tumors need active antineoplastic agents that can evoke better outcomes without intolerable morbidity. To that end, it is necessary to critically review the clinical experience with current antineoplastic agents, address known mechanisms for resistance to these agents, and consider alternative therapeutic approaches to systemic therapy.

SYSTEMIC CHEMOTHERAPEUTICS, BY CLASS OF AGENT

Antimetabolites

Antimetabolites encompass compounds that have sufficient structural similarity to naturally occurring intermediates critical to the synthesis of key molecules, such as RNA and DNA, as to interfere with normal metabolism and take advantage of metabolic differences between normal and malignant cells for therapeutic specificity. Although most antimetabolite chemotherapeutic agents are nucleoside analogs, interfering with nucleic acid synthesis, some may also interfere with other critical cellular processes, such as glycosylation, organelle activities, or phospholipid synthesis. These drugs have proven most useful in hematological malignancies. Pyrimidine analogs, hindering the synthesis of cytidine, thymidine, or uridine, include the fluoropyrimidines (notably 5-fluorouracil) and cytidine analogs (cytarabine and gemcitabine). There is some preclinical single agent activity with these compounds in anaplastic thyroid carcinomas, but somewhat greater promise for their contribution to combination chemotherapy. Purine analogs, interfering with adenosine and guanosine synthesis, include the thiopurines (6-mercaptopurine and 6-thioguanine) and the adenosine analogs (fludarabine, pentostatin, and cladribine); however, these agents have not proven useful in solid tumors. Methotrexate is the most clinically useful antifolate compound, although agents such as raltitrexed (ZD1694) and edatrexate have been showing promise. These agents inhibit dihydrofolate reductase, depleting cells of reduced folates and resulting in decreased purines, thymidylate, amino acids (methionine and serine), and effects on gene methylation (4, 5).

Among the pyrimidine analogs, the only agent with any clinical experience in thyroid carcinoma is 5-fluorouracil. In all cases, it was used as part of a drug combination, with dacarbazine in advanced medullary thyroid carcinoma for modest partial responses in three of five patients (6), in combination with many drugs for a rare partial response in anaplastic carcinoma patients (7), and with three other agents in 49 patients with poorly-differentiated non-anaplastic thyroid cancers resulting in negligible clinical activity (8). This poor effect was presaged in preclinical studies using poorly differentiated or anaplastic thyroid cancer cell lines (9), although concomitant Bcl-2 antisense nucleotides (10), but not radioiodine (11), seem to enhance antineoplastic effects. Initial anaplastic thyroid cancer monolayer studies with gemcitabine were promising (12, 13) but were not followed by confirmatory reports using xenograft model systems, suggesting this agent to be less impressive than originally suggested. These deficiencies may be remedied by using a novel multimeric gemcitabine preparation (14); however, confirmatory studies have not been published for at least three years. Likewise, an early cell culture study using (E)-2′-fluoromethylene-2′-deoxycytidine (MDL-101,731) in anaplastic cells (15) has no documented follow-up. Methotrexate is not usually considered to have clinically useful activity, although two clinical reports of its benefit in anaplastic thyroid cancer were made up to thirty years ago (16, 17). Unique cell lines may exhibit monolayer inhibition (18) but antifolate therapy is not usually considered useful for these tumors, even in combination therapy.

Alkylating agents

The first alkylating agent was the nitrogen mustard mechlorethamine, based on serendipitous observations made on sulfur mustard gas used in World War I. This class of drugs encompasses a wide range of structures with a common endpoint of forming covalent adducts on cellular DNA (5). Many of these agents differ sufficiently in their properties as to prove useful in combination with other agents of the same class. They are generally considered to be cell cycle phase non-specific, although the more rapidly proliferating cells are most sensitive. The group of nitrogen mustards, besides mechlorethamine, includes cyclophosphamide, melphalan, chlorambucil, and ifosfamide. Although a preclinical xenograft study suggested single agent cyclophosphamide to have significant activity against ATC (19), this has not been seen in clinical trials (8, 20), despite rare activity in combination with 5-fluorouracil and bleomycin (21, 22). Nitrosoureas comprise another group within this class, including BCNU (carmustine), CCNU (lomustine), MeCCNU (semustine), and streptozotocin. As with the nitrogen mustards, these agents are not useful in ATC as single agents and have only rare partial responses in combination with multiple additional chemotherapeutic drugs (23, 24). The next group of alkylating agents, the aziridines, includes triethylenemelamine, thio-tepa, mitomycin C, hexamethylmelamine, and diaziquone, as well as the related compounds, procarbazine, dacarbazine (DTIC), and temozolomide. This group is notable for the absence of published information regarding activity of these compounds in any thyroid cancer, aside from dacarbazine for medullary carcinomas. The remaining agents are classified as alkyl sulfphonates and consist of busulfan and treosulfan, neither of which is associated with treatment of thyroid cancers.

Platinum-based agents

Cisplatin has been in clinical use as an antitumor agent for over 30 years. Although the precise mechanistic pathways of activity are still unclear, the primary target is DNA. This agent has proven effective in a number of solid tumors, particularly in combination with other agents. Additional analogs include carboplatin and oxaliplatin, as well as other drugs in development. There is some evidence that failure of expression of wild-type p53, a tumor suppressor gene usually mutated or not-expressed in poorly-differentiated thyroid cancers, results in resistance to cisplatin therapy (25, 26). This may be part of the explanation for the absence of significant benefit of monotherapy with this class of agents in anaplastic thyroid carcinomas. Cell culture studies show minimal antineoplastic activity in ATC cell lines, except for sequential application after gemcitabine (13). One veterinary study of cisplatin monotherapy for canine thyroid cancer suggested reasonable antineoplastic activity (27); however, translation of this to human disease is problematic. Consequently, most clinical application of platinum-based agents for ATC involve combination therapy, most often with doxorubicin-related drugs (24, 28–31). One possible factor affecting tumor sensitivity may relate to proliferation rate, possibly accounting for increased responsiveness of poorly differentiated thyroid cancers when patients were mildly hypothyroid causing thyrotropin stimulation of tumors (32). However, few solid tumors proliferate as rapidly as ATC and tumor dedifferentiation often results in loss of thyrotropin-dependent growth control. Although overall response was low, one study suggests enhanced response of advanced thyroid cancers to the combination of cisplatin with doxorubicin compared with doxorubicin monotherapy (31). Newer modes of delivery, using liposomal platinum complexes, will need to be assessed in clinical trials, since it may be that drug delivery and distribution problems underlie the failure to achieve significant levels of clinical response.

Topoisomerase inhibitors

Topoisomerases are critical nuclear enzymes that cut DNA strands, permitting adjustment of their topological structure during transcription, replication and recombination. Single DNA strands are cut by topoisomerase I and double strand cuts are made by alpha and beta isotypes of topoisomerase II. Inhibition of these enzymes leads to cellular death. Antitumor drugs, which inhibit one or more topoisomerase types, are among the most useful clinical agents.

There are three groups of topoisomerase II inhibitors, arranged by mechanism of activity (4). Group 1 consists of DNA intercalating compounds (anthracyclines, amsacrines, and ellipticines) that stabilize the cleavable complex of cut DNA strands but prevent religation. Group 2 agents do the same, without intercalating into DNA (epipodophyllotoxins), while group 3 compounds inhibit topoisomerase II activity, but do not intercalate into DNA nor stabilize the cleavable complex (including: dioxopiperazine, mebarone, and suramin). Generally, the level of topoisomerase II expression in a tumor positively correlates with the response of the tumor to these agents. Topoisomerase I inhibitors inhibit the religation of the cut DNA strand, trapping the enzyme in a covalent complex with DNA. These agents include camptothecin, irenotecan (CPT-11), and topotecan.

Anthracyclines, particularly doxorubicin, have been used often in thyroid carcinomas, particularly in poorly-differentiated tumors and ATC. Although some older published reports suggested this to be an active agent (20, 33–35), complete responses are rare, with partial responses achieved at the expense of significant toxicity. Anthracycline monotherapy is most often used in the context of doxorubicin radiosensitization for external beam radiotherapy, based upon early reports on ATC patients (36, 37). Doxorubicin is more typically employed in the context of combination chemotherapy, frequently administered with cisplatin (20, 24, 31, 38, 39). Other anthracycline agents have also been tested as single agents in thyroid carcinoma patients, but have not proven effective (40) and are most commonly used, as for doxorubicin, in combination with other agents (32, 41).

Mitoxantrone is another group 1 topoisomerase II inhibitor that belongs to the class of anthracenedione antibiotics and seems to have similar toxicities as the anthracyclines. As a single agent, mitoxantrone has little activity in ATC (42), although it may have some benefit as part of combination chemotherapy (43). An additional group 1 agent, actinomycin D, has been evaluated by in vitro testing in ATC cell lines, suggesting that this agent is active in some lines (44), but it has not proven noteworthy in clinical studies.

The podophyllotoxins, particularly etoposide (VP-16) and teniposide, constitute much of the group 2 topoisomerase II inhibitors. Analysis of the expression of topoisomerase II alpha, a target of these inhibitors, shows higher levels in ATC, tall cell variant papillary carcinomas, and Hurthle cell carcinomas than in less aggressive varieties of thyroid cancer (45). This seems to suggest that podophyllotoxins would be useful for these types of thyroid cancer however, aside from rare complete responses (17), these agents have not proven active as single agents or in combination therapy (8, 46). Suramin is the only member of the group 3 topoisomerase II inhibitors that has been evaluated in ATC. Despite potent activity in monolayer and spheroid cell cultures, the same cell lines grown as xenografts had enhanced growth with suramin treatment (47) making this an unlikely candidate for clinical trials.

Topoisomerase I inhibitors inhibit the DNA religation step which traps topoisomerase I in a covalent complex and results in cytotoxicity. These are derived from camptothecin and include topotecan and CPT-11 (irinotecan). Oncologic investigations suggest that these agents work best in combination with cisplatin or its analogs; however there are no studies evaluating these agents or the combination in thyroid carcinomas.

Additional antitumor antibiotics

Bleomycin has effective tumor cytotoxic activity caused by its ability to fragment DNA. There is a long history of clinical use of this agent in aggressive and poorly differentiated thyroid carcinomas. Although there is some activity, it has not proven sufficient to suffice for single agent therapy (34, 48, 49). The most useful combination therapies have included bleomycin with doxorubicin, either by themselves (50, 51), with cisplatin (24, 52), with vincristine (17), or with vincristine and melphalan (53). Mitomycin C is an antibiotic agent that is a bioreductive alkylating compound with no effective application to thyroid carcinoma therapy.

Antimicrotubule agents

Compounds that bind tubulin have proven quite effective as antineoplastic agents. They cause mitotic arrest, even at doses too low to affect tubulin polymerization (54). Agents that stabilize microtubules are taxanes, paclitaxel (taxol) and docetaxel (taxatere), and epothilones A and B. Microtubule-destabilizing agents include the Vinca alkaloids (vincristine, vinblastine, vindesine, and vinorelbine), dolastatins, and combretastatins (combretastatin A4 phosphate).

Paclitaxel, a taxane, has proven to be the most effective single agent in ATC. This was first demonstrated in preclinical trials using ATC monolayers and xenografts (55), then in a phase 2 clinical trial (56). When administered as a weekly intravenous infusion of 175 mg/m^2 over one hour, response rates to paclitaxel exceed 50 percent. Unfortunately, although this has prolonged survival, it has not been sufficient to prevent the eventual lethality of this disease. There have not been any published clinical reports of combination chemotherapy for ATC that includes taxanes. In preclinical studies of ATC cell lines, the combination of manumycin, a farnesyltransferase inhibitor, and paclitaxel causes increased cytotoxicity more than either agent alone (57). Later evaluation in xenograft models suggests that manumycin inhibits tumor vascularity as a component of its antineoplastic activity (58). Epothilones have not been evaluated in ATC, with the exception of an apparent enhancement of epothilone B uptake and cytotoxicity in ATC xenografts treated with imatinib mesylate (STI571) (59). This is likely consequent to imatinib effects upon tumor vasculature (60, 61) rather than a direct effect of this tyrosine kinase inhibitor on ATC cells (KB Ain, unpublished data).

The Vinca alkaloids, first extracted from the Madagascar periwinkle, bind to both high and low affinity binding sites on tubulin that are distinct from taxane binding sites and cause inhibition of microtubule assembly. This causes inhibition of mitotic spindle function and results in a block in metaphase, although it is likely to involve additional mechanisms (5). None of these compounds have proven useful as monotherapy; however, vincristine in combination with doxorubicin and bleomycin (17, 62), with melphalan added to the combination (53), in combination with doxorubicin and 5-fluorouracil (63), or in combination with cisplatin and mitoxantrone (43) seems to have some moderate clinical activity. The only other agent of this group to be studied in thyroid cancer, vindesine, had no appreciable activity in combination with doxorubicin and cisplatin (29).

Additional microtubule-destabilizing drugs include the dolastatins and combretastatins. Dolastatin 10 and dolastatin 15, including some analogs, have been used in clinical trials, but have not been included in published trials in thyroid cancers. On the other hand, combretastatin A4 phosphate has been associated with an unexpected durable complete response in a patient with anaplastic thyroid carcinoma (64), prompting further evaluation and trials (reports pending). This drug has primary antineoplastic effects in ATC similar to those of paclitaxel (65) and likely has an additional mechanism of activity as a vascular targeting agent to disrupt the irregular vessels that feed tumor growth (66).

MECHANISMS OF RESISTANCE TO CHEMOTHERAPEUTIC AGENTS

Drug efflux proteins

Increased efflux of chemotherapeutic agents from tumor cells is a well-characterized mechanism of resistance to these agents. Membrane protein pumps, responsible for drug efflux, are typically members of the ATP-binding cassette (ABC) superfamily. These proteins are capable of transporting a wide range of compounds, serving a physiological role in benign tissues and, when over-expressed in malignancies, a contribution towards chemotherapy resistance. P-glycoprotein, a product of the *MDR1* gene on chromosome 7, is found in many normal human tissues serving to pump hydrophobic amphipathic drugs and metabolites (67). High levels of expression are seen in tumors derived from tissues which normally express P-glycoprotein (68) as well as in tumors from other tissues, particularly those expressing Ras and mutant p53 proteins (69). Inhibitors of P-glycoprotein activity, such as verapamil, are capable of restoring the cytotoxicity of chemotherapy drugs in these tumors at dosages previously without such effect (70). The next major subset of the ABC superfamily includes the Multidrug Resistance Protein (MRP) group, consisting of 6 identifiable homologous members (MRP1—MRP6). These are organic anion transporters physiologically expressed in a range of normal human tissues (71). MRP1 and MRP2 are clearly over-expressed in a number of malignant tissues, high expression of MRP3 and MRP5 can be found by screening panels of different tumor cell lines (72), malignant over-expression of MRP4 can be seen in lung cancers (73), but similar studies of MRP6 have not been reported. Recent investigations suggest that high levels of MRP4 (74) and MRP5 (75) expression result in resistance to nucleoside analog drugs; however, the efflux of a wide range of glutathione-conjugated chemotherapy drugs, via MRP1 and MRP2 (also known as cMOAT, the canalicular multispecific organic anion transporter), has been well-characterized for over a decade. Lung resistance related protein, LRP (also known as the human major vault protein), is a transporter of chemotherapeutic drugs into intracytoplasmic vaults and is also associated with resistance to these drugs (76).

Normal thyroid tissues are known to express both MRP1 and LRP transporters, but not P-glycoprotein (77). This pattern of expression is similar to the one seen in multiple ATC cell lines and tissues with nearly all having MRP1 and LRP transporters, but P-glycoprotein being rarely expressed (78–81). This pattern of expression may account for the greater sensitivity of ATC to paclitaxel, since MRP1 is less effective at transporting paclitaxel than P-glycoprotein (82). There are no published reports on ATC expression of any other MRP analogs to MRP1.

Additional mediators of drug resistance

Decreased expression of topoisomerases or mutations of its genes may be responsible for resistance to topoisomerase inhibitors. Evaluation of topoisomerase II alpha expression and gene sequences in 10 ATC cell lines and 3 tumor samples failed to find any evidence of reduced expression or gene mutation (81), making this an unlikely cause of multidrug resistance. Alternatively, increased chemotherapy drug metabolism by glutathione S-transferase, may contribute to multidrug resistance (83). A recent study suggests that enhanced activity of this enzyme in thyroid carcinoma patients may contribute to their chemotherapy drug resistance (84).

The tumor suppressor gene, p53, is a critical mediator of tumor cell apoptosis in response to DNA damage from cytotoxic agents. Mutations of the p53 gene, or epigenetic loss of expression, are extremely common in poorly differentiated thyroid carcinomas, particularly ATC (25, 85). Experimental transfection of wild-type p53 into ATC cell lines with adenovirus vectors has been shown to significantly enhance sensitivity to a variety of chemotherapeutic agents (86, 87). Likewise, targeting Bcl-2 gene expression in ATC cells by transfection with antisense oligonucleotides, removes a potent inhibitor of the BAX protein, a critical component of p53-mediated apoptosis. This also served to enhance chemosensitivity of these cells to paclitaxel, cisplatin, docetaxel, doxorubicin, mitomycin C, and 5-fluorouracil (10). Effects of alterations of the p53 pathway are not always predictable and related interventions may not always provide expected results (88).

THE FUTURE

Anaplastic thyroid carcinomas are almost always distantly metastatic by the time the primary tumor is discovered. For this reason, despite heroic efforts with primary surgery and radiotherapy, mortality is usually inevitable. Any hope for success at enhancing survival is contingent upon effective systemic chemotherapies. At this time, high-dose taxanes are the most useful agents; however, they are insufficient to alter eventual disease mortality. Although much progress is being made with antiangiogenic and tumor vascular-targeting agents, it seems unlikely to effect major benefits without new potent cytotoxic drugs. A two-pronged approach, attacking chemotherapy resistance mechanisms and developing new antineoplastic drugs, appears to be critical. In the meantime, ATC patients should be enrolled, whenever possible, in sufficient phase 1 and 2 clinical trials to permit accurate assessment of potential new therapies. Likewise, considering the rapid lethality of these tumors and cross-applications to other aggressive malignancies, ATC is an appropriate cancer model for creative translational research programs. These approaches provide hope for eventual successful therapeutic strategies.

REFERENCES

1. Ain KB 2000 Management of undifferentiated thyroid cancer. Baillieres Best Pract Res Clin Endocrinol Metab 14:615–29.
2. Ain KB 1999 Anaplastic thyroid carcinoma: a therapeutic challenge. Sem Surg Oncol 16:64.
3. Ain KB 1998 Anaplastic thyroid carcinoma: behavior, biology, and therapeutic approaches. Thyroid 8:715–726.
4. Alison M 2002 The cancer handbook. Nature Pub. Group; Distributed in the U.S. by Grove's Dictionaries, London, New York.
5. Souhami RL 2002 Oxford textbook of oncology, 2nd ed. Oxford University Press, Oxford ; New York.
6. Orlandi F, Caraci P, Berruti A, et al. 1994 Chemotherapy with dacarbazine and 5-fluorouracil in advanced medullary thyroid cancer. Ann Oncol 5:763–765.
7. Tallroth E, Wallin G, Lundell G, Löwhagen T, Einhorn J 1987 Multimodality treatment in anaplastic giant cell thyroid carcinoma. Cancer 60:1428–1431.
8. Droz JP, Schlumberger M, Rougier P, Ghosn M, Gardet P, Parmentier C 1990 Chemotherapy in metastatic nonanaplastic thyroid cancer: experience at the Institut Gustave-Roussy. Tumori 76:480–3.
9. Nederman T 1984 Effects of vinblastine and 5-fluorouracil on human glioma and thyroid cancer cell monolayers and spheroids. Cancer Res 44:254–6.
10. Kim R, Tanabe K, Uchida Y, Emi M, Toge T 2003 Effect of Bcl-2 antisense oligonucleotide on drug-sensitivity in association with apoptosis in undifferentiated thyroid carcinoma. Int J Mol Med 11:799–804.
11. Misaki T, Iwata M, Iida Y, Kasagi K, Konishi J 2002 Chemo-radionuclide therapy for thyroid cancer: initial experimental study with cultured cells. Ann Nucl Med 16:403–8.
12. Ringel MD, Greenberg M, Chen X, et al. 2000 Cytotoxic activity of $2',2'$-difluorodeoxycytidine (gemcitabine) in poorly differentiated thyroid carcinoma cells. Thyroid 10:865–9.
13. Voigt W, Bulankin A, Muller T, et al. 2000 Schedule-dependent antagonism of gemcitabine and cisplatin in human anaplastic thyroid cancer cell lines. Clin Cancer Res 6:2087–93.

14. Kotchetkov R, Groschel B, Gmeiner WH, et al. 2000 Antineoplastic activity of a novel multimeric gemcitabine-monophosphate prodrug against thyroid cancer cells in vitro. Anticancer Res 20: 2915–22.
15. Kotchetkov R, Krivtchik AA, Cinatl J, Kornhuber B, Cinatl J, Jr. 1999 Selective cytotoxic activity of a novel ribonucleoside diphosphate reductase inhibitor MDL-101,731 against thyroid cancer in vitro. Folia Biol (Praha) 45:185–91.
16. Jereb B, Stjernswärd J, Löwhagen T 1975 Anaplastic giant-cell carcinoma of the thyroid: a study of treatment and prognosis. Cancer 35:1293–1295.
17. Hoskin PJ, Harmer C 1987 Chemotherapy for thyroid cancer. Radiother Oncol 10:187–94.
18. Palyi I, Peter I, Daubner D, Vincze B, Lorincz I 1993 Establishment, characterization and drug sensitivity of a new anaplastic thyroid carcinoma cell line (BHT-101). Virchows Arch B Cell Pathol Incl Mol Pathol 63:263–9.
19. Yoshida A, Fukazawa M, Aiyoshi Y, Soeda S, Ito K 1990 The biological characteristics and chemosensitivity of anaplastic thyroid carcinoma transplanted into nude mice. Jpn J Surg 20:690–5.
20. Asakawa H, Kobayashi T, Komoike Y, et al. 1997 Chemosensitivity of anaplastic thyroid carcinoma and poorly differentiated thyroid carcinoma. Anticancer Res 17:2757–2762.
21. Tallroth E, Wallin G, Lundell G, Lowhagen T, Einhorn J 1987 Multimodality treatment in anaplastic giant cell thyroid carcinoma. Cancer 60:1428–31.
22. Andersson T, Biorklund A, Landberg T, Akerman M, Aspegren K, Ingemansson S 1977 Combined therapy for undifferentiated giant and spindle cell carcinoma of the thyroid. Acta Otolaryngol 83: 372–7.
23. Bernhardt B 1981 Follicular thyroid carcinoma: response to chemotherapy. Am J Med Sci 282: 45–6.
24. De Besi P, Busnardo B, Toso S, et al. 1991 Combined chemotherapy with bleomycin, adriamycin, and platinum in advanced thyroid cancer. J Endocrinol Invest 14:475–80.
25. Farid NR 2001 P53 mutations in thyroid carcinoma: tidings from an old foe. J Endocrinol Invest 24:536–45.
26. van der Zee AG, Hollema HH, de Bruijn HW, et al. 1995 Cell biological markers of drug resistance in ovarian carcinoma. Gynecol Oncol 58:165–78.
27. Fineman LS, Hamilton TA, de Gortari A, Bonney P 1998 Cisplatin chemotherapy for treatment of thyroid carcinoma in dogs: 13 cases. J Am Anim Hosp Assoc 34:109–12.
28. Ekman ET, Lundell G, Tennvall J, Wallin G 1990 Chemotherapy and multimodality treatment in thyroid carcinoma. Otolaryngol Clin NA 23:523–527.
29. Scherubl H, Raue F, Ziegler R 1990 Combination chemotherapy of advanced medullary and differentiated thyroid cancer. Phase II study. J Cancer Res Clin Oncol 116:21–3.
30. Schlumberger M, Parmentier C, Delisle MJ, Couette JE, Droz JP, Sarrazin D 1991 Combination therapy for anaplastic giant cell thyroid carcinoma. Cancer 67:564–6.
31. Shimaoka K, Schoenfeld DA, DeWys WD, Creech RH, DeConti R 1985 A randomized trial of doxorubicin versus doxorubicin plus cisplatin in patients with advanced thyroid carcinoma. Cancer 56:2155–60.
32. Santini F, Bottici V, Elisei R, et al. 2002 Cytotoxic effects of carboplatinum and epirubicin in the setting of an elevated serum thyrotropin for advanced poorly differentiated thyroid cancer. J Clin Endocrinol Metab 87:4160–5.
33. Ahuja S, Ernst H 1987 Chemotherapy of thyroid carcinoma. J Endocrinol Invest 10:303–310.
34. Poster DS, Bruno S, Penta J, Pina K, Catane R 1981 Current status of chemotherapy in the treatment of advanced carcinoma of the thyroid gland. Cancer Clin Trials 4:301–7.
35. Gottlieb JA, Hill CS, Jr 1974 Chemotherapy of thyroid cancer with Adriamycin. Experience with 30 patients. N Engl J Med 290:193–7.
36. Kim JH, Leeper RD 1983 Treatment of anaplastic giant and spindle cell carcinoma of the thyroid gland with combination adriamycin and radiation therapy: A new approach. Cancer 52:954–57.
37. Kim JH, Leeper RD 1987 Treatment of locally advanced thyroid carcinoma with combination doxorubicin and radiation therapy. Cancer 60:2372–75.
38. Shade RJ, Pisters KM, Huber MH, et al. 1998 Phase I study of paclitaxel administered by ten-day continuous infusion. Invest New Drugs 16:237–43.
39. Williams SD, Birch R, Einhorn LH 1986 Phase II evaluation of doxorubicin plus cisplatin in advanced thyroid cancer: a Southeastern Cancer Study Group trial. Cancer Treat Rep 70:405–7.
40. Benjamin RS, Keating MJ, Swenerton KD, Legha S, McCredie KB 1979 Clinical studies with rubidazone. Cancer Treat Rep 63:925–9.

41. Di Bartolomeo M, Bajetta E, Bochicchio AM, et al. 1995 A phase II trial of dacarbazine, fluorouracil and epirubicin in patients with neuroendocrine tumours. A study by the Italian Trials in Medical Oncology (I.T.M.O.) Group. Ann Oncol 6:77–9.
42. Schlumberger M, Parmentier C 1989 Phase II evaluation of mitoxantrone in advanced non anaplastic thyroid cancer. Bull Cancer 76:403–406.
43. Kober F, Heiss A, Keminger K, Depisch D 1990 [Chemotherapy of highly malignant thyroid tumors]. Wien Klin Wochenschr 102:274–6.
44. Osawa Y, Yoshida A, Asaga T, Kawahara S, Yanoma S 1996 [In vitro chemosensitivity test for seven undifferentiated thyroid carcinoma cell lines using MTT assay]. Gan To Kagaku Ryoho 23:471–6.
45. Lee A, LiVolsi VA, Baloch ZW 2000 Expression of DNA topoisomerase IIalpha in thyroid neoplasia. Mod Pathol 13:396–400.
46. Leaf AN, Wolf BC, Kirkwood JM, Haselow RE 2000 Phase II study of etoposide (VP-16) in patients with thyroid cancer with no prior chemotherapy: an Eastern Cooperative Oncology Group Study (E1385). Med Oncol 17:47–51.
47. Ain KB, Ishizawar RC, Taylor KD Suramin inhibits growth of differentiated and anaplastic human thyroid carcinomas in monolayer and spheroid cultures with disparate effects *in vivo*. 76th Annual Meeting of the Endocrine Society, Anaheim, CA, 1994.
48. Harada T, Nishikawa Y, Suzuki T, Ito K, Baba S 1971 Bleomycin treatment for cancer of the thyroid. Am J Surg 122:53–7.
49. Hayat M 1977 Où en est la chimiothérapie des cancers de lo thyroïde? (Status of chemotherapy for thyroid carcinomas). Ann Radiol 20:807–9.
50. Benker G, Hackenberg K, Hoff HG, et al. 1977 [Combined doxorubicin and bleomycin treatment of metastasising thyroid carcinoma: results in 21 patients (author's transl)]. Dtsch Med Wochenschr 102:1908–13.
51. Busnardo B, Daniele O, Pelizzo MR, et al. 2000 A multimodality therapeutic approach in anaplastic thyroid carcinoma: study on 39 patients. J Endocrinol Invest 23:755–61.
52. Spanos GA, Wol KD, Desner MR, et al. 1982 Preoperative chemotherapy for giant cell carcinoma of the thyroid. Cancer 50:2252–6.
53. Bukowski RM, Brown L, Weick JK, Groppe CW, Purvis J 1983 Combination chemotherapy of metastatic thyroid cancer: phase II study. Am J Clin Oncol (CCT) 6:579–81.
54. Jordan MA, Wilson L 1998 Microtubules and actin filaments: dynamic targets for cancer chemotherapy. Curr Opin Cell Biol 10:123–30.
55. Ain KB, Tofiq S, Taylor KD 1996 Antineoplastic activity of taxol against human anaplastic thyroid carcinoma cell lines in vitro and in vivo. J Clin Endocrinol Metab 81:3650–3.
56. Ain KB, Egorin MJ, DeSimone PA 2000 Treatment of anaplastic thyroid carcinoma with paclitaxel: phase 2 trial using ninety-six-hour infusion. Collaborative Anaplastic Thyroid Cancer Health Intervention Trials (CATCHIT) Group. Thyroid 10:587–94.
57. Yeung SC, Xu G, Pan J, Christgen M, Bamiagis A 2000 Manumycin enhances the cytotoxic effect of paclitaxel on anaplastic thyroid carcinoma cells. Cancer Res 60:650–6.
58. Xu G, Pan J, Martin C, Yeung SC 2001 Angiogenesis inhibition in the in vivo antineoplastic effect of manumycin and paclitaxel against anaplastic thyroid carcinoma. J Clin Endocrinol Metab 86:1769–77.
59. Pietras K, Stumm M, Hubert M, et al. 2003 STI571 enhances the therapeutic index of epothilone B by a tumor-selective increase of drug uptake. Clin Cancer Res 9:3779–87.
60. Frasca F, Vigneri P, Vella V, Vigneri R, Wang JY 2001 Tyrosine kinase inhibitor STI571 enhances thyroid cancer cell motile response to Hepatocyte Growth Factor. Oncogene 20:3845–56.
61. Pietras K, Rubin K, Sjoblom T, et al. 2002 Inhibition of PDGF receptor signaling in tumor stroma enhances antitumor effect of chemotherapy. Cancer Res 62:5476–84.
62. Sokal M, Harmer CL 1978 Chemotherapy for anaplastic carcinoma of the thyroid. Clin Oncol 4:3–10.
63. Alexieva-Figusch J, Van Gilse HA, Treurniet RE 1977 Chemotherapy in carcinoma of the thyroid: retrospective and prospective. Ann Radiol 20:810–13.
64. Dowlati A, Robertson K, Cooney M, et al. 2002 A phase I pharmacokinetic and translational study of the novel vascular targeting agent combretastatin a-4 phosphate on a single-dose intravenous schedule in patients with advanced cancer. Cancer Res 62:3408–16.
65. Dziba JM, Marcinek R, Venkataraman G, Robinson JA, Ain KB 2002 Combretastatin a4 phosphate has primary antineoplastic activity against human anaplastic thyroid carcinoma cell lines and xenograft tumors. Thyroid 12:1063–70.
66. Griggs J, Metcalfe JC, Hesketh R 2001 Targeting tumor vasculature: the development of combretastatin A4. The Lancet Oncology 2:82–87.

67. Gottesman MM, Pastan I 1993 Biochemistry of multidrug resistance mediated by the multidrug transporter. Annu Rev Biochem 62:385–427.
68. Fojo AT, Ueda K, Slamon DJ, Poplack DG, Gottesman MM, Pastan I 1987 Expression of a multidrug-resistance gene in human tumors and tissues. Proc Natl Acad Sci U S A 84:265–9.
69. Chin KV, Ueda K, Pastan I, Gottesman MM 1992 Modulation of activity of the promoter of the human MDR1 gene by Ras and p53. Science 255:459–62.
70. Pauli-Magnus C, von Richter O, Burk O, et al. 2000 Characterization of the major metabolites of verapamil as substrates and inhibitors of P-glycoprotein. J Pharmacol Exp Ther 293:376–82.
71. Borst P, Evers R, Kool M, Wijnholds J 2000 A family of drug transporters: the multidrug resistance-associated proteins. J Natl Cancer Inst 92:1295–302.
72. Kool M, de Haas M, Scheffer GL, et al. 1997 Analysis of expression of cMOAT (MRP2), MRP3, MRP4, and MRP5, homologues of the multidrug resistance-associated protein gene (MRP1), in human cancer cell lines. Cancer Res 57:3537–47.
73. Young LC, Campling BG, Voskoglou-Nomikos T, Cole SP, Deeley RG, Gerlach JH 1999 Expression of multidrug resistance protein-related genes in lung cancer: correlation with drug response. Clin Cancer Res 5:673–80.
74. Zelcer N, Reid G, Wielinga P, et al. 2003 Steroid and bile acid conjugates are substrates of human multidrug-resistance protein (MRP) 4 (ATP-binding cassette C4). Biochem J 371:361–7.
75. Wijnholds J, Mol CA, van Deemter L, et al. 2000 Multidrug-resistance protein 5 is a multispecific organic anion transporter able to transport nucleotide analogs. Proc Natl Acad Sci U S A 97:7476–81.
76. Scheffer GL, Schroeijers AB, Izquierdo MA, Wiemer EA, Scheper RJ 2000 Lung resistance-related protein/major vault protein and vaults in multidrug-resistant cancer. Curr Opin Oncol 12:550–6.
77. Sugawara I, Akiyama S, Scheper RJ, Itoyama S 1997 Lung resistance protein (LRP) expression in human normal tissues in comparison with that of MDR1 and MRP. Cancer Lett 112:23–31.
78. Sekiguchi M, Shiroko Y, Arai T, et al. 2001 Biological characteristics and chemosensitivity profile of four human anaplastic thyroid carcinoma cell lines. Biomed Pharmacother 55:466–74.
79. Sugawara I, Masunaga A, Itoyama S, Sumizawa T, Akiyama S, Yamashita T 1995 Expression of multidrug resistance-associated protein (MRP) in thyroid cancers. Cancer Lett 95:135–8.
80. Yamashita T, Watanabe M, Onodera M, et al. 1994 Multidrug resistance gene and P-glycoprotein expression in anaplastic carcinoma of the thyroid. Cancer Detect Prev 18:407–13.
81. Satake S, Sugawara I, Watanabe M, Takami H 1997 Lack of a point mutation of human DNA topoisomerase II in multidrug-resistant anaplastic thyroid carcinoma cell lines. Cancer Letters 116:33–39.
82. Loe DW, Deeley RG, Cole SPC 1996 Biology of the multidrug resistance-associated protein, MRP. Eur J Cancer 32A:945–957.
83. Niitsu Y, Takahashi Y, Ban N, et al. 1998 A proof of glutathione S-transferase-pi-related multidrug resistance by transfer of antisense gene to cancer cells and sense gene to bone marrow stem cell. Chem Biol Interact 111-112:325–32.
84. Dincer Y, Akcay T, Celebi N, Uslu I, Ozmen O, Hatemi H 2002 Glutathione S-transferase and O6-methylguanine DNA methyl transferase activities in patients with thyroid papillary carcinoma. Cancer Invest 20:965–71.
85. Shahedian B, Shi Y, Zou M, Farid NR 2001 Thyroid carcinoma is characterized by genomic instability: evidence from p53 mutations. Mol Genet Metab 72:155–63.
86. Blagosklonny MV, Giannakakou P, Wojtowicz M, et al. 1998 Effects of p53-expressing adenovirus on the chemosensitivity and differentiation of anaplastic thyroid cancer cells. J Clin Endocrinol Metab 83:2516–22.
87. Nagayama Y, Yokoi H, Takeda K, et al. 2000 Adenovirus-mediated tumor suppressor p53 gene therapy for anaplastic thyroid carcinoma in vitro and in vivo. J Clin Endocrinol Metab 85:4081–6.
88. Ceraline J, Deplanque G, Noel F, Natarajan-Ame S, Bergerat JP, Klein-Soyer C 2003 Sensitivity to cisplatin treatment of human K1 thyroid carcinoma cell lines with altered p53 function. Cancer Chemother Pharmacol 51:91–5.

21. GENE THERAPY FOR THYROID CANCER

YUJI NAGAYAMA, M.D.

Department of Pharmacology 1, Graduate School of Biomedical Sciences, Nagasaki University, Nagasaki 852–8523 Japan (TEL) 81+95-849-7042 (FAX) 81+95-849-7044 (email) nagayama@net.nagasaki-u.ac.jp

INTRODUCTION

The original concept of gene therapy is to treat and cure diseases caused by a known monogenic defect by introducing and expressing a normal copy of the mutated or deleted gene into the host cells. In this regard, gene therapy for cancer should be aimed at correcting gene alternations in cancer cells, that is, replacement of tumor suppressor genes and inactivation of oncogenes. However, cancer gene therapy has evolved in somewhat different directions. These include (i) transfer of suicide genes that convert inactive prodrugs into cytotoxic compounds, (ii) transfer of genes coding immuno-stimulators such as cytokines and chemokines to enhance anti-tumor immunity, (iii) transfer of genes coding anti-angiogenic factors to inhibit angiogenesis in solid tumors, (iv) transfer of drug resistant genes into normal hematopoietic stem cells to render them resistant to high-dose myelosuppressive chemotherapeutic agents. These strategies do not constitute "gene-replacement therapy" as defined above, and might instead be called "DNA therapeutics" for instance (1). Cancer gene therapy can be defined simply as "the transfer of nucleic acids into cancer or normal cells to eliminate or reduce tumor burden".

Genes can be introduced into target cells *ex vivo* and placed back into the host or directly into target cells (*in vivo*). Viral or non-viral vectors are used to facilitate the transfer of genes into target cells. This chapter discusses recent advances in gene therapy of the thyroid cancer field. Attention is focused on the therapeutic genes used.

STRATEGIES USED FOR THYROID CANCER GENE THERAPY

Silencing of oncogenes

According to the original concept of gene therapy, that is, "gene-replacement therapy", we may speculate that correction of a mutated or an aberrantly overexpressed oncogene might reverse malignant phenotype. On the other hand, some may contend that since cancers generally arises as the culmination of a multiple process that involves a variety of somatic gene alternations (see Chapter 1 for more detail), it is impossible to correct all the genetic abnormalities, as neither to restore normal gene function in every cancer cells with currently available vectors.

Several mutations or overexpression of oncogenes have been identified in thyroid cancers. The former includes RAS mutations and RET gene rearrangements in follicular and papillary carcinomas, respectively (2), and the latter overexpression of c-myc and high mobility group I (Y) protein [HMG I (Y)] in some thyroid cancers with highly malignant phenotypes (3, 4). Theoretically, suppression of gene expression can possibly be achieved with antisense, ribozyme, intracellular single-chain antibodies or RNA interference. For instance, suppression by antisense method of expression of c-myc and HMG I (Y) protein is reported to induce growth inhibition and cell death, respectively, in thyroid cancer cell lines with overexpression of a respective gene (3, 4).

Replacement of tumor suppressor gene

Among numerous mutations in different tumor suppressor genes so far identified in distinct types of cancers, the gene for tumor suppressor p53 (5) is well known to be frequently mutated in anaplastic, not well-differentiated, thyroid carcinoma (6–8). These mutations are closely associated with de-differentiation of thyroid cancer, and therefore thought to be the late event in thyroid carcinogenesis.

One can expect that introduction of wild type (wt)-p53 gene into thyroid cancer cells defective in normal p53 might reverse malignant phenotype or induce re-differentiation. Indeed it has been reported that reintroduction of wt-p53 by stable transfection into p53-defective follicular cell-derived thyroid cancer cell lines and a medullary thyroid cancer (MTC) cell line led to cell cycle arrest and growth inhibition (presumably the cells expressing p53 at relatively low levels survived) (9–16). Re-expression of wt-p53 is accompanied by chemosensitization, radiosensitization and re-appearance of the differentiated markers such as TPO, TSHR and PAX8 (9–11, 14, 15). Besides, of interest, despite *in vitro* cell growth inhibitory, not cell-killing, effect of wt-p53 in an anaplastic thyroid cancer cell line FRO, FRO cells stably expressing wt-p53 exhibits poor tumorigenicity in nude mice (16). Thus, tumors can not grow more than a few mm in a diameter. Tumors are found to be in an angiogenesis-restricted dormant state, that is, growth of FRO cells is counterbalanced with apoptotic cell death induced by anti-angiogenic effect of wt-p53. Wt-p53 appears to exert more complex anti-cancer actions than expected from *in vitro* data.

In contrast, however, high level expression of wt-p53 achieved with recombinant adenovirus clearly induces apoptotic cell death *in vitro* (17, 18). Furthermore, in *in vivo* experiments in nude mice, intratumoral injection of adenovirus expressing wt-p53

(1×10^9 pfu/tumor) into pre-established FRO tumors almost completely inhibited tumor growth and induced a small but significant tumor reduction when combined with doxorubicin (18). Of interest, it has recently been shown that a histone deacetylase inhibitor (depsipeptide) increases p53 transcriptional activity and thereby p21 expression, a downstream target of p53, and leads to enhancement of p53's anti-tumor effect (19). Since anaplastic thyroid cancer is highly aggressive and refractory to conventional treatments, p53 gene therapy may be a promising new strategy for this type of cancer.

Suicide gene/prodrug

Genes whose products convert a relatively nontoxic prodrug into its toxic form are referred as "suicide genes" (20). Herpes simplex virus-thymidine kinase (HSV-TK), a most widely used suicide gene product, phosphorylates a prodrug ganciclovir (GCV) ~1000-fold more efficiently than mammalian TK. The resultant GCV monophosphate is further phosphorylated by the mammalian enzyme to GCV triphosphate, which inhibits DNA polymerase and is thus cytotoxic. *E. coli* Cytosine deaminase converts nontoxic 5-fluorocytosine to toxic 5-fluorouracil (5-FU) by deamination, which blocks thymidylate synthetase and mRNA transcription. Deoxycytidine kinase phosphorylates and activates a number of anti-neoplastic nucleotide analogues including cytosine arabinoside (Ara-C). *E. coli* Nitroreductase converts a prodrug CB 1954 to its toxic form. The *in vitro* efficacy of all these combinations was confirmed in several thyroid cancer cell lines (21, 22). Nishihara *et al.* (21) have also demonstrated HSV-TK/GCV-mediated radiosensitization in thyroid cancer cells. Although it is impossible to transduce a therapeutic gene into every cancer cells *in vivo* with currently available vectors, non-transduced cells can be killed by neighboring transduced cells, a phenomenon called "bystander effect". Phosphorylated GCV can be transferred from transduced cells to adjacent non-transduced cells through gap junctions and phagocytosis of apoptotic vesicles of dead cells by live tumor cells. Induction of active, local immune response against tumors may participate in *in vivo* bystander effect. In addition, 5-FU, phosphorylated Ara-C and toxic CB1954 can also be secreted and taken up by surrounding cells. In this regard, these latter three combinations seem to be more efficacious than HSV-TK/GCV (22). Nevertheless, most of thyroid cancer gene therapy has been performed with HSV-TK/GCV.

HSV-TK and GCV system exerts their cytotoxic effect on not only proliferating cells (including cancer cells) but also metabolically active, non-proliferating cells such as normal thyroid cells (23, 24). It is therefore necessary to target expression of HSV-TK to cancer cells. One of the methods for targeting is transcriptional control of therapeutic gene expression. Although no thyroid cancer-specific promoter has been identified, several tissue-specific promoters are available [thyroglobulin (Tg), calcitonin (CT), *etc.*]. The preliminary experiments suggesting the potential usefulness of Tg promoter for thyroid cancer gene therapy have been performed *in vitro* with normal, differentiated rat thyroid cell line FRTL5 by Zeiger *et al.* (25). Subsequently with the retrovirus vector and transformed rat FRTC cells, a model for differentiated thyroid cancer cells, Braiden *et al.* (26) have demonstrated the feasibility of Tg promoter and

HSV-TK/GCV system *in vitro* and *in vivo*. Zhang et al. (27, 28) have recently demonstrated not only the efficacy but also the safety of Tg promoter with adenovirus *in vivo*. Thus intravenous (i.v.) injection of adenovirus containing HSV-TK gene under the control of Tg promoter did not induce liver damage (the main target organ for i.v. adenovirus).

However, the activities of tissue-specific promoters are generally weaker than those of constitutive viral promoters [*eg.,* human cytomegalovirus (CMV) promoter]. To overcome this drawback, use of Cre-*lox*P system is one option (29). In this study, two adenovirus vectors were constructed; one contained the expression cassette of Tg promoter and Cre recombinase gene, and the other of CMV promoter and HSV-TK gene which were interrupted with two *lox*P sequences flanking the neomycin-resistance gene. When these two adenoviruses were co-infected into the cells in which Tg promoter is active, Cre was expressed from Tg promoter in the first vector, and excised the neomycin-resistance sequence and placed HSV-TK gene under the control of the CMV promoter in the second vector, which exhibited the enhanced therapeutic effect as compared with the combination of Tg promoter and HSV-TK gene. However, it should be noted here that the need of double infection might curtail the therapeutic efficacy when multiplicity of infection (MOI) is low or tumor cells are resistant to adenovirus infection. In addition, Takeda *et al.* (30) have reported the higher efficacy of a tandemly repeated Tg promoters.

Another problem for use of tissue-specific promoters is loss of tissue-specific promoter activities in poorly differentiated and anaplastic thyroid cancer, making Tg promoter useless for treatment of these types of thyroid cancer. Two studies suggest the potential usefulness of thyroid-related transcription factors to re-activate Tg promoter in thyroid cancer cell lines with no Tg expression, but data are somewhat different (30, 31). Chun *et al.* (31) have shown enhancement of Tg promoter by co-transfection of thyroid transcription factor-1 (TTF-1) and PAX-8, while TTF-1 alone was sufficient in studies by Shimura *et al.* (32). The different cell lines used (ARO and WRO cells *versus* FRT and BHP15-3 cells) may explain these different results. Further studies will be necessary to clarify this controversy, a very important point considering clinical trial in the future.

Furthermore, Kitazono *et al.* (33, 34) have found that histone deacetylase inhibitors (depsipeptide and sodium butyrate) enhanced activity of Tg promoter or Tg enhancer/promoter and this effect was further augmented by a cAMP analogue in thyroid cancer cell lines with no Tg expression.

Similar studies with HSV-TK/GCV and a tissue-specific promoter (CT promoter) have also been performed in MTC with a rat MTC cell line, 6–23 (clone 6), and a human MTC cell line, TT, *in vitro* and with 6–23 cells *in vivo* (35, 36).

Finally, Soler *et al.* (37) have used nitric oxide synthase II (NOS II) gene as a suicide gene for treatment of MTC. NOS II produces NO which is the main mediator of the tumoricidal action of activated macrophage. Despite an extremely low gene transfer efficiency (~1 %), injection of the naked plasmid containing CMV promoter and NOS II cDNA into orthotopically established MTC tumors led to tumor growth inhibition, suggesting marked bystander effect probably due to NO diffusion. Thus NOS II gene can also be used as a suicide gene in cancer gene therapy.

Enhancement of tumor immunity

Cancer cells can be recognized as a foreign by host immune system. However, this anti-tumor immune response is usually not strong enough to eradicate tumors. The mechanisms of insufficient anti-tumor immunity include loss of expression of major histocompatibility complex (MHC) antigens and/or co-stimulatory molecules on cancer cells, and secretion of immuno-suppressive cytokine(s) (*e.g.*, TGF-β) from cancer cells. Systemic administration of cytokine(s) can be used to enhance immune response to tumor antigens, but is always accompanied by undesirable side effects. To overcome these problems, cDNAs coding cytokines, MHC or co-stimulatory molecules have been introduced into tumor cells to make tumor cells more immunogenic and reduce the toxicity. Two approaches are usually employed; immunization with transduced (and irradiated) autologous tumor cells or *in situ* gene delivery into an established tumor mass.

To my knowledge, the first article describing immune-gene therapy against thyroid cancer is one by Lausson *et al.* (38). They showed that rat MTC cells stably expressing interleukin-2 (IL-2) injected subcutaneously or orthotopically were completely rejected in syngeneic rats. This anti-tumor effect appeared to involve the recruitment of CD8+ T lymphocytes. Subsequently, DeGroot and his colleagues performed extensive studies on immuno-gene therapy for MTC with cytokines in rat and mouse MTC models. Tumorigenicity of mouse MTC cells infected with adenovirus harboring IL-2 gene (under the control of CMV promoter) was shown very poor in syngeneic immuno-competent mice (39). Established long lasting immunity was demonstrated by re-challenge with parental MTC cells in protected mice. Cell-mediated cytotoxic assays showed that both cytotoxic T lymphocytes and NK cells play a role. Loss of tumorigenesis of MTC cells infected with adenovirus expressing IL-2 in severe combined immune deficiency mice also indicates involvement of NK cells in this anti-tumor immunity (39). In *in vivo* situations where adenovirus expressing IL-2 (1×10^9 pfu in mice and 2×10^9 pfu in rat) was injected into pre-established MTC tumors, 70% and 43%, respectively, of the small tumors (<30 mm^3 in mice and <100 mm^3 in rat) were eradicated, but all the large tumors (>30 mm^3 in mice and >100 mm^3 in rat) showed stabilization in size (40, 41). They have also addressed the safety issue of intratumoral inoculation of adenovirus harboring IL-2 gene under the control of constitutive CMV promoter (41). Despite detection of dissemination of inoculated adenovirus from tumor to liver, no liver dysfunction was observed except mild pathological change (lymphocyte infiltration) even when constitutive viral promoter was used to drive IL-2 expression, suggesting that direct injection of adenovirus expressing IL-2 (and presumably other cytokines) can be safe. Their recent studies have demonstrated that IL-12 appears to be more efficacious than IL-2 (42). In a rat MTC model, the cure rate was 100% in smaller tumors (<100 mm^3) injected with 1×10^9 pfu adenovirus expressing IL-12, *versus* 43% complete eradication with 2×10^9 pfu adenovirus expressing IL-2 in the aforementioned report (41). Seventy-eight % of large tumors (>100 mm^3) was also eradicated (*versus* 0% in case of IL-2). Furthermore, they showed intravenous injection of adenovirus coding IL-12 was safe when IL-12 gene expression was confined to MTC tumors (and thyroid parafollicular C cells) by using the modified CT promoter comprised of two tandemly arranged tissue-specific enhancer elements and a minimal proximal CT promoter (43). More recently the efficacy of adenovirus expressing IL-12 has also been shown in thyroid follicular cancer (44).

In addition, enhanced effect of the combined HSV-TK/GCV and IL-2 has also been demonstrated by three groups (45–47). For example, in studies by DeGroot's group (46), the complete eradication of pre-established MTC tumors was induced in 63% of mice treated with adenovirus expressing HSV-TK and IL-2, 38% with adenovirus expressing IL-2 and 12% with adenovirus expressing HSV-TK (all 2×10^9 pfu).

Finally, although no thyroid tumor rejection antigens have yet been identified, the possibility of preprocalcitonin ((PPCT) as a tumor rejection antigen in MTC has been investigated by a means of DNA immunization (48). Co-delivery of PPCT and granulocyte-macrophage colony-stimulating factor genes induced cellular and humoral immune responses against PPCT, suggesting a potential of DNA immunization as a novel immunotherapeutic treatment for MTC.

Selectively replicative virus (Oncolytic virus)

As shown above, recombinant adenovirus is being widely used as a vehicle for gene delivery in cancer gene therapy. *In vivo* therapeutic efficacy of non-replicative adenovirus is however limited mainly because of its low infectivity and poor gene delivery to a solid tumor. Use of replicative adenovirus is thus a potential candidate to overcome this issue (49). ONYX-015 is such an adenovirus with a deletion in E1B 55 kD gene and reportedly replicates selectively in the cells defective in p53 gene (50), although this p53 mutation-selective replication has been disputed (49). Intratumorally (or i.v.) injected ONYX-015 first infects to a small fraction of tumor cells, in which virus replicates and induces cell death (cytopathic effect), and then virus progeny released infects to surrounding tumor cells. Portella *et al.* (51) have recently demonstrated anti-tumor effect and chemosensitivity of ONYX-015 in several thyroid cancer cell lines defective in wt-p53. They have also addressed the safety of this virus using a rat normal thyroid cell line PC Cl3. However, one should be cautious for these data, because human adenovirus does not usually replicate well in non-human (*eg.*, rodent) cells. Indeed we have previously found that selectively replicative adenovirus can replicate and produce progeny in normal human thyroid cells in culture. Further, there is no difference in viral replication between anaplastic thyroid cancer cell line FRO and FRO cells stably expressing wt-p53, suggesting that adenovirus replication appears independent from p53 status (our unpublished data). These data does not exclude the use of replicative adenovirus for thyroid cancer treatment, rather indicate that this type of oncolytic virus can be used for both differentiated and anaplastic thyroid cancers. In this case, there is a need to strictly control virus replication in order to avoid undesired viral spread. For example, we have used Cre-*lox*P system and p53-responsive promoter to control E1A protein expression, which is essential for adenovirus replication (52). This may be a promising means to restrict virus replication to anaplastic thyroid cancer. Tg promoter can also be used to express E1A proteins in differentiated thyroid cancer (53).

However, it is usually impossible to completely eradicate tumors with replicative adenovirus alone. Therefore, multimodality treatment with other antitumor agents might be necessary. Indeed, replicative adenovirus has also been reported to work synergistically with chemotherapy. Also replicative adenovirus can be armed with a therapeutic gene such as a suicide or a cytokine gene (54).

Antiangiogenic factors

It is well known that solid tumors can not growth more than a few mm^3 without oxygen and nutrient supplied from blood (55), suggesting that new vessel formation (called angiogenesis) is a prerequisite for solid tumor growth. Therefore, inhibition of angiogenesis might be a promising strategy for cancer treatment. Numerous antiangiogenic factors have so far been isolated such as angiostatin, endostatin, *etc*. Since these agents act basically on normal vascular endothelial cells, resistance to these agents can not be easily induced. To my knowledge, only one study describes the effect of an antiangiogenic factor gene on thyroid cancer; thrombomodulin-1 inhibits angiogenesis and growth of FRO tumors (16). As mentioned above, this article also demonstrates the ability of wt-p53 to induce anti-angiogenesis-mediated dormancy.

Iodide transporter

Active influx and efflux of iodide in the thyroid gland are mediated by sodium iodide symporter (NIS) and chloride-iodide transporter (Pendrin), respectively (56, 57). Failure of iodide concentration in some differentiated and most anaplastic thyroid cancers are generally due to decreased or loss of NIS expression. Therefore, targeted expression of NIS gene in thyroid cancers with no or little NIS expression (and also non-thyroid cancers) would offer the possibility of radioiodide therapy (58, 59). Shimura *et al.* (60) have first shown the significant iodide concentration in transformed rat thyroid cancer cells genetically engineered to express NIS. However, no or weak efficacy was demonstrated in *in vivo* studies (61, 62) because of rapid efflux of iodide. Co-expression of thyroid peroxidase has recently been demonstrated to augment iodide retention in the cells by iodide organification (63). In addition, a histone deacetylase inhibitor (Trichostatin A) has been reported to increase NIS expression and decrease Pendrin expression (64). In contrast, expression of endogenous NIS in breast cancer can be diagnostically and therapeutically useful (65). Further studies will be needed to investigate the possibility of NIS gene for cancer gene therapy.

CONCLUSIONS

I here summarized the recent articles regarding gene therapy for thyroid cancer. Although there have been tremendous progresses in this field in the last decade, there is unfortunately no published report on clinical trial of gene therapy for thyroid cancer [except one patient treated with ONYX-015 (66)]. Patients with thyroid cancer, particularly those with anaplastic and medullary cancers, will hopefully benefit from gene therapy approach in the near future.

REFERENCES

1. Roth J.A., Cristiano R.J. Gene therapy for cancer: what have we done and where are we going? J Natl Cancer Inst 1997; 89: 21–39.
2. Fagin J.A. Perspective: lesson learned from molecular genetic studies of thyroid cancer – insights into pathogenesis and tumor-specific therapeutic targets. Endocrinology 2002; 143: 2025–2028.
3. Scala S., Portella G., Fedele M., Chiappetta G., Fusco A. Adenovirus-mediated suppression of HMG(Y) protein synthesis as potential therapy of human malignant neoplasias. Proc Natl Acad Sci USA 2000; 97: 4256–4261.
4. Cerutti J., Trapasso F., Battaglia C., Zhang L., Martelli M.L., Visconti R., Berlingieri M.T., Fagin J.A., Santoro M., Fusco A. Block of c-myc expression by antisense oligonucleotides inhibits proliferation of human thyroid carcinoma cell lines. Clin Cancer Res 1996; 2:119–126.
5. Levine A.J. p53, the cellular gatekeeper for growth and division. Cell 1997; 88: 323–331.
6. Fagin J.A., Matsuo K., Karmakar A., Chen D.L., Tang S.H., Koeffler H.P. High prevalence of mutations of the p53 gene in poorly differentiated human thyroid carcinomas. J Clin Invest 1993; 91: 179–184.
7. Donghi R., Longoni A., Pilotti S., Michieri P., Porta G.D., Pierotti M.A. Gene p53 mutations are restricted to poorly differentiated and undifferentiated carcinomas of the thyroid gland. J Clin Invest 1993; 91: 1753–1760.
8. Ito T., Seyama T., Mizuno T., Tsuyama N., Hayashi T., Hayashi Y., Dohi K., Nakamura N., Akiyama M. Unique association of p53 mutations with undifferentiated but not differentiated carcinomas of the thyroid. Cancer Res 1992; 52: 1369–1371.
9. Battista S., Martelli S., Fedele M., Chiappetta G., Trapasso F., De Vita G., Battaglia C., Santoro M., Viglietto G., Fagin J.A. A mutated p53 gene alters thyroid cell differentiation. Oncogene 1995; 16: 2029–2037.
10. Fagin J.A., Tang S.H., Zeki K., Lauro R., Fusco A., Gonsky R. Reexpression of thyroid peroxidase in a derivative of an undifferentiated thyroid carcinoma cell line by introduction of wild-type p53. Cancer Res 1996; 56: 765–771.
11. Morreti F., Farsetti A., Soddu S., Misiti S., Crescenzi M., Filetti S., Andreoli M., Sacchi A., Pontecorvi A. p53 re-expression inhibits proliferation and restores differentiation of human thyroid anaplastic carcinoma cells. Oncogene 1997; 14: 729–740.
12. Yang T.-T., Namba H., Hara T., Takamura N., Nagayama Y., Fukata S., Ishikawa N., Kuma K., Ito K., Yamashita S. p53 induced by ionizing radiation mediates DNA end-jointing activity, but not apoptosis of thyroid cells. Oncogene 1997; 14: 1511–1519.
13. Velasco J.A., Medina D.L., Romero J., Mato M.E., Santisteban P. Introduction of p53 induces cell-cycle arrest in p53-deficient human medullary thyroid-carcinoma cells. Int J Cancer 1997; 73: 449–455.
14. Kim S.-B., Ahn I.-M., Park H.-J., Park J.-S., Cho H.-J., Gong G., Suh C., Lee J.-S., Kim W.-K., Kim S.-H. Growth inhibition and chemosensitivity of poorly differentiated human thyroid cancer cell line (NPA) transfected with p53 gene. Head & Neck 2001; 23: 223–229.
15. Narimatsu M., Nagayama Y., Akino K., Yasuda M., Yamamoto T., Yang T.-T., Ohtsuru A., Namba H., Ayabe H., Yamashita S., Niwa M. Therapeutic usefulness of wild-type *p53* gene introduction in a *p53*-null anaplastic thyroid carcinoma cell line. J Clin Endocrinol Metab 1998; 83: 3668–3672.
16. Nagayama Y., Shigematsu K., Namba H., Zeki K., Yamashita S., Niwa M. Inhibition of angiogenesis and tumorigenesis, and induction of dormancy by p53 in a p53-null thyroid carcinoma cell line in vivo. Anticancer Res 2000; 20: 2723–2728.
17. Blagosklonny M.V., Giannakakou P., Wojtowicz M., Romanova L.Y., Ain K.B., Bates S.E., Fojo T. Effects of p53-expressing adenovirus on the chemosensitivity and differentiation of anaplastic thyroid cancer cells. J Clin Endocrinol Metab 1998; 83: 2516–2522.
18. Nagayama Y., Yokoi H., Takeda K., Hasegawa M., Nishihara E., Namba H., Yamashina S., Niwa M. Adenovirus-mediated tumor suppressor *p53* gene therapy for anaplastic thyroid carcinoma *in vitro* and *in vivo*. J Clin Endocrinol Metab 2000; 85: 4081–4086.
19. Imanishi R., Ohtsuru A., Iwamatsu M., Iioka T., Namba H., Seto S., Yano K., Yamashita S. A histone deacetylase inhibitor enhances killing of undifferentiated thyroid carcinoma cells by p53 gene therapy. J Clin Endocrinol Metab 2002; 87: 4821–4824.
20. Davis B.M., Koc O.N., Lee K., Gerson S.L. Current progress in the gene therapy of cancer. Cur Opin Oncol 1996; 8: 499–508.
21. Nishihara E., Nagayama Y., Watanabe M., Narimatsu M., Namba H., Niwa M., Yamashita S. Treatment of thyroid carcinoma cells with four different suicide gene/prodrug combinations *in vitro*. Anticancer Res 1998; 18: 1521–1526.

22. Nishihara E., Nagayama Y., Mawatari F., Tanaka K., Namba H., Niwa M., Yamashita S. Retrovirus-mediated herpes simplex virus thymidine kinase gene transduction renders human thyroid carcinoma cell lines sensitive to ganciclovir and radiation *in vitro* and *in vivo*. Endocrinology 1997; 138: 4577–4583.
23. van der Eb M.M., Cramer S.J., Vergouwe Y., Schagen F.H., van Krieken J.H., van der Eb A.J., Rinkers I.H., van de Velde C.J., Hoeben R.C. Severe hepatic dysfunction after adenovirus-mediated transfer of the herpes simplex virus thymidine kinase gene and ganciclovir administration. Gene Ther 1998; 5: 451–458.
24. Wallace H., Ledent C., Vassart G., Bishop J.O., Al-Shawi R. Specific ablation of thyroid follicle cells in adult transgenic mice. Endocrinology 1991; 129: 3217–3226.
25. Zeiger M., Takiyama Y., Bishop J.O., Ellison A.R., Saji M., Levine M.A. Adenoviral infection of thyroid cells: a rationale for gene therapy for metastatic thyroid carcinoma. Surgery 1996; 120: 921–925.
26. Braiden V., Nagayama Y., Iitaka M., Namba H., Niwa M., Yamashita S. Retrovirus-mediated suicide gene/prodrug therapy targeting thyroid carcinoma using a thyroid-specific promoter. Endocrinology 1998; 139: 3996–3999.
27. Zhang R., Straus F., DeGroot L.J. Adenoviral-mediated gene therapy for thyroid carcinoma using thymidine kinase controlled by thyroglobulin promoter demonstrates high specificity and low toxicity. Thyroid 2001; 11: 115–123.
28. Zhang R., Straus F.H., DeGroot L.J. Cell-specific viral gene therapy of a Hurthle cell tumor. J Clin Endocrinol Metab 2002; 87:1407–14.
29. Nagayama Y., Nishihara E., Iitaka M., Namba H., Yamashita S., Niwa M. Enhanced efficacy of transcriptionally targeted suicide gene/prodrug therapy for thyroid carcinoma with the Cre-*lox*P system. Cancer Res 1999 59: 3049–3052.
30. Takeda T., Yamazaki M., Minemura K., Imai Y., Inaba H., Suzuki S., Miyamoto T., Ichikawa K., Kakizawa T., Mori J., DeGroot L.J., Hashizume K. A tandemly repeated thyroglobulin core promoter has potential to enhance efficacy for tissue-specific gene therapy for thyroid carcinoma. Cancer Gene Ther 2002; 9: 864–874.
31. Chun Y.S., Saji M., Zeiger M.A. Overexpression of TTF-1 and PAX-8 restores thyroglobulin gene promoter activity in ARO and WRO cell lines. Surgery 1998; 124: 1100–1105.
32. Shimura H., Suzuki H., Miyazaki A., Furuya F., Ohta K., Haraguchi K., Endo T., Onaya T. Transcriptional activation of the thyroglobulin promoter directing suicide gene expression by thyroid transcription factor-1 in thyroid cancer cells. Cancer Res 2001; 61: 3640–3646.
33. Kitazono M., Chuman Y., Aikou T., Fojo T. Construction of gene therapy vectors targeting thyroid cells: enhancement of activity and specificity with histone deacetylase inhibitors and agents modulating the cyclic adenosine 3',5'-monophosphate pathway and demonstration of activity in follicular and anaplastic thyroid carcinoma cells. J Clin Endocrinol Metab 2001; 86: 834–840.
34. Kitazono M., Chuman Y., Aikou T., Fojo T. Adenovirus HSV-TK construct with thyroid-specific promoter: enhancement of activity and specificity with histone deacetylase inhibitors and agents modulating the cAMP pathway. Int J Cancer 2002; 99: 453–459.
35. Zhang R., DeGroot L.J. Gene therapy of established medullary thyroid carcinoma with herpes simplex viral thymidine kinase in a rat tumor model: relationship of bystander effect and antitumor efficacy. Thyroid 2000; 10: 313–319.
36. Minemura K., Takeda T., Minemura K., Nagasawa T., Zhang R., Leopardi R., DeGroot L.J. Cell-specific induction of sensitivity to ganciclovir in medullary thyroid carcinoma cells by adenovirus-mediated gene transfer of herpes simplex virus thymidine kinase. Endocrinology2000; 1814–1822.
37. Soler M.N., Bobe P., Benohoud K., Lemaire G., Roos B.A., Lausson S. Gene therapy of rat medullary thyroid cancer by naked nitric oxide synthase II DNA injection. J Gene Med 2000; 2: 344–352.
38. Lausson S., Fournes B., Borrel C., Milhaud G., Treilhou-Lahille F. Immune response against medullary thyroid carcinoma (MTC) induced by parental and/or interleukin-2-secreting MTC cells in a rat model of human familial MTC. Cancer Immunol Immunother 1996; 43: 116–123.
39. Zhang R., Baunoch D., DeGroot L.J. Genetic immunotherapy for medullary thyroid carcinoma: destruction of tumors in mice by *in vivo* delivery of adenovirus vector transducing the murine interleukin-2 gene. Thyroid 1998; 8: 1137–11464.
40. Zhang R., Minemura K., DeGroot L.J. Immunotherapy for medullary thyroid carcinoma by a replication-defective adenovirus transducing murine IL-2. Endocrinology 1998; 139: 601–608.
41. Zhang R., Straus F.H., DeGroot L.J. Effective genetic therapy of established medullary thyroid carcinomas with murine interleukin -2: dissemination and cytotoxicity studies in a rat model. Endocrinology 1999; 140: 2152–2158.

42. Zhang R., DeGroot L.J. Genetic immunotherapy of established tumours with adenovirus vectors transducing murine interleukin-12 subunits in a rat medullary thyroid carcinoma model. Clin Endocrinol 2000; 52: 687–694.
43. Yamazaki M., Zhang R., Straus F.H., Messina M., Robinson B.G., Hashizume K., DeGroot L.J. Effective gene therapy for medullary thyroid carcinoma using recombinant adenovirus inducing tumor-specific expression of interleukin-12. Gene Therapy 2002; 9: 64–74.
44. Zhang R., DeGroot L.J. Gene therapy of a rat follicular thyroid carcinoma model with adenoviral vectors transducing murine interleukin-12. Endocrinology 2003; 144:1393–8.
45. Soler M.N., Milhaud G., Lekmine F., Treilhou-Lahille F., Klatzmann D., Lausson S. Treatment of medullary thyroid carcinoma by combined expression of suicide and interleukin-2 genes. Cancer Immunol Immunother 1999; 48: 91–99.
46. Zhang R., DeGroot L.J. An adenoviral vector expressing functional heterologous proteins herpes simplex viral thymidine kinase and human interleukin-2 has enhanced *in vivo* antitumor activity against medullar thyroid carcinoma. Endocr Relat Cancer 2001; 8: 315–325.
47. Barzon L., Bonaguro R., Castagliuolo I., Chilosi M., Franchin E., Del Vecchio C., Giaretta I., Boscaro M., Palu G. Gene therapy of thyroid cancer via retrovirally-driven combined expression of human interleukin-2 and herpes simplex virus thymidine kinase. Eur J Endocrinol 2003; 148: 73–80.
48. Haupt K., Siegel F., Lu M., Yang D., Hilken G., Mann K., Roggendorf M., Saller B. Induction of a cellular and humoral immune response against preprocalcitonin by genetic immunization: a potential new treatment for medullary thyroid carcinomas. Endocrinology 2001; 142: 1017–1023.
49. Heise C., Kirn D.H. Replication-selective adenoviruses as oncolytic agents. J Clin Invest 2000; 105: 847–851.
50. Bischoff J.R., Kirn D.H., Willimas A., Heise C., Horn S., Muna M., Ng L., Nye J.A., Sampson-Johannes A., Fattaey A., McCormick F. An adenovirus mutant that replicates selectively in p53-deficient human tumor cells. Science 1996; 274: 373–376.
51. Portella G., Scala S., Vitagliano D., Vecchio G., Fusco A. ONYX-015, an E1B gene-defective adenovirus, induces cell death in human anaplastic thyroid carcinoma cell lines. J Clin Endocrinol Metab 2002; 87: 2525–2531.
52. Nagayama Y., Nishihara E., Namba H., Yokoi H., Hasegawa M., Mizuguchi H., Hayakawa T., Yamashita S., Niwa M. Targeting the replication of adenovirus to *p53*-defective thyroid carcinoma with a *p53*-regulated Cre-*lox*P system. Cancer Gene Ther 2001; 8: 36–44.
53. Prabakaran I., Kesmodel S.B., Menon C., Molnar-Kimber K., Fraker D.L. A replication-selective adenoviral vector driven by the human Tg promoter-enhancer is selective for Tg+ thyroid cancer cells. Abstract for 93rd Annual Meeting of American Association for Cancer Research 2002;43: #3782.
54. Hermiston T.W., Kuhn I. Armed therapeutic viruses: strategies and challenges to arming oncolytic viruses with therapeutic genes. Cancer Gene Ther 2002; 9: 1022–1035.
55. Kong H.-L., Crystal R.G. Gene therapy strategies for tumor antiangiogenesis. J Natl Cancer Inst 1998; 90: 273–286.
56. Dai G., Levy O., Carrasco N. Cloning and characterization of the thyroid iodide transporter. Nature 1996; 379: 458–460.
57. Scott V.C., Wang R., Kreman T.M., Sheffield V.C., Karnishki L.P. The Pendred syndrome gene encodes a chloride-iodide transporter. Nat Genet 1999; 21: 440–443.
58. Spitzweg C., Harrington K.J., Pinke L.A., Vile R.G., Morris J.C. The sodium iodide symporter and its potential role in cancer therapy. J Clin Endocrinol Metab 2001; 86: 3327–3335.
59. Heufelder A.E., Morgenthaler N., Schipper M.L., Joba W. Sodium iodide symporter-based strategies for diagnosis and treatment of thyroid and nonthyroid malignancies. Thyroid 2001; 11: 839–847.
60. Shimura H., Haraguchi K., Miyazaki A., Endo T., Onaya T. Iodide uptake and experimental ^{131}I therapy in transplanted undifferentiated thyroid cancer cells expressing the Na$^+$/I$^-$ symporter gene. Endocrinology 1997; 138: 4493–4496.
61. Spitzweg C., O'Connor M.K., Bergert E.R., Tindall D.J., Young C.Y.F., Morris J.C. Treatment of prostate cancer by radioiodine therapy after tissue-specific expression of the sodium iodide symporter. Cancer Res 2000; 60: 6526–6530.
62. Cho J.-Y., Shen D.H.Y., Yang W., Williams B., Buckwalter T.L.F., La Perle K.M.D., Hinkle G., Pozderac R., Kloos R., Nagaraja H.N., Barth R.F., Jhiang S.M. In vivo imaging and radioiodide therapy following sodium iodide symporter gene transfer in animal model of intracerebral gliomas. Gene Ther 2002; 9: 1139–1145.
63. Huang M., Batra R.K., Kogai T., Lin Y.Q., Hershman J.M., Lichtenstein A., Sharma S., Zhu L.X., Brent G.A., Dubinett S.M. Ectopic expression of the thyroperoxidase gene augments radioiodide uptake

and retention mediated by the sodium iodide symporter in non-small cell lung cancer. Cancer Gene Ther 2001; 8: 612–618.
64. Zarnegar R., Brunaud L., Kanauchi H., Wong M., Fung M., Ginzinger D., Duh Q.Y., Clark O.H. Increasing the effectiveness of radioactive iodine therapy in the treatment of thyroid cancer using Trichostatin A, a histone deacetylase inhibitor. Surgery 2002; 132: 984–90.
65. Tazebay U.H., Wapnir I.L., Levy O., Dohan O., Zuckier L.S., Hhua Zhao Q., Fu Deng H., Amenta P.S., Fineberg S., Pestell R.G., Carrasco N. The mammary gland iodide transporter is expressed during lactation and in breast cancer. Nat Med 2000; 6: 871–878.
66. Nemunaitis J., Cunningham C., Buchanan A., Blackburn A., Edelman G., Maples P., Netto G., Tong A., Randlev B., Olson S., Kirn D. Intravenous infusion of a replication-selective adenovirus (ONYX-015) in cancer patients: safety, feasibility and biological activity. Gene Ther 2001; 8: 746–759.

22. FAMILIAL PAPILLARY THYROID CARCINOMA

CARL D. MALCHOFF, M.D., PH.D. AND DIANA M. MALCHOFF, PH.D.
University of Connecticut Health Center, 263 Farmington Avenue Farmington, CT 06030

INTRODUCTION

Prior to 2000 papillary thyroid carcinoma (PTC) was considered by most to be a sporadic disorder without familial predisposition. In contrast to this traditional teaching and as understood early on by Dr. Nadir Farid [1], approximately 5 percent of all PTC are familial. The evidence that supports this familial susceptibility is reviewed here and potential clinical implications are discussed. In addition, PTC may be a relatively infrequent component of other familial tumor syndromes. Although recent findings strongly support a familial PTC predisposition, the final proof will require the identification of the susceptibility genes. There is not yet convincing evidence to suggest that other nonmedullary thyroid carcinomas (follicular thyroid carcinoma, anaplastic thyroid carcinoma, and insular thyroid carcinoma) are familial.

EVIDENCE FOR AN INHERITED SUSCEPTIBILITY TO PTC

It is reasonable to suggest that any malignancy may have a familial predisposition. Cancer is caused by multiple gene mutations that are acquired over time by the cancer progenitor cell. Although these are usually somatic mutations, it would not be surprising if the first gene mutation was inherited (germline mutation). Family members possessing this hypothetical gene mutation would be at increased risk for developing PTC. Such a hypothetical susceptibility gene could persist in the population. It takes years to decades for the thyroid cancer progenitor cell to develop into a malignancy, since it must acquire other necessary gene mutations. Even then the malignancy is slow growing. If such an inherited gene mutation did not disrupt other essential functions, then those individuals carrying this susceptibility gene mutation would not be at any reproductive disadvantage. By chance alone the gene mutation could persist within a population. Therefore, one can make a theoretical argument that a familial predisposition to PTC may occur.

Epidemiological studies, pedigree analysis, and pathology studies all provide evidence for a familial susceptibility to PTC. Although no single type of study is sufficient to prove a familial susceptibility, taken as a whole, the evidence is strong. This evidence led investigators with access to large kindreds to perform linkage studies that further support a familial predisposition to this disorder. Interestingly, the linkage studies suggest that familial PTC (fPTC) is a heterogeneous disorder caused by more than one susceptibility gene.

Epidemiologic studies have consistently found that first-degree relatives of those with PTC have a 4 to 10 fold increased risk of PTC [2–7]. Most other malignancies in these same studies do not show this familial association. Therefore, it seems unlikely that the observed PTC association is due to an ascertainment bias. Other interpretations of this association include a predisposition caused by an environmental exposure. It seems unlikely that this would be an unusual environmental factor such as radioactive iodine released from nuclear tests, since the association has been observed in multiple studies on different continents and is not limited to populations with the greatest exposure to radiation. This does not exclude the possibility that the susceptibility gene may act by increasing the risk of malignancy as a result of exposure to a more common environmental factor.

A number of large kindreds with fPTC have been described [8–15]. These kindreds are further evidence for a familial predisposition to PTC. Against this interpretation, it can be argued that these kindreds represent the rare association of multiple sporadic thyroid carcinomas, and that the number of affected family members has been exaggerated by ascertainment bias. That is, once two family members have been identified an aggressive search for thyroid carcinoma in other family members may identify microscopic (<1 cm) papillary thyroid carcinomas that have no clinical significance, and, as opposed to large PTC (>1 cm), are relatively common at post mortem examination. However, this is probably not the case, since the PTC within kindreds differs from sporadic PTC in two subtle characteristics. First, fPTC generally presents at a younger age than sporadic disease [16]. Second, there is a greater prevalence of multifocal disease in fPTC than in sporadic PTC [16, 17]. Multifocal disease within the thyroid suggests that a predisposing factor (possibly an inherited genetic susceptibility) is present. Finally, analyses of large kindreds with genetic linkage studies have identified statistically significant associations of PTC with specific chromosomal regions, and these are discussed in the next section. For all these reasons it seems likely the familial association of PTC does not represent the rare association of sporadic PTC, but represents a true familial predisposition.

In summary, the epidemiologic observation of an increased incidence of PTC in first degree relatives of PTC subjects, the presence of large kindreds in which affected members have a tendency to develop PTC at a relatively young age, and the pathologic finding of multifocality taken together suggest that some cases of PTC are caused by an inherited susceptibility gene mutation. It should be noted that others have interpreted these results to suggest that the familial clustering of PTC indicates that fPTC is a polygenic disease caused by relatively more common but less disruptive gene polymorpisms when the associate by chance in a single kindred [18]. These two hypotheses are not mutually exclusive.

LINKAGE ANALYSIS AND THE CHROMOSOMAL LOCI OF PUTATIVE FPTC SUSCEPTIBILITY GENES

Many tumor susceptibility genes are discovered through the genetic analysis of large kindreds. Genetic analysis is particularly useful for identifying tumor susceptibility genes that were of unknown function. The first step in this genetic analysis is to determine the chromosomal location of the tumor susceptibility gene by linkage analysis.

Linkage analysis has been applied to large fPTC kindreds and statistically significant linkage of fPTC to specific chromosomal regions has been identified (Table 1). In linkage studies a statistically significant association is generally agreed to occur when the odds ratio of the probability of affected subjects carrying the same genetic polymorphism and unaffected subjects not carrying this polymorphism is one in one thousand or greater. The results are summarized as a log of the odds ratio or LOD score, so that a LOD score of 3.0 or greater is considered statistically significant. Interestingly the results between studies are discordant suggesting more than one susceptibility gene.

A large kindred with fPTC and benign thyroid nodules with the distinct pathologic finding of eosinophilia (TCO) has been mapped to 19p13.2 with a maximum LOD score of 3.0 [19]. Eosinophilia refers to the staining of the cytosol by eosin, is often caused by a large cytoplasmic population of mitochondria, and in the thyroid these are often referred to as Hurthle cells. Interestingly, other fPTC kindreds also link to this region (19p13), but the fPTC in these kindreds were not associated with eosinophilia [20]. Since the tumors of these fPTC kindreds are pathologically distinct, it is possible that there are two different susceptibility genes at this locus. Alternatively, there may be a single susceptibility gene this locus and an additional modifier gene contributes to the eosinophilia in one kindred.

Table 1. Familial papillary thyroid carcinoma—summary of linkage analyses

Disorder	Clinical description	Linkage locus	Reference
TCO	Oxyphilic PTC and benign oxyphilic nodules Autosomal Dominant with Partial Penetrance	19p13.2	[19]
PTC at 19p13	PTC without oxyphilia Autosomal dominant	19p13	[20]
FNMTC	Autosomal Dominant with Partial Penetrance	2q21	[21]
fPTC/PRN	PTC enriched with PRN Autosomal Dominant with Partial Penetrance	1q21	[22]

In another group of 80 fPTC kindreds a familial nonmedullary thyroid cancer susceptibility gene referred to as *FNMTC* has been mapped to the long arm of chromosome 2 (2q21). The maximum multipoint LOD score in all families was 3.07, and this increased to 4.17, when the 17 pedigrees with the follicular variant of PTC were analyzed alone [21]. As with the previous linkage analysis, the susceptibility gene at this locus has not been identified.

Our studies identified the familial association of PTC and papillary renal neoplasia PRN (both adenomas and carcinomas) in a large kindred. This disorder, which is designated fPTC/PRN (OMIM #605642), has been mapped to the long arm of chromosome 1 (1q21) with a multipoint single kindred LOD score of 3.58 [22]. Therefore, this syndrome is both clinically and genetically distinct from other fPTC disorders. There are a number of other neoplasms in this large kindred including benign thyroid adenomas, germ cell neoplasms premenopausal breast carcinomas and renal oncocytoma that occur in subjects that carry the affected allele. Unfortunately there are not enough genetically affected individuals to determine if these non-PTC neoplasms are components of the fPTC/PRN syndrome with low penetrance, or if they are just sporadic events in a large kindred. In this regard, it is of interest that epidemiology studies have identified an increased incidence of premenopausal breast carcinoma in PTC subjects [23]. One interpretation of this finding is that the use of I-131 in thyroid carcinoma subjects predisposes to breast carcinoma. Alternatively, our results support the hypothesis that an inherited susceptibility is responsible for this association. It may be that the *fPTC/PRN* gene predisposes to other malignancies.

Frequently sporadic tumors and familial tumors may be caused by mutations of the same susceptibility genes. For example, activating *RET* mutations are inherited in multiple endocrine neoplasia type 2 and develop spontaneously in sporadic medullary thyroid carcinoma. We have reviewed of the gene abnormalities of sporadic PTC to determine if these occur in genes that map to the linkage regions of the familial PTC syndromes. The neurotrophic tyrosine kinase receptor type 1 (NTRK1; *TRK; TRKA*) that is located at 1q23.1 and *RET* that is located at 10q11.2 are both rearranged in sporadic PTC. These rearrangements effect illicit expression of these tyrosine kinases in the thyroid follicular cell. Activating *BRAF* (7q34) mutations also occur in sporadic PTC [24] and activating mutations of *hRAS* occur in sporadic follicular thyroid neoplasms [25]. Other genes contributing to the pathogenesis of follicular neoplasms include *PTEN* (10q23.31), *PAX8* (2q13), and *PPARG1* (3p25). Of these seven genes, *PAX8*, *hRAS* and *TRK* are potential candidates for fPTC based upon their chromosomal location. The sequence analysis of *PAX8* in the FNMTC kindreds that map to 2q21 has not been reported. Completion of the human genome project indicates that *TRK* is telomeric to the *fPTC/PRN* locus. Therefore, it is not the *fPTC/PRN* susceptibility gene. Sequence analysis of *hRAS* in fPTC/PRN indicates that the known activating mutation of *hRAS* does not cause this disorder [26]. Interestingly LOH, normally a rare event in PTC, has been observed in about 10 percent of sporadic PTC in the region near 1q21 [27]. This finding suggests that there may be a tumor suppressor gene for

PTC at the *fPTC/PRN* locus at 1q21. In summary, the genes causing sporadic PTC are not located within the fPTC loci, suggesting that the fPTC genes are distinct from the genes that cause sporadic PTC.

CLINICAL FEATURES OF fPTC AND IMPLICATIONS FOR PATIENT CARE

The clinical features of fPTC are beginning to emerge and are compared with the clinical features of sporadic PTC in Table 2. Loh first summarized the clinical features based upon a review of available published kindreds [16]. A more recent study from Japan has reported similar results [17]. Although these results are probably reliable, final confirmation of their accuracy must await the identification of the fPTC susceptibility genes, so that the genetically affected individuals can be unequivocally distinguished from those that are genetically unaffected.

The evaluation of large kindreds suggests that inheritance is autosomal dominant with partial penetrance, although it is possible that modifying genes play an important role. As with sporadic PTC, women are affected more frequently than men. Multifocal disease is more common in fPTC than in sporadic PTC, and the age of onset is somewhat younger in fPTC (mean = 38 y) than in sporadic PTC (mean = 48 y) [16, 28]. However, Uchino did not find an age difference between familial and sporadic PTC [17]. There seems to be a greater incidence of benign thyroid nodules associated with fPTC than with sporadic PTC [17]. There may be other malignancies associated with fPTC. Epidemiologic studies suggest an increased incidence of breast carcinoma in individuals with PTC [23], and one large kindred with fPTC is enriched in PRN and possibly other malignancies [9]. Although it has been, suggested that fPTC may be more aggressive than sporadic PTC [30], the differences on a whole seem to be modest. There are occasional kindreds in which fPTC seems to be more aggressive than sporadic PTC with some subjects dieing from this disorder. A more recent study does suggest a greater incidence of recurrent disease with fPTC than with sporadic PTC, but no increased incidence of death [17].

Two known familial tumor syndromes are associated with an increased incidence of PTC [29]. The frequency of PTC in familial adenomatous polyposis (FAP) is about

Table 2. Clinical characteristics of familial and sporadic papillary thyroid carcinoma (approximate ratios and percentages)

Characteristic	Familial PTC	Sporadic PTC
Age of Onset	mean = 38 [16]	mean 45–50 [28]
	mean = 49.1	mean 48.5 [17]
Female:Male Ratio	2:1 [16]	3:1 [16]
Multifocal PTC	41% [17]	29% [17]
Recurrence	16% [17]	10% [17]
Death	rare	rare
Benign thyroid nodules	42% [17]	30% [17]
Associated malignancies	papillary renal neplasia (selected kindreds) [29]	? breast carcinoma [23]

10 times as great as the incidence expected for sporadic PTC. In the Cowden syndrome (multiple hamartoma syndrome) there is an increased incidence breast carcinoma, follicular thyroid carcinoma, and to a lesser degree PTC.

The clinical characteristics of fPTC may modify the evaluation and treatment of fPTC patients. Clinicians should review the family history carefully in subjects with PTC, since it is anticipated that about 5 percent of all PTC subjects will have a familial predisposition to this disorder. FAP and the Cowden syndrome should be excluded. There is no role for prophylactic thyroidectomy as there is in the MEN2 syndromes, since fPTC usually is a relatively slow growing malignancy rate and since asymptomatic carriers cannot be unequivocally identified. Unfortunately, except in the very largest kindreds, genetic studies will not help to identify asymptomatic carriers. We do know that any kindred members with affected first-degree relatives are at 50 percent risk of carrying the susceptibility gene. There is debate as to how aggressively these individuals at risk should be followed. Children do not need to be followed closely, since PTC rarely occurs before puberty. After puberty, yearly neck examinations are a reasonable screening tool. Some clinicians prefer to perform an ultrasound examination of the thyroid in addition to the physical examination. The disadvantage of this approach is that it is likely to identify minor abnormalities that have little clinical significance, but, because of a strong family history, may lead to unnecessary thyroidectomy. For now, the use of ultrasound for screening should be left to the discretion of the individual clinician.

SUMMARY AND CONCLUSIONS

Over the last decade, several lines of evidence have been accumulated that support the existence of fPTC susceptibility genes. Preliminary clinical characteristics of fPTC have been identified, and linkage studies have identified the chromosomal locations of putative fPTC susceptibility genes. A logical clinical approach to fPTC is emerging.

REFERENCES

1. Farid, N.R., Y. Shi, and M. Zou, 1994, Molecular basis of thyroid cancer. Endo Rev, 15: 202–232.
2. Galanti, M.R., A. Ekbom, L. Grimelius, and J. Yuen, 1997, Parental cancer and risk of papillary and follicular thyroid carcinoma. British J of Cancer, 75: 451–456.
3. Goldgar, D.E., D.F. Easton, L.A. Cannon-Albright, and M.H. Skolnick, 1994, Systematic population-based assessment of cancer risk in first-degree relatives of cancer probands. J Natl Cancer Inst, 86: 1600–1608.
4. Hemminki, K. and C. Dong, 2000, Familial relationships in thyroid cancer by histolopathological type. Int J Cancer, 85: 201–205.
5. Pal, T., F.D. Vogl, P.O. Chappuis, R. Tsang, J. Brierley, H. Renard, K. Sanders, T. Kantemiroff, S. Bagah, D.E. Goldgar, S.A. Narod, and W.D. Foulkes, 2001, Increased risk for nonmedullary thyroid cancer in the first degree relatives of prevalent cases of nonmedullary thyroid cancer: A hospital-based study. J Clin Endocrinol Metab, 86: 5307–5312.
6. Ron, E., R.A. Kleinerman, J.D. Boice, V.A. LiVolsi, J.T. Flannery, and J.F. Fraumeni, 1987, A population-based case-control study of thyroid cancer. J Natl Cancer Inst, 79: 1–12.
7. Hrafnkelsson, J., H. Tulinius, J.G. Jonasson, G.U. Olafsdottir, and H. Sigvaldason, 2001, Familial nonmedullary thyroid cancer in iceland. J Med Genet, 38: 189–192.
8. Stoffer, S.S., D.L. Van Dyke, J.V. Bach, W. Szpunar, and L. Weiss, 1986, Familial papillary carcinoma of the thyroid. Am. J. Med. Genet., 25: 775–782.

9. Malchoff, D., M. Sarfarazi, B. Tendler, F. Forouhar, G. Whalen, and C. Malchoff, 1999, Familial papillary thyroid carcinoma is genetically distinct from familial adenomatous polyposis coli. Thyroid, 9: 247–252.
10. Lote, K., K. Andersen, E. Nordal, and I.O. Brennhovd, 1980, Familial occurrence of papillary thyroid carcinoma. Cancer, 46: 1291–1297.
11. Fischer, D.K., M.D. Groves, S.J. Thomas, and P.C. Johnson, 1989, Papillary carcinoma of the thyroid: Additional evidence in support of a familial component. Cancer Investigation, 7: 323–5.
12. Flannigan, G.M., R.P. Clifford, M. Winslet, D.A.S. Lawrence, and R.V. Fiddian, 1983, Simultaneous presentation of papillary carcinoma of thyroid in a father and son. Br J Surg, 70: 181–2.
13. Kobayashi, K., Y. Tanaka, S. Ishiguro, T. Mori, Y. Mitani, and C. Shigemasa, 1995, Family with nonmedullary thyroid neoplasms. J Surg Oncology 7, 58: 274–77.
14. Burgess, J.R., A. Duffield, S.J. Wilkinson, R. Ware, T.M. Greenaway, J. Percival, and L. Hoffman, 1997, Two families with an autosomal dominant inheritance pattern for papillary carcinoma of the thyroid. J Clin Endocrinol Metab, 82: 345–348.
15. Ozaki, O., K. Ito, K. Kobayashi, A. Suzuki, Y. Manabe, and Y. Hosoda, 1988, Familial occurrence of differentiated, nonmedullary thyroid carcinoma. World J Surg, 12: 565–71.
16. Loh, K.-C., 1997, Familial nonmedullary thyroid carcinoma: A meta-review of case series. Thyroid, 7: 107–113.
17. Uchino, S., S. Noguchi, H. Kawamoto, S. Watanabe, H. Yamashita, and S. Shutok, 2002, Familial nonmedullary thyroid carcinoma characterized by multifocality and a high recurrence rate in a large study population. World J Surg., 26: 897–902.
18. Links, T., K. van Tol, G. Meerman, and E. de Vries, 2001, Differentiated thyroid carcinoma: A polygenic disease. Thyroid, 11: 1135–40.
19. Canzian, F., P. Amati, R. Harach, J.-L. Kraimps, F. Lesueur, J. Barbier, P. Levillain, G. Romeo, and D. Bonneau, 1998, A gene predisposing to familial thyroid tumors with cell oxyphilia maps to chromosome 19p13.2. Am J Hum Genet, 63: 1743–1748.
20. Bevan, S., T. Pal, C.R. Greenberg, H. Green, J. Wixey, G. Bignell, S.A. Narod, W.D. Foulkes, M.R. Stratton, and R.S. Houlston, 2001, A comprehensive analysis of mng1, tco1, fPTC, pten, tshr and trka in familial nonmedullary thyroid cancer: Confirmation of linkage to tco1. J Clin Endocrinol Metab, 86: 3701–3704.
21. McKay, J.D., F. Lesueur, L. Jonard, A. Pastore, J. Williamson, L. Hoffman, J. Burgess, A. Duffield, M. Papotti, M. Stark, H. Sobol, B. Maes, A. Murat, H. Kaariainen, M. Bertholon-Gregoire, M. Zini, M.A. Rossing, M.-E. Toubert, F. Bonichon, M. Cavarec, A.-M. Bernard, A. Boneu, F. Leprat, O. Haas, C. Lasset, M. Schlumberger, F. Canzian, D.E. Goldgar, and R. Romeo, 2001, Localization of a susceptibility gene for familial nonmedullary thyroid carcinoma to chromosome 2q21. Am J Hum Genet, 69: 440–446.
22. Malchoff, C.D., M.S. Sarfarazi, B. Tendler, F. Forouhar, G. Whalen, V. Joshi, A. Arnold, and D.M. Malchoff, 2000, Papillary thyroid carcinoma associated with papillary renal neoplasia: Genetic linkage analysis of a distinct heritable tumor syndrome. J Clin Endocrinol Metab, 85: 1758–1764.
23. Chen, A.Y., L. Levy, H. Goepfert, B.W. Brown, M.R. Spitz, and R. Vassilopoulou-Sellin, 2001, Development of breast carcinoma in women with thyroid carcinoma. Cancer, 92: 225–231.
24. Kimura, E.T., M.N. Nikiforova, Z. Zhu, J.A. Knauf, Y.E. Nikiforov, and J.A. Fagin, 2003, High prevalence of braf mutations in thyroid cancer. Cancer Research, 63: 1454–1457.
25. Suarez, H.G., J.A. du Villard, M. Severino, B. Caillou, M. Schlumberger, M. Tubiana, C. Parmentier, and R. Monier, 1990, Presence of mutations in all three ras genes in human thyroid tumors. Oncogene, 5: 565–570.
26. Malchoff, D.M., V. Joshi, B. Tendler, G. Whalen, and C.D. Malchoff. The syndrome of familial papillary thyroid carcinoma with papillary renal neoplasia: Evaluation of linked candidate genes. in The Endocrine Society's 82nd annual Meeting. 2000. Toronto, Ontario: The Endocrine Society Press.
27. Bieche, I., E. Ruffet, A. Zweibaum, F. Vilde, R. Lidereau, and B. Franc, 1997, Muc1 mucin gene transcripts, and protein in adenomas and papillary carcinomas of the thyroid. Thyroid, 7: 725–31.
28. Schlumberger, M.J., 1998, Papillary and follicular thyroid carcinoma. New Engl J Med, 338: 297–306.
29. Malchoff, C.D. and D.M. Malchoff, 2002, Genetics of familial nonmedullary thyroid carcinoma. J Clin Endocrinol Metab, 87: 2455–59.
30. Grossman, R.F., S.-H. Tu, Q.-Y. Duh, A.E. Siperstein, F. Novosolov, and O.H. Clark, 1995, Familial nonmedullary thyroid cancer: An emerging entity that warrants aggressive treatment. Arch. Surg., 130: 892–899.

23. RET ACTIVATION IN MEDULLARY CARCINOMAS

MARCO A. PIEROTTI, ELENA ARIGHI, DEBORA DEGL'INNOCENTI,
MARIA GRAZIA BORRELLO

Istituto Nazionale Tumori, Department of Experimental Oncology Operative Unit #3.
Via G. Venezian, 1 20133 Milan Italy

INTRODUCTION

RET gene encodes a receptor tyrosine kinase acting as the subunit of a multimolecular complex that binds four distinct ligands and activates a signaling network crucial for neural and kidney development.

Different alterations of *RET* are associated to five diseases. *RET* is the susceptibility gene for the inherited cancer syndrome multiple endocrine neoplasia type 2 (MEN2), which includes MEN2A, MEN2B and familial medullary thyroid carcinoma (FMTC), as well as a major susceptibility gene for the syndrome characterized by the congenital absence of enteric ganglia, the Hirschsprung's disease (HSCR). Finally, somatic tumor-specific rearrangements of RET gene, which originate constitutively activated fused proteins, have been found in a consistent fraction of papillary thyroid carcinomas.

This review focuses on *RET* alterations in medullary thyroid carcinoma, a rare malignancy of thyroid gland present either in sporadic or MEN2-associated hereditary forms.

RET

RET gene and RET proteins

The human *RET* gene is located on chromosome 10q11.2 (Ishizaka, Y. et al., 1989) and comprises 21 exons. Homologues of *RET* have been identified in higher and lower vertebrates, as well as in *Drosophila melanogaster* (Hahn, M. et al., 2001).

Table 1. *RET* related pathologies

Disease	Genetic alteration	Pathogenic mechanism
PTCs	Chromosomal rearrangements	Constitutive TK activity
MEN2A	Germline point mutations in the Cys-rich domain	Constitutive disulfide linked dimerization
MEN2B	Germline point mutations in RET TK domain	Altered substrate specificity Constitutive TK activity
FMTC	Germline point mutations: – in the Cys-rich domain – in RET TK domain	 Constitutive dimerization Constitutive TK activity? Altered substrate specificity?
HSCR	Germline mutations (deletions, insertions, frame shift, nonsense or missense): – in RET extracellular domain – in RET TK domain – in RET C-terminus	 Impairment of RET cell surface expression Partial loss of RET TK activity Impairment of binding of docking proteins

RET gene was identified in 1985 as a novel oncogene, following transfection of NIH3T3 cells with DNA from a human T-cell lymphoma (Takahashi, M. et al., 1985). The transforming gene resulted from a recombination event between two unlinked DNA sequences, which occurred during the transfection process; hence the name *RET*, for '*re*arranged during *t*ransfection'. The resulting chimaeric gene encoded a fusion protein comprising an amino-terminal region that displayed a putative zinc finger motif fused to a tyrosine kinase domain. Subsequently, the name *RET* has been retained to designate the gene coding for the tyrosine kinase protein of the fused oncogene. Rearrangements of *RET* with different genes are found frequently in papillary thyroid carcinomas (RET/PTCs) (Grieco, M. et al., 1990; Santoro, M. et al., 1992). On the other hand gain-of-function mutations of *RET* cause sporadic thyroid and adrenal cancers (Lindor, N. M. et al., 1994; Beldjord, C. et al., 1995; Komminoth, P. et al., 1996) as well as cancer syndromes, such as multiple endocrine neoplasia types 2A and 2B (MEN2A and MEN2B) and familial medullary thyroid carcinoma (FMTC) (reviewed in Mulligan, L. M. et al., 1995a; Goodfellow, P. J. et al., 1995; Pasini, B. et al., 1996). Interestingly, loss-of-function mutations of the same RET gene cause Hirschsprung's disease (HSCR) or colonic aganglionosis (reviewed in Amiel, J. et al., 2001) (Table 1).

RET encodes a transmembrane tyrosine kinase displaying a structure similar to that of other receptor tyrosine kinases (RTKs), comprising extracellular, transmembrane and cytoplasmic domains.

The large extracellular portion, preceded by a typical cleavable signal sequence of 28 aminoacids, has no similarity with other RTKs and contains a conserved cysteine-rich region close to the cellular membrane and a more distal region with homology to the cadherin family of cell adhesion molecules (Takahashi, M. et al., 1988; Schneider, R., 1992; Iwamoto, T. et al., 1993; Takahashi, M. et al., 1989). Cadherins are Ca^{2+}-dependent cell—cell adhesion proteins and their adhesive properties depend on a domain of about 110 amino acids tandemly repeated in the extracellular region. RET

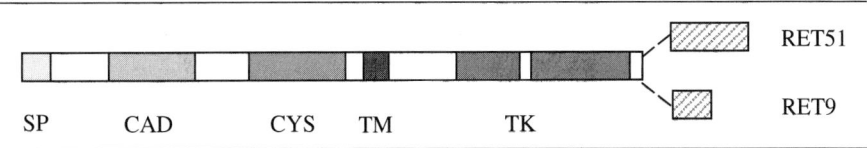

Figure 1. RET protein.
Schematic representation of the two RET isoforms, RET9 and RET51, with the signal peptide (SP), cadherin-like (CAD), cysteine-rich (CYS), transmembrane (TM), and tyrosine kinase (TK) domains.

comprises four tandemly repeated cadherin-like domains and binds specifically to Ca^{2+} ions (Anders, J. et al., 2001), supporting the hypothesis of RET as a distant member of the cadherin superfamily. RET is the only member of this superfamily containing an intrinsic tyrosine kinase domain, suggesting that RET may have arisen by the recombination of an ancestral cadherin with a protein-tyrosine kinase (Anders, J. et al., 2001).

Twenty seven of 28 cysteine (Cys) residues in the cysteine-rich domain are conserved among species suggesting a critical role for these residues in formation of intramolecular disulfide bonds and thus in determining the tertiary structure of RET proteins (Takahashi, M. et al., 1988; Iwamoto, T. et al., 1993). A single transmembrane domain of RET is followed by an evolutionary conserved tyrosine kinase (TK) domain, which is interrupted by a 27 amino acids kinase insert (Takahashi, M. et al., 1987).

The *RET* gene is alternatively spliced to yield two main protein isoforms of 1072 (RET9 or short isoform) or 1114 (RET51 or long isoform) amino acids (Tahira, T. et al., 1990) differing at the C-terminus region, by displaying 9 or 51 unrelated aminoacids (Figure 1). The RET9 and RET51 isoforms are evolutionary highly conserved over a broad range of species, suggesting that distinct isoforms can exert different roles in physiological functions of RET (Carter, M. T. et al., 2001).

RET is the signaling component of a multiprotein receptor complex involving members of two distinct groups of proteins: a soluble ligand belonging to the glial cell line-derived neurotrophic factor (GDNF) family and a glycosyl-phosphatidylinositol (GPI)-membrane anchored co-receptor belonging to GDNF family receptor α (GFRα). RET remained an orphan receptor until 1996 when GDNF was identified as the ligand of RET (Durbec, P. et al., 1996; Trupp, M. et al., 1996; Vega, Q. C. et al., 1996; Treanor, J. J. et al., 1996). Four members in the GDNF family ligands have now been characterized: Glial cell line-derived neurotrophic factor (GDNF), neurturin (NRTN), artemin (ARTN) and persephin (PSPN) (Figure 2). They represent a new subclass of the transforming growth factor-β (TGF-β) superfamily. They are secreted as disulfide-linked dimers, function as homodimers and are all neuronal survival factors (reviewed in Baloh, R. H. et al., 2000; Saarma, M., 2000). GFRα molecules do not display intracellular domains but are anchored to the cell membrane via a glycosyl-phosphatidylinositol (GPI) linkage. The ligands GDNF, neurturin, artemin and persephin use GFRα1, GFRα2, GFRα3 and GFRα4, as the preferred receptors, respectively (reviewed in Airaksinen, M. S. et al., 2002).

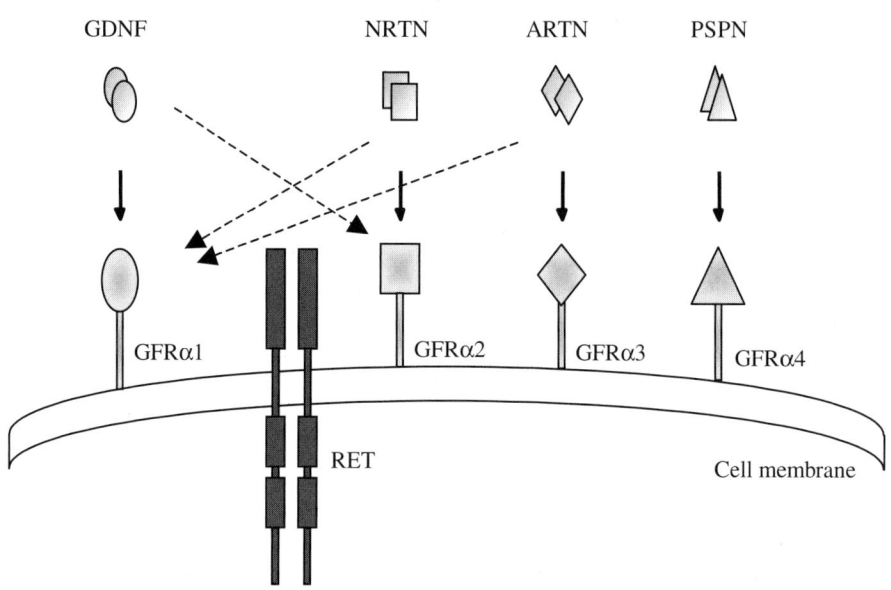

Figure 2. GDNF family ligands with their receptors.
Homodimeric GDNF family ligands activate the transmembrane RET tyrosine kinase by binding with high affinity to different GPI-linked GFRα receptors. Binding of ligand-GFRα complex to RET triggers its homodimerization, phosphorylation and intracellular signaling. The complete lines represent preferred functional binding; dotted lines may not be significant *in vivo*.

The GDNF and GFRα family members show both distinct and overlapping expression patterns (Baloh, R. H. et al., 2000), suggesting that activation of RET by formation of ligand-receptor complexes is a tightly regulated process. GDNF can also signal via GFRα1 in a RET-independent manner (Poteryaev, D. et al., 1999; Trupp, M. et al., 1999). It was recently demonstrated that in hippocampal and cortical neurons GDNF/GFRα1 make a complex with neural cell adhesion molecule (NCAM) and induce activation of Fyn and FAK promoting migration and axonal growth independently of RET (Paratcha, G. et al., 2003).

Role of RET signaling during development

The RET signaling has a critical role in the development of the enteric nervous system (ENS) and kidney, as attested by the similar and peculiar phenotype of mice with null mutations in *RET, GDNF* and *GFRα* genes. They all show severe defects in enteric innervation and renal differentiation (Schuchardt, A. et al., 1994; Sanchez, M. P. et al., 1996; Cacalano, G. et al., 1998). During vertebrate embryogenesis *RET* is expressed in the developing excretory system, in all lineages of the peripheral nervous system (PNS) and in motor and catecholaminergic neurons of the central system (CNS), including ventral midbrain dopaminergic neurons (Avantaggiato, V. et al., 1994; Durbec, P. et al., 1996; Marcos, C. et al., 1996; Pachnis, V. et al., 1993; Trupp, M. et al., 1997; Tsuzuki, T.

et al., 1995; Young, H. M. et al., 1998). Despite the widespread expression of *RET* in the nervous system of vertebrates, mutations of this locus affect, albeit drastically, only a subset of PNS ganglia. Thus, loss of function mutations of *RET* in humans lead to Hirschsprung's disease, a condition characterized by the absence of enteric ganglia from the terminal colon (Edery, P. et al., 1994; Romeo, G. et al., 1994).

Organ culture experiments and transgenic approaches have shown that RET signaling triggered by GDNF is essential for the initial ureteric budding and subsequent branching of kidney during mammalian embryogenesis (reviewed in Sariola, H. et al., 1999). In the mammalian kidney, the ureteric bud (UB), which expresses RET, induces epithelial differentiation of the nephrogenic mesenchyme, which expresses GDNF and, in turn, promotes branching of the bud. The co-receptor GFRα is expressed by both the nephrogenic mesenchyme and the UB. Thus, GDNF/RET signaling regulates the reciprocal inductive interactions between the UB and the nephrogenic mesenchyme. Recent data indicate that only RET9 seems to be critically important for kidney morphogenesis and enteric nervous system development, whereas RET51 appears dispensable (de Graaff, E. et al., 2001). However, RET51 has been suggested to be related to differentiation events in later kidney organogenesis (Lee, D. C. et al., 2002). Besides neuronal tissues and kidney, GDNF was recently implicated in sperm differentiation. GDNF is expressed by Sertoli cells, and RET and GFRα are displayed by a subset of spermatogonia including the stem cells for spermatogenesis (Meng, X. et al., 2000). Gene-targeted mice with one *GDNF*-null allele show depletion of spermatogenic stem cells, whereas mice overexpressing GDNF accumulate undifferentiated spermatogonia. Thus, GDNF contributes to the paracrine regulation of spermatogonial self-renewal and differentiation. The regulatory functions of GDNF/RET signaling in kidney morphogenesis and spermatogenesis indicate that the dosage of GDNF has both quantitative (e.g. number of branches from the UB) and qualitative (e.g. cell lineage determination of spermatogonia) dose-dependent effects in the target tissue. Thus, the expression of RET and GFRα on a cell defines the target cell type for GDNF, while the quality and nature of the response are regulated by the dosage of the ligand (reviewed in Sariola, H., 2001).

RET signaling

Ligand stimulated wild-type RET, as well as constitutive active oncogenic RET mutants, are phosphorylated at specific cytoplasmic tyrosine residues (Liu, X. et al., 1996; Coulpier, M. et al., 2002). Tyrosine autophosphorylation is required for downstream RET signaling. Recent studies have shown differences between the two isoforms, RET9 and RET51, in the intracellular signaling (Lorenzo, M. J. et al., 1997; Borrello, M. G. et al., 2002; Tsui-Pierchala, B. A. et al., 2002) as well as in the ligand-induced activation of RET inside or outside the lipid rafts (Paratcha, G. et al., 2001), which are detergent-insoluble sphingolipid and cholesterol-rich lipid microdomains that exist as phase-separated "rafts" in the plasma membrane (reviewed in Simons, K. et al., 1997; Brown, D. A. et al., 1998). Lipid rafts may be considered highly specialized signaling organelles, which assist to compartmentalize different sets of signaling molecules at both sides of the plasma membrane allowing them to interact

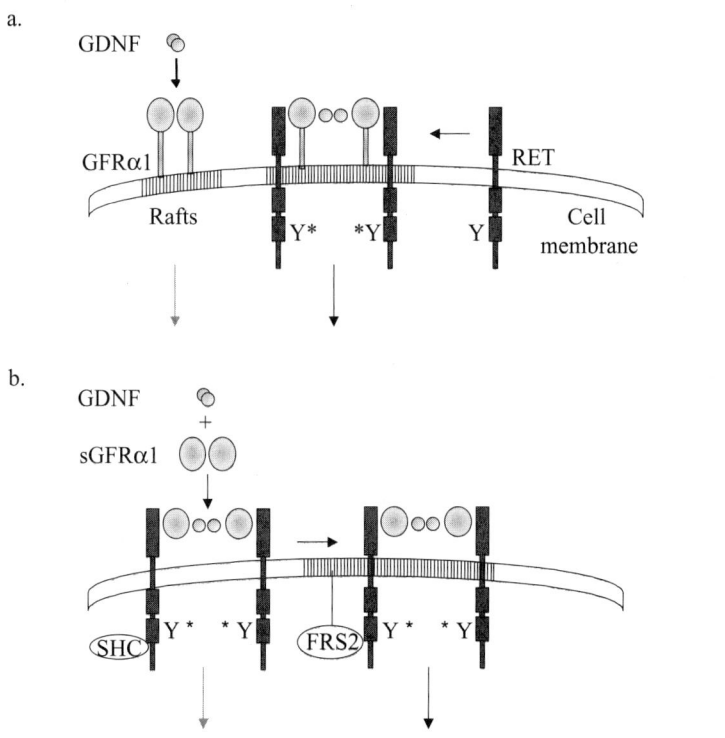

Figure 3. *Cis versus trans* signaling of RET activation.
(a) In the *cis* model of RET activation, GPI-anchored GFRα dimers, located into lipid rafts, first bind a GDNF dimer with high affinity. RET is then recruited to the GDNF-GFRα complex within the raft compartment. (b) GDNF binds to soluble GFRα in the *trans* model of RET activation. The GDNF-GFRα complex is then presented to RET, triggering RET activation. Activated RET preferentially associates with SHC outside the rafts, and predominantly associates with FRS2 within the rafts. Unphosphorylated (Y) and phosphorylated (Y*) tyrosine residues are indicated.

in a strictly regulated manner. GPI-linked GFRα proteins cluster into lipid rafts and recruit RET to lipid rafts after GDNF stimulation (Figure 3a). This recruitment of RET to rafts (through *cis* signaling) is independent on RET kinase activity. An alternative model for RET activation has been suggested by Paratcha and coworkers (Paratcha, G. et al., 2001; Manie, S. et al., 2001) (Figure 3b). Previously, soluble forms of GFRα were shown to be able to bind GDNF family ligands and to activate RET *in trans* (Jing, S. et al., 1996; Treanor, J. J. et al., 1996). A biologically active, soluble form of GFRα has been detected in the conditioned medium of neuronal and glial cell cultures (Worley, D. S. et al., 2000; Paratcha, G. et al., 2001). In the alternative pathway for RET activation, GDNF binds to soluble GFRα. The GDNF-GFRα complex is then presented to RET, triggering RET activation (through *trans* signaling). Transactivated RET is located initially outside the raft compartment and subsequently recruited to the lipid compartment through a process requiring the catalytic activity of the receptor. Of note, this differential compartmentalization of activated RET can trigger different signaling pathways. Raft-located RET preferentially associates with the adaptor FRS2 leading to sustained ERK activation, whereas RET located outside the rafts associates with SHC and leads to transient activation of ERK and activation of PI3K/AKT pathway (Paratcha, G. et al., 2001).

The intracellular domain of RET contains 14 tyrosine residues in the long and 12 in the short isoform, the latter lacking two tyrosine residues in the C-terminus. Interactions of RET with a number of downstream targets have been identified (Figure 4).

Phosphorylated tyrosine residues Tyr905, Tyr1015 and Tyr1096, the latter long isoform-specific, have been identified as docking sites for the adaptor proteins GRB7/GRB10, Phospholipase-Cγ and GRB2, respectively (Pandey, A. et al., 1995; Pandey, A. et al., 1996; Borrello, M. G. et al., 1996; Alberti, L. et al., 1998). Tyr1062 is a multidocking site interacting with a number of transduction molecules: SHC, FRS2, IRS1/2, DOK proteins, ENIGMA and PKCα (Durick, K. et al., 1996; Arighi, E. et al., 1997; Lorenzo, M. J. et al., 1997; Kurokawa, K. et al., 2001; Melillo, R. M. et al., 2001; Hennige, A. M. et al., 2000; Grimm, J. et al., 2001; Andreozzi, F. et al., 2003). The binding of SHC, FRS2, IRS1/2 and DOK to Tyr1062 is dependent on phosphorylation of this residue and is mediated by PTB or SH2 phosphotyrosine binding

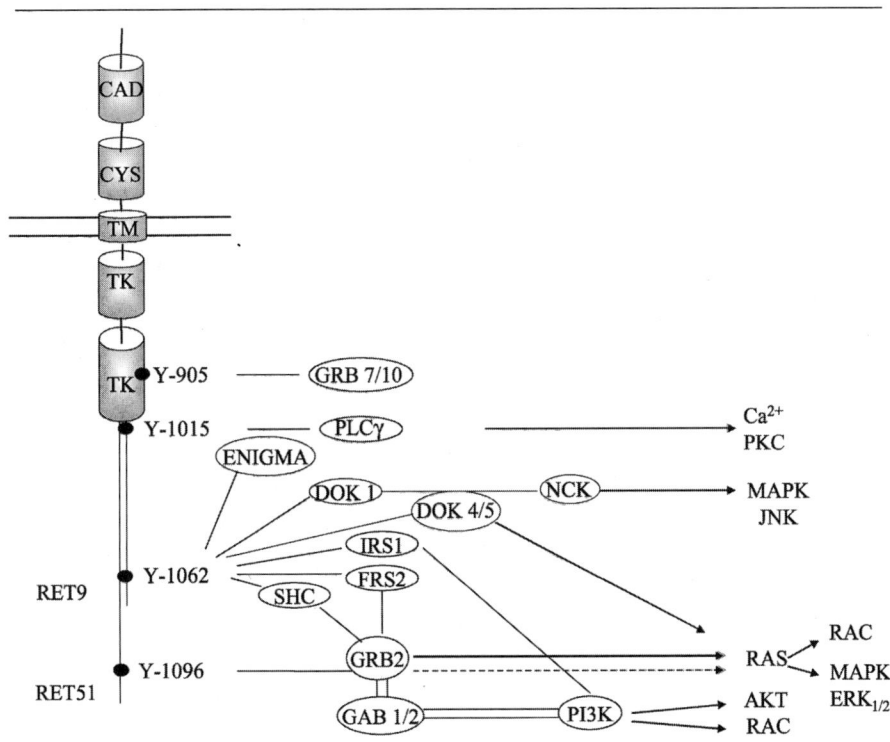

Figure 4. RET signaling pathways.

domains. In contrast, the binding to Tyr1062 of ENIGMA, a PDZ-LIM protein, is phospho-independent. Furthermore, ENIGMA binds specifically RET9, since short isoform-specific aminoacid residues +2 to +4 to Tyr1062 are required for interaction with ENIGMA (Borrello, M. G. et al., 2002).

Tyr1062-associated adaptor proteins contribute to activation of several downstream signaling pathways such as the RAS/ERK, PI3K/AKT, p38MAPK, JNK and ERK5 (Besset, V. et al., 2000; Hayashi, H. et al., 2000; Hayashi, Y. et al., 2001; Segouffin-Cariou, C. et al., 2000; Kurokawa, K. et al., 2003).

Tyr1096 is the most C-terminal phosphorylated tyrosine residue and it is unique to the long isoform (Liu, X. et al., 1996). The Tyr1062 multidocking site, although common to both isoforms, is only two residues amino-terminal to the C-terminal RET splice site, which alters the context of this residue between RET9 and RET51. Accordingly, Tyr1062 in short and long isoform does appear to have differential interactions with SHC and ENIGMA proteins (Lorenzo, M. J. et al., 1997; Borrello, M. G. et al., 2002). In addition, the two isoforms, though sharing identical extracellular domains, do not associate with each other and show different tyrosine phosphorylated associated proteins in sympathetic neurons (Tsui-Pierchala, B. A. et al., 2002).

MEDULLARY THYROID CARCINOMA

Medullary thyroid carcinoma (MTC) is a rare tumor of the thyroid gland. It was recognized as an unique entity by Hazard in 1959 (Hazard, J. B. et al., 1959); previously it was often classified as undifferentiated thyroid carcinoma.

MTC comprises approximately 5–10% of all thyroid malignancies. At variance with other thyroid malignancies, deriving from the follicular thyroid cells, MTC arises from parafollicular C cells (Williams, E. D., 1966). C cells derive from the neural crest and are able to secrete the hormone calcitonin (CT), a specific tumor marker for MTC. Calcitonin is in fact a useful marker in the follow up of treated patients and was used for screening the individuals predisposed to the hereditary form of the disease. RET analysis has now replaced CT testing to diagnose MEN2 carrier state.

About 75–80% of MTCs are sporadic (sMTC) and the remainder 20–25% are hereditary (hMTC) (Farndon, J. R. et al., 1986). In contrast to the sporadic cases which are characterized by a unifocal clonal tumor cell population, the heritable variants generally emerge from a multifocal origin (reviewed in Eng, C., 1999; Hazard, J. B., 1977).

In 1959, Hazard and coworkers first recognized medullary thyroid carcinoma as a distinct tumor (Hazard, J. B. et al., 1959). Sipple first described the association of medullary thyroid cancer, pheochromocytoma and parathyroid adenoma in 1961 (Sipple, J. H., 1961), and the syndrome was later termed "multiple endocrine neoplasia type 2" by Steiner and coworkers (Steiner, A. L. et al., 1968). The association between medullary thyroid carcinoma, pheochromocytoma, and multiple mucosal neuromas was described by Williams and Pollock in 1966 (Williams, E. D. et al., 1966) and confirmed by others. This syndrome was named MEN2B in 1975 by Chong and coworkers to be distinguished from the Sipple's syndrome (now called MEN2A) (Chong, G. C. et al., 1975).

Table 2. Clinical subtypes of MEN2

Disease	Characteristic features
MEN2A	Thyroid C-cells tumor
	Pheochromocytoma
	Parathyroid hyperplasia/adenoma
FMTC	Thyroid C-cells tumor
MEN2A with cutaneous lichen amyloidosis	MEN2A and cutaneous lesions
MEN2A/FMTC with Hirschsprung's disease	MEN2A/FMTC with intestinal aganglionosis
MEN2B	Thyroid C-cells tumor
	Pheochromocytoma
	Intestinal/mucosal ganglioneuromatosis
	Habitus marfanoid

Three clinically different types of MEN2 are now distinguished: MEN2A, MEN2B, and familial medullary thyroid carcinoma (FMTC), all transmitted in autosomal dominant fashion (Table 2).

They vary in aggressiveness of MTC and spectrum of disturbed organs. Their common feature is the thyroidal C cell hyperfunction with the occurrence of medullary thyroid carcinoma. MTC that occurs in hereditary forms is usually multifocal and bilateral. MEN type 2A is characterized by medullary thyroid carcinoma (MTC), pheocromocytoma in about 50% of cases, and parathyroid hyperplasia or adenoma in about 20–30% of cases. MEN2A accounts for over 75% of MEN2 (Eng, C. et al., 1996a; Ponder, B. A. J., 2001). MEN2B is the most distinctive and aggressive of the MEN2 variants and it is characterized by earlier age of tumor onset and by developmental abnormalities which include intestinal ganglioneuromatosis, atypical facies and marphanoid habitus. FMTC is characterized by the presence of MTC alone in at least four family members. FMTC is considered the least aggressive of the three MEN2 subtypes. In MTC families in fact, the tumor usually develops at a later stage of life and its course is more benign (Farndon, J. R. et al., 1986).

Several rare variants of MEN2 include MEN2A with cutaneous lichen amyloidosis (Nunziata, V. et al., 1989; Donovan, D. T. et al., 1989), and MEN2A or FMTC with Hirschsprung's disease (Verdy, M. et al., 1982).

RET ACTIVATION IN INHERITED AND SPORADIC MEDULLARY THYROID CARCINOMAS

RET mutations in MEN2 syndromes

In 1991, genetic linkage analyses mapped putative loci for MEN2 syndrome to a small interval on chromosome 10q11.2 and few years later *RET* gene was identified as the susceptibility gene for these syndromes (Donis-Keller, H. et al., 1993; Mulligan, L. M. et al., 1993b; Carlson, K. M. et al., 1994; Eng, C. et al., 1994; Hofstra, R. M. et al., 1994). Unlike other cancer syndromes, which are associated with inactivation of tumor suppressor genes, MEN2 arises as a result of activating mutations of the *RET* gene. This was the first time that predisposition to a cancer syndrome was associated with the activation of an oncogene rather than inactivation of a tumor suppressor gene (reviewed in Frischauf, A. M., 1993).

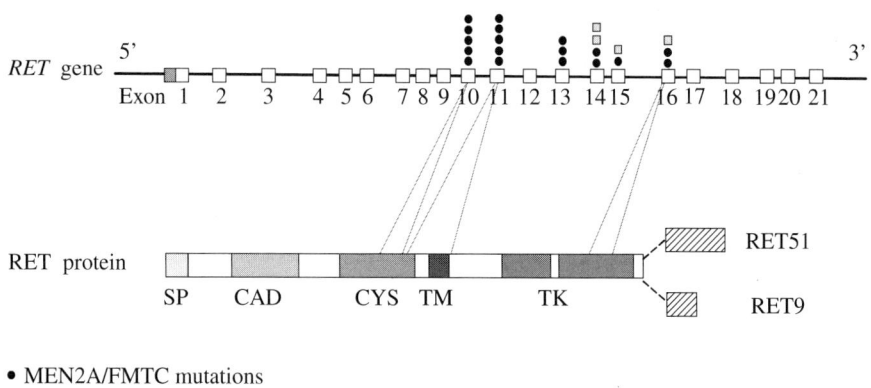

Figure 5. Schematic diagram of the *RET* gene and RET protein showing the location of MEN2 mutations.

Germline point mutations of *RET* are responsible for the inheritance of all the autosomal dominant MEN2 cancer syndromes MEN2A, MEN2B and FMTC (Figure 5 and Table 3).

The correlation between the various RET mutations and the development of thyroid carcinomas has been proved in fibroblast (Santoro, M. et al., 1995; Borrello, M. G. et al., 1995) and in a variety of different transgenic models (Asai, N. et al., 1995; Michiels, F. M. et al., 1997; Reynolds, L. et al., 2001; Acton, D. S. et al., 2000).

RET in multiple endocrine neoplasia type 2A (MEN2A)

Missense mutations of the RET gene have been found in the constitutional DNA of virtually all MEN2A families. These mutations affect the cysteine-rich extracellular domain of RET, each converting a critical cysteine residue (Cys) to another aminoacid at codons 609, 611, 618, 620, (exon 10) or at codons 630, 634 (exon 11) (see references in Table 3). They account for 98% of all mutations associated with MEN2A; the most common mutation, accounting for over 80% of all mutations associated with MEN2A, affects codon 634 and converts this cysteine into an arginine in about half of cases. Rarer duplication/insertion mutations associated with MEN2A have been described in exon 11 (Hoppner, W. et al., 1997; Hoppner, W. et al., 1998) resulting in the insertion of three or four aminoacids including a cysteine residue within the cysteine-rich domain. *De novo* cases of MEN2A have been associated with two new germline mutations (at both codon 634 and 640) on the same RET allele (Tessitore, A. et al., 1999).

RET-MEN2A oncoproteins display constitutive kinase activity consequent to ligand-independent dimerization. It is postulated that the cysteine residues are normally involved in intramolecular disulfide bonds. The disruption of a Cys by mutation may render the partner Cys available for aberrant disulfide bonding with other mutant

Table 3. *RET* mutations in MEN2 syndromes and sMTC

Exon	Codon number	Amino acid change	Phenotype	Reference
10	603	Lys to Gln	sMTC	Rey JM, 2001
	609	Cys to Arg	MEN2A/FMTC	Mulligan LM, 1995b; Eng C, 1996
		Cys to Tyr	MEN2A	Mulligan LM, 1994
		Cys to Ser	MEN2A	Igaz P, 2002
	611	Cys to Tyr	MEN2A	Mulligan LM, 1995b; Eng C, 1996
		Cys to Trp	MEN2A/FMTC	Donis-Keller H, 1993
		Cys to Gly	FMTC	Mulligan LM, 1995b; Eng C, 1996
		Cys to Ser	MEN2A/FMTC	Nishikawa M, 2003
	618	Cys to Phe	MEN2A	Mulligan LM, 1995b; Eng C, 1996
		Cys to Ser	MEN2A/FMTC	Donis-Keller H, 1993; Morita H, 1996
		Cys to Gly	MEN2A	Mulligan LM, 1995b; Eng C, 1996
		Cys to Arg	MEN2A/FMTC	Donis-Keller H, 1993; Marsh DJ, 1994
		Cys to Tyr	MEN2A/FMTC	Donis-Keller H, 1993
		Cys to Stop	MEN2A	Mulligan LM, 1995b; Eng C, 1996
	620	Cys to Arg	MEN2A/FMTC	Donis-Keller H, 1993
		Cys to Tyr	MEN2A	Donis-Keller H, 1993
		Cys to Phe	MEN2A	Mulligan LM, 1995b; Eng C, 1996
		Cys to Ser	MEN2A	Oishi S, 1995
		Cys to Gly	MEN2A	Mulligan LM, 1993b
11	630	Cys to Phe	FMTC	Komminoth P, 1995
	634	Cys to Arg	MEN2A	Donis-Keller H, 1993; Mulligan LM, 1994
		Cys to Tyr	MEN2A/FMTC	Mulligan LM, 1994
		Cys to Phe	MEN2A/FMTC	Mulligan LM, 1994
		Cys to Gly	MEN2A	Mulligan LM, 1993b
		Cys to Trp	MEN2A	Mulligan LM, 1994
		Cys to Ser	MEN2A/FMTC	Mulligan LM, 1993b; Eng C, 1996
	634 and 640	Cys to Arg and Ala to Gly	*de novo* MEN2A	Tessitore A, 1999
	639 and 641	Ala to Gly and Ala to Arg	sMTC	Kalinin VN, 2001
13	768	Glu to Asp	FMTC/sMTC	Eng C, 1995
	790	Leu to Phe	MEN2A/FMTC	Berndt I, 1998
	791	Tyr to Phe	FMTC	Berndt I, 1998
14	804	Val to Leu	FMTC	Bolino A, 1995
		Val to Met	FMTC	Fattoruso O, 1998
	804 and 806	Val to Met and Tyr to Cys	*de novo* MEN2B	Miyauchi A, 1999
	778 and 804	Val to Ile and Val to Met	FMTC	Kasprzak L, 2001
15	883	Ala to Phe	*de novo* MEN2B	Smith DP, 1997
	891	Ser to Ala	FMTC	Hofstra RMW, 1997
16	918	Met to Thr	MEN2B	Carlson KM, 1994
			sMTC	Eng C, 1994; Hofstra RMW, 1994
	922	Ser to Phe	sMTC	Kalinin VN, 2001

Exon	Base pairs duplication	Codon number	Amino acids inserted	Phenotype	Reference
8	9 bp	531–532	EEC	hFMTC	Pigny P, 1999
11	12 bp	634–635	HELC	hMEN2A	Hoppner W, 1997
	9 pb	636–637	CRT	MEN2A	Hoppner W, 1998

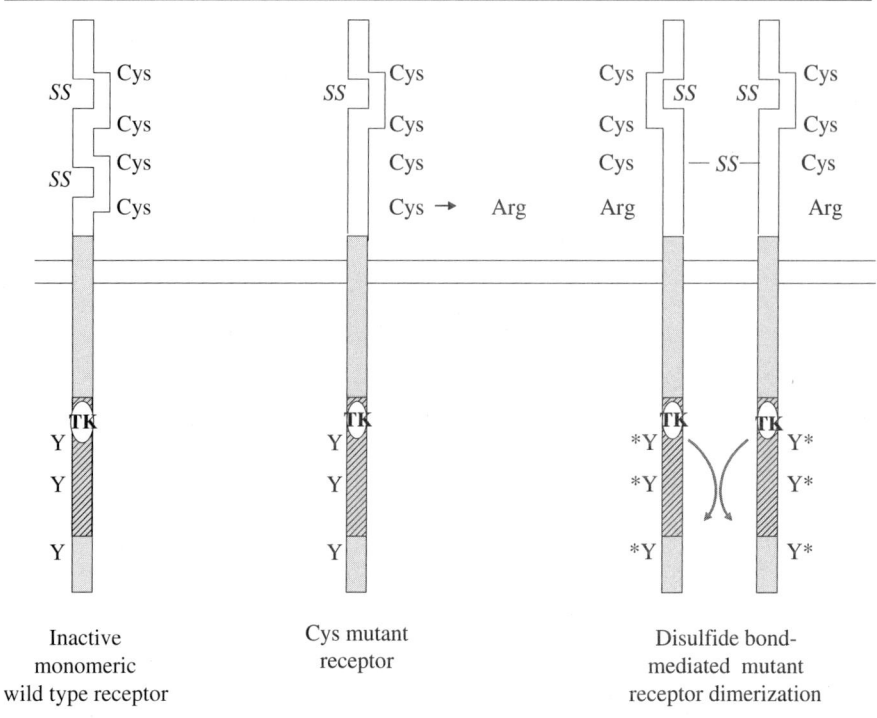

Figure 6. Mechanism of disulfide bond-mediated RET dimerization. Intramolecular and intermolecular disulfide bonds (SS), unphosphorylated (Y) and phosphorylated (Y*) tyrosine residues are indicated.

RET molecules thus leading to constitutive receptor dimerization and hence activation (Figure 6) (Asai, N. et al., 1995; Santoro, M. et al., 1995; Borrello, M. G. et al., 1995).

Accordingly, transgenic mice in which the *RET9* gene carrying the MEN2A-C634R mutation was expressed under the control of the human calcitonin promoter or under the MoMuLv LTR, developed C-cell tumors resembling human MTC (Michiels, F. M. et al., 1997; Kawai, K. et al., 2000).

RET mutations at codons 609, 618, and 620 lead to constitutive RET activity by causing ligand-independent disulfide-bridged homodimerization as "classical" RET-C634R mutation but, in addition, they markedly decrease the cell surface expression of RET (Carlomagno, F. et al., 1997; Chappuis-Flament, S. et al., 1998; Ito, S. et al., 1997).

Some tumors in MEN2 display a second hit, a somatic mutation involving the *RET* gene in the tumor clone precursor cell; the activated *RET* allele is amplified by chromosome 10 duplication in some tumors, or the normal *RET* allele is deleted in some others (Huang, S. C. et al., 2000).

RET in multiple endocrine neoplasia type 2B (MEN2B)

Most MEN2B cases (95%) are caused by the M918T mutation (exon 16) (Carlson, K. M. et al., 1994). Other rarer (5%) intracellular mutations involve codon 883 (exon 15) in the RET tyrosine kinase domain (Smith, D. P. et al., 1997).

The M918T substitution is also found in sporadic MTC (reviewed in Jhiang, S. M., 2000), with M918T mutation-positive tumors often displaying a more aggressive phenotype. Recently, a double mutation at codons 804 and 806 has been found in a Japanese patient that had clinical features characteristic of MEN2B (Miyauchi, A. et al., 1999). The M918T mutation does not cause constitutive dimerization but activates RET by an intramolecular mechanism (Santoro, M. et al., 1995). The methionine at codon 918 is highly conserved in receptor tyrosine kinases and it maps in the P+1 loop of the kinase domain that is predicted to interact with the protein substrate. A threonine is found at the equivalent position in cytosolic tyrosine kinases, and the two kinase classes (receptorial and cytosolic) have different signaling specificity (Marengere, L.E. et al., 1994). Accordingly, it was demonstrated that the MEN2B-M918T mutation changes the substrate specificity of RET kinase. Indeed, RET-MEN2B displays phosphorylation of intracellular proteins as well as autophosphorylation sites different from RET-MEN2A (Santoro, M. et al., 1995). Thus, the shift of RET autophosphorylation sites and of RET intracellular substrates, rather than the modest rise of RET kinase activity (Borrello, M. G. et al., 1995), may be crucial for the oncogenic activity of RET-MEN2B and responsible for its specific neoplastic activity (Santoro, M. et al., 1995). Furthermore, GDNF stimulation seems to be necessary for the full activation of RET-MEN2B (Bongarzone, I. et al., 1998).

It is not known how the A883F affects RET function. However, residue 883 is located in a subdomain of RET that defines substrate preference (Smith, D.P. et al., 1997) thus suggesting that the alteration of substrate specificity may be the common etiologic thread that underlies the pathogenesis of MEN2B. The production of a mouse model of MEN2B by introduction of the corresponding mutation into the *RET* gene demonstrated that heterozygous mutant mice displayed several features of the human disease, including C-cell hyperplasia and pheochromocytoma, while homozygous displayed more severe thyroid adrenal disease as well as male infertility. Only homozygous mice did develop ganglioneuromas of the adrenal medulla and enlargement of the associated sympathetic ganglia (Smith-Hicks, C.L. et al., 2000).

RET in familial medullary thyroid carcinoma (FMTC)

FMTC mutations can be found either in the extracellular or in the tyrosine kinase domain of RET. The ones occurring in the extracellular RET domain are the same mutations also associated with MEN2A: substitution of cysteines 609, 611, 618, 620 (exon 10), 630 and 634 (exon 11). The mutations in the tyrosine kinase domain occur at residues 768, 790, 791 (exon 13), 804, 844 (exon 14) or 891 (exon 15) (see references in

Table 3). Rare mutations have been recently reported, such as a 9-base pair duplication in exon 8 in a FMTC family (Pigny, P. et al., 1999) or mutations at codons 778 and 804 on the same RET allele which are associated with both FMTC and prominent corneal nerves (Kasprzak, L. et al., 2001). FMTC mutations occurring in the intracellular RET domain were thought to be infrequent and only a few number of families bearing the RET mutation within exons 13, 14 and 15 have been described. However, in the past two years the frequency of detection of these mutations has increased (Niccoli-Sire, P. et al., 2001) due to more accurate analysis and screening. No data are yet available on the mechanisms of activation of FMTC mutations occurring in RET tyrosine kinase domain. Patients with RET mutations in exons 13, 14 and 15 exhibit a mild C-cell disease phenotype (Berndt, I. et al., 1998; Fattoruso, O. et al., 1998) confirmed by *in vitro* studies. In fact, mutant RET proteins carrying mutations at residues 768, 804 or 891 display lower transforming activity (Pasini, A. et al., 1997; Iwashita, T. et al., 1999) compared with RET substitutions at codons 634, 918 or 883 strongly associated with MEN2A and MEN2B, respectively. Computer modeling has suggested that the E768D substitution modifies the kinase activity of the receptor by altering the substrate specificity or the ATP-binding capacity (Pasini, A. et al., 1997). As for its location, also the substitution at position 804 may exert an activating effect by altering the kinetics of interactions with normal cellular substrates or by modifying the range of substrates that are phosphorylated (Bolino, A. et al., 1995; Eng, C. et al., 1995; Iwashita, T. et al., 1999; Pasini, A. et al., 1997).

Recent studies (Feldman, G. L. et al., 2000; Brauckhoff, M. et al., 2002) have reported cases of patients harboring RET germline mutations in exons 14 and 15 (at codons 790, 791, 804) resulting in papillary microcarcinoma. Rey and colleagues (Rey, J. M. et al., 2001) also described the case of a kindred in which a novel single point germline RET mutation (K603E in exon 10) cosegregates with medullary and papillary thyroid carcinomas (PTCs). Despite the low number, these observations suggest that there might be a correlation between the occurrence of PTC and RET germline mutations in exons 13 and 14 that may play a role in pathogenesis of PTC. Of note, PTC seems to be present just in patients with low penetrance RET germline mutations. It remains an open question whether the simultaneous occurrence of inherited MTC and PTC is coincidental or the result of partly common pathogenic pathways. Reynolds and coworkers (Reynolds, L. et al., 2001) found the co-existence of MTC and PTC in transgenic mice expressing the long isoform of RET MEN2A and suggested that this might be due to the possible existence of an ultimobranchial stem cell of endodermal origin, which gives rise to a subset of both thyroid follicular cells and C-cells (Kovacs, C. S et al., 1994).

MEN2/HSCR paradox: the same mutation of RET with both gain and loss of function

In 20 to 30% of families with a mutation at cysteine residues 609, 611, 618 or 620 and no additional mutations within the coding sequence of *RET*, MEN2A and FMTC associate with HSCR (Mulligan, L.M. et al., 1994; Attie, T. et al., 1995; Borst, M. J. et al., 1995; Nishikawa, M. et al., 2003). The occurrence of HSCR in MEN2A/FMTC pedigrees is difficult to be explained with a gain-of-function mutation in RET, which is typical for the MEN 2 mutations. RET proteins containing these specific cysteine mutations have been shown to translocate to the cell surface with low efficiency (Ito, S. et al., 1997; Chappuis-Flament, S. et al., 1998). Moreover, a kinase activity under the threshold required for cell survival (Takahashi, M. et al., 1999), or an inability to respond to GDNF, and protect RET-expressing cells from apoptosis (Mograbi, B. et al., 2001) have also been proposed as explanations. The mutation of each cysteine involved in MEN2A/FMTC promotes the aberrant formation of disulfide-linked RET homodimers, causing a constitutive activation of RET. However, mutation of Cys634 is approximately fivefold more strongly activating than mutations of cysteine 609, 611, 618, or 620 (Chappuis-Flament, S. et al., 1998). As a result, the low level of the RET covalent dimers resulting from mutations of cysteine 609, 611, 618, or 620, might be sufficient to activate the RET signaling pathways in the thyroid C-cell and chromaffin cell, leading to hyperplasia or tumor formation. On the other hand, insufficient RET protein is available in the developing enteric nervous system, thereby leading to HSCR. However, the fact that HSCR and MEN2A/FMTC are associated in only a fraction of families with a mutation at codon 609, 611, 618, or 620, indicates that other genetic or environmental factors might influence the clinical expression of the enteric phenotype (Mulligan, L. M. et al., 1994; Decker, R. A. et al., 1998).

RET in sporadic MTC (sMTC)

The majority of MTC cases (75%) have no associated family history. However, it has been found recently that 3–7% of sporadic cases represent occult or *de novo* MEN2 cases as determined by finding germline RET mutations (Wohllk, N. et al., 1996).

Somatic RET mutations are found, however, in 30 to 70% of true sporadic medullary thyroid carcinomas and, rarely, in pheochromocytomas. Mutation at the codon 918 is largely predominant but also mutations at the cysteine codons 609, 611, 620, 630, 634 were found in sporadic MTC cases. Recently three new somatic missense mutations (at codons 639, 641 and 922) of the *RET* gene associated with sporadic MTC have been described (Kalinin, V. N. et al., 2001). The functional significance of RET mutations, however, is unclear. They have been shown to be present heterogeneously, suggesting that they have occurred during tumor evolution rather than being the initiating step (Eng, C. et al., 1996b). In addition, loss of heterozygosity (LOH) has been found in up to 30% of tumors on chromosomes 1p, 3p, 3q, 11p, 13q, 17p, 22q (Mulligan, L. M. et al., 1993a).

RET-MEN2A and RET-MEN2B signaling

The functions of RET in normal and tumorigenic cells are mediated by a complex series of downstream interactions. RET-activated pathways, such as AKT pathway, have been shown to be important for cell signaling mediated by both ligand-dependent and -independent activation of RET and to have a role in cell survival, proliferation and oncogenic transformation by all RET oncogenic forms (reviewed in Manie, S.

et al., 2001). However, RET-MEN2A is considered a constitutively activated kinase, whereas RET-MEN2B appears to be an activated kinase with in addition altered catalytic properties (Santoro, M. et al., 1995; Borrello, M. G. et al., 1995). Consistent with this fact, differences in cell signaling triggered by each of these oncogenic forms have been emerging. Phosphorylation of Tyr864 and Tyr952 is crucial for transformation triggered by RET-MEN2B while Tyr905 phosphorylation is essential for transformation promoted by RET-MEN2A (Iwashita, T. et al., 1996). Mutation of Tyr1062 multidocking site markedly impaired the transforming activity of all MEN2 mutants (Iwashita, T. et al., 1996). However it was reported that the level of phosphorylation of Tyr1062 is increased in cells expressing RET-MEN2B compared to those expressing RET-MEN2A, resulting in enhancement of activation of ERK and PI3K/AKT pathways (Salvatore, D. et al., 2001). In addition, DOK1, a Tyr1062-associated docking protein activating JNK pathways, more strongly binds RET-MEN2B than RET-MEN2A protein (Murakami, H. et al., 2002). Consequently, enhanced signaling via Tyr1062 has been suggested to be involved in MEN2B phenotype. Furthermore, recent studies obtained by differential display analysis of gene expression in cells expressing either RET-MEN2A or RET-MEN2B mutant proteins identified genes predominantly induced by either mutations (Watanabe, T. et al., 2002).

DIAGNOSIS AND MANAGEMENT OF MEN2

MEN2 gives a unique model for early prevention and cure of cancer and for stratified roles of mutation-based diagnosis of carriers. MTC is the first neoplastic manifestation in most MEN2 kindreds because of its earlier and overall higher penetrance. In older MEN2A series, with treatment initiated after the identification of a thyroid nodule, MTC progressed and showed 15–20% mortality (Kakudo, K. et al., 1985). The impact of carrier diagnosis before adulthood has been proven in long-term studies with measurement of serum calcitonin (CT). Early thyroidectomy has lowered the mortality from hMTC to less than 5%. However, the longest follow-up period for prospective CT screening is less than 25 years (Gagel, R. F. et al., 1988). Moreover, it is probable that improved management of pheochromocytoma has decreased the rate of premature mortality in MEN2 even more than has the improved management of MTC. Syndromic morbidity is more severe, and mortality is earlier in MEN2B than in MEN2A. Recognition of the most highly aggressive MTC in MEN2B and recognition of the possibility for early carrier detection have led to thyroidectomy in MEN2B far earlier than before. Like pheochromocytoma in MEN2A, pheochromocytoma in MEN2B has been virtually eliminated as a major cause of death because of improved management.

Multifocal C-cell hyperplasia is a precursor lesion to hMTC; the progression from C-cell hyperplasia to microscopic MTC is variable and may take many years (Papotti, M. et al., 1993). Metastasis may be in the central and lateral, cervical, and mediastinal lymph nodes or more distantly in lung, liver, or bone. The aggressiveness of MTC correlates with the MEN2 variant syndrome and with the mutated *RET* codon. The primary secretory product of MTC is CT, which is important only as an excellent tumor marker (Gagel, R. F. et al., 1988; Pacini, F. et al., 1994). CT values (basal or stimulated by pentagastrin, calcium, or both) are nearly always elevated with MTC. Similarly, elevated CT values after surgery are generally the first sign of persistent or recurrent disease.

Prevention or cure of MTC is by surgery; success is mainly dependent upon the adequacy of the initial operation. Therefore, surgery for MTC should be performed, if possible, before the age of possible malignant progression. Unfortunately, standard chemotherapeutic regimens have not been proven beneficial in patients with metastatic MTC, and the tumors are not very sensitive to x-ray or thermal radiation therapy (reviewed in Brandi, M. L. et al., 2001).

MEN2 carrier determination is one of the few examples of a genetic test that mandates a highly effective clinical intervention. Consensus was reached at the MEN97 Workshop that the decision to perform thyroidectomy in MEN2 should be based predominantly on the result of *RET* mutation testing, rather than on CT testing (Lips, C. J., 1998). Sequencing of DNA for *RET* mutations is indeed effective and widely available. 98% of MEN2 index cases have an identified *RET* mutation, and testing in no MEN2 family has excluded the *RET* locus. A limited number of MEN2-associated mutations, involving *RET* exons 10, 11, 13, 14, 15, and 16, have been identified. Thus, only these exons must be tested routinely. If this is negative, the remaining 15 exons should be sequenced.

RET inactivating mutations account for approximately half of cases of familial Hirschsprung's disease (HSCR). It is thus surprising that activating mutations of *RET* codons 609, 618, and 620 have also been associated, albeit rarely, with MEN2A and HSCR. In addition, there have been rare cases of HSCR with exon 10 mutations identical to those found in hMTC. Germline mutation analysis of *RET* (containing codons 609, 618, and 620) is indicated in all children with HSCR. In those rare cases with potential activating mutation at one of these codons, consideration should be given to prophylactic thyroidectomy, and parents and other first degree relatives should be screened. *RET* codon 918 mutations, like those in MEN2B, have been reported in several children with colonic ganglioneuromatosis. In children with this disorder and a codon 918 mutation or other *RET* activating mutation, consideration should be given to prophylactic thyroidectomy.

The specifically mutated codon of *RET* correlates with the MEN2 variant, including the aggressiveness of MTC. Children with MEN2B and/or *RET* codon 883, 918, or 922 mutation are classified as level 3 or as having the highest risk from aggressive MTC and should have thyroidectomy within the first 6 months and preferably within the first month of life.

Children with any *RET* codon 611, 618, 620, or 634 mutation are classified as level 2 or as having a high risk for MTC and should have thyroidectomy performed before the age of 5 years. Total thyroidectomy should be performed.

Children with *RET* codon 609, 768, 790, 791, 804, and 891 mutations are classified as level 1 or as having the least high risk among the three *RET* codon mutation stratification categories. They, too, should have a total thyroidectomy. The biological behavior of MTC in patients with these mutations is variable, but, in general, MTC grows more slowly and develops at a later age than with the high risk mutations. Variations between members of the same family regarding the clinical presentation of the MEN2 disease and the age at onset might be related to factors such as polymorphisms that increase susceptibility to the syndrome including variation in pathological phenotype. Identification of these factors is one of the key problems in medical genetics. Recently, the two *RET* polymorphisms G691S and S904S have been suggested to have a role as a low penetrance risk factor of MEN2A (Robledo, M. et al., 2003).

Therefore, because of DNA-based testing, many MEN2 carriers should undergo total thyroidectomy before expressing MTC. However, basal and stimulated CT testing are still useful indexes of tumor mass to screen for or monitor MTC before or after thyroid surgery.

Gene therapeutic approaches for inhibition of oncogenic RET signaling

In recent years, new therapeutic approaches as alternative strategy in MTC surgical treatment have been investigated. The inhibition of tyrosine kinase activity by small cell-permeable molecules is a promising tool to target oncoproteins and has already reached clinical application for Erb/HER subgroup of receptor (reviewed in Mendelsohn, J. et al., 2000; Dancey, J. E. et al., 2001). The availability of inhibitors specific for RET oncoproteins might provide new tools to highlight the physiologically and pathologically activated pathways involved. The tyrosine kinase inhibitors STI571, genistein, and allyl-geldanamycin selectively inhibited cell growth and RET tyrosine kinase activity of MTC cells *in vitro* in a dose manner (Cohen, M. S. et al., 2002). Carlomagno and colleagues (Carlomagno, F. et al., 2002) showed that the pyrazolo-pyrimidine PP1 blocks tumorigenesis induced by RET/PTC cytoplasmic oncoproteins by inhibiting RET enzymatic activity and its transforming effects. Carniti and coworkers (Carniti, C. et al., 2003) additionally demonstrated that along with the inhibition of tyrosine phosphorylation, PP1 induces proteosomal destruction of the activated membrane-bound RET receptors associated with MEN2 syndrome.

Another approach is to generate molecular mimetics directed toward specific mutations of the RET oncogene. The soluble ectodomain of RET carrying the C634Y-MEN2A substitution has been recently shown to inhibit *in vitro* the membrane-bound RET-MEN2A receptor by interfering with its dimerization and to compete with the wild-type RET for ligand binding (Cerchia, L. et al., 2003).

As another option for MTC treatment by gene therapeutic means, the transductional targeting of vectors to tumor cells might provide promising new alternatives in terms of selectivity and safety. The feasibility of efficient introduction of toxic transgenes into tumor cells by adenoviral (Ad) vectors would allow new aspects in tumor treatment, either alone or in combination with established therapeutic approaches. Infection of human MTC-derived cells with adenoviral-dominant-negative RET (Ad-dn-RET) were shown to inhibit oncogenic RET signaling and growth of MTC cells (Drosten, M. et al., 2002). Moreover, using transplanted human MTC cells as an *in vivo* MTC model in nude mice, adenoviral transduction of dn-RET was shown to be sufficient to achieve a strong inhibition of tumor growth accompanied by a significant increase in animal survival (Drosten, M. et al., 2003b). Modified vector capsid would allow lower viral loads to be administered and thereby reducing virus-related toxicity (reviewed in Wickham, T. J., 2003). The development of selective peptides for different tumor cell types and their incorporation into the vector capsid demonstrate the eligibility of this approach (reviewed in Nicklin, S. A. et al., 2002).

Taken together, multiple possibilities have been and continue to be employed for improving gene therapy for inhibition of oncogenic RET signaling and, in general, for MTC. It is hard to judge whether gene therapy will totally replace surgical intervention as the primary treatment for MTC, especially after early-stage diagnosis of inherited disease. However, recurrent or metastatic disease is difficult to manage, and in these cases gene therapy may soon lead to an improvement in standard therapies. With some improvements in vector design in terms of safety and efficacy, gene therapy may soon help to overcome many obstacles in cancer therapy, especially with the emerging knowledge of molecular mechanisms of cancer (reviewed in Drosten, M. et al., 2003a).

REFERENCES

1. Acton D.S., Velthuyzen D., Lips C.J., Hoppener J.W. Multiple endocrine neoplasia type 2B mutation in human RET oncogene induces medullary thyroid carcinoma in transgenic mice. Oncogene 2000; 19:3121–3125.
2. Airaksinen M.S., Saarma M. The GDNF family: signalling, biological functions and therapeutic value. Nat Rev Neurosci 2002; 3:383–394.
3. Alberti L., Borrello M.G., Ghizzoni S., Torriti F., Rizzetti M.G., Pierotti M.A. GRB2 binding to the different isoforms of RET tyrosine kinase. Oncogene 1998; 17:1079–1087.
4. Amiel J., Lyonnet S. Hirschsprung disease, associated syndromes, and genetics: a review. J Med Genet 2001; 38:729–739.
5. Anders J., Kjar S., Ibanez C.F. Molecular modeling of the extracellular domain of the RET receptor tyrosine kinase reveals multiple cadherin-like domains and a calcium-binding site. J Biol Chem 2001;
6. Andreozzi F., Melillo R.M., Carlomagno F., Oriente F., Miele C., Fiory F., Santopietro S., Castellone M.D., Beguinot F., Santoro M., Formisano P. Protein kinase Calpha activation by RET: evidence for a negative feedback mechanism controlling RET tyrosine kinase. Oncogene 2003; 22:2942–2949.
7. Arighi E., Alberti L., Torriti F., Ghizzoni S., Rizzetti M.G., Pelicci G., Pasini B., Bongarzone I., Piutti C., Pierotti M.A., Borrello M.G. Identification of SHC docking site on Ret tyrosine kinase. Oncogene 1997; 14:773–782.
8. Asai N., Iwashita T., Matsuyama M., Takahashi M. Mechanism of activation of the *ret* proto-oncogene by multiple endocrine neoplasia 2A mutations. Mol Cell Biol 1995; 15, No. 3:1613–1619.
9. Attie T., Pelet A., Edery P., Eng C., Mulligan L.M., Amiel J., Boutrand L., Beldjord C., Nihoul-Fekete C., Munnich A., et al. Diversity of RET proto-oncogene mutations in familial and sporadic Hirschsprung disease. Human Molec Genet 1995; 4:1381–1386.
10. Avantaggiato V., Dathan N.A., Grieco M., Fabien N., Lazzaro D., Fusco A., Simeone A., Santoro M. Developmental expression of the *RET* protooncogene. Cell Growth Diff 1994; 5:305–311.
11. Baloh R.H., Enomoto H., Johnson E.M., Jr., Milbrandt J. The GDNF family ligands and receptors—implications for neural development. Curr Opin Neurobiol 2000; 10:103–110.
12. Beldjord C., Desclaux-Arramond F., Raffin-Sanson M., Corvol J.C., De Keyzer Y., Luton J.P., Plouin P.F., Bertagna X. The RET protooncogene in sporadic pheochromocytomas: frequent MEN 2-like mutations and new molecular defects. J Clin Endocrinol Metab 1995; 80:2063–2068.
13. Berndt I., Reuter M., Saller B., Frank-Raue K., Groth P., Grussendorf M., Raue F., Ritter M.M., Hoppner W. A new hot spot for mutations in the ret protooncogene causing familial medullary thyroid carcinoma and multiple endocrine neoplasia type 2A. J Clin Endocrinol Metab 1998; 83:770–774.
14. Besset V., Scott R.P., Ibanez C.F. Signaling complexes and protein-protein interactions involved in the activation of the Ras and P13K pathways by the c-Ret receptor tyrosine kinase. J Biol Chem 2000; 275:39159–39166.
15. Bolino A., Schuffenecker I., Luo Y., Seri M., Silengo M., Tocco T., Chabrier G., Houdent C., Murat A., Schlumberger M., Tourniaire J., Lenoir G.M., omeo G. RET mutations in exons 13 and 14 of FMTC patients. Oncogene 1995; 10:2415–2419.

16. Bongarzone I., Vigano' E., Alberti L., Borrello M.G., Pasini B., Greco A., Mondellini P., Smith D.P., Ponder B.A.J., Romeo G., Pierotti M.A. Full activation of MEN2B mutant RET by an additional MEN2A mutation or by ligand (GDNF) stimulation. Oncogene 1998; 16:2295–2301.
17. Borrello M.G., Smith D.P., Pasini B., Bongarzone I., Greco A., Lorenzo M.J., Arighi E., Miranda C., Eng C., Alberti L., Bocciardi R., Mondellini P., Scopsi L., Romeo G., Ponder B.A.J., Pierotti M.A. RET activation by germline MEN2A and MEN2B mutations. Oncogene 1995; 11:2419–2427.
18. Borrello M.G., Alberti L., Arighi E., Bongarzone I., Battistini C., Bardelli A., Pasini B., Piutti C., Rizzetti M.G., Mondellini P., Radice M.T., Pierotti M.A. The full oncogenic activity of Ret/ptc2 depends on tyrosine 539, a docking site for phospholipase Cgamma. Mol Cell Biol 1996; 16, No. 5:2151–2163.
19. Borrello M.G., Mercalli E., Perego C., Degl'Innocenti D., Ghizzoni S., Arighi E., Eroini B., Rizzetti M.G., Pierotti M.A. Differential interaction of Enigma protein with the two RET isoforms. Biochem Biophys Res Commun 2002; 296:515–522.
20. Borst M.J., VanCamp J.M., Peacock M.L., Decker R.A. Mutational analysis of multiple endocrine neoplasia type 2A associated with Hirschsprung's disease. Surgery 1995; 117:386–391.
21. Brandi M.L., Gagel R.F., Angeli A., Bilezikian J.P., Beck-Peccoz P., Bordi C., Conte-Devolx B., Falchetti A., Gheri R.G., Libroia A., Lips C.J., Lombardi G., Mannelli M., Pacini F., Ponder B.A., Raue F., Skogseid B., Tamburrano G., Thakker R.V., Thompson N.W., Tomassetti P., Tonelli F., Wells S.A., Jr., Marx S.J. Guidelines for diagnosis and therapy of MEN type 1 and type 2. J Clin Endocrinol Metab 2001; 86:5658–5671.
22. Brauckhoff M., Gimm O., Hinze R., Ukkat J., Brauckhoff K., Dralle H. Papillary Thyroid Carcinoma in Patients with RET Proto-Oncogene Germline Mutation. Thyroid 2002; 12:557–561.
23. Brown D.A., London E. Functions of lipid rafts in biological membranes. Annu Rev Cell Dev Biol 1998; 14:111–36.:111–136.
24. Cacalano G., Farinas I., Wang L., Hagler K., Forgie A., Moore M., Armanini M., Phillips H., Ryan A.M., Reichardt L., et al. GFRa1 is an essential receptor component for GDNF in the developing nervous system and kidney. Neuron 1998; 21:53–62.
25. Carlomagno F., Salvatore G., Cirafici A.M., De Vita G., Melillo R.M., de, Franciscis V., Billaud M., Fusco A., Santoro M. The different RET-activating capability of mutations of cysteine 620 or cysteine 634 correlates with the multiple endocrine neoplasia type 2 disease phenotype. Cancer Res 1997; 57:391–395.
26. Carlomagno F., Vitagliano D., Guida T., Napolitano M., Vecchio G., Fusco A., Gazit A., Levitzki A., Santoro M. The kinase inhibitor PP1 blocks tumorigenesis induced by RET oncogenes. Cancer Res 2002; 62:1077–1082.
27. Carlson K.M., Dou S., Chi D., Scavarda N.J., Toshima K., Jackson C.E., Wells S.A.Jr., Goodfellow P., Donis-Keller H. Single missense mutation in the tyrosine kinase catalytic domain of the RET protooncogene is associated with multiple endocrine neoplasia type 2B. Proc Natl Acad Sci USA 1994; 91:1579–1583.
28. Carniti C., Perego C., Mondellini P., Pierotti M.A., Bongarzone I. PP1 inhibitor induces degradation of RETMEN2A and RETMEN2B oncoproteins through proteosomal targeting. Cancer Res 2003; 63:2234–2243.
29. Carter M.T., Yome J.L., Marcil M.N., Martin C.A., Vanhorne J.B., Mulligan L.M. Conservation of RET proto-oncogene splicing variants and implications for RET isoform function. Cytogenet Cell Genet 2001; 95:169–176.
30. Cerchia L., Libri D., Carlomagno M.S., de F., V. The soluble ectodomain of RetC634Y inhibits both the wild-type and the constitutively active Ret. Biochem J 2003; 372:897–903
31. Chappuis-Flament S., Pasini A., De Vita G., Segouffin-Cariou C., Fusco A., Attie T., Lenoir G.M., Santoro M., Billaud M. Dual effect on the RET receptor of MEN 2 mutations effecting specific extracytoplasmic cysteines. Oncogene 1998; 17:2851–2861.
32. Chong G.C., Beahrs O.H., Sizemore G.W., Woolner L.H. Medullary carcinoma of the thyroid gland. Cancer 1975; 35:695–704.
33. Cohen M.S., Hussain H.B., Moley J.F. Inhibition of medullary thyroid carcinoma cell proliferation and RET phosphorylation by tyrosine kinase inhibitors. Surgery 2002; 132:960–966.
34. Coulpier M., Anders J., Ibanez C.F. Coordinated activation of autophosphorylation sites in the RET receptor tyrosine kinase: importance of tyrosine 1062 for GDNF mediated neuronal differentiation and survival. J Biol Chem 2002; 277:1991–1999.
35. Dancey J.E., Schoenfeldt M. Clinical trials referral resource. Epidermal growth factor receptor inhibitors in clinical trials. Oncology (Huntingt) 2001; 15:748.

36. de Graaff E., Srinivas S., KilKenny C., D'Agati V., Mankoo B.S., Costantini F., Pachnis V. Differential activities of the RET tyrosine kinase receptor isoforms during mammalian embryogenesis. Genes Dev 2001; 15:2433–2444.
37. Decker R.A., Peacock M.L., Watson P. Hirschsprung disease in MEN 2A: increased spectrum of RET exon 10 genotypes and strong genotype-phenotype correlation. Hum Mol Genet 1998; 7:129–134.
38. Donis-Keller H., Dou S., Chi D., Carlson K.M., Toshima K., Lairmore T.C., Howe J.R., Moley J.F., Goodfellow P., Wells S.A.Jr. Mutations in the RET proto-oncogene are associated with MEN 2A and FMTC. Human Molec Genet 1993; 2:851–856.
39. Donovan D.T., Levy M.L., Furst E.J., Alford B.R., Wheeler T., Tschen J.A., Gagel R.F. Familial cutaneous lichen amyloidosis in association with multiple endocrine neoplasia type 2A: a new variant. Henry Ford Hosp Med J 1989; 37:147–150.
40. Drosten M., Frilling A., Stiewe T., Putzer B.M. A new therapeutic approach in medullary thyroid cancer treatment: inhibition of oncogenic RET signaling by adenoviral vector-mediated expression of a dominant-negative RET mutant. Surgery 2002; 132:991–997.
41. Drosten M., Putzer B.M. Gene therapeutic approaches for medullary thyroid carcinoma treatment. J Mol Med 2003a; 81:411–419.
42. Drosten M., Stiewe T., Putzer B.M. Antitumor capacity of a dominant-negative RET proto-oncogene mutant in a medullary thyroid carcinoma model. Hum Gene Ther 2003b; 14:971–982.
43. Durbec P., Marcos-Gutierrez C.V., KilKenny C., Grigoriou M., Wartiowaara K., Suvanto P., Smith D., Ponder B., Costantini F., Saarma M., Sariola H., Pachnis V. GDNF signalling through the Ret receptor tyrosine kinase. Nature 1996; 381:789–793.
44. Durick K., Wu R.Y., Gill G.N., Taylor S.S. Mitogenic signaling by Ret/ptc2 requires association with enigma via a LIM domain. J Biol Chem 1996; 271:12691–12694.
45. Edery P., Lyonnet S., Mulligan L.M., Pelet A., Dow E., Abel L., Holder S., Nihoul-Fekete' C., Ponder B.A.J., Munnich A. Mutations of the RET proto-oncogene in Hirschsprung's disease. Nature 1994; 367:378–380.
46. Eng C., Smith D.P., Mulligan L.M., Nagai M.A., Healey C.S., Ponder M.A., Gardner E., Scheumann G.F.W., Jackson C.E., Tunnacliffe A., Ponder B.A.J. Point mutation within the tyrosine kinase domain of the RET proto-oncogene in multiple endocrine neoplasia type 2B and related sporadic tumours. Human Molec Genet 1994; 3:237–241.
47. Eng C., Smith D.P., Mulligan L.M., Healey C.S., Zvelebil M.J., Stonehouse T.J., Ponder M.A., Jackson C.E., Waterfield M.D., Ponder B.A.J. A novel point mutation in the Tyrosine kinase domain of the RET proto-oncogene in sporadic medullari thyroid carcinoma and in a family with FMTC. Oncogene 1995; 10:509–513.
48. Eng C., Clayton D., Schuffenecker I., Lenoir G., Cote G., Gagel R.F., Van, Amstel H.K., Lips C.J., Nishisho I., Takai S.I., Marsh D.J., Robinson B.G., Frank-Raue K., Raue F., Xue F., Noll W.W., Romei C., Pacini F., Fink M., Niederle B., Zedenius J., Nordenskjold M., Komminoth P., Hendy G.N., Mulligan L.M. The relationship between specific RET proto-oncogene mutations and disease phenotype in multiple endocrine neoplasia type 2. International RET mutation consortium analysis. JAMA 1996a; 276:1575–1579.
49. Eng C., Mulligan L.M., Healey C.S., Houghton C., Frilling A., Raue F., Thomas G.A., Ponder B.A. Heterogeneous mutation of the RET proto-oncogene in subpopulations of medullary thyroid carcinoma. Cancer Res 1996b; 56:2167–2170.
50. Eng C. RET proto-oncogene in the development of human cancer. J Clin Oncol 1999; 17:380–393.
51. Farndon J.R., Leight G.S., Dilley W.G., Baylin S.B., Smallridge R.C., Harrison T.S., Wells S.A., Jr. Familial medullary thyroid carcinoma without associated endocrinopathies: a distinct clinical entity. Br J Surg 1986; 73:278–281.
52. Fattoruso O., Quadro L., Libroia A., Verga U., Lupoli G., Cascone E., Colantuoni V. A GTG to ATG novel point mutation at codon 804 in exon 14 of the RET proto-oncogene in two families affected by familial medullary thyroid carcinoma. Hum Mutat 1998; Suppl 1:167–71.
53. Feldman G.L., Edmonds M.W., Ainsworth P.J., Schuffenecker I., Lenoir G.M., Saxe A.W., Talpos G.B., Roberson J., Petrucelli N., Jackson C.E. Variable expressivity of familial medullary thyroid carcinoma (FMTC) due to a RET V804M (GTG−>ATG) mutation. Surgery 2000; 128:93–98.
54. Frischauf A.M. Positional cloning uncovers a new old oncogene. Hum Mol Genet 1993; 2:847–848.
55. Gagel R.F., Tashjian A.H., Jr., Cummings T., Papathanasopoulos N., Kaplan M.M., Delellis R.A., Wolfe H.J., Reichlin S. The clinical outcome of prospective screening for multiple endocrine neoplasia type 2a. An 18-year experience. N Engl J Med 1988; 318:478–484.

56. Goodfellow P.J., Wells S.A., Jr. RET gene and its implications for cancer. J Natl Cancer Inst 1995; 87:1515–1523.
57. Grieco M., Santoro M., Berlingieri M.T., Melillo R.M., Donghi R., Bongarzone I., Pierotti M.A., Della Porta G., Fusco A., Vecchio G. PTC is a novel rearranged form of the ret proto-oncogene and is frequently detected in vivo in human thyroid papillary carcinomas. Cell 1990; 60:557–563.
58. Grimm J., Sachs M., Britsch S., Di Cesare S., Schwarz-Romond T., Alitalo K., Birchmeier W. Novel p62dok family members, dok-4 and dok-5, are substrates of the c-Ret receptor tyrosine kinase and mediate neuronal differentiation. J Cell Biol 2001; 154:345–354.
59. Hahn M., Bishop J. Expression pattern of Drosophila ret suggests a common ancestral origin between the metamorphosis precursors in insect endoderm and the vertebrate enteric neurons. Proc Natl Acad Sci U S A 2001; 98:1053–1058.
60. Hayashi H., Ichihara M., Iwashita T., Murakami H., Shimono Y., Kawai K., Kurokawa K., Murakumo Y., Imai T. Characterization of intracellular signals via tyrosine 1062 in RET activated by glial cell line-derived neurotrophic factor. Oncogene 2000; 14:4469–4475.
61. Hayashi Y., Iwashita T., Murakamai H., Kato Y., Kawai K., Kurokawa K., Tohnai I., Ueda M., Takahashi M. Activation of BMK1 via tyrosine 1062 in RET by GDNF and MEN2A mutation. Biochem Biophys Res Commun 2001; 281:682–689.
62. Hazard J.B. The C cells (parafollicular cells) of the thyroid gland and medullary thyroid carcinoma. A review. Am J Pathol 1977; 88:213–250.
63. Hazard J.B., Hawk W.A., Crile G. Medullary (solid) carcinoma of the thyroid—a clinicopathologic entity. J Clin Endocrinol Metab 1959; 19:152–161.
64. Hennige A.M., Lammers R., Arlt D., Hoppner W., Strack V., Niederfellner G., Seif F.J., Haring H., Kellerer M. Ret oncogene signal transduction via a IRS-2/PI 3-kinase/PKB and SHC/Grb-2 dependent pathway: possible implication for transforming activity in NIH3T3 cells. Mol Cell Endocrinol 2000; 167:69–76.
65. Hofstra R.M., Landsvater R.M., Ceccherini I., Stulp R.P., Stelwagen T., Luo Y., Pasini B., Hoppner J.W.M., Ploos van Hamstel H.K., Romeo G., Lips C.J.M., Buys C.H.C.M. A mutation in the RET proto-oncogene associated with multiple endocrine neoplasia type 2B and sporadic medullary thyroid carcinoma. Nature 1994; 367:375–376.
66. Hofstra R.M., Fattoruso O., Quadro L., Wu Y., Libroia A., Verga U., Colantuoni V., Buys C.H. A novel point mutation in the intracellular domain of the ret protooncogene in a family with medullary thyroid carcinoma. J Clin Endocrinol Metab 1997; 82:4176–4178.
67. Hoppner W., Ritter M.M. A duplication of 12 bp in the critical cysteine rich domain of the RET proto-oncogene results in a distinct phenotype of multiple endocrine neoplasia type 2A. Human Molec Genet 1997; 6:587–590.
68. Hoppner W., Dralle H., Brabant G. Duplication of 9 base pairs in the critical cysteine-rich domain of the RET proto-oncogene causes multiple endocrine neoplasia type 2A. Hum Mutat 1998; Suppl 1:S128-30.:S128–S130.
69. Huang S.C., Koch C.A., Vortmeyer A.O., Pack S.D., Lichtenauer U.D., Mannan P., Lubensky I.A., Chrousos G.P., Gagel R.F., Pacak K., Zhuang Z. Duplication of the mutant RET allele in trisomy 10 or loss of the wild-type allele in multiple endocrine neoplasia type 2-associated pheochromocytomas. Cancer Res 2000; 60:6223–6226.
70. Igaz P., Patocs A., Racz K., Klein I., Varadi A., Esik O. Occurrence of pheochromocytoma in a MEN2A family with codon 609 mutation of the RET proto-oncogene. J Clin Endocrinol Metab 2002; 87:2994.
71. Ishizaka Y., Itoh F., Tahira T., Ikeda I., Sugimura T., Tucker J., Fertitta A., Carrano A.V., Nagao M. Human ret proto-oncogene mapped to chromosome 10q11.2. Oncogene 1989; 4:1519–1521.
72. Ito S., Iwashita T., Asai N., Murakami H., Iwata Y., Sobue G., Takahashi. Biological properties of Ret with cysteine mutations correlate with multiple endocrine neoplasia type 2A, familial medullary thyroid carcinoma, and Hirschsprung's disease phenotype. Cancer Res 1997; 57:2870–2872.
73. Iwamoto T., Taniguchi M., Asai N., Ohkusu K., Nakashima I., Takahashi M. cDNA cloning of mouse ret proto-oncogene and its sequence similarity to the cadherin superfamily. Oncogene 1993; 8:1087–1091.
74. Iwashita T., Asai N., Murakami H., Matsuyama M., Takahashi M. Identification of tyrosine residues that are essential for transforming activity of the RET proto-oncogene with MEN2A or MEN2B mutation. Oncogene 1996; 12:481–487.
75. Iwashita T., Kato M., Murakami H., Asai N., Ishiguro Y., Ito S., Iwata Y., Kawai K., Asai M., Kurokawa K., Kajita H., Takahashi M. Biological and biochemical properties of Ret with kinase

domain mutations identified in multiple endocrine neoplasia type 2B and familial medullary thyroid carcinoma. Oncogene 1999; 18:3919–3922.
76. Jhiang S.M. The RET proto-oncogene in human cancers. Oncogene 2000; 19:5590–5597.
77. Jing S., Wen D., Yu Y., Holst P.L., Luo Y., Fang M., Tamir R., Anatonio L., Hu Z., Cupples R., Louis J.-C., Hu S., Altrock B.W., Fox G.M. GDNF-induced activation of the Ret protein tyrosine kinase is mediated by GDNFR-alpha, a novel receptor for GDNF. Cell 1996; 85:1113–1124.
78. Kakudo K., Carney J.A., Sizemore G.W. Medullary carcinoma of thyroid. Biologic behavior of the sporadic and familial neoplasm. Cancer 1985; 55:2818–2821.
79. Kalinin V.N., Amosenko F.A., Shabanov M.A., Lubchenko L.N., Hosch S.B., Garkavtseva R.F., Izbicki J.R. Three novel mutations in the RET proto-oncogene. J Mol Med 2001; 79:609–612.
80. Kasprzak L., Nolet S., Gaboury L., Pavia C., Villabona C., Rivera-Fillat F., Oriola J., Foulkes W.D. Familial medullary thyroid carcinoma and prominent corneal nerves associated with the germline V804M and V778I mutations on the same allele of RET. J Med Genet 2001; 38:784–787.
81. Kawai K., Iwashita T., Murakami H., Hiraiwa N., Yoshiki A., Kusakabe M., Ono K., Ida K., Nakayama A., Takahashi M. Tissue-specific carcinogenesis in transgenic mice expressing the RET proto-oncogene with a multiple endocrine neoplasia type 2A mutation. Cancer Res 2000; 60:5254–5260.
82. Komminoth P., Kunz E.K., Matias-Guiu X., Hiort O., Christiansen G., Colomer, A, Roth J., Heitz P.U. Analysis of RET protooncogene point mutations distinguishes heritable from nonheritable medullary thyroid carcinomas. Cancer 1995; 76:479–489.
83. Komminoth P., Roth J., Muletta-Feurer S., Saremaslani P., Seelentag W.K., Heitz P.U. RET protooncogene point mutations in sporadic neuroendocrine tumors. J Clin Endocrinol Metab 1996; 81:2041–2046.
84. Kovacs C.S., Mase M., Kovacs K., Nguyen G.K., Chik C. Thyroid medullary carcinoma with thyroglobulin immunoreactivity in sporadic multiple endocrine neoplasia type 2-B. Cancer 1994; 74:928–932.
85. Kurokawa K., Iwashita T., Murakami H., Hayashi H., Kawai K., Takahashi M. Identification of SNT/FRS2 docking site on RET receptor tyrosine kinase and its role for signal transduction. Oncogene 2001; 20:1929–1938.
86. Kurokawa K., Kawai K., Hashimoto M., Ito Y., Takahashi M. Cell signalling and gene expression mediated by RET tyrosine kinase. J Intern Med 2003; 253:627–633.
87. Lee D.C., Chan K.W., Chan S.Y. RET receptor tyrosine kinase isoforms in kidney function and disease. Oncogene 2002; 21:5582–5592.
88. Lindor N.M., Honchel R., Kosla S., Thibodeau S.N. Mutations in the RET proto-oncogene in sporadic pheocromocytomas. J Clin Endocrin Metab 1994; 80:627–629.
89. Lips C.J. Clinical management of the multiple endocrine neoplasia syndromes: results of a computerized opinion poll at the Sixth International Workshop on Multiple Endocrine Neoplasia and von Hippel-Lindau disease. J Intern Med 1998; 243:589–594.
90. Liu X., Vega Q.C., Decker R.A., Pandey A., Worby C.A., Dixon J.E. Oncogenic RET receptors display different autophosphorylation sites and substrate binding specificities. J Biol Chem 1996; 271:5309–5312.
91. Lorenzo M.J., Gish G.D., Houghton C., Stonehouse T.J., Pawson T., Ponder B.A.J., Smith D.P. RET alternate splicing influences the interaction of activated RET with the SH2 and PTB domains of Shc, and the SH2 domain of Grb2. Oncogene 1997; 14:763–771.
92. Manie S., Santoro M., Fusco A., Billaud M. The RET receptor: function in development and dysfunction in congenital malformation. Trends Genet 2001; 17:580–589.
93. Marcos C., Pachnis V. The effect of the ret-mutation on the normal development of the central and parasympathetic nervous systems. Int J Dev Biol 1996; Suppl 1:137S–138S.:137S–138S.
94. Marengere L.E., Songyang Z., Gish G.D., Schaller M.D., Parsons J.T., Stern M.J., Cantley L.C., Pawson T. SH2 domain specificity and activity modified by a single residue. Nature 1994; 369:502–505.
95. Marsh D.J., Robinson B.G., Andrew S., Richardson A.L., Pojer R., Schnitzler M., Mulligan L.M., Hyland V.J. A rapid screening method for the detection of mutations in the RET proto-oncogene in multiple endocrine neoplasia type 2A and familial medullary thyroid carcinoma families. Genomics 1994; 23:477–479.
96. Melillo R.M., Carlomagno F., De Vita G., Formisano P., Vecchio G., Fusco A., Billaud M., Santoro M. The insulin receptor substrate (IRS)-1 recruits phosphatidylinositol 3-kinase to Ret: evidence for a competition between Shc and IRS-1 for the binding to Ret. Oncogene 2001; 20:209–218.
97. Mendelsohn J., Baselga J. The EGF receptor family as targets for cancer therapy. Oncogene 2000; 19:6550–6565.

98. Meng X., Lindahl M., Hyvonen M.E., Parvinen M., de Rooij D.G., Hess M.W., Raatikainen-Ahokas A., Sainio K., Rauvala H., Lakso M., Pichel J.G., Westphal H., Saarma M., Sariola H. Regulation of cell fate decision of undifferentiated spermatogonia by GDNF. Science 2000; 287:1489–1493.
99. Michiels F.M., Chappuis S., Caillou B., Pasini A., Talbot M., Monier R., Lenoir G.M., Feunteun J., Billaud M. Development of medullary thyroid carcinoma in transgenic mice expressing the RET protooncogene altered by a multiple endocrine neoplasia type 2A mutation. Proc Natl Acad Sci U S A 1997; 94:3330–3335.
100. Miyauchi A., Futami H., Hai N., Yokozawa T., Kuma K., Aoki N., Kosugi S., Sugano K., Yamaguchi K. Two germline missense mutations at codons 804 and 806 of the RET proto-oncogene in the same allele in a patient with multiple endocrine neoplasia type 2B without codon 918 mutation. Jpn J Cancer Res 1999; 90:1–5.
101. Mograbi B., Bocciardi R., Bourget I., Juhel T., Farahi-Far D., Romeo G., Ceccherini I., Rossi B. The sensitivity of activated cys ret mutants to glial cell line-derived neurotrophic factor is mandatory to rescue neuroectodermic cells from apoptosis. Mol Cell Biol 2001; 21:6719–6730.
102. Morita H., Daidoh H., Nagata K., Okano Y., Sudoh Y., Maruyama T., Sarui H., Ishizuka T., Akagi K., Nishisho I., Yasuda K. A family of multiple endocrine neoplasia type 2A: genetic analysis and clinical features. Endocrine J 1996; 43:25–30.
103. Mulligan L.M., Gardner E., Smith B.A., Mathew C.G., Ponder B.A. Genetic events in tumour initiation and progression in multiple endocrine neoplasia type 2. Genes Chrom Cancer 1993a; 6:166–177.
104. Mulligan L.M., Kwok J.B.J., Healey C.S., Elsdon M.J., Eng C., Gardner E., Love D.R., Mole S.E., Moore J.K., Papi L., Ponder M.A., Telenius H., Tunnacliffe A., Ponder B.A.J. Germ-line mutations of the RET proto-oncogene in multiple endocrine neoplasia type 2A. Nature 1993b; 363:458–460.
105. Mulligan L.M., Eng C., Attie T., Lyonnet S., Marsh D.J., Hyland V.J., Robinson B.G., Frilling A., Verellen-Dumoulin C., Safar A. Diverse phenotypes associated with exon 10 mutations of the RET proto-oncogene. Hum Mol Genet 1994; 3:2163–2167.
106. Mulligan L.M., Ponder B.A. Genetic basis of endocrine disease: multiple endocrine neoplasia type 2. J Clin Endocrinol Metab 1995a; 80:1989–1995.
107. Mulligan L.M., Marsh D.J., Robinson B.G., Schuffenecker I., Zedenius J., Lips C.J., Gagel R.F., Takai S.I., Noll W.W., Fink M., . Genotype-phenotype correlation in multiple endocrine neoplasia type 2: report of the International RET Mutation Consortium. J Intern Med 1995b; 238:343–346.
108. Murakami H., Yamamura Y., Shimono Y., Kawai K., Kurokawa K., Takahashi M. Role of Dok1 in cell signaling mediated by RET tyrosine kinase. J Biol Chem 2002; 277:32781–32790.
109. Niccoli-Sire P., Murat A., Rohmer V., Franc S., Chabrier G., Baldet L., Maes B., Savagner F., Giraud S., Bezieau S., Kottler M.L., Morange S., Conte-Devolx B., The French Calcitonin Tumors Group (GETC). Familial medullary thyroid carcinoma with noncysteine ret mutations: phenotype-genotype relationship in a large series of patients. J Clin Endocrinol Metab 2001; 86:3746–3753.
110. Nicklin S.A., Baker A.H. Tropism-modified adenoviral and adeno-associated viral vectors for gene therapy. Curr Gene Ther 2002; 2:273–293.
111. Nishikawa M., Murakumo Y., Imai T., Kawai K., Nagaya M., Funahashi H., Nakao A., Takahashi M. Cys611Ser mutation in RET proto-oncogene in a kindred with medullary thyroid carcinoma and Hirschsprung's disease. Eur J Hum Genet 2003; 11:364–368.
112. Nunziata V., Giannattasio R., Di Giovanni G., D'Armiento M.R., Mancini M. Hereditary localized pruritus in affected members of a kindred with multiple endocrine neoplasia type 2A (Sipple's syndrome). Clin Endocrinol (Oxf) 1989; 30:57–63.
113. Oishi S., Sato T., Takiguchi-Shirahama S., Nakamura Y. Mutations of the RET proto-oncogene in multiple endocrine neoplasia type 2A. Endocrine J 1995; 42:527–536.
114. Pachnis V., Mankoo B., Costantini F. Expression of the c-ret proto-oncogene during mouse embryogenesis. Development 1993; 119:1005–1017.
115. Pacini F., Fontanelli M., Fugazzola L., Elisei R., Romei C., Di Coscio G., Miccoli P., Pinchera A. Routine measurement of serum calcitonin in nodular thyroid diseases allows the preoperative diagnosis of unsuspected sporadic medullary thyroid carcinoma. J Clin Endocrinol Metab 1994; 78:826–829.
116. Pandey A., Duan H., Di Fiore P.P., Dixit V.M. The Ret receptor protein tyrosine kinase associates with the SH2-containing adapter protein Grb10. J Biol Chem 1995; 270:21461–21463.
117. Pandey A., Liu X., Dixon J.E., Di Fiore P.P., Dixit V.M. Direct association between the Ret receptor tyrosine kinase and the Src homology 2-containing adapter protein Grb7. J Biol Chem 1996; 271:10607–10610.

118. Papotti M., Botto M.F., Favero A., Palestini N., Bussolati G. Poorly differentiated thyroid carcinomas with primordial cell component. A group of aggressive lesions sharing insular, trabecular, and solid patterns. Am J Surg Pathol 1993; 17:291–301.
119. Paratcha G., Ledda F., Baars L., Coulpier M., Besset V., Anders J., Scott R., Ibanez C.F. Released GFRalpha1 potentiates downstream signaling, neuronal survival, and differentation via a novel mechanism of recruitment of c-Ret to lipid rafts. Neuron 2001; 29:171–184.
120. Paratcha G., Ledda F., Ibanez C.F. The neural cell adhesion molecule NCAM is an alternative signaling receptor for GDNF family ligands. Cell 2003; 113:867–879.
121. Pasini A., Geneste O., Legrand P., Schlumberger M., Rossel M., Fournier L., Rudkin B., Schuffenecker I., Lenoir G., Billaud M. Oncogenic activation of RET by two distint FMTC mutations affetting the tirosine kinase domain. Oncogene 1997; 15:393–402.
122. Pasini B., Ceccherini I., Romeo G. RET mutations in human disease. TIG 1996; 12:138–144.
123. Pigny P., Bauters C., Wemeau J.L., Houcke M.L., Crepin M., Caron P., Giraud S., Calender A., Buisine M.P., Kerckaert J.P., Porchet N. A novel 9-base pair duplication in RET exon 8 in familial medullary thyroid carcinoma. J Clin Endocrinol Metab 1999; 84:1700–1704.
124. Ponder BAJ. Multiple endocrine neoplasia type 2. In: Scriver C, Beaudet AL, Sly W, Valle D, editors. The metabolic and molecular bases of inherited disease. New York: 2001: 931–942.
125. Poteryaev D., Titievsky A., Sun Y.F., Thomas-Crusells J., Lindahl M., Billaud M., Arumae U., Saarma M. GDNF triggers a novel Ret-independent Src kinase family-coupled signaling via a GPI-linked GDNF receptor a1. FEBS 1999; 463:63–66.
126. Rey J.M., Brouillet J.P., Fonteneau-Allaire J., Boneu A., Bastie D., Maudelonde T., Pujol P. Novel germline RET mutation segregating with papillary thyroid carcinomas. Genes Chrom Cancer 2001; 32:390–391.
127. Reynolds L., Jones K., Winton D.J., Cranston A., Houghton C., Howard L., Ponder B.A.J., Smith D.P. C-cell and thyroid apithelial tumours and altered follicular development in transgenic mice expressing the long isoform of MEN 2A RET. Oncogene 2001; 20:3986–3994.
128. Robledo M., Gil L., Pollan M., Cebrian A., Ruiz S., Azanedo M., Benitez J., Menarguez J., Rojas J.M. Polymorphisms G691S/S904S of RET as genetic modifiers of MEN 2A. Cancer Res 2003; 63:1814–1817.
129. Romeo G., Ronchetto P., Luo Y., Barone V., Seri M., Ceccherini I., Pasini B., Bocciardi R., Lerone M., Kaariainen H., Martucciello G. Point mutations affecting the tyrosine kinase domain of the *RET* proto-oncogene in Hirschsprung's disease. Nature 1994; 367:377–378.
130. Saarma M. GDNF–a stranger in the TGF-beta superfamily? Eur J Biochem 2000; 267:6968–6971.
131. Salvatore D., Melillo R.M., Monaco C., Visconti R., Fenzi G., Vecchio G., Fusco A., Santoro M. Increased in vivo phosphorylation of ret tyrosine 1062 is a potential pathogenetic mechanism of multiple endocrine neoplasia type 2B. Cancer Res 2001; 61:1426–1431.
132. Sanchez M.P., Silos-Santiago I., Frisen J., He B., Lira S.A., Barbacid M. Renal agenesis and the absence of enteric neurons in mice lacking GDNF. Nature 1996; 382:70–73.
133. Santoro M., Carlomagno F., Hay I.D., Herrmann M.A., Grieco M., Melillo R., Pierotti M.A., Bongarzone I., Della Porta G., Berger N., Peix J.L., Paulin C., Fabien N., Vecchio G., Jenkins R.B., Fusco A. Ret oncogene activation in human thyroid neoplasms is restricted to the papillary cancer subtype. J Clin Invest 1992; 89:1517–1522.
134. Santoro M., Carlomagno F., Romano A., Bottaro D.P., Dathan N.A., Grieco M., Fusco A., Vecchio G., Matoskova B., Kraus M.H., Di Fiore P.P. Activation of *RET* as a dominant transforming gene by germline mutations of MEN2A and MEN2B. Science 1995; 267:381–383.
135. Sariola H. The neurotrophic factors in non-neuronal tissues. Cell Mol Life Sci 2001; 58:1061–1066.
136. Sariola H., Saarma M. GDNF and its receptors in the regulation of the ureteric branching. Int J Develop Biol 1999; 43:413–418.
137. Schneider R. The human protooncogene ret: a communicative cadherin? Trends Biochem Sci 1992; 17:468–469.
138. Schuchardt A., D'Agati V., Larsson-Blomberg L., Costantini F., Pachnis V. Defects in the kidney and enteric nervous system of mice lacking the tyrosine kinase receptor Ret. Nature 1994; 367:380–383.
139. Segouffin-Cariou C., Billaud M. Transforming ability of MEN2A-RET requires activation of the phosphatidylinositol 3-kinase/AKT signaling pathway. J Biol Chem 2000; 275:3568–3576.
140. Simons K., Ikonen E. Functional rafts in cell membranes. Nature 1997; 387:569–572.
141. Sipple J.H. The association of pheochromocytoma with carcinoma of the thyroid gland. Am J Med 1961; 31:163–166.

142. Smith D.P., Houghton C., Ponder B.A. Germline mutation of RET codon 883 in two cases of de novo MEN 2B. Oncogene 1997; 15:1213–1217.
143. Smith-Hicks C.L., Sizer K.C., Powers J.F., Tischler A.S., Costantini F. C-cell hyperplasia, pheochromocytoma and sympathoadrenal malformation in a mouse model of multiple endocrine neoplasia type 2B. EMBO J 2000; 19:612–622.
144. Steiner A.L., Goodman A.D., Powers S.R. Study of a kindred with pheochromocytoma, medullary thyroid carcinoma, hyperparathyroidism and Cushing's disease: multiple endocrine neoplasia, type 2. Medicine (Baltimore) 1968; 47:371–409.
145. Tahira T., Ishizaka Y., Itoh F., Sugimura T., Nagao M. Characterization of ret proto-oncogene mRNAs encoding two isoforms of the protein product in a human neuroblastoma cell line. Oncogene 1990; 5:97–102.
146. Takahashi M., Buma Y., Hiai H. Isolation of Ret proto-oncogene cDNA with an amino-terminal signal sequence. Oncogene 1989; 4:805–806.
147. Takahashi M., Buma Y., Iwamoto T., Inaguma Y., Ikeda H., Hiai H. Cloning and expression of the ret proto-oncogene encoding a tyrosine kinase with two potential transmembrane domains. Oncogene 1988; 3:571–578.
148. Takahashi M., Cooper G.M. Ret transforming gene encodes a fusion protein homologous to tyrosine kinases. Mol Cell Biol 1987; 7:1378–1385.
149. Takahashi M., Iwashita T., Santoro M., Lyonnet S., Lenoir G.M., Billaud M. Co-segregation of MEN2 and Hirschsprung's disease: the same mutation of RET with both gain and loss-of-function?. Hum Mutat 1999; 13:331–336.
150. Takahashi M., Ritz J., Cooper G.M. Activation of a novel human transforming gene, ret, by DNA rearrangement. Cell 1985; 42:581–588.
151. Tessitore A., Sinisi A.A., Pasquali D., Cardone M., Vitale D., Bellastella A., Colantuoni V. A novel case of multiple endocrine neoplasia type 2A associated with two de novo mutations of the RET protooncogene. J Clin Endocrinol Metab 1999; 84:3522–3527.
152. Treanor J.J., Goodman L., de Sauvage F., Stone D.M., Poulsen K.T., Beck C.D., Gray C., Armanini M.P., Pollock R.A., Hefti F., Phillips H.S., Goddard A., Moore M.W., Buj-Bello A., Davies A.M., Asai N., Takahashi M., Vandlen R., Henderson C.E., Rosenthal A. Characterization of a multicomponent receptor for GDNF. Nature 1996; 382:80–83.
153. Trupp M., Arenas E., Fainzilber M., Nilsson A.S., Sieber B.A., Grigoriou M., KilKenny C., Salazar-Grueso E., Pachnis V., Arumae U. Functional receptor for GDNF encoded by the c-ret proto-oncogene. Nature 1996; 381:785–788.
154. Trupp M., Belluardo N., Funakoshi H., Ibanez C.F. Complementary and overlapping expression of glial cell line-derived neurotrophic factor (GDNF), c-ret proto-oncogene, and GDNF receptor-a indicates multiple mechanisms of trophic actions in the adult Rat CNS. J Neurosci 1997; 17:3554–3567.
155. Trupp M., Scott R., Whittemore S.R., Ibanez C.F. Ret-dependent and -independent mechanisms of glial cell line-derived neurotrophic factor signaling in neuronal cells. J Biol Chem 1999; 274:20885–20894.
156. Tsui-Pierchala B.A., Ahrens R.C., Crowder R.J., Milbrandt J., Johnson E.M.Jr. The long and short isoforms of Ret function as independent signaling complexes. J Biol Chem 2002; 277:34618–34625.
157. Tsuzuki T., Takahashi M., Asai N., Iwashita T., Matsuyama M., Asai J. Spatial and temporal expression of the RET proto-oncogene product in embryonic, infant and adult rat tissues. Oncogene 1995; 10:191–198.
158. Vega Q.C., Worby C.A., Lechner M.S., Dixon J.E., Dressler G.R. Glial cell line-derived neurotrophic factor activates the receptor tyrosine kinase RET and promotes kidney morphogenesis. Proc Natl Acad Sci USA 1996; 93:10657–10661.
159. Verdy M., Weber A.M., Roy C.C., Morin C.L., Cadotte M., Brochu P. Hirschsprung's disease in a family with multiple endocrine neoplasia type 2. J Pediatr Gastroenterol Nutr 1982; 1:603–607.
160. Watanabe T., Ichihara M., Hashimoto M., Shimono K., Shimoyama Y., Nagasaka T., Murakumo Y., Murakami H., Sugiura H., Iwata H., Ishiguro N., Takahashi M. Characterization of gene expression induced by RET with MEN2A or MEN2B mutation. Am J Pathol 2002; 161:249–256.
161. Wickham T.J. Ligand-directed targeting of genes to the site of disease. Nat Med 2003; 9:135–139.
162. Williams E.D. Histogenesis of medullary carcinoma of the thyroid. J Clin Pathol 1966; 19:114–118.
163. Williams E.D., Pollock D.J. Multiple mucosal neuromata with endocrine tumours: a syndrome allied to von Recklinghausen's disease. J Pathol Bacteriol 1966; 91:71–80.

164. Wohllk N., Cote G.J., Bugalho M.M., Ordonez N., Evans D.B., Goepfert H., Khorana S., Schultz P., Richards C.S., Gagel R.F. Relevance of RET proto-oncogene mutations in sporadic medullary thyroid carcinoma. J Clin Endocrinol Metab 1996; 81:3740–3745.
165. Worley D.S., Pisano J.M., Choi E.D., Walus L., Hession C.A., Cate R.L., Sanicola M., Birren S.J. Developmental regulation of GDNF response and receptor expression in the enteric nervous system. Development 2000; 127:4383–4393.
166. Young H.M., Hearn C.J., Ciampoli D., Southwell B.R., Brunet J.F., Newgreen D.F. A single rostrocaudal colonization of the rodent intestine by enteric neuron precursors is revealed by the expression of Phox2b, Ret, and p75 and by explants grown under the kidney capsule or in organ culture. Dev Biol 1998; 202:67–84.

24. FROM GENES TO DECISIONS

EVOLVING VIEWS OF GENOTYPE-BASED MANAGEMENT IN MEN 2

LOIS M. MULLIGAN
Queen's University

INTRODUCTION

The genomic revolution of the past 20 years has led to the identification of the genetic mechanisms that are responsible for a wide variety of human cancers, and has made a huge impact on our ability to recognize, diagnose and, more recently, treat patients with these diseases. Genetic diagnosis of heritable forms of cancer holds out the potential for presymptomatic detection in familial cases and raises the possibility of prophylactic treatments that would decrease morbidity and mortality and improve the quality of life for those affected. While the potential impact of these advances is huge, to date, our understanding of the underlying genetic events that contribute to the familial cancers has only allowed us to significantly modify our management of the disease in a few instances. The paradigm for such genetically based molecular management is the multiple endocrine neoplasia type 2 (MEN 2) syndromes.

Multiple endocrine neoplasia type 2 (MEN 2)

As described in previous chapters(1), MEN 2 is an inherited cancer syndrome characterized by medullary thyroid carcinoma (MTC) and its precursor lesion, C-cell hyperplasia. These phenotypes are clinically recognizable in >90% of all cases (2). Traditionally, MEN 2 has been divided into three disease subtypes, based on the presence of other associated phenotypes. The most common subtype, MEN 2A accounts for about 85% of MEN 2 cases. In addition to MTC, MEN 2A is characterized by pheochromocytoma (PC), tumours of the adrenal chromaffin cells, in about 50% of cases, and hyperparathyroidism (HPT) in 15–30% of individuals. The most aggressive of the MEN 2 subtypes, MEN 2B, occurs in about 5% of cases and has a median age of tumour onset that is 10 years earlier than other forms of MEN 2 (<10 years)(3, 4). Approximately 50% of MEN 2B are *de novo* cases with no previous family history (5). As in MEN 2A, PC occurs in about 50% of individuals with MEN 2B but HPT is rare and patients also have a variety of other developmental anomalies such as buccal neuromas, marfanoid habitus, ganglioneuromas of the gut, and thickened corneal nerves (3, 6). The final disease subtype, familial MTC (FMTC) is characterized only by thyroid tumors and has no other associated anomalies. This disease form is the least aggressive MEN 2 subtype and may have a lower penetrance and later disease onset (7). As a result, FMTC families are frequently small and may be phenotypically quite difficult to distinguish from MEN 2A families in which cases of PC or HPT have not yet manifested. Because of this, stringent definitions have been suggested in which the diagnosis of FMTC requires a minimum of 4 (8, 9) or even 10 (10) family members with MTC in the absence of other phenotypes.

RET and the genetics of MEN 2

MEN 2 is inherited as an autosomal dominant disease and, as a result, all first-degree relatives of an affected individual are at 50% risk of inheriting the disease causing mutation. Although they differ in phenotype and aggressiveness, all three MEN 2 subtypes are caused by mutations of the *RET* (Rearranged in Transfection) oncogene (8, 9). *RET* encodes a cell surface receptor tyrosine kinase normally required for development of neuroendocrine cell types, the peripheral nervous system, and kidney (1, 11). *RET* mutations are identified in more than 95% of all MEN 2 families and there is no evidence of families in which the MEN 2 phenotype is not linked to *RET*. In each case, RET mutations are single amino acid substitutions that result in inappropriate activation of the RET receptor (12, 13). Mutations are clustered in "hot spots" in the extracellular domain (exons 10 and 11) or in the tyrosine kinase domain (exons 13–16) of the receptor (8, 9) (Figure 1).

Because >99% of mutations occur in only 10 codons of RET, direct DNA testing in MEN 2 is simple, widely available, and very efficient and is recommended for all at-risk individuals (Discussed below).

Although all MEN 2 subtypes are associated with *RET* mutations, specific mutations confer much higher risks for some phenotypes. For example, mutations of *RET* codon 634 are strongly correlated with HPT and PC and thus, not surprisingly, represent 85% of MEN 2A mutations (14, 15). In MEN 2A, mutations generally alter specific cysteine residues in the extracellular domain of RET (residues 609, 611, 618, 620, 634), resulting in a ligand-independent constitutively activated molecule (Figure 1). The mutations found in patients with FMTC have a broader range of functional effects, and may include both the same type of mutations as those seen in MEN 2A as well as mutations in the tyrosine kinase domain (residues 768, 804, 891) that appear to alter ATP binding (16). More than 95% of MEN 2B patients share the same amino acid substitution (Met918Thr) in the binding pocket of the RET kinase

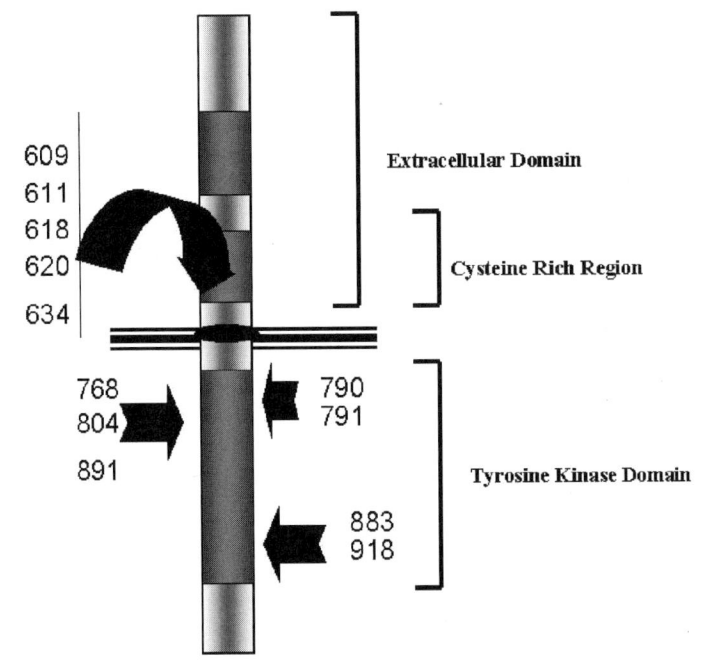

Figure 1. Schematic diagram of the RET receptor showing the relative positions of the more common mutations found in MEN 2.

domain (8, 9), although rare mutations of codon 883 are also detected (17, 18). Both mutations appear to alter the substrates of RET, thereby changing the downstream signals it sends (16) (Figure 1). The strong associations of specific mutations with each of the disease phenotypes can provide us with an additional tool for predicting patient prognosis and guiding management strategies (Discussed below).

In contrast to the activating *RET* mutations found in MEN 2, inactivating mutations of RET are identified in patients with Hirschsprung disease (HSCR), a congenital abnormality of gut innervation[19]. HSCR mutations are found throughout the *RET* gene and result in reduced levels of functional RET protein (20, 21). In rare cases, both the MEN 2 and HSCR phenotypes are associated with a single *RET* mutation (22, 23). These are generally single amino acid substitutions found in cysteine residues in the extracellular domain of RET (exon 10) (22). These oncogenic mutations may be as frequent as 1% in the HSCR population (24).

Diagnosis and prediction of MEN 2

Diagnosis in the "pre-genotyping" era

Before the identification of disease causing mutations in *RET*, MEN 2 disease status in at-risk individuals was established by biochemical screening. Generally, this involved measurement of calcitonin peptide release by C-cells in response to a provocative agent, such as pentegastrin or calcium (25). Elevated levels of calcitonin indicated the presence of an increased number of C-cells (C-cell hyperplasia) or of MTC and these individuals would be offered prophylactic thyroidectomy. This strategy, while clinically important, had several drawbacks, not the least of which was that diagnosis was dependent on identification of early hyperplastic changes and frequently was not made until MTC or even metastatic disease was already present (26, 27). Further, a negative screen result did not indicate that a patient did not carry the MEN 2 disease mutation, only that they had no detectable disease at that time. Thus, repeated screening of all at-risk individuals was required annually, or at regular intervals, in order to detect all MEN 2 cases. As a result, 50% of at-risk individuals who had no MEN 2 mutation would be repeatedly and unnecessarily screened. Because every at-risk individual needed to be repeatedly tested, biochemical screening for MEN 2 was a relatively costly strategy. Further, after several negative tests compliance could be a significant issue. For those undergoing regular testing, borderline or difficult to interpret biochemical screening results occasionally resulted in unnecessary thyroidectomy in individuals who did not carry the MEN 2 mutation (28). The incidence of false positives may have been as high as 5–10% (10).

In individuals with a confirmed diagnosis of MEN 2 additional screening for other associated phenotypes such as PC and HPT was required. Patients would be screened for PC on a regular basis by measurement of plasma metanephrines or levels of catecholamines or metanephrines in 24 h urine collection (29). A positive screen would lead to unilateral or, if necessary bilateral adrenalectomy. In general, prophylactic adrenalectomy would not be recommended due to risks from adrenal insufficiency (30). HPT is rarely symptomatic in MEN 2 but can be detected by measurement of calcium or parathyroid hormone levels. Biochemical screening for PC and HPT is recommended annually for individuals diagnosed with MEN 2.

MEN 2 and *RET* mutation testing

The identification of *RET* mutations as the underlying cause of MEN 2 has changed the management of the individual and family with MEN 2 significantly. Genetic testing, scanning the *RET* codons known to be frequently mutated, is now the preferred method for confirming the clinical diagnosis of MEN 2 and is considered the standard of good practice (9, 10, 31). The rate of false negative (2–5%) (10) and false positive (<0.1%) results in DNA testing is a dramatic improvement over biochemical screening methods. Individuals at-risk for MEN 2 should now be screened at birth or at the earliest possible time for *RET* mutations and the results should provide the basis for recommending thyroidectomy. Prophylactic thyroidectomy for individuals carrying a germline *RET* mutation has dramatically reduced morbidity and mortality due to MTC, and perceived quality of life is much better in individuals at risk for MTC than for those at risk of other cancers where diagnosis and management are less clear cut (32).

Because the basis and expectations associated with genetic testing need to be clearly understood in order for at-risk individuals to understand the implications of a *RET* mutation test and for them to use that information to make informed decisions about disease management, it is essential that all DNA testing be accompanied by appropriate genetic counseling. This would generally take the form of pretest counseling to explain the implications and risks of the test and one or more post-test counseling sessions involving delivery of results and discussion of their implications as necessary.

INDICATIONS FOR *RET* MUTATION TESTING. Screening for *RET* mutations is now the basis of all management strategies for MEN 2, replacing reliance on biochemical screening. In families where the disease causing mutation has already been established by previous screening of affected individuals, all at-risk individuals should be genetically screened for the familial mutation. Individuals who do not carry this mutation are not at risk of MEN 2 and can be excluded from further testing. Individuals with the mutation are at high risk for MEN 2 phenotypes and should be managed accordingly. If diagnosis is made in a child, thyroidectomy should be performed before age 5 for MEN 2A and FMTC families and before age 6 months in individuals with MEN 2B mutations which are associated with earlier tumour development (10).

Early, genetically based identification of mutation carriers permits surgery before the usual onset of malignant disease and carries the optimal possibility of preventing metastatic disease. Older patients diagnosed with *RET* mutations will be offered thyroidectomy as soon as possible accompanied by biochemical monitoring for the presence of metastatic disease. Mutation positive individuals will be monitored throughout life for other tumour types or anomalies associated with their specific MEN 2 subtype, as described above. The regime for these screening protocols may, in theory, be modified based on the occurrence and age of onset of these phenotypes in other family members. However, variability in these, even within a single family, suggests that caution should be used when relaxing screening protocols (33, 34).

If an individual represents a new case/family diagnosed for MEN 2, *RET* mutation screening should be performed in a known affected family member. This also holds true for all individuals diagnosed with apparently sporadic MTC, as 1–7% of these have germline *RET* mutations and represent new MEN 2 families (35). Interestingly, early studies had suggested that germline *RET* mutations were very rare in sporadic PC but recent studies showing they may occur in up to 5% of cases (36) have suggested that all patients with these tumours should also be screened for *RET* mutations (10). Initial screening must include *RET* exons in which mutations are most frequently found, (exons 10, 11, 13–16) however these may be prioritized based on the patient phenotype. For example, 85% of MEN 2A families have mutations in exon 11 and almost 95% of MEN 2B cases have mutations of codon 918 in exon 16. If mutations of these exons are not identified a broader screen, including all *RET* exons may be necessary. Once a *RET* mutation is identified, all other at-risk family members may be screened specifically for that change and individuals carrying the mutation are managed as described above.

In a few instances, a *RET* mutation may not be identified in a putative MEN 2 individual. These cases are rare and frequently, although not always, involve families that are quite small with few or a single affected individual. In the past, some of these families may have resulted from conservative diagnosis of FMTC in families that did not have clear features of MEN 2. For example, studies have shown that up to 5% of the population may have C-cell hyperplasia but do not have *RET* mutations nor a true MEN 2 phenotype (28). Recent studies suggest that at least some of these cases may be related to mutations of the succinate dehydrogenase subunit D gene (chromosome 11q23) and not to *RET* (37).

This highlights the necessity of accurate and unambiguous clinical diagnosis in cases where *RET* mutations have not been identified. If families with clearly defined MEN 2 but no *RET* mutation have sufficient confirmed affected family members available, linkage analysis using polymorphic sites in or near the *RET* gene (chromosome 10q11.2) may provide an alternative to direct mutation detection. In this method, a haplotype for a series of polymorphisms over the region of *RET* which presumably includes a disease mutation may be constructed based on the genotype of multiple affected family members (38–41). Inheritance of this "disease haplotype" can be used to identify individuals who have also inherited the predicted *RET* mutation and are therefore assumed to be MEN 2 carriers. This method is less amenable to diagnosis than is direct mutation testing since it is dependent on the availability of a suitable family structure, the participation of multiple family members and relies on the assumption that the clinical diagnosis is correct in suggesting MEN 2.

Where suitable family members are not available, or a haplotype cannot be constructed, MEN 2 families without *RET* mutations will be treated as they were before the advent of DNA mutation testing, using repeated biochemical screening of all at-risk individuals and offering surgery at the first sign of a positive test result.

WHO SHOULD BE OFFERED SCREENING? *RET* mutation screening is considered the standard of care for all individuals at-risk for MEN 2, irrespective of their age. Ideally, at-risk individuals in known MEN 2 families would be screened for *RET* mutations at birth or shortly thereafter. This is somewhat different from mutation testing in many other cancer syndromes where minors are not automatically screened. In the case of MEN 2, the penetrance of the disease is very high (>90% have clinically detectable disease) and onset is very young, the earliest recognition of MEN 2B being reported in children under age 5 (24, 42, 43) necessitating very early detection to allow presymptomatic intervention. Further, unlike many other cancer syndromes of childhood, there are clear, well tolerated, prophylactic options available which are demonstrably valuable in decreasing the burden of the disease in affected individuals. The advent of early childhood mutation detection has greatly reduced the incidence of MTC in families with known MEN 2 and will, with time, virtually eliminate the morbidity and mortality associated with metastatic disease in known MEN 2 families.

RET mutation screening is also recommended for individuals with sporadic MTC and also PC, although there has been no indications that RET mutations contribute to sporadic HPT (44). In each case, it is important to remember that RET mutations can occur somatically in these tumours (45–49) and that these should not be confused with germline MEN 2-RET mutations.

Approximately 1% of individuals with HSCR have a RET mutation in exon 10 which may also confer risk for MEN 2 phenotypes (24). While this may seem rare, RET mutations in HSCR are widely distributed throughout the gene and exon 10 mutations, primarily in codons 609, 618 and 620, represent one of the largest clusterings of mutations. Because of the oncogenic risk associated with these mutations, RET exon 10 mutation screening is recommended for all children diagnosed with HSCR. Individuals identified with any of these mutations should be treated as a potential MEN 2 case and screening of at-risk family members and surgical intervention should be offered.

Diagnosis and management: The evolving genetic contribution

While the advent of genetic testing for RET mutations has significantly improved our ability to manage patients and families with MEN 2, the potential exists for additional refinement that may improve the prospects even further. Several exciting options for this refinement are currently being evaluated and the accumulating body of experience with RET genotype and phenotype are allowing us to improve the accuracy of disease prediction.

Genotype-phenotype associations in genetically based management

Our 10 year experience of RET mutation and MEN 2 disease phenotype correlation has shown us that not all RET mutations carry equal associated risk and that the traditional definitions of disease phenotype may in future not be as useful to us as genetically or mutation based disease risk estimates.

We have long known that some RET mutations conferred higher risk of PC (e.g. Cys634Arg or Met918Thr) (8, 9) while others are associated with a less aggressive disease phenotype (e.g. Glu768Arg or Val804Met). Recent studies have begun to investigate the potential of using specific RET mutation data to guide management strategies. Three general categories of high, medium, and low risk RET mutations may be defined based on their relative penetrance, the specific disease phenotypes associated with them, and the aggressiveness of these phenotypes (Table 1) (10, 31). Mutations in the highest disease risk group include those found in MEN 2B (Met 918Thr, Ala883Phe). The lowest risk mutations are those found most frequently in FMTC and those associated with later disease onset (Table 1) (50).

These risk groupings are an attractive tool to supplement clinical diagnosis for defining individuals with high risk who need early thyroidectomy and/or stringent biochemical screening regimes. By defining a subgroup of higher risk patients genetically predisposed to more, or more severe, disease phenotypes we may be able to focus health care resources more effectively and reduce patient stress associated with disease management. In future, the specific RET mutation found in a patient is likely to act

Table 1. Relative risk groups in MEN 2 associated with specific *RET* mutations

Relative risk	Mutant RET codons	Disease phenotype	MTC characteristics	Recommended MTC management
High	918, 883	MEN 2B	Earliest onset Aggressive tumours	Thyroidectomy < 6 months
Moderate	611, 618, 620, 634	FMTC, MEN 2A	Early onset	Thyroidectomy <3 years
Lowest	609, 768, 804, 891	FMTC, MEN 2A	Later onset, relatively indolent	Thyroidectomy <3 years[1]

[1]Management of this risk group remains controversial (10). In some centers, later surgery is recommended based on the age of onset seen in other family members.

as a guide to determine the frequency of screening required and the age at which surgery should be offered to mutation carriers. We may, for example, be able to reduce the frequency of screening for PC in individuals with mutations rarely associated with PC (e.g. Glu768Arg or Val804Met), or use a more relaxed age for thyroidectomy in patients with mutations and a family history consistent with later onset tumours. Such genotype-based management must be used with caution however, as there is still some variability in clinical presentation of MEN 2, even in families/individuals carrying the identical *RET* mutation. Aggressive, early onset cases can occur in families with mutations that have elsewhere been shown to be quite indolent (33, 34). It is clear that genotype-based management strategies will still rely heavily on the clinical diagnosis and the specific pattern of the disease within a family to optimize a program of surgery and biochemical screening appropriate to the specific genotype and phenotype of each patient.

Disease associated RET haplotypes in sporadic MTC and PC

The genotype at the *RET* locus may, in future, also provide us with some predictive information on the occurrence of sporadic tumours. The majority of MTC and PC (>75%) occur sporadically, without any associated family history (36, 51). However, recent studies have suggested that some haplotypes for polymorphic variants surrounding the *RET* locus are associated with increased risk for these sporadic tumours (39, 52). These risk haplotypes may reflect a combination of variants that themselves confer risk or may be a simple marker for another risk contributing gene lying upstream of *RET* and not yet identified. In the future, this information may be useful in predicting individuals at risk for sporadic tumours or in establishing the risk of recurrence in family members of individuals with sporadic disease.

SUMMARY CONCLUSIONS

Diagnosis and management of MEN 2 has evolved considerably since the identification of the underlying disease mutations in the *RET* proto-oncogene. Presymptomatic detection and prophylactic surgical intervention are now the accepted standard of care. The strong correlation of disease phenotype and mutation genotype has already also allowed us to develop mutation-guided management strategies to optimize time of intervention and schedule follow-up and management. As our understanding of the depth of these correlations increases we look forward to better refining our management regimes to fit both the best care requirements and the quality of life needs of the MEN 2 patient.

REFERENCES

1. Pierotti, M. A. RET Activation in Medullary carcinomas. *In:* N. Farid (ed.), Molecular Basis of Thyroid Cancer: Kluwar Academic Publishers, In Press.
2. Easton, D. F., Ponder, M. A., Cummings, T., Gagel, R. F., Hansen, H. H., Reichlin, S., Tashjian, A. H., Telenius-Berg, M., Ponder, B. A. J., and Cancer Research Campaign Medullary Thyroid Group The clinical and screening age-at-onset distribution for the MEN-2 syndrome. Am J Hum Genet, *44*: 208–215, 1989.
3. Gorlin, R. J., Sedano, H. O., Vickers, R. A., and Cervenka, J. Multiple mucosal neuromas, pheochromocytoma and medullary carcinoma of the thyroid—a syndrome. Cancer, *22*: 293–299, 1968.
4. Leboulleux, S., Travagli, J. P., Caillou, B., Laplanche, A., Bidart, J. M., Schlumberger, M., and Baudin, E. Medullary thyroid carcinoma as part of a multiple endocrine neoplasia type 2B syndrome: influence of the stage on the clinical course. Cancer, *94*: 44–50, 2002.
5. Carlson, K., Bracamontes, J., Jackson, C., Clark, R., Lacroix, A., Wells, S., and Goodfellow, P. Parent-of-origin effects in multiple endocrine neoplasia type 2B. Am J Hum Genet, *55*: 1076–1082, 1994.
6. Carney, J. A., Go, V. L., Sizemore, G. W., and Hayles, A. B. Alimentary-tract ganglioneuromatosis. A major component of the syndrome of multiple endocrine neoplasia, type 2b. N Engl J Med, *295*: 1287–1291, 1976.
7. Farndon, J. R., Leight, G. S., Dilley, W. G., Baylin, S. B., Smallridge, R. C., Harrison, T. S., and Wells, S. A. Familial medullary thyroid carcinoma without associated endocrinopathies: a distinct clinical entity. Br J Surg, *73*: 278–281, 1986.
8. Mulligan, L. M., Marsh, D. J., Robinson, B. G., Schuffenecker, I., Zedenius, J., Lips, C. J. M., Gagel, R. F., Takai, S.-I., Noll, W. W., Fink, M., Raue, F., Lacroix, A., Thibodeau, S. N., Frilling, A., Ponder, B. A. J., Eng, C., and International *RET* Mutation Consortium Genotype-phenotype correlation in multiple endocrine neoplasia type 2: report of the International *RET* Mutation Consortium. J Intern Med, *238*: 343–346, 1995.
9. Eng, C., Clayton, D., Schuffenecker, I., Lenoir, G., Cote, G., Gagel, R. F., Ploos van Amstel, H.-K., Lips, C. J. M., Nishisho, I., Takai, S.-I., Marsh, D. J., Robinson, B. G., Frank-Raue, K., Raue, F., Xu, F., Noll, W. W., Romei, C., Pacini, F., Fink, M., Niederle, B., Zedenius, J., Nordenskjöld, M., Komminoth, P., Hendy, G., Gharib, H., Thibodeau, S., Lacroix, A., Frilling, A., Ponder, B. A. J., and Mulligan, L. M. The relationship between specific *RET* proto-oncogene mutations and disease phenotype in multiple endocrine neoplasia type 2: International *RET* Mutation Consortium. JAMA, *276*: 1575–1579, 1996.
10. Brandi, M. L., Gagel, R. F., Angeli, A., Bilezikian, J. P., Beck-Peccoz, P., Bordi, C., Conte-Devolx, B., Falchetti, A., Gheri, R. G., Libroia, A., Lips, C. J., Lombardi, G., Mannelli, M., Pacini, F., Ponder, B. A., Raue, F., Skogseid, B., Tamburrano, G., Thakker, R. V., Thompson, N. W., Tomassetti, P., Tonelli, F., Wells, S. A., Jr., and Marx, S. J. Guidelines for diagnosis and therapy of MEN type 1 and type 2. J Clin Endocrinol Metab, *86*: 5658–5671, 2001.
11. Schuchardt, A., D'Agati, V., Larsson-Blomberg, L., Costantini, F., and Pachnis, V. Defects in the kidney and enteric nervous system of mice lacking the tyrosine kinase receptor Ret. Nature, *367*: 380–383, 1994.
12. Santoro, M., Carlomagno, F., Romano, A., Bottaro, D. P., Dathan, N. A., Grieco, M., Fusco, A., Vecchio, G., Matoskova, B., Kraus, M. H., and Di Fiore, P. P. Activation of *RET* as a dominant transforming gene by germline mutations of MEN2A and MEN2B. Science, *267*: 381–383, 1995.
13. Asai, N., Iwashita, T., Matsuyama, M., and Takahashi, M. Mecahanism of activation of the *ret* proto-oncogene by multiple endocrine neoplasia 2A mutations. Mol Cell Biol, *15*: 1613–1619, 1995.
14. Mulligan, L. M., Eng, C., Healey, C. S., Clayton, D., Kwok, J. B. J., Gardner, E., Ponder, M. A., Frilling, A., Jackson, C. E., Lehnert, H., Neumann, H. P. H., Thibodeau, S. N., and Ponder, B. A. J. Specific mutations of the *RET* proto-oncogene are related to disease phenotype in MEN 2A and FMTC. Nature Genet, *6*: 70–74, 1994.

15. Schuffenecker, I., Virally-Monod, M., Brohet, R., Goldgar, D., Conte-Devolx, B., Leclerc, L., Chabre, O., Boneu, A., Caron, J., Houdent, C., Modigliani, E., Rohmer, V., Schlumberger, M., Eng, C., Guillausseau, P. J., and Lenoir, G. M. Risk and penetrance of primary hyperparathyroidism in multiple endocrine neoplasia type 2A families with mutations at codon 634 of the RET proto-oncogene. Groupe D'etude des Tumeurs a Calcitonine. J Clin Endocrinol Metab, *83*: 487–491, 1998.
16. Iwashita, T., Kato, M., Murakami, H., Asai, N., Ishiguro, Y., Ito, S., Iwata, Y., Kawai, K., Asai, M., Kurokawa, K., Kajita, H., and Takahashi, M. Biological and biochemical properties of Ret with kinase domain mutations identified in multiple endocrine neoplasia type 2B and familial medullary thyroid carcinoma. Oncogene, *18*: 3919–3922, 1999.
17. Smith, D. P., Houghton, C., and Ponder, B. A. J. Germline mutation of *RET* codon 883 in two cases of *de novo* MEN 2B. Oncogene, *15*: 1213–1217, 1997.
18. Gimm, O., Marsh, D. J., Andrew, S. D., Frilling, A., Dahia, P. L. M., Mulligan, L. M., Zajac, J. D., Robinson, B. G., and Eng, C. Germline dinucleotide mutation in codon 883 of the *RET* proto-oncogene in multiple endocrine neoplasia type 2B without codon 918 mutation. J Clin Endocrinol Metab, *82*: 3902–3904, 1997.
19. Edery, P., Lyonnet, S., Mulligan, L. M., Pelet, A., Dow, E., Abel, L., Holder, S., Nihoul-Fékété, C., Ponder, B. A. J., and Munnich, A. Mutations of the *RET* proto-oncogene in Hirschsprung's disease. Nature, *367*: 378–380, 1994.
20. Pasini, B., Borrello, M. G., Greco, A., Bongarzone, I., Luo, Y., Mondellini, P., Alberti, L., Miranda, C., Arighi, E., Bocciardi, R., Seri, M., Barone, V., Radice, M. T., Romeo, G., and Pierotti, M. A. Loss of function effect of *RET* mutations causing Hirschsprung disease. Nature Genet, *10*: 35–40, 1995.
21. Iwashita, T., Murakami, H., Asai, N., and Takahashi, M. Mechanisms of Ret dysfunction by Hirschsprung mutations affecting its extracellular domain. Hum Molec Genet, *5*: 1577–1580, 1996.
22. Mulligan, L. M., Eng, C., Attié, T., Lyonnet, S., Marsh, D. J., Hyland, V. J., Robinson, B. G., Frilling, A., Verellen-Dumoulin, C., Safar, A., Venter, D. J., Munnich, A., and Ponder, B. A. J. Diverse phenotypes associated with exon 10 mutations of the *RET* proto-oncogene. Hum Mol Genet, *3*: 2163–2167, 1994.
23. Takahashi, M., Iwashita, T., Santoro, M., Lyonnet, S., Lenoir, G. M., and Billaud, M. Co-segregation of MEN2 and Hirschsprung's disease: the same mutation of RET with both gain and loss-of-function? Hum Mutat, *13*: 331–336, 1999.
24. Torre, M., Martucciello, G., Ceccherini, I., Lerone, M., Aicardi, M., Gambini, C., and Jasonni, V. Diagnostic and therapeutic approach to multiple endocrine neoplasia type 2B in pediatric patients. Pediatr Surg Int, *18*: 378–383, 2002.
25. Heshmati, H. M., Gharib, H., van Heerden, J. A., and Sizemore, G. W. Advances and controversies in the diagnosis and management of medullary thyroid carcinoma. Am J Med, *103*: 60–69, 1997.
26. Wells, S., Chi, D., Toshima, K., Dehner, L., Coffin, C., Dowton, B., Ivanovich, J., DeBenedetti, M., Dilley, W., Moley, J., Norton, J., and Donis-Keller, H. Predictive DNA testing and prophylactic thyroidectomy in patients at risk for multiple endocrine neoplasia type 2A. Ann Surg, *220*: 237–250, 1994.
27. Dralle, H., Gimm, O., Simon, D., Frank-Raue, K., Gortz, G., Niederle, B., Wahl, R. A., Koch, B., Walgenbach, S., Hampel, R., Ritter, M. M., Spelsberg, F., Heiss, A., Hinze, R., and Hoppner, W. Prophylactic thyroidectomy in 75 children and adolescents with hereditary medullary thyroid carcinoma: German and Austrian experience. World J Surg, *22*: 744–750; discussion 750–741, 1998.
28. Lips, C. J. M., Landsvater, R. M., Höppener, J. W. M., Geerdink, R. A., Blijham, G., Jansen-Schillhorn van Veen, J. M., van Gils, A. P. G., de Wit, M. J., Zewald, R. A., Berends, M. J. H., Beemer, F. A., Brouwers-Smalbraak, J., Jansen, R. P. M., Ploos van Amstel, H. K., van Vroonhoven, T. J. M. V., and Vroom, T. M. Clinical screening as compared with DNA analysis in families with multiple endocrine neoplasia type 2A. N Engl J Med, *331*: 828–835, 1994.
29. Frank-Raue, K., Kratt, T., Hoppner, W., Buhr, H., Ziegler, R., and Raue, F. Diagnosis and management of pheochromocytomas in patients with multiple endocrine neoplasia type 2-relevance of specific mutations in the RET proto-oncogene. Eur J Endocrinol, *135*: 222–225, 1996.
30. Lee, J. E., Curley, S. A., Gagel, R. F., Evans, D. B., and Hickey, R. C. Cortical-sparing adrenalectomy for patients with bilateral pheochromocytoma. Surgery, *120*: 1064–1070; discussion 1070–1061, 1996.
31. Yip, L., Cote, G. J., Shapiro, S. E., Ayers, G. D., Herzog, C. E., Sellin, R. V., Sherman, S. I., Gagel, R. F., Lee, J. E., and Evans, D. B. Multiple endocrine neoplasia type 2: evaluation of the genotype-phenotype relationship. Arch Surg, *138*: 409–416, 2003.
32. Freyer, G., Ligneau, B., Schlumberger, M., Blandy, C., Contedevolx, B., Trillet-Lenoir, V., Lenoir, G. M., Chau, N., and Dazord, A. Quality of life in patients at risk of medullary thyroid carcinoma

and followed by a comprehensive medical network: trends for future evaluations. Ann Oncol, *12*: 1461–1465, 2001.
33. Feldman, G. L., Edmonds, M. W., Ainsworth, P. J., Schuffenecker, I., Lenoir, G. M., Saxe, A. W., Talpos, G. B., Roberson, J., Petrucelli, N., and Jackson, C. E. Variable expressivity of familial medullary thyroid carcinoma (FMTC) due to a RET V804M (GTG–>ATG) mutation. Surgery, *128*: 93–98, 2000.
34. Lombardo, F., Baudin, E., Chiefari, E., Arturi, F., Bardet, S., Caillou, B., Conte, C., Dallapiccola, B., Giuffrida, D., Bidart, J. M., Schlumberger, M., and Filetti, S. Familial medullary thyroid carcinoma: clinical variability and low aggressiveness associated with RET mutation at codon 804. J Clin Endocrinol Metab, *87*: 1674–1680, 2002.
35. Eng, C., Mulligan, L. M., Smith, D. P., Healey, C. S., Frilling, A., Raue, F., Neumann, H. P. H., Ponder, M. A., and Ponder, B. A. J. Low frequency of germline mutations in the *RET* proto-oncogene in patients with apparently sporadic medullary thyroid carcinoma. Clin Endocrinol, *43*: 123–127, 1995.
36. Neumann, H. P., Bausch, B., McWhinney, S. R., Bender, B. U., Gimm, O., Franke, G., Schipper, J., Klisch, J., Altehoefer, C., Zerres, K., Januszewicz, A., Eng, C., Smith, W. M., Munk, R., Manz, T., Glaesker, S., Apel, T. W., Treier, M., Reineke, M., Walz, M. K., Hoang-Vu, C., Brauckhoff, M., Klein-Franke, A., Klose, P., Schmidt, H., Maier-Woelfle, M., Peczkowska, M., and Szmigielski, C. Germ-line mutations in nonsyndromic pheochromocytoma. N Engl J Med, *346*: 1459–1466, 2002.
37. Lima, J., Teixeira-Gomes, J., Soares, P., Maximo, V., Honavar, M., Williams, D., and Sobrinho-Simoes, M. Germline succinate dehydrogenase subunit D mutation segregating with familial non-RET C cell hyperplasia. J Clin Endocrinol Metab, *88*: 4932–4937, 2003.
38. Sancandi, M., Griseri, P., Pesce, B., Patrone, G., Puppo, F., Lerone, M., Martucciello, G., Romeo, G., Ravazzolo, R., Devoto, M., and Ceccherini, I. Single nucleotide polymorphic alleles in the 5' region of the RET proto-oncogene define a risk haplotype in Hirschsprung's disease. J Med Genet, *40*: 714–718, 2003.
39. Borrego, S., Wright, F. A., Fernandez, R. M., Williams, N., Lopez-Alonso, M., Davuluri, R., Antinolo, G., and Eng, C. A Founding Locus within the RET Proto-Oncogene May Account for a Large Proportion of Apparently Sporadic Hirschsprung Disease and a Subset of Cases of Sporadic Medullary Thyroid Carcinoma. Am J Hum Genet, *72*: 88–100, 2003.
40. Griseri, P., Pesce, B., Patrone, G., Osinga, J., Puppo, F., Sancandi, M., Hofstra, R., Romeo, G., Ravazzolo, R., Devoto, M., and Ceccherini, I. A rare haplotype of the RET proto-oncogene is a risk-modifying allele in hirschsprung disease. Am J Hum Genet, *71*: 969–974, 2002.
41. Burzynski, G. M., Nolte, I. M., Osinga, J., Ceccherini, I., Twigt, B., Maas, S. M., Brooks, A. S., Verheij, J. B. G. M., Menacho, I. P., Buys, C. H. C. M., and Hofstra, R. M. W. Mapping a putative mutation as the major contributor to the development of sporadic Hirschsprung diseae to the *RET* genomic sequence between the promoter region and exon 2. Eur J Hum Genet, In press.
42. Skinner, M. A., DeBenedetti, M. K., Moley, J. F., Norton, J. A., and Wells, S. A., Jr. Medullary thyroid carcinoma in children with multiple endocrine neoplasia types 2A and 2B. J Pediatr Surg, *31*: 177–181; discussion 181–172, 1996.
43. Stjernholm, M. R., Freudenbourg, J. C., Mooney, H. S., Kinney, F. J., and Deftos, L. J. Medullary carcinoma of the thyroid before age 2 years. J Clin Endocrinol Metab, *51*: 252–253, 1980.
44. Padberg, B.-C., Schröder, S., Jochum, W., Kastendieck, H., Roth, J., Heitz, P. U., and Komminoth, P. Absence of *RET* proto-oncogene point mutations in sporadic hyperplastic and neoplastic lesions of the parathyroid gland. Am J Pathol, *147*: 1600–1607, 1995.
45. Eng, C., Crossey, P. A., Mulligan, L. M., Healey, C. S., Houghton, C., Prowse, A., Chew, S. L., Dahia, P. L. M., O'Riordan, J. L. H., Toledo, S. P. A., Smith, D. P., Maher, E. R., and Ponder, B. A. J. Mutations in the *RET* proto-oncogene and the von Hippel-Lindau disease tumour suppressor gene in sporadic and syndromic phaeochromocytomas. J Med Genet, *32*: 934–937, 1995.
46. Eng, C., Mulligan, L. M., Smith, D. P., Healey, C. S., Frilling, A., Raue, F., Neumann, H. P. H., Pfragner, R., Behmel, A., Lorenzo, M. J., Stonehouse, T. J., Ponder, M. A., and Ponder, B. A. J. Mutation of the *RET* protooncogene in sporadic medullary thyroid carcinoma. Genes Chrom Canc, *12*: 209–212, 1995.
47. Hofstra, R. M. W., Landsvater, R. M., Ceccherini, I., Stulp, R. P., Stelwagen, T., Luo, Y., Pasini, B., Höppener, J. W. M., Ploos van Amstel, H. K., Romeo, G., Lips, C. J. M., and Buys, C. H. C. M. A mutation in the *RET* proto-oncogene associated with multiple endocrine neoplasia type 2B and sporadic medullary thyroid carcinoma. Nature, *367*: 375–376, 1994.

48. Blaugrund, J. E., Johns, M. M., Eby, Y. J., Ball, D. W., Baylin, S. B., Hruban, R. H., and Sidransky, D. *RET* proto-oncogene mutations in inherited and sporadic medullary thyroid cancer. Hum Mol Genet, *3*: 1895–1897, 1994.
49. Beldjord, C., Desclaux-Arramond, F., Raffin-Sanson, M., Corvol, J. C., De Keyser, Y., Luton, J. P., Plouin, P. F., and Bertagna, X. The *RET* protooncogene in sporadic pheochromocytomas: frequent MEN 2-like mutations and new molecular defects. J Clin Endocrinol Metab, *80*: 2063–2068, 1995.
50. Machens, A., Gimm, O., Hinze, R., Hoppner, W., Boehm, B. O., and Dralle, H. Genotype-phenotype correlations in hereditary medullary thyroid carcinoma: oncological features and biochemical properties. J Clin Endocrinol Metab, *86*: 1104–1109, 2001.
51. Gimm, O. Multiple Endocrine Neoplasia Type 2: Clinical Aspects. *In:* P. L. Dahia and C. Eng (eds.), Genetic Disorders of Endocrine Neoplasia, 1 edition, Vol. 28, pp. 103–130. Basel: Karger, 2001.
52. McWhinney, S. R., Boru, G., Binkley, P. K., Peczkowska, M., Januszewicz, A. A., Neumann, H. P., and Eng, C. Intronic single nucleotide polymorphisms in the RET protooncogene are associated with a subset of apparently sporadic pheochromocytoma and may modulate age of onset. J Clin Endocrinol Metab, 88 : 4911–4916, 2003.

INDEX

AA (arachidonic acid) 241
ABC (ATP-binding cassette) 362
absence of enteric ganglia 393
activating RET mutations 384
acute myelogenous leukemia 95
acute myeloid leukaemia 209
additional antitumor antibiotics 361
adenocarcinomas 282
adenoma 27, 275, 278
  histopathological diagnosis of 47
adenomatoid nodules 25
adenosine analog 358
adenovirus
  recombinant 370
  replication, essential for 374
  vector 372
adenylyl cyclase 242
adrenal chromaffin cells 417
adrenal medulla ganglioneuromas of the 401
adrenal tumors 50
adrenomedullin 267
age exposure 115
AIT (apical iodide transporter) 230
AKT 10
AKT2 11
alkyl sulfphonate 359
alkylating agent 359
allyl-geldanamycin 406
allythiourea 274

ALT (alternative lengthening of telomeres) 6, 12
  malignant transformation in 12
amphiregulin 122
analogs include carboplatin analog 359
anaplastic (small cell) carcinoma 81, 49–53, 113, 153, 300, 302, 397
  differential diagnosis 81
  diagnosis of 52
anaplastic large cell lymphoma 71
  ALK in 210
anaplastic thyroid cancer 359, 362, 370
  cell line FRO 370
anaplastic thyroid carcinoma 50, 52, 90, 269, 317, 357, 358, 364, 381
  agents 359
  cell lines (HTH74 and C643) 167
anaplastic tumor 16
aneuploidy 13
angiogenesis 14, 179, 358, 375
angiostatin 14
anthracyclines 360
  agent 364
  factor 375
  proteins 14
anticancer radiotherapy 233
anticancer therapy MMP inhibition in 186
antimetabolite 358–59
antimicrotubule agent 3 361–62

antineoplastic therapy pathobiology of 357–64
anti-tumor immunity 369
APC (adenomatous polyposis coli) 2
APC (adenomatous polyposis colonic) gene 113
apoptosis 5, 150–51
  cell cycle dregulation and 140–41
apoptotic cascade
  akt cascade 7
  bcl-2 cascade 7
  caspases cascade 7
ARF gene 150
aromatic amines and azo dyes tumor induction by 282
arthritis 180
ARTN (artemin) 391
associated sympathetic ganglia, enlargement of 401
ataxia telangiectasia 13
ATC 359–61
  agent 362
  combination chemotherapy for 362
  derived cell line ARO 251
  monolayers 362
  primary antineoplastic effects in 362
  xenografts treatment cytotoxicity in 362
attention-deficit hyperactivity disorder 170
atypical adenomas 26
atypical Hurthle cell adenoma 45
autoradiography 227
aziridines 359

BAX 152
  proapoptotic moiety 251
  protein potent inhibitor 364
BBF2H7 87
B-catenin and p53 mutation 94
B-cell lymphomas 8, 266
Bcl-2 (for B-cell lymphoma leukemia-2) family 250
Bcl-x (anti-apoptotic moiety) 251
BCNU (carmustine) 359
benign 274
  adenoma 268
  conditions radiotherapy for 191
  follicular adenomas 24, 134
  lesions 32
  nodule 296
  thyroid adenoma 240, 384
  thyroid nodules incidence of 385
  thyroid tumors 245
  tumor 275, 276, 279, 280
    follicular adenoma 276
    growth 297
    light-cell solid adenoma 276
    microfollicular adenoma 276
    papillary adenoma 276
    polymorphofollicular adenoma 276
    simple solid adenoma 276
    squamous cell (epideroid) cystadenoma 276
    trabecular adenoma 276
beta emitting Y-90 334
bFGF (basic fibroblast growth factor) 122, 245
BHP18-21 metastasis of tumor 172
bleomycin 361
blind therapy of 131I 325
BMP (bone morphogenetic proteins) 251
B-Raf 301–02
BRAF gene 11, 111, 200, 201
BRAF mutation 93, 116, 142, 209, 247
brain tumor 152
breast
  cancer 8, 15, 165, 207, 209, 233, 266, 302
    see also endocrine cancer
    HER2/NEU amplification in 9
  carcinomas 11, 386
  tumor 113
BTC (betacellin) 122
Burkitt's like lymphoma 79
Burkitt's lymphoma 304
bystander effect 371
b-ZIP (leucine zipper) DNA binding proteins 243

CA 19-9 303
ca 70-amino acid hydrophilic carboxy terminus 222
cAMP-dependent protein kinase C 227
camptothecin 360, 361
cancer
  cell lines 4
  gene therapy 187, 369
  genetic requirements for 2
  invasion, process of 179
  metastasis 180
    process of 179
  modeling method of 4
  origin of 1–16
  understanding and treatment of 14
canine thyroid cancer cisplatin monotherapy for 360
carboxy terminus 227
carcinoma 275
carcinosarcoma 276
CARD (caspase recruitment domain) 249
casein kinase-2 227
caused sporadic genetic disease 241
C-cell hyperplasia 56, 401, 420, 422
CCNU (lomustine) 359
CD15 (Leu-M1) 303
CD30 304
CD8+ T lymphocytes recruitment of 373
CDK4 8
CEA (carcinoembryonic antigen) 55, 337
cell adhesion 267
cell cycle deregulation and apoptosis 140–41
cell cyle regulators 149–60
cell genome 15 15
cell proliferation 122
cellular atypia 27

cellular process
    adipogenesis 172
    apoptosis 172
    atherosclerosis 172
    carcinogenesis 172
    cell cycle control 172
    inflammation 172
cellular RAS activity 132
cellular RAS in thyroid cells, role of 135–37
centroblastic appearing cell 72, 77
ceruloplasmin 302
cervical adenopathy 307
cervical cancer 9, 152
cervical carcinomas 9
CGRP (calcitonin gene-related peptide) 55
charge reversal mutagenesis 351
chemical carcinogens 281–83
    aromatic amines and azodyes 282
    nitrosamines 282
    nitrosoureas 283
chemical carcinogens, thyroid tumorigenesis induced by, 281–83
chemokines 369
chemosensitization 370
chemotherapeutic agents mechanisms of resistance 362–64
chemotherapies, effective systemic, 364
chemotherapy 16
    cytotoxicity of 363
    drug resistance 363
    drugs glutathione-conjugated 363
chimeric oncogenes 207, 209
Chinese hamster ovary cells 352
CHK1 13
CHK2 13
chlorambucil 359
chloride-iodide transporter (pendrin) 375
CHO (Chinese hamster ovary) 348, 352
    A81K 350
    G73K 350
    N64K 350
    P16K 349
    Q13K 349
    Q20K 349
    S64K 350
cholesterol clefts 24
chromaffin cell 403
chromosomal instability 15
chromosome 11q23 422
chronic hypercalcemia 56
chronic lymphocytic thyroiditis 44, 70
chronic thyroiditis 69
CIPA (congenital insensitivity to pain with anhidrosis) 207, 208
cisplatin 360, 361, 364
    mitoxantrone combination with 362
    therapy 359
CK2 214

"classic" competitive inhibitor perchlorate 222
classic papillary carcinoma 93
"classical" RET-C634R mutation 400
clear cell carcinoma 50
clinical application 334–35
    papillary and follicular thyroid carcinoma 334–35
    medullary thyroid carcinoma 335
clinical features of fPTC 385
cloning in Xenopus laevis oocytes 222
cluster analysis 266
cMOAT (canalicular multispecific organic anion transporter) 363
CMV (human cytomegalovirus) 372
CNS glioblastomas 125
collagen peptidomimetics 186
collumnar cell carcinoma 42
colon cancer
    cell 15
    pathogenesis 3
    tumor suppressor in 231
colorectal carcinoma 2, 10, 209
colorectal carcinoma development 3
combination chemotherapy 360–61
combination factors 283–84
combination therapies 361
combretastatin 361–62
combretastatin A4 phosphate 361–62
composite binding domain 346
computed tomography 306
congenital absence of enteric ganglia 389
Cowden syndrome 386
Cowden's disease 113, 248
Cox-2 (cyclooxygenase type 2) 304
CPI/KIP family 157
CPT-11 (irenotecan) 360, 361
    anthracyclines 360
    topotecan 360
CRAB1 (cellular retinoic aid binding protein) 269
Cre 372
CREB (cAMP-responsive element binding protein) 242, 243
CREB3L2 87
Cre-loxP, use of 372
CREM (cAMP-responsive element modulator) 243
cribriform-morular variant 41
CT (calcitonin) 371
cultured human follicular thyroid carcinoma 184
cycle arrest and apoptosis 150
cyclic nucleotide phosphodiesterase activity of 243
cyclin A 159
cyclin B1 159
cyclin cdc2 159
cyclin D1 157
cyclin E 9
cyclin E overexpression 9
cycline-kinase inhibitors 157

cyclins 157
cyclooxygenase-2 304–05
cyclophosphamide 359
Cys634 mutations of 403
cystic papillary thyroid cancer 296
cytogenetic deformities 13
cytogenetics biology 80–81
cytokeratin 38, 40, 303
  staining 80
cytokine signaling 249
cytokines 369
cytologic atypia 38

DD (death domain) 249
decoxycytidine kinase phosphorylates 371
decreased weight 170
DED (death effector domain) 249
diagnostic scintigraphy 323–24
diagnostic131I WBS 322
diaziquone 359
differential diagnosis 23
differentiated thyroid carcinoma 229
diffuse sclerosish variant 40
diffuse thyroid hyperplasia 113 113
dioxopiperazine 360
dipeptidylpeptidase IV 267
DIPN (diisopropanolnitrosamine) 282
disseminated medullary thyroid carcinoma 358
distant metastases detection of 306–07
DIT (diiodotyrosine) 319
DLBCL (diffuse large B cell lymphoma) 71, 76, 79
DMSA-V 331, 336
DNA damage 7
  elements 15
DNA microarrays 265–66
  application 266
DNA religation step 361
DNA therapeutics 369
DNMT (DNA mehtyltransferases) 15
docetaxel 364
dolastatin 361–62
dolastatin10 362
dolastatin15 362
doxorubicin 360, 361, 364
  5-fluorouracil combination with 362
  bleomycin vincristine in combination with 362
  cisplatin combination with 362
doxorubicin monotherapy 360
drug efflux proteins 362–63
drug resistance additional mediators of 363–64
drug resisting gene into normal hematopoietic stem cells, transfer of 369
DTC (differentiated thyroid carcinoma) 319
DTIC (dacarbazine) 359
dysphagia 70
dysplasis 4
dyspnoea 70

E2F 158
E7 oncoprotein sequesters 9
early hyperthyroidism 113
E-CDK2 8
ECM (extracellular matrix) 179, 184
EGF (epidermal growth factor) 10, 122, 124, 181, 245
EGFR (epidermal growth factor receptor) 10, 122
ELISA 186
ellipticine 360
EMA (epithelial membrane antigen) 51, 304
embryogenesis 179
EMMPRIN (extracellular matrix metalloproteinase inducer) 184, 267, 268
endemic goitre 53
endocrine cancers 165
endocrine cell regulation 122
endocrine tumor 295
  breast cancer 174
  prostate cancer 174
endometrium 165
endometrium cancer 165 see also endocrine cancers
endostatin 14
ENIGMA proteins 396
ENS (enteric nervous system), development of 392
enzymatic activity 12
enzyme-coupled membrane receptor systems 245–52
eosinophil-derived neurotoxin 269
eosinophilia 383
epidermal growth factor 122
epigenetic alterations 15
epigenetic phenomena 15
epipodophyllotoxin 360
epithelial cancer 96
epithelial membrane antigen 304
epithelial thyroid tumor rearrangements 108
epithelial thyroid tumorigenesis 117
epothilones A 361
epothilones B 361
erbβ-2/neu in thyroid neoplasia 123
erbβ-3 122
erbβ-4 122
ERK (extrcellular signal-regulated kinase) 246
estrogen and progesteron receptors, abnormal expression of, 166
estrogen stimulation 122
ETS transcription 183
ETU (ethylenethiourea) 278
evolving genetic contribution 423
external beam radiotheray 32
external X-ray irradiation tumor induction after 281

familial nonmedullary thyroid cancer susceptibility gene 384

familial papillary thyroid carcinoma 381–86
    clinical characteristics of 385
    FNMTC 383
    fPTC/PRN 383
    PTC at 19p13 383
    TCO 383
FAP (familial adenomatous polyposis) 2, 385
    syndrome 41
farnesyltransferase inhibitor 362
fatty acid binding 267
    protein 269
FDG (FluoroDeoxyGlucose) 317, 326
    clinical application 326
    general mechanism 327
    medullary thyroid cancer 327–29
    papillary and follicular thyroid cancer 327–28
    PET tracers 328
    scan method 329
18F-DOPA 329
FGF (fibroblast growth factors) 124–25
FGF1 (fibroblast growth factor) 117
FGF-2 125
FGFR (fibroblast growth factor receptor) 125
FGFR1 125
FHIT 156
fibromyxoid sarcoma 89
fibrosis 24
fibrous variant 48
FISH technology 30
FLICE-inhibitory proteins (FLIP) 250
5-fluorouracil 364, 371
FLT3 mutation 95
FMTC (familial medullary thyroid carcinoma) 55, 389, 390, 418
    diagnosis of 422
    mutations, activation of 402
    RET in 401
FNA (fine needle aspiration) 295
focal necrosis 24
follicular adenoma 24, 26–27, 29, 90, 92, 123, 185, 275, 300, 303
follicular and papillary carcinomas mutations and RET gene, rearrangements in 370
follicular cancer 303, 308
follicular carcinoma 26–32, 50, 90, 123, 134, 136, 300, 301
    carcinosarcoma 276
    clincial and pathological characteristics of 90
    external beam radiotherapy 43
    incidence of 32
    light-cell solid carcinoma 276
    microfollicular carcinoma 276
    minimally invasive 28
    mixed tumors 276
    NIS immunohistochemistry in 225
    papillary carcinoma 276
    polymorphofollicular carcinoma 276
    polymorphous solid carcinoma 276
    sarcomas 276
    small cell carcinoma 276
    solid carcinoma 276
    TSH as initiator 171
    unencapsulated 29
    vasculoinvasive 29
    widely invasive 28
follicular epithelium, normal thyroid 30
follicular hyperplasia-like proliferation 92
follicular lesion 28
    diagnosis of 26
    malignancy in thyroid diagnosis of 31
follicular lymphoma 71, 79
follicular neoplasms pathogenesis of 384
follicular nodules 24
follicular thyroid cancer 306, 327
follicular thyroid carcinogenesis 170
follicular thyroid carcinoma 113, 171, 330, 334, 381, 386
    development and progression of 174
    follicular thyroid carcinoma, PPARγ gene rearrangements in 88
follicular thyroid tumor 113, 215
    K-RAS and H-RAS mutations 92
    molecular events 85–96
    molecular pathways in 89
follicular tumorigenesis 112
follicular tumors 267–68, 282
follicular variant 37
FOS 183
    clinical characteristics of 386
    evaluation and treatment of 386
    susceptibility gene, existence of 386
    susceptibility genes identification of 385
frank carcinoma 2
FRO 370
    growth of 370
    tumors pre-established 371
FRTL5 371

G protein mutation 93
G2-M 159
GADD45 152
galectin3 267, 298
    use of 29
GAP (GTPase activating proteins) 10
GAPDH (glyceraldehyde-3-phosphate-dehydrogenase) 309, 310
GCV (prodrug ganciclovir) 371
GDNF (glial cell line derived neurotrophic factor) 391, 192, 393
    null mutations in 392
GDP (G-proteins bind guanosine diphosphate) 240
GEF (guanine nucleotide exchange factor) 10
gemcitabine 360
gene coding immunostimulators transfer of 369

gene mutation 363
gene rearrangement 30
gene therapy, concept of 369, 370
gene transcription 252
gene-replacement therapy 369, 370
generic environmental cellular insults 239
genes in particular cancers 4 4
genetic abnormalities 113–14
genetic instability 12–14
genetic mutation 53
genetic predisposition 114
genistein 406
genomic instability 5
   RAS and 139–40
germ cell neoplasms premenopausal breast carcinoma 384
germline mutations role of 170
GFR a genes null mutations in 392
GGF (glial growth factor) 122
Ghrelin 244
GHS-R1a (growth hormone secretagogue-receptor) 244
giant cell variant 50
gland embryogenesis 275
glioblastome multiforme cancer 9
Glu768Arg 423
Glut 1 303
GLUT-1transporter 327
glutathione S-transferase 363
glycoprotein hormones
   FSH 346
   hCG 346
   LH 346
glycoproteins
   elastin 180
   fibronectin 180
   laminin 180
   proteoglycans 180
   tenascin 180
   vitronectin 180
glycosilation sites 214
glycosylation 358
goitre thyroiditis 47
goitrogenic drugs 274
goitrogen-induced tumors 278
GPCR (G-protein coupled receptor) 238
   systems 240
G-protein 240
granulation tissue 24
Graves' disease 25, 44
   NIS immunohistochemistry in 225
GRK (G-proteins-coupled kinase) 240
ground glass 34
growth factors and receptors 121–23
   amphiregulin 122
   basic fibroblast 122
   BTC 122
   EFG 122

EGF (epidermal growth factor) family 122
erbβ-3 122
erbβ-4 122
GGF 122
HB-EGF 122
heregulin 122
IGF-I 122
IGF-II 122
NDF 122
platelet-derived 122
TGFα 122
TGF-α 122
TGF-β 122
Gsα 26
GTPase activity 241

haemorrhage 24
haemosiderin deposition 24
hAIT (human apical iodide transporter) 230
hAIT gene 231
HAMA (human anti-mouse antibody) 337
Hashimoto's disease 48
Hashimoto's thyroiditis 39, 48, 70, 80, 81, 158
   development of 250
   nodules associated 47
HB-EGF (heparin-binding EGF-like growth factor) 122
HBME-1 29, 303–04
hCG (human chorionic gonadotopin) 346
healthy thyroid gland 228
hearing abnormalities 170
hemangioendothelioma 50
hemangioma 276
hematologic cancer 96
hematological malignanci 358
heregulins 122
heterocomplex formation 123
heterozygosity loss of 8
hexamethylmelamine 359
hexokinase isoenzyme 327
HGFR system 246
hierarchical clustering 266, 269
high-dose taxanes 364
highly malignant phenotypes 370
high-molecular-weight glycoproteins 300
Hirschsprung's disease 393
HMGA 140
HMGI(Y) Mrna 302
HNGI(Y) [high mobility group I(Y)] 302
hoarseness 70
Hodgkin's disease 71, 304
housekeeping gene 309, 311
HPT (hyperparathyroidism) 418
HPV (humsn papillomaviruses) 9
H-RAS 10
H-RAS mutation 131
HSCR 423
HSCR (Hirschsprung's disease) 389, 390, 405

HSV-TK (herpes simplex virus-thymidine kinase) 371
HSV-TK gene 372
HSV-TK/GCV 371, 372
HSV-TK/GCV-mediated radiosensitization in thyroid cancer cells 371, 72
HTA (hyalinizing trabecular adenoma) 39
HTC (hyalinizing trabecular carcinoma) 39
hTERT 5, 6
HTERT mRNA 297
HTT (hyalinizing trabecular tumors) 39
human cancer
   development 15
   pathogenesis 2
human cell immortalization 6
human cell transformation 6
human cellular immortalization 4–6
human colon carcinoma 208
human hepatocellular carcinoma 168
human malignancies 266
human neuroblastoma 209
human papillary thyroid carcinoma 172
human papilloma virus 152
human prostate carcinoma cell 229
human tumor 2, 208
human undifferentiated thyroid carcinoma cells irradiation of 195
Hurthel cell 157, 383
   adenomas 44
   carcinoma 91, 267
   follicular carcinomas 44
   follicular variant papillary carcinoma, diagnosis of 47
   hyperplasia 44
   lesion 43, 44, 49
   neoplasm 44
   papillary carcinoma 46, 47
      diagnosis of 44
   tumors 44, 45, 276
hyalinizing trabecular tumor 39
hydrolysis, phosphatidylinositol 4, 5-biphasphate, 243
hypermethylation-mediated silencing 15
hyperplasia 24, 247, 403
hyperplastic nodule 24, 32
hypothyroidism 70, 319
   non-autoimmune autosomal dominant 94
   thyroiditis 47
hypoxia 7, 239

ICE (interleukin-1β-converting enzyme) 250
identity-specific signaling systems 238
ifosfamide 359
IGFBP (IGF-1-binding proteins) 245
IGF-I (insulin-like growth factors-I) 122
IGF-II (insulin-like growth factors-II) 122
IL-2 (interleukin-2) 373

imatinib mesylate 362
immunoblot analysis 224
immunoglobulins 25
immunohistochemical makers 29
immunohistochemical staining 55
immunohistochemistry 51, 79–80, 123, 166
immuno-suppressive cytokine, secretion of 373
indeterminate malignancy tumor *see* atypical Hurthle cell adenoma
indium-111 DTPA-PHE-octreotide 333–35
   general mechanism 333
   isotope characteristic 333
   scan method 333
inflammation mediator 244
inflammatory bowel disease 154
ingenetically based management genotype-phenotype associations 423
inherited and sporadic medullary thyroid carcinomaRET activation in 397–07
inherited genetic susceptibility 382
inherited susceptibility gene mutation 383
inhibitors groups
   allipticines 360
   amsacrines 360
   anthracyclines 360
   camptothecin 360
   dioxopiperazine 360
   epipodophyllotoxins 360
   irenotecan 360
   mebarone 360
   suramin 360
   topotecan 360
INK4 family 157
insufficient anti-tumor immunity mehanisms of 373
insular carcinoma 49, 53
insular carcinoma, recognition of 57
insular thyroid carcinoma 381
insulin and IGF-1 (insulin-like growth factor-1) 245
intergrin-dependent cel adhesion 248
internal radio-iodine application tumor growth following 280
intracellular signaling pathway, defects in 110
intraglandular lymphatic dissemination 34
intravascular lymphomatosis 71
iodide retention 357
iodide transporter 375
iodine 318–26
   blind therapy of131I 318
   characteristics of 319
   clinical application 318–21
   deficiency 279
   diagnostic 131IWBC 319
   general mechanism 319–21
   isotope 319–21
   lithium 321–22
   patient preparation 322

iodine (cont.)
   post therapeutic diagnostic scintigraphy 322–26
   pretherapeutic diagnostic scintigraphy 322
   radioactive 323–24
   retinoic acid 325
   rhTSH 324
   scan method 325
   sodium iodide sympoter 325
   stunning 325
   WHO recommendations 325–26
iodine-123 320
iodine-124 320–21
iodine-125 321
iodine-131 320
ionizing radiation 279–81
   external X-ray irradiation 281
   tumor growth following interanl radioiodine application 280–81
ionizing radiation, tumor induction by, 279
isotope characteristic 329, 331, 33
^{131}I WBC
   interpretation 322
   scanning techniqe 322

Jak (Janus kinases) activation of 249
JAK-STAT pathway 249
JUN 183

karyotypic abnormalities 5
keratin-19 267
keratinocytes 208
K-RAS 10
K-RAS mutation 131
K-RAS transformed cell 138

LCA (leukocyte common antigen) 53
leiomyoma 276
lentiviral vector transcriptionally targeted 229
Leu-7 (CD57) 304
Li-Fraumeni syndrome 3
light-cell solid adenoma 276
light-cell solid carcinoma 276
Lindsay tumor 276
lipid moleties 247
lithium 325
liver tumor 282
LOH (loss of heteroygocity) 299
LRP transporters 363
lung cancer 9
   cell 15
lung carcinoma 10
lymph node recurrence 305–06
lymphocytes 208
lymphocytic thyroiditis 47, 73
lymphoepithelial lesion 72, 80
lymphoma 276
lymphoplasmacytoid lymphocyte 72, 74

Madagascar periwinkle 362
magnetic resonance imaging 306
malignancy, diagnostis of 29
malignant cell 1
malignant follicular 24
   carcinomas 24
   neoplasm 296
malignant melanoma 111, 306
   cell proliferation 125
malignant thyroid
   cell expression in 186
   tumor 153, 245, 279, 300, 155, 157
      Rb immunoreactivity in 157
malignant transformation 2, 6, 238
malignant tumor 276, 280
malignant tumorous growth 274
MALT (mucosa associated lymphoid tissue) 69–72
MALT ball 76
MALT type, MZBL of 71–72, 81, 82
MALT-lymphoma 79–81
   relationship between low and high grade 81
mantle cell lymphomas 9
manumycin 362
MAPK (mitogen-activated protein kinase) 10, 183, 208, 242, 246
MAPK kinase/MARKpathway 246
masacrines 360
matrix metalloproteinases 179–87
matrix metalloproteinases groups 182
McCune-Albright syndrome 94
   thyroid manifestations of 241
MDM2 159, 152, 150
MDR1 gene 363
meatstatic follicular thyroid cancer treatment for 221
mebarone 360
MeCCNU (semustine) 359
mechlorethamine 359
medullary cancer 306
medullary carcinoma 52–56, 277
   thyroglobulin by 57
medullary thyroid cancer 186, 328
medullary thyroid carcinoma 48, 330, 335, 396–97
   diagnosis of 55
   onset of 56
mehionine 358
MEK (MAP/ERK kinase) 246
melanoma 8, 266
melphalan 359, 361, 362
MEN (multiple endocrine neoplasia) type ILA 55
MEN IIB 56 56
MEN2 (multiple endocrine neoplasia type 2) 417–18, 16
   cancer syndrome 389
   clinical subtypes 397

FMTC 397
MEN2 397
MEN2A with cutaneous lichen amyloidosis 397
MEN2A/FMTC with Hirschsprung's disease 397
MEN2B 397
diagnosis and management of 404–06
diagnosis and prediction of 419–20
genetics of 418-19
genotype-based management in 417–25
mutations, location of 398
syndromes 386
syndromes RET mutations in 397–99
RET mutation testing 420
MEN2A (multiple endocrine neoplasia type 2A)
RET in 398, 390
cancer syndrome 389
MEN2B (multiple endocrine neoplasia type 2B)
RET in 390, 401
cancer syndrome 389
thyroidectomy in 404
clinical features characteristic of 401
MEN2/HSCR paradox 402–03
mental retardation 170
mercury-201 329
MET oncogene 110, 211–12
metastasis 14
disease 310
lung of RRfiPV/PV 171
melanoma 306
metastatic papillary thyroid cancer treatment for 221
metastatic thyroid cancer 305, 325
metastatic tumor 56, 134
Methoxy-Isobutyl-Isonitrile 331
methylation 15
MHC 373
MIBG (meta-iodobenzylguanidin) 331, 335–36
application 335
general mechanism 335–36
scan method 336
microarray technology 266
microcarcinomas 34
microcarcinomas size 36
microcomal antigen 47
microfollicular adenoma
microfollicular carcinoma 276
microtubule-destabilizing agent 361, 362
mild sialadenitis 221
mimic papillary carcinoma 48
minimal immunoglobulin promoter control of 230
missense mutation 209
MIT (monoiodotyrosine) 319
mitochondrial DNA variant of 43
mitogen 244

mitogenic stimulation 9
mitogenic stimuli 9–12
mitomucin C 359, 361, 364
mitotic spindle function, inhibition of 362
mitoxantrone 361
mixed follicular-C cell lesions 57
mixed follicular-parafollicular cell carcinoma 57
mixed MZBL 76
mixed tumors 276
MLH1 13
MMAC1/TEP1 gene enode 248
MMP (matric metalloproteinase) 179 181, 184
activity regulation of 180
family and structure
collagenase 180
gelatinase 180
membranne-type 180
novel MMPs 180
stromelys 180
MMP-2 183
MMP-11 183
MMP-14 183
MMP-28 183
MNG (multinodular goitre) 268
model malignancy 252
molecular biology 80–81
monocytoid B-lymphocyte 72
montoxic prodrug 371
mRNA 167
MRP (multidrug resistance protein) 363
MRP1-MRP6 363
MRP4 malignant over-expression of 363
MSH2 13
MTC (medullary thyroid cancer) 337
PAX8 370
TPO 370
TSHR 370
MTC (medullary thyroid carcinoma) 417
treatment 372
MTU 279
mucoepidermoid carcinoma 358
multicentric C-cell hyperplasia 56
multifocal C-cell hyperplasia 404
multinodular goitre 268
multiple endocrine neoplasia type 2 396
multiple gene mutations 381
multiple hamartoma 113
syndrome 386
multiple sporadic thyroid carcinomas association of 382
mutant p53 proteins 363
mutation combination of 8
mutations 122
MUTS 13
myeloid leukemia 95, 96
MZBL (marginal zone B-cell lymphomas) 70–72, 81

NCAM (neural cell adhesion molecule) 392
NDF (neu differentiation factor) 122
neoplasia 24, 274–75
neoplastic formation 15, 16
neovascularization 14
NER (nucleotide excision repair proteins) 13
neural crest origin malignant tumors of 11
neurogenous tumor 276
neurotrophin 207
NF1 (neurofibromin loss) 10
NGF (nerve growth factor) 126, 207, 245
NHEJ (non-homologous end joining) 215
NIS (intracellular concentration of iodide) 357
NIS (sodium iodide symporter) 318, 325, 238, 375
  expressing Xenopus laevis oocytes 222
  function and structure of 222
  immunohistochemical analysis of 224
  localization indirect immunofluorescence analysis of 225
  localized in the intracellular membrane 225
  mediates the active accumulation 222, 228
  oligomerization 222
  phosphorylation 226–27
  plasma membrane localization 225
  regulation of 227
  regluation in health and disease 224
  subcellular distribution regulation of 227
  transcriptional level 224
nitrogen mustards 359
  mechlorthamine 359
nitrosamines tumor growth induced by 282
nitrosoureas 359
  tumor suppressor gene 302
NMU (N-nitroso-N-methylurea) 283
NMU injection 284
nodular goitre 24–26, 44, 53 273
non-medullary thyroid carcinoma 54
non-metastic encapsulated follicular carcinoma, morbidity and mortality for 31
normal colonic epithelium 2
NOS II (nitric oxide synthase) 372
novel mutimeric gemcitabine preparation 359
Noxa 151 151–52
N-RAS 10
N-RAS mutation 131
NRTN (neurturin) 391
N-TRK 110
NTRK1 (neurotrophic tyrosine receptor kinase type 1) 126, 209, 214–15, 110
  deregulation of 207
  gene 207
  in human disease 208–09
  kinase inhibitors 209
  oncogenic rearrangement, genomic features of 214
  proto-oncogene 207–08
  rearrangement 92

NTRK2 (TRKB) 207
NTRK3 (TRKC) 207
nuclear atypia 27, 44, 27
nuclear receptor
  ligands 96
  abnormalities of 165–74
nucleoside analog drugs 363

oncocytic follicular carcinoma 54
oncocytic papillary carcinomas 46
oncocytic tumours 46
oncofetal fibronectin 300
oncogenes 121
  activation of 15
  and thyroid tumor 107–14
  inactivation of 369
  mutations or overexpression of 370
  silencing of 370
    met 107–10
    ret/PTC 108–09
    TRK 110
    tyrosine kinase receptors 110
  TRK 207–16
oncogenesis 12
oncogenic mutation 419
oncogenic RAS 9
oncogenic RET signaling gene therapeutic approaches for inhibition of 406
oncogenic transformation process 237
oncolytic virus 374–75
oncoproteins 5
oncoproteins with TK activity 248
ONXY-015 374, 375
organ morphogenesis 179
organification 230
osteosarcomas cancer 9
ovarian 165
  cancer 15 *see also* endocrine cancer
  carcinomas 11
  tumor 11
oxaliplatin analog 359
oxyphilic metaplasia 48

P110α gene 11
P13K 11
P14ARF 8
p16INK4A 8, 9
p21CIP1 8
p27KIP1 8
p53 6, 7, 9, 149–60
  A1P1 151, 152
  gene mutations 116, 363
  gene therapy 371
  in human cancers 151–52
  in thyroid tumors, abundance of 154
  mediated apoptosis component of 364
  mutation 8, 52, 56, 117, 154, 200
  network 149–50

tumor suppressor 5
tumor suppressor gene 6–8, 359
tumor suppressor pathways 7
p53R2 152
paclitaxel 362, 364
paediatric thyroid cancers 41
palpable thyroid nodule 23
pancreatic cancer 9
pancreatic carcinoma 10
papillary (follicular variant) carcinoma 90
papillary adenoma 32, 276
papillary cancer 296
papillary cancers (stage IV) 302
parafollicular C-cells 277
partial thyroidectomy tumor growth after 279
pathetic ganglia 401
patient care implication for 385
PAX3 gene 89
PAX7 gene 89
PAX8 gene 87, 165
  analysis of 384
Pax8-PPARfi 301
PAX8-PPARfi rearrangement 198–99
PAX8-PPARfi1 fusion gene 111
PAX8-PPARγ 165
  fusion gene 215
PC (pheochromocytoma) 417
PCK isoenzyme 244
PCR 309
PDGFR (platelet-derived growth facrto receptor) 246
PDS (pendred syndrome) 318, 319
  gene defective in 230
  organification defect characteristic of, 230
pendrin 230
pentavalent 99m technetium dimercaptosuccinic acid 336–37
  clinical application 336
  general mechanism 337
  scan method 337
periodontal disease 180
peroxisom proliferator-activated receptor
  abnormalities of 172
PET (positron emission tomography) 317, 319, 329
PGH2 (generation of prostaglandin H2) 241
P-glycoprotein 363
  inhibitors of 363
PHD (pleckstrin homology domains) 248
pheochromocytoma 401
phospholipase C 243
phospholipids signaling dependent on 247
phosphorylated Ara-C 371
phosphorylates GCV 371
PI3 (Phosphatidyl Inositol 3) 113
PI3 kinase, (phosphatidylinositol-3-phospokinases) 243
PI3K (phosphatidylinositol 3-kinase) 208
PIDD 151

PIP2 243
PKA catalytic subunit of 225
PKC (protein kinase C) 214, 243
plasminogen activator ihibitors 185
PLAT (paraganglioma-like adenoma of thyroid) 39
platelet-derived growth factor 122
platinum-based agents 359–60
PNS (peripheral nervous system) 392
PNS ganglia 393
podophyllotoxins 361
polymorphofollicular carcinoma 276
polymorphous solid carcinoma 276
polypeptides 121
poorly differentiated carcinoma 48, 57
positron emissions tomography 306
post-translational modifications 15
potent vasoconstrictor 244
PPARγ (peroxisome proliferator-activated receptor
  amma) 30, 31, 91, 165, 171–74, 268
  down reulation of 268
  mRNA 172, 173
  rearrangement 87–90
  1/PAX8 mutations 116
  1/PAX8 translocation 116
PPCT (preprocalcitonin) tumor rejection antigen 374
PPRE (peroxisome proliferator-activated receptor
  reponse element) 172
pRB 8
pretherapeutic diagnostic scintigraphy 322
primarily activating AC (adenylyl cyclase) 240
primary thyroid lymphoma
  procarbazine 359
  staging of 71
  type of 70–71
promyelocytic leukemia 96
prophylactic adrenalectomy 420
prostaglandin-endoperoxide H synthose-2 241
prostate 165
prostate carcinoma 207
prostate cells 208
prostatic carcinoma 209
protein kinase 227
protein kinase A 242
protein kinase C 243
protein phosphorylated region of 222
PSPN (persephin) 391
PTC (papillary thyroid carcinoma) 108, 192, 209, 381
  familial susceptibilty to 382
  inherited susceptibility to 381–83
PTEN gene 248
PTEN tumor suppressor gene 11
PTTG (pituitary tumor transforming gene) 125
pump hydrophobic amphipathic drugs and
  metabolites 363
purative fPTC susceptibility genes, chromosomal
  locations of 386

purine analog 358
putative fPTC susceptibility gene linkage analysis and the chromosomal loci of 383
putative phosphorylation 214
putative tumor suppressor gene TSG101 155
pyrazolo-pyrimidine PP1 blocks tumorigenesis 406
pyrimidine analog 358

qualitative thyroid mRNA assays 307
quantitative thyroid mRNA assays 309–10

RAC 10
RAD53 13
radiation iodine-dependent changes after 288
radiation molecular pathways induced by 191–201
radiation related thyroid cancer, mutations in 153
radiation-associated carcinoma 92
radiation-associated thyroid tumors 114–16
    genetic predisposition 114–15
    genetic abnormalities 115
    age at exposure 115–16
radiation-associated tumor 116
radiation-induced carcinogenesis 201
radiation-induced thyroid cancer 195
radiation-induced thyroid tumors 199
radiation-induced tumor 38
    neural 114
    parathyroid 114
    salivary 114
    thyroid 114, 199
radioactive iodide 319
radioiodide therapy 230, 231, 375
    effectiveness of 224–28
    specific considerations related to 228–31
radioiodine 319
    ablative therapy 307
    therapy 43, 324
radiolabeled anti carcinoembryonic antigen antibody
    clinical application 337
    general mechanism 337–38
    scan method 338
RALGDS 10
RAR 167
RARa- immunostaining 167
RARa- mRNA 167
RAS 6, 246, 363
    activating point mutations of 10
    and genomic instability 139–40
    and thyroid cell survival 138
    gene 87, 201
        H- 110
        K- 110
        N- 110
    genes, activating mutations in 116
    mutations 2, 92–93, 116, 119–200
        prevalence of 199
    oncogenes 2
    regulation and signaling 132
    stimulated DNA synthesis 138
    stimulation of PI3K (phosphatidylinositol 3-kinases) 10
    thyroid cells, biology of 131–43
RAS-GTP 10
RAS-MAPK (mitogen-activated protein kinase) 245
rat hepatocarcinoma 211
rayleigh distribution 197
RB 9
    genes 149
    pathways 5–7
    protein 8
readiosensitization 370
REAL (Revised European-American Lymphoma) 70
receptor-activated signal cascade kinase 246
recombinant human TSH 348
recurrent thyroid cancer 325
REG-RET fusion proteins 91
renal oncocytoma 384
renal tumors 50
replicative senescence 4
reproduction 179
responder genes 9
RET 215
RET 418–19
RET gene 389
RET germline mutation 402
RET in sMTC (sporadic MTC) 403
RET mutation screening 422, 423
RET mutation testing, indications for 421
RET mutations, correlation between 398
RET null mutations in 392
RET proteins 389, 391
RET proto-oncogene 192, 424
RET rearrangement 90, 91, 92
RET related pathologies 390
RET signaling 392, 393–96
RET, alterations of 389
RET-MEN2A 403–04
RET-MEN2A oncoproteins 398
RET MEN2B signaling 403
RET/PTC generation after radiaation exposure potential mechanisma of 196
RET/PTC oncogene 108–09, 192–4, 300–301
RET/PTC rearrangements
    frequency of 109
    molecular basis of 108
RET/PTC1 108
RET/PTC2 108
RET/PTC3 108
RET/PTC-RAS-BRAF signaling pathway 11
retinoblastoma see RB
retinoic acid 325
retinoic acid receptor in thyroid cancer altered expression of 167

rheumatoid arthritis 154
rhTSH 324
rhTSH (recombinant human TAH) 321
RIP (receptor-interacting protein) 250
rodent cell
   E1a/RAS 4
   immortalization 6
   Myc/RAS 4
   transformation 4
rodent systems 4
rodents
   E2f 9
   Rb 9
RSK-B (ribosome protein S6 kinase-B) 247
RTH (resistance to thyroid hormone) 170
RTK (receptor-tyrosine kinases) and downstream effectors 245
RTK oncogenes, oligomerization of 213
RT-PCR (reverse transcriptase-polymerase chain reaction) 296, 298, 309, 311
RT-PCR, oncofetal fibronectin 300
RXRα (retinoid X receptor alpha) 111

SAPK (stress-activated protein kinase) 250
sarcoma 152, 276
scanning techniques of 322
SCFR (stem-cell factor receptor) 246
secreted frizzled related protein 269
selectively replicative virus 374–75
senescence program 6
serine 358
serum calcitonin 337
serum formed monolayers 228
SH2-binding sites 214
SH3-binding sites 214
SHC proteins 396
signal transduction 267
signaling, RAS regulation and 132–33
simple solid adenoma 276
Sipple's syndrome 396
SMAD-1 to-8 (cytoplasmic SMAD proteins) 251
small cell carcinomas 53, 69, 276
small cell lymphomas 53
small cell tumor 9
sMTC RET mutations in 399
SNP (single nucleotide polymorphisms) 183
sodium butyrate treatment 232
sodium/iodide symporter 30
solid carcinoma 276
solitary follicular nodules 26
somatic arrangement 90
somatic gene alternations 370
somatic mutation 1, 2, 43, 200, 381
somatic rearrangements in gene encoding 87
somatostatin receptor 333
spindle cell, anaplastic carcinoma 50
spontaneous thyroid tumors 276–77

sporadic and radiation-associated tumors RET/PTC prevalence in 194
sporadic carcinogenesis 201
sporadic medullary carcinomas 56
sporadic medullary thyroid carcinoma 403
sporadic MTC and PC disease associated RET haplotypes in 423–24
sporadic nodular goitre 24, 26, 32
sporadic papillary thyroid carcinoma 109
sporadic papillary thyroid carcinoma, clinical characteristics of
   age of onset 385
   associated malignancies 385
   benign thyroid nodules 385
   female:male ratio 385
   multifocal PTC 385
   recurrence death 385
squamoid variant 50
squamous cell (epidermoid) cystadenoma 276
squamous cell carcinoma 276
STAT (signal transducer and activator of transcription) 249
STI571 406
STK (serine-threonine kinase) receptors 251
streptozotocin 359
struma reticulosa 69
stunning 231, 324
suicide gene/prodrug 371–73
SUMO-1 150
suramin 360, 361
susceptibility gene mutation 382
susceptibility gene, identification of 381
sustained RAS activity 137–38
SV40 early region 6
Syrian hamsters 277
systemic chemotherapeutic 358–62

T cell ALL cancer 9
T cell lymphoma 71
T oncoprotein 6
T3, cytomel (L-triiodothyronine) 321
T4 (thyroxine) 318
T5 (triiodothyronine) 318
tachycardia 170
tall cell variant 42
tall cell variant papillary carcinoma 361
taxane 361, 362
taxane binding 362
taxatere (docetaxel) 361
taxol (paclitaxel) 361
Tc-99m furifosmin 332
Tc-99m pertechnate 332
Tc-99m tetrofosmin 332
Tc-99m-sestamibi 331
Tc-DMSA see DMSA-V 336

technetium-99m-sestamibi 331 *see also*
    methoxy-isobutyl-isonitrile
  clinical application 331
  general mechanism 331
  isotope characteristic 332
  scan method 332
telomerase 12, 296–98
telomerase expression 6
telomeres, function of 12
temozolomide 359
teniposide 361
teratoma 276
TFG gene 214
Tg (thyroglobulin) 371
Tg (thyroglobulin) loss of 238
TGF-α (transforming growth factor α) 10, 122, 245
TGF-β (transforming growth factor β) 122, 124
TGI (thyroid growth-stimulating immunoglobulins) 47
thallium-201 chloride
  clinical application 330–31
  general mechanism 329
  isotope characteristic 329–30
  medullary thyroid cancer 330–31
  papillary and follicular thyroid cancer 330
  scan mehod 330
therapeutic gene expression 371
thiocyanate 222
thio-tepah 359
thyrocyte hyperplasia 241
thyroglobulin 30, 239, 325, 357
  immunoassays 308
  molecule 228
  mRNA 309
thyroid adenoma 279
thyroid cancer 6, 9, 57, 155, 304
  cAMP analogs in 372
  correlation of telomere length to telomerase activity 12
  diagnostic molecular markers in 295–311
  distinction of 48
  formation, histologic-molecular 86 87
  gene therapy for 369–75
  gene therapy strategies used for 370–75
  genesis and treatment 121–27
  imaging 317–38
  improving I- transport in 231–33
  less aggressive varieties of 361
  MDM2 in 155
  molecular epidemiology of 107–17
  molecular signaling in 237–52, 317
  NIS expression in 223–24
  progression and metastasis MMPs and TIMPS in 184–86
  pathology of 23–57
  p53 mutations in 152

radioiodide treatment of 221
RAS mutations in 134
treatment of 359
typical follicular architecture 229
thyroid carcinogenesis 109, 173, 213, 289
thyroid carcinoma 8, 10, 38, 53, 95, 96
  differentiated 32, 91
  enzyme in 363
  management of 345
  metastases 231
  proliferation of 166
  Rb in 156
  therapy effective application to 361
  type of 37
tRa (trans-retinoic acid) treatment in 232
thyroid carcinogenesis 273–89
thyroid C-cell 403
thyroid cell proliferation 137–38
thyroid cell survival, RAS and 138–39
thyroid cells effect of spatial organization of 228
thyroid cells effects of adenosine on cAMP accumulation in 244
thyroid differentiation 138
thyroid disease, pathogenesis of 57
thyroid epithelial cells apical-basolateral polarization of 228
thyroid epithelium 215
thyroid follicular cancer, adenovirus expressing IL-12 374
thyroid follicular hyperplasia 24–32
thyroid follicular neoplasia 24–32
thyroid follicular nodular disease 56
thyroid FRTL-5 cells extracellualr adenosin triphosphate (ATP) in 241
thyroid function 285
thyroid goiters, hyperplastic nodules from 94
thyroid hormone biosythesis 222, 227
thyroid hormone receptor 159, 168
thyroid hyperplasis 282
thyroid lymphoma 69–82
  clinical presentation 69–70
  gross pathology 70
  historical aspect 70
  incidence 70
  light microscopy 71
  nomenclature and terminology 71
  pathology 71
  staging 71
thyroid malignancies 115
thyroid malignancy, radiation-associated 191
thyroid metabolism 267
thyroid nodules 273
  benign and malignant 23
  diagnostic criteria 23
  management of patients 23
  multiple 23
  non-neoplastic and neoplastic 23

numerous entities 23
  preoperative evaluation of 295–96
  solitary 24
thyroid oncogenes 123
thyroid peroxidase 375
thyroid strom 24
thyroid TRK oncogenes 209–11
thyroid tumor 85
  aneuploidy aberrations 87–90, 94–95
  B-catenin mutations 90–91
  benign and malignant 131
  BRAF mutations 92
  chromosomal aberration 92–93, 94–95
  diagnosis 85
  G protein mutation
  gene expression in 265–70
  histologic-molecular model
  hormone receptor 93–94
  induction 277–89
  NTRK1 rearrangements 93–94
  p53 mutations 94
  PPARγ rearrangements 94
  radiation-induced 191
  RAS mutations 94–95
  RET rearrangements 94–95
  spectrum of 268–69
thyroid tumorigenesis 30, 95, 122, 166
thyroidal iodide transport 221–33
thyroid-derived fibroblasts 186
thyroidectomy 307
thyroidectomy and radioactive iodine therapy 32
thyroidectomy therapy 43
thyroiditis 56
thyroid-specific gene rearrangement 92
thyroid-specific monitoring 307
thyroperoxidase 30
thyrotimulin 354
thyrotropin-dependent growth control 360
TIMP (tissue inhibitors of meatalloproteinases) 179, 184
TIMP-2 183
tissue resorption and remodeling 179
TKAR (tyrosin kinase (TK)-associated receptors) 249
TMTU (tetramethylthioura) 278
TNF (tumor necrosis factor) 249
TNF and apoptosis-related molecule 249
TNF receptor 208
TNFR activation of 250
topoisomerase DNA strands cut by 360
topoisomerase I 361
topoisomerase II
  alpha isotype 360
  beta isotype 360
  evaluation of 363
topoisomerase inhibitors 360–61
toposimerase II 361

topotecan 361
toxic CB1954 371
TPM3 gene 209, 211
TPO (thyroid peroxidase) 299–300
TPO mRNA 310
TR in thyroid carcinoma, mutation of 159, 168–69
trabecular adenoma
trabecular cell variant 42
TRADD (TNFR1-associated death domain protein) 249–50
transfection of NIH3T3 cells with DNA 390
transformation process from normal cell to malignant 1
transforming growth factor-α 122
TRAP 298
TRAP (Telemeric Repeat Amplification Protocol) 297
TRβ 165
Trfi gene in thyroid cancer germline mutations of 169–72
Trichostatin A (histone deacetylase inhibitor) 375
triethylenemelamine 359
triggering crisis 5
TRK oncogenes 110, 126, 210, 215
TRK oncogenic activation, role of activating sequences in 211–14
TRK oncoproteins 210
TRK rearrangement 116
TRK tyrosine kinase receptor 9
TRKA see NTRK1
TRK-T1 110
TRK-T1 oncogenes 212
TRK-T2 110
TRK-T2 oncogene 215
TRK-T3 110
TRK-T3 oncogenic activation 212
TRK-T3 protein 213
tropomyosin gene 208
tryosine residues (Y90, Y670, Y674, Y675 and Y785) 208
TSH (thyroid-stimulating hormone) 171, 186, 273, 277, 282, 289, 319, 321, 345–54
TSH analogs
  clinical application 345
  general mechanism 345
  mehanism of enhanced bioactivity of 350–52
  scan method 345
TSH dicovery phase 345
TSH elevation 277–79
  goitrogen-induced tumors 278
  low-iodine intake 278–79
  tumor growth after partial thyrodectomy 279
TSH optimization phase 345
TSH receptor, hypermethylation of 305

TSH stimulation pathway, defects in 112
TSH structure-function 345–47
TSH superactive analogs
  dicovery of 353
  optimization of 348, 350
  uses of 348, 350
TSH tumor induction by elevation of 277–79
TSH-independent G-protein-mediated signaling pathways 244
TSHR (thyroid stimulating hormone receptor) 93–94
TSHR (TSH receptor) 240
TSH-receptor gene and gsp oncogene mutation 112–13
TSH-stimulated proliferation 136
TSH-TSHR complex 352
TSP-1 (thrombospondin-1) 14
TTAGGG 296
tubulin polymerization 361
tumor cell invasion and metastasis 179
tumor classification 274–76
tumor cytotoxic activity 361
tumor formation 403
tumor growth 209
tumor immunity enhancement of 373
tumor induction by low-iodine intake 278
tumor invasion 185
tumor progression 14
tumor recurrence or progression molecular markers of 305–11
tumor sites on thyroid scintigraphic scan presence of "cold nodules" 222
tumor suppressor 8
tumor suppressor gene 2, 8, 113–14, 121, 149, 155, 267, 363
  DCC 3
  DPC4 3
  Hdm2 8
  JV18 3
  network 159
  P53 3, 370
  replacement of 369, 370
  silencing of 15
tumor vascularity 362
tumor vascular-targeting agent 364
tumorigenesis 41
tumor-inducing factors combination 283–84
tumors thyrotropin stimulation of 360
tumor size 35
tumor-specific mRNA assays 310–11
TXA2 (thromboxane A2) 241
Tyr1062 mutation of 404
Tyr864 and Tyr952 phosphorylation of 404
tyrosine autophosphorylation 393

tyrosine kinase activation 212
tyrosine kinase inhibitor 96, 406
tyrosine kinase receptors 107–10
tyrosine phosphorylation 132

ultrasound 306
ultrasound, detection of palpable thyroid nodule 23
undifferentiated carcinoma see also anaplastic carcinoma 50
undifferentiated spermatogonia 393
undifferentiated thyroid cancer 115
undifferentiated thyroid cancer, pathobiology of 357–64
undifferentiated thyroid carcinoma 396

Val804Met 423
variants 37–43
vectors viral non-viral 369
VEGF (vascular endothelial cell geowth factor) 14, 117, 245
VEGFR 246
ventral midbrain dopamiunergic neurons 392
v-erbA 168
VGEF 151
vinca alkaloid 361–362
  vinblastine 361
  vincristine 361
  vindesine 361
  vinorelbine 361
VIP (vasoactive intestinal peptide) 245
viral oncoproteins
  human papillomavirus E6 and E7 oncoproteins 5
  SV40 large T antigen 5
VP-16 (etoposide) 361

Warthin-like variants 157
WHAFFT 38
Wilmsí tumors 1
WRT (Wistar rat thyroid) 136
wt (wild type)-p53 370
wt-p53 reintroduction of 370

xenograft
  evaluation in 362
  model systems 358
  study 359
  tumors 231
xenografted human glioma cells 229
Xeroderma pigmentosum 13
X-ray irradiation, therapeutic 194
X-ray therapy 191

Yttrium-90 334